Operative Treatment of Elbow Injuries

Springer
*New York
Berlin
Heidelberg
Barcelona
Hong Kong
London
Milan
Paris
Singapore
Tokyo*

Champ L. Baker, Jr., M.D.
The Hughston Sports
  Medicine Foundation
Columbus, Georgia

Kevin D. Plancher, M.D.
Plancher Orthopaedic
  Associates
New York, NY

Editors

Operative Treatment of Elbow Injuries

Foreword by Bernard F. Morrey, M.D.

With 499 Illustrations, 17 in Full Color

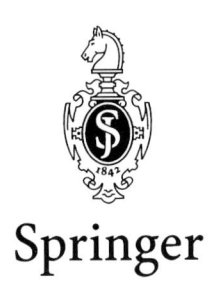

Springer

Champ L. Baker, Jr., M.D.
The Hughston Sports Medicine Foundation
6262 Veterans Parkway
P.O. Box 9517
Columbus, GA 31909
USA

Kevin D. Plancher, M.D.
Plancher Orthopaedic Associates
111 East 88th Street, Suite 1A
New York, NY 10128
USA

♦

Operative Treatment
of
Elbow Injuries
is dedicated to my family
— CLB

♦

Cover illustration by Carolyn M. Capers.

Library of Congress Cataloging-in-Publication Data
Operative treatment of elbow injuries / editors, Champ L. Baker, Jr., Kevin D. Plancher.
    p. ; cm.
  Includes bibliographical references and index.
  ISBN 0-387-98905-6 (h/c : alk. paper)
    1. Elbow—Surgery.   2. Elbow—Wounds and Injuries—Treatment.   3. Arthroscopy.
  I. Baker, Champ L.   II. Plancher, Kevin D.
    [DNLM: 1. Elbow—surgery.   2. Arthroscopy—methods.   3. Elbow—injuries.   4. Elbow Joint—injuries.   5. Elbow Joint—surgery.   WE 820 O61 2001]
  RD558.O64   2001
  617.5′74—dc21   00-067910

Printed on acid-free paper.

© 2002 Springer-Verlag New York, Inc.
All rights reserved. This work may not be translated or copied in whole or in part without the written permission of the publisher (Springer-Verlag New York, Inc., 175 Fifth Avenue, New York, NY 10010, USA), except for brief excerpts in connection with reviews or scholarly analysis. Use in connection with any form of information storage and retrieval, electronic adaptation, computer software, or by similar or dissimilar methodology now known or hereafter developed is forbidden.
The use of general descriptive names, trade names, trademarks, etc., in this publication, even if the former are not especially identified, is not to be taken as a sign that such names, as understood by the Trade Marks and Merchandise Marks Act, may accordingly be used freely by anyone.
While the advice and information in this book are believed to be true and accurate at the date of going to press, neither the authors nor the editors nor the publisher can accept any legal responsibility for any errors or omissions that may be made. The publisher makes no warranty, express or implied, with respect to the material contained herein.

Production coordinated by WordCrafters Editorial Services, Inc., and managed by Lesley Poliner; manufacturing supervised by Joe Quatela.
Typeset by Matrix Publishing Services, Inc., York, PA.
Printed and bound by Maple-Vail Book Manufacturing Group, York, PA.
Printed in the United States of America.

9 8 7 6 5 4 3 2 1

ISBN 0-387-98905-6   SPIN 10738477

Springer-Verlag New York Berlin Heidelberg
A member of BertelsmannSpringer Science+Business Media GmbH

Foreword

This outstanding text is the most comprehensive to date focusing on athletic and other injuries to the elbow. The book is very well organized, with a considerable amount of material providing a background and foundation for the procedures that are subsequently described. This text fills a void in the orthopaedic surgeon's library with regard to the detailed treatment of sports injuries. The book has been thoroughly edited to avoid redundancies and to provide a uniformity of style. This is reflected in the chapter length, the number of references, and the artwork. A distinctive order and homogeneity are reflected in the care with which the book was conceived and edited. The subject matter is treated in a thorough manner, and adequate emphasis is placed on technique. Overall, this text is one that will be extremely worthwhile to surgeons managing elbow injuries, and it is relevant also for surgeons who are just beginning training and for increasing understanding in those who are more experienced. The editors have done an excellent job of satisfying their stated goals in writing this text.

Bernard F. Morrey, M.D.
Rochester, Minnesota
May, 2001

Preface

Keeping up with the medical literature is a difficult task. Stacks of journals collect on desks, and the number of textbooks on bookshelves grows while the time to read them shrinks. At the same time, we feel the pressure to stay current in our areas of interest because our patients expect and deserve informed doctors. A good reference book can be of great value to the busy surgeon. It is my hope that this book is a useful compilation of the most effective management of elbow injuries and is a useful tool for the busy practitioner. The text also contains a thorough description of the anatomy and physical examination of the elbow. With its excellent illustrations, I believe this timely volume will be extremely useful to the orthopaedic surgeon and the sports medicine specialist regarding the specific aspects of surgical technique.

I am indebted to the diverse group of physicians who shared their expertise regarding their most successful methods of treating elbow and upper extremity injuries. It is they who have made this textbook an important step in the continued advancement of the treatment of these disorders. I am particularly indebted to Carol Binns and Carol Capers of the Hughston Sports Medicine Foundation. Their untiring efforts and expertise in medical writing and medical illustration, respectively, have made this book a reality.

Champ L. Baker, M.D.
Columbus, Georgia
May, 2001

Contents

Foreword		v
Preface		vii
Contributors		xi
1	Anatomy of the Elbow Joint and Surgical Approaches	1
	GREGORY I. BAIN AND JANAK A. MEHTA	
2	Biomechanics of the Elbow and Throwing Mechanisms	29
	STEVEN W. BARRENTINE, GLENN S. FLEISIG, CHARLES J. DILLMAN, AND JAMES R. ANDREWS	
3	History and Physical Examination of the Elbow	41
	CHAMP L. BAKER AND GRANT L. JONES	
4	Magnetic Resonance Imaging of the Elbow	55
	RUSSELL C. FRITZ	
5	Little League Elbow	69
	STEPHEN J. AUGUSTINE, GEORGE M. MCCLUSKEY III, AND LUIS MIRANDA-TORRES	
6	Lateral and Medial Epicondylitis	79
	GEORGE M. MCCLUSKEY III AND MICHAEL S. MERKLEY	
7	Ulnar Collateral Ligament Injuries	89
	NATHAN M. BREAZEALE AND DAVID W. ALTCHECK	
8	Lateral Collateral Ligament Reconstruction	101
	MARK S. COHEN	
9	Biceps Tendon and Triceps Tendon Ruptures	109
	BRUCE M. LESLIE AND HELEN RANGER	
10	Valgus Extension Overload Syndrome	123
	JAMES R. ANDREWS AND ERIC P. LAUNER	

11	Cubital Tunnel Syndrome	131
	GLENN C. TERRY AND TODD E. ZEIGLER	
12	Pronator Syndrome	141
	N. GEORGE KASPARYAN AND ANDREW J. WEILAND	
13	Radial Nerve Compression about the Elbow	149
	DAVID C. REHAK	
14	Arthroscopy of the Elbow	157
	ARLON H. JAHNKE JR. AND NICHOLAS YOKAN	
15	Diagnostic Arthroscopy of the Elbow	163
	MATTHEW L. RAMSEY AND R. JOHN NARANJA	
16	Arthroscopic Removal of Loose Bodies in the Elbow	171
	MARK S. SCHICKENDANTZ	
17	Arthroscopic Treatment of Ankylosis of the Elbow	177
	FELIX H. SAVOIE III, LARRY D. FIELD, AND CHARLES W. HARTZOG, JR.	
18	Arthroscopic Radial Head Resection	185
	LARRY D. FIELD AND FELIX H. SAVOIE, III	
19	Problem Fractures of the Distal Humerus	195
	ARNOLD-PETER C. WEISS AND HILL HASTINGS II	
20	Radial Head Fractures	207
	FRANCES SHARPE AND STUART H. KUSCHNER	
21	Supracondylar Fractures of the Humerus in Children	223
	W. DAVID BRUCE AND HUGH P. BROWN	
22	Pediatric Lateral Condylar Fractures	245
	MICHAEL EHRLICH AND DONNA PACICCA	
23	Elbow Dislocation	253
	STUART H. KUSCHNER AND FRANCES SHARPE	
24	Treatment of Olecranon, Coronoid, and Proximal Ulnar Fracture–Dislocation	259
	JAMES B. BENNETT AND THOMAS L. MEHLHOFF	
25	Nonunions of the Elbow	271
	DAVID RING AND JESSE B. JUPITER	
26	Elbow Contracture Release: Open Operative Strategies	285
	KENNETH J. FABER AND GRAHAM J.W. KING	
27	Tumors of the Elbow	295
	DEMPSEY S. SPRINGFIELD AND STEPHANIE SWEET	
28	Olecranon Bursitis	303
	CHAMP L. BAKER, JR. AND PETER W. HESTER	
29	Rehabilitation of Elbow Injuries in Overhead-Throwing Athletes	309
	KEVIN E. WILK AND TERESE CHMIELEWSKI	
Index		321

Contributors

DAVID W. ALTCHEK, M.D.
 Associate Professor of Clinical Surgery
Department of Orthopaedics
Weill Medical College of Cornell University
1300 York Avenue
New York, NY 10021
 Orthopaedic Surgeon
Sports Medicine and Shoulder Service
Hospital for Special Surgery
535 East 70th Street
New York, NY 10021, USA

JAMES R. ANDREWS, M.D.
 Medical Director
American Sports Medicine Institute
1313 13th Street South
Birmingham, AL 35205
 Orthopaedic Surgeon
Alabama Sports Medicine and Orthopaedic Center
1201 11th Avenue South
Birmingham, AL 35205, USA

STEPHEN J. AUGUSTINE, D.O.
 Assistant Professor
Department of Orthopaedic Surgery
University of Florida
Shands Jacksonville
655 West 8th Street
Jacksonville, FL 32209, USA

GREGORY IAN BAIN, FRACS
 Clinical Lecturer
Department of Orthopaedic Trauma
University of Adelaide
North Terrace
Adelaide, SA, 5005
 Senior Visiting Orthopaedic Surgeon
Department of Orthopaedic Surgery and Trauma
Royal Adelaide Hospital
North Terrace
Adelaide, SA, 5000
AUSTRALIA

CHAMP L. BAKER, JR., M.D.
 Staff Physician
The Hughston Sports Medicine Foundation
6262 Veterans Parkway
Columbus, GA 31909
 Clinical Assistant Professor
Department of Orthopaedic Surgery
Tulane University School of Medicine
New Orleans, Louisiana 70112, USA

STEVE W. BARRENTINE, M.S.
 Biomechanics Lab Coordinator
American Sports Medicine Institute
1313 13th Street South
Birmingham, AL 35205, USA

JAMES B. BENNETT, M.D.
  Clinical Professor
Department of Orthopaedic Surgery
U.T. Health Science Center at Houston
  Chief of Staff
Texas Orthopedic Hospital
7401 South Main Street
Houston, TX 77030, USA

NATHAN M. BREAZEALE, M.D.
Austin Sports Medicine
900 West 38th #300
Austin, TX 78705, USA

HUGH P. BROWN, M.D.
  Associate Professor
Department of Orthopaedic Surgery
University of Tennessee at Chattanooga
975 East Third Street
Chattanooga, TN 37403
  Spine Surgery Associates, P.-C.
979 East Third Street, Suite C-0225
Chattanooga, TN 37403, USA

W. DAVID BRUCE, M.D.
  Clinical Professor
Pediatric Orthopaedics
University of Tennessee at Chattanooga
975 East Third Street
Chattanooga, TN 37403
  Chattanooga Bone and Joint Surgeons, P.-C.
1809 Gunbarrel Road, Suite 101
Chattanooga, TN 37421, USA

TERESE L. CHMIELEWSKI, M.A., P.T.
  Doctoral Student
Department of Physical Therapy
University of Delaware
301 McKinly Lab
Newark, DE 19716, USA

MARK S. COHEN, M.D.
  Associate Professor
  Director, Orthopedic Education
  Director, Hand and Elbow Program
Department of Orthopedic Surgery
Rush-Presbyterian-St. Luke's Medical Center
1725 West Harrison Street, Suite 1063
Chicago, IL 60612, USA

CHARLES J. DILLMAN, Ph.D.
  President & CEO
Znetix
600 University Street, Suite 2500
Seattle, WA 98101, USA

MICHAEL G. EHRLICH, M.D.
  Professor and Chairman
Department of Orthopaedics
Brown Medical School
  Surgeon-in-Chief
Department of Orthopaedics
Rhode Island Hospital
593 Eddy Street
Providence, RI 02903, USA

KENNETH J. FABER, M.D., F.R.C.S.C.
  Assistant Professor
Department of Surgery
University of Western Ontario
  Consultant
Department of Surgery
Hand and Upper Limb Centre
St. Joseph's Health Care London
268 Grosvenor Street
London ON N6A 4L6
CANADA

LARRY D. FIELD, M.D.
  Co-Director, Upper Extremity Service
Mississippi Sports Medicine Center
1325 East Fortification Street
Jackson, MS 39202, USA

GLENN S. FLEISIG, Ph.D.
  Adjunct Professor
Department of Biomedical Engineering
The University of Alabama at Birmingham
370 Hoehn Engineering Building
1075 13th Street South
Birmingham, AL 35294
  Smith & Nephew Chair of Research
American Sports Medicine Institute
1313 13th Street South
Birmingham, AL 35205, USA

RUSSELL C. FRITZ, M.D.
  Medical Director
National Orthopedic Imaging Associates
1260 South Eliseo Drive
Greenbrae, CA 94904, USA

CHARLES W. HARTZOG, JR., M.D.
  Orthopaedic Surgeon
Department of Surgery
Jackson Hospital
1725 Pine Street
Montgomery, AL 36106
  Alabama Orthopaedic Specialists
4294 Lomac Street
Montgomery, AL 36106, USA

HILL HASTINGS II, M.D.
　Clinical Associate Professor of Orthopaedic Surgery
Department of Orthopaedic Surgery
Indiana University School of Medicine
Indianapolis, IN
　The Indiana Hand Center
8501 Harcourt Road
Indianapolis, IN 46280-0434, USA

PETER W. HESTER, M.D.
　Fellow in Orthopaedic Sports Medicine
The Hughston Clinic
6262 Veterans Parkway
Columbus, GA 31909, USA

ARLON H. JAHNKE JR., M.D.
　Associate Clinical Professor
Department of Surgery
Medical College of Georgia
Augusta, GA 30912
　Augusta Orthopaedic Specialists
PO Box 14039
Augusta, GA 30919, USA

GRANT L. JONES, M.D.
　Assistant Professor of Clinical Orthopaedics
Department of Orthopaedic Surgery
The Ohio State University
410 West 10th Avenue
Columbus, OH 43210, USA

JESSE B. JUPITER, M.D.
　Professor
Department of Orthopaedic Surgery
Harvard Medical School
10 Shattuck Street
Boston, MA
　Director, Hand Surgery
Department of Orthopaedics
Massachusetts General Hospital
ACC 527, 15 Parkman Street
Boston, MA 02114, USA

NURHAN GEORGE KASPARYAN, M.D., Ph.D.
　Assistant Professor of Orthopaedic Surgery
Boston University School of Medicine
One BMC Place
Boston, MA 02118
　Senior Staff Surgeon
Department of Orthopaedics
Lahey Clinic
41 Mall Road
Burlington, MA 01805, USA

GRAHAM KING, M.D., F.R.C.S.C.
　Associate Professor
University of Western Ontario
Hand and Upper Limb Centre
St. Joseph's Health Care
268 Grosvenor Street
London, ON N6A 4L6
CANADA

STUART H. KUSCHNER, M.D.
　Clinical Associate Professor of Orthopedics
Department of Orthopedics
Keck School of Medicine
University of Southern California
2025 Zonal Avenue
Los Angeles, CA 90089-9312
　Active Staff
Division of Orthopedics
Department of Surgery
Cedars-Sinai Medical Center
8700 Beverly Boulevard
Los Angeles, CA 90048-1865, USA

ERIC P. LAUNER, M.D.
　Clinical Fellow
Cincinnati Sports Medicine and Orthopaedic Center
311 Straight Street
Cincinnati, OH 45219, USA

BRUCE M. LESLIE, M.D.
　Hand Surgeon
Suite 343
Newton Wellesley Hospital
2000 Washington Street
Newton, MA 02462, USA

GEORGE M. MCCLUSKEY III, M.D.
　Clinical Assistant Professor
Department of Orthopaedic Surgery
Tulane University School of Medicine
New Orleans, LA 70112
　Chief, Shoulder Surgery
The Hughston Clinic
Hughston Sports Medicine Hospital
Columbus, GA 31909, USA

THOMAS L. MEHLHOFF, M.D.
　Assistant Clinical Professor
Department of Orthopedic Surgery
Baylor College of Medicine
　Team Physician, Houston Astros
Texas Orthopedic Hospital
7401 South Main
Houston, TX 77030, USA

JANAK A. MEHTA, M.B.B.S.Ms (ORTH)
  Clinical Lecturer
Orthopaedic Surgery and Trauma
NT Clinical School
Flinders University
Royal Darwin Hospital
Casuarina, NT, 5006
  Registrar
Department of Orthopaedics
Modbury Public Hospital
Smart Road
Modbury, SA, 5092
Adelaide
AUSTRALIA

MICHAEL S. MERKLEY, M.D.
  Midwest Orthopedic Center
2805 N. Knoxville Avenue
Peoria, IL 61604
  Department of Orthopedic Surgery
St. Francis Hospital
530 NE Glen Oak Avenue
Peoria, IL 61637, USA

LUIS A. MIRANDA-TORRES, M.D.
  Instituto de Ortopedia de Caguas
201 Avenue Gautier Benitez
Caguas, PR 00725
  Director
Department of Orthopaedics
Hospital Menonita—Cayey
PO Box 373130
Cayey, PR 00737-3130

R. JOHN NARANJA, JR., M.D.
  Clinical Assistant Professor of Surgery
Department of Surgery
University of North Dakota School of Medicine
Grand Forks, ND 58202
  Chief of Medical Staff
Department of Orthopaedics
5th Medical Group, USAF
10 Missile Avenue
Minot AFB, ND 58705, USA

DONNA M. PACICCA, M.D.
  Assistant Professor
Department of Orthopaedic Surgery and Pediatrics
Boston University School of Medicine
715 Albany Street
Boston, MA 02118
  Attending Surgeon
Department of Orthopaedic Surgery
Boston Medical Center
850 Harrison Avenue, Dowling 2-N
Boston, MA 02118, USA

MATTHEW L. RAMSEY, M.D.
  Assistant Professor
Department of Orthopaedic Surgery
Penn Orthopaedic Institute
Presbyterian Medical Center
One Cupp Pavilion, 39th and Market Streets
Philadelphia, PA 19104
  Assistant Professor
Department of Orthopaedic Surgery
University of Pennsylvania
3400 Spruce Street
Philadelphia, PA 19104, USA

HELEN E. RANGER, M.S., P.T., C.H.T.
  Hand Therapy Service Coordinator
Rehabilitation Services
Newton Wellesley Hospital
2014 Washington Street
Newton, MA 02462, USA

DAVID C. REHAK, M.D.
  Orthopaedic/Hand Surgeon
The Hughston Clinic
6262 Veterans Parkway
Columbus, GA 31909, USA

DAVID RING, M.D.
  Instructor
Department of Orthopaedic Surgery
Harvard Medical School
  Hand Surgery Service
Department of Orthopaedic Surgery
Massachusetts General Hospital
ACC 527, 15 Parkman Street
Boston, MA 02114, USA

FELIX H. SAVOIE III, M.D.
  Co-Director, Upper Extremity Service
Mississippi Sports Medicine Center
1325 East Fortification Street
Jackson, MS 39202, USA

MARK S. SCHICKENDANTZ, M.D.
  Orthopedic Surgeon
Horizon Orthopedic
Lutheran Hospital
2709 Franklin Boulevard
Cleveland, OH 44113, USA

FRANCES SHARPE, M.D.
  Staff Physician
Kaiser-Permanente
9985 Sierra Avenue
Fontana, CA 92335, USA

DEMPSEY SPRINGFIELD, M.D.
　Professor and Chairman
Department of Orthopaedics
Mount Sinai School of Medicine
　Chief of Staff
Department of Orthopaedics
Mount Sinai Hospital
1 Gustave L. Levy Place
New York, NY 10029, USA

STEPHANIE SWEET
　Philadelphia Hand Center
Thomas Jefferson University
Clinical Assistant Professor
Department of Orthopaedic Surgery
834 Chestnut Street, Suite G114
Philadelphia, PA 19107, USA

GLENN C. TERRY, M.D.
　Assistant Clinical Professor
Department of Orthopaedic Surgery
Tulane University School of Medicine
New Orleans, LA 70112
　Staff Physician
The Hughston Clinic
6262 Veterans Parkway
Columbus, GA 31909, USA

ANDREW J. WEILAND, M.D.
　Professor
Department of Orthopaedics and Plastic Surgery
Weill Medical College
1300 York Avenue
New York, NY 10021
　Attending Orthopaedic Surgeon
Hospital for Special Surgery
535 East 70th Street
New York, NY 10021, USA

ARNOLD-PETER C. WEISS, M.D.
　Professor
Department of Orthopaedics
Brown Medical School
　Hand and Elbow Surgeon
University Orthopedics
2 Dudley Street
Providence, RI 02905, USA

KEVIN E. WILK, P.T.
　Adjunct Associate Professor
Department of Physical Therapy
Marquette University
Milwaukee, WI
　National Director of Research and Clinical Education
HealthSouth Rehabilitation
1201 11th Avenue South, #100
Birmingham, AL 35205, USA

NICHOLAS YOKAN, M.D.
　Chief of Orthopaedic Surgery
Moncrief Army Community Hospital
PO Box 485
Fort Jackson, SC 29207-5728, USA

TODD E. ZEIGLER, M.D.
　North Georgia Orthopaedic Specialists
555 Old Norcross Road, Suite 100
Lawrenceville, GA 30045, USA

CHAPTER 1

Anatomy of the Elbow Joint and Surgical Approaches

Gregory I. Bain and Janak A. Mehta

INTRODUCTION

The art of surgery lies in the reconstruction of diseased or injured tissues with minimal additional destruction. Surgery (from the Greek *chirur* + *erg* = hands + work) is not just handiwork and certainly not carpentry in the case of orthopedics. It is the masterly expression of the superior functions of the mind, eyes, hands, and heart working in flawless coordination. The knowledge of anatomy defines the extent, precision, and safety of surgery. Approaches to any joint or structure in the body are developed on this foundation. Familiarity with the intricate anatomy of and multiple approaches to the elbow allows the surgeon to embark confidently toward the repair or reconstruction of any injury or disorder of the joint.

CLINICAL ANATOMY

The elbow is a compound uniaxial synovial joint comprising three articulations: the ulnotrochlear, radiocapitellar, and proximal radioulnar joints. The ulnohumeral joint is a ginglymus (hinge) joint, whereas the radiocapitellar and the proximal radioulnar joints are gliding joints (Fig. 1.1).

The clinical significance of the three-joint concept is that injuries or arthritis involving the elbow can affect the flexion arc and the rotation of the forearm. Infection near, but not involving, the elbow joint can restrict flexion or extension, but it may not affect forearm rotation.

We conceptualize the elbow and upper limb as the surgeon would encounter them, with the scalpel proceeding from the skin to the deeper layers. The upper limb is a cylinder enveloped by the skin. Beneath the skin lies the subcutaneous adipose tissue that contains the superficial veins, cutaneous nerves, and superficial lymphatics. Next, the investing layer of the deep fascia encircles the muscles with their accompanying neurovascular structures. The long bones and the elbow joint lie beneath these structures.

The Subcutaneous Plane

The subcutaneous plane consists mainly of adipose tissue that is abundant except over each epicondyle and on the subcutaneous border of the ulna and olecranon. This plane contains the veins, which are predominantly anterior and drain into the cephalic (lateral) and basilic (medial) veins (Fig. 1.2). The subcutaneous plane also contains the cutaneous nerves, which are located in the depth of the subcutaneous fat and just superficial to the investing fascia.[1]

The **lateral cutaneous nerve of the forearm** (C5, C6) lies adjacent to the cephalic vein and is at risk for injury during surgery on the lateral aspect of the elbow.[2,3] It pierces the brachial fascia 3.2 cm proximal to the lateral epicondyle and passes 4.5 cm medial to the lateral epicondyle. Its anterior and posterior branches supply the anterolateral and posterolateral surfaces of the forearm. The **medial cutaneous nerve of the forearm** (C8, T1) is also at risk of injury during elbow surgery on the medial aspect of the elbow.[4,5] The posterior branch divides into two or three branches that cross anywhere from 6 cm proximal to 6 cm distal to the medial epicondyle[6] (see Fig. 1.2A). Because the cutaneous nerves lie just superficial to the deep fascia, they are protected if the surgeon

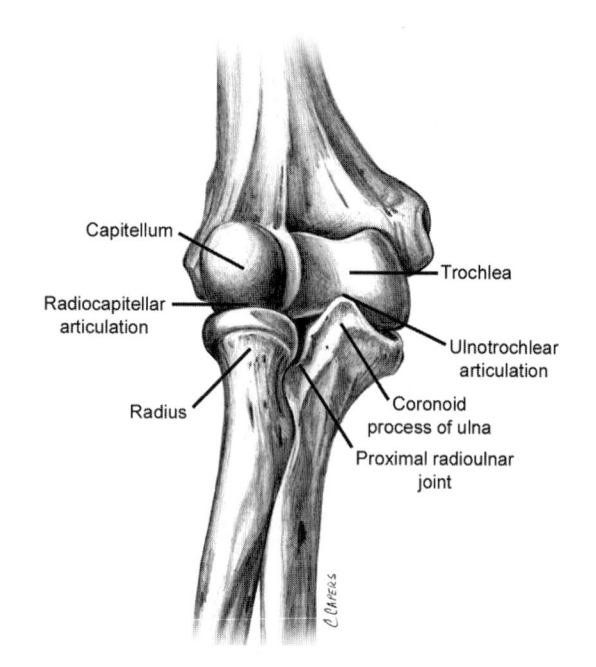

FIGURE 1.1. Three articulations of the elbow joint: the ulnotrochlear, radiocapitellar, and proximal radioulnar joints.

creates full-thickness skin flaps.[1] The anterior and posterior cutaneous nerve distribution of the upper limb is shown in Figures 1.2B and C, respectively.

The superficial **lymphatics** of the upper limb follow the superficial veins. Some of the lymphatics of the hand follow the basilic vein to the supratrochlear node, which is located just proximal to the medial epicondyle. Patients who have disorders of the hand may present with a tender or enlarged supratrochlear lymph node.[7]

The Deep Fascia of the Upper Limb

The next layer encountered is the investing layer of deep fascia, which is strongest posteriorly where it covers the triceps muscle. Below the insertion of the deltoid, it is thickened on each side by a strong intermuscular septum that stabilizes the fascia to the respective supracondylar ridge and epicondyle. The intermuscular septa separate the posterior triceps muscle from the muscles of the anterior compartment of the arm and provide attachment for both.

The radial nerve and the anterior descending branch of the profunda brachii artery perforate the **lateral intermuscular septum** (Fig. 1.3) 10 cm proximal to the lateral epicondyle. The ulnar nerve and the ulnar collateral artery perforate the **medial intermuscular septum** 8 cm above the medial epicondyle. Excision or division of this septum is recommended when performing anterior transposition of the ulnar nerve. The **bicipital aponeurosis** (lacertus fibrosis) (Fig. 1.4) is a thickening of the deep fascia that extends from the biceps brachii tendon to the subcutaneous border of the ulna and can be palpated on the medial aspect of the taut biceps tendon.

The Muscular Layer

Beneath the deep fascia lies the muscular layer, which is interspersed with the major neurovascular structures. An understanding of the various intermuscular intervals is critical to safely performing elbow surgery. A few muscles are of particular surgical importance to the elbow and are described in detail (Table 1.1). **Hilton's law** states that the motor nerve to a muscle that crosses a joint gives a branch to that joint and the skin over the joint.[8]

Triceps Brachii Muscle

The triceps brachii constitutes the entire musculature of the posterior compartment of the arm (Fig. 1.5). The long head of this muscle originates at the infraglenoid tuberosity of the scapula. The lateral head has a linear origin proximal and lateral to the spiral groove that separates it from the medial head. The medial head (or the deep head) is deep to the other two heads; it originates below and medial to the spiral groove and widens to include the adjacent intermuscular septa.[8] Thus, each head takes origin distal to the other, with progressively larger areas of origin.

The long and lateral heads are superficial and blend in the midline to form a common superficial tendon that inserts into the posterior surface of the proximal olecranon and the adjacent deep fascia[9] (Fig. 1.6). The deep medial head is fleshy and inserts mainly into the deep surface of the common tendon, with the remainder inserting into the olecranon and joint capsule.[10] Insertion into the capsule prevents impingement of the capsule in the olecranon fossa. The triceps muscle does not insert into the proximal tip of the olecranon, but is separated by the subtendinous olecranon bursa.

Proximal to the spiral groove, the radial nerve provides muscular branches to the long and medial heads. Within the spiral groove, muscular branches supply the lateral and medial heads. This second branch to the medial head traverses it to supply the anconeus and is at risk of injury during some surgical approaches.[11–13]

The medial head is active in all phases of extension, while the long and lateral heads are minimally active except in resisted extension.[13] An anomalous musculotendinous slip of the triceps can run through the groove behind the medial epicondyle in extension and snap forward in flexion to produce a "snapping triceps tendon."[10] This condition can be confused with a snapping ulnar nerve.

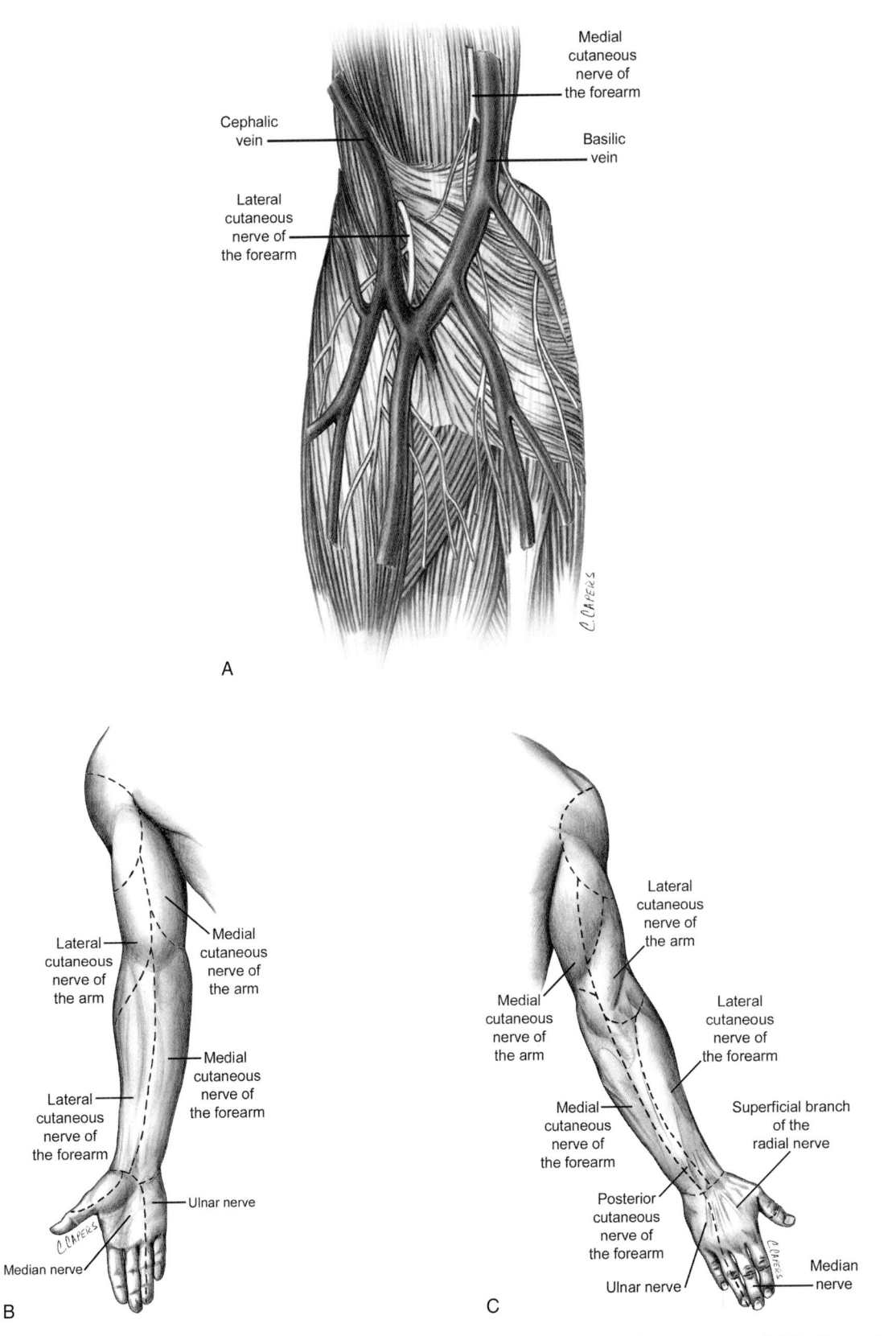

FIGURE 1.2. (A) Subcutaneous nerves and veins around the elbow. Anterior view. (B) Sensory nerve distribution pattern. Anterior view. (C) Sensory nerve distribution pattern. Posterior view.

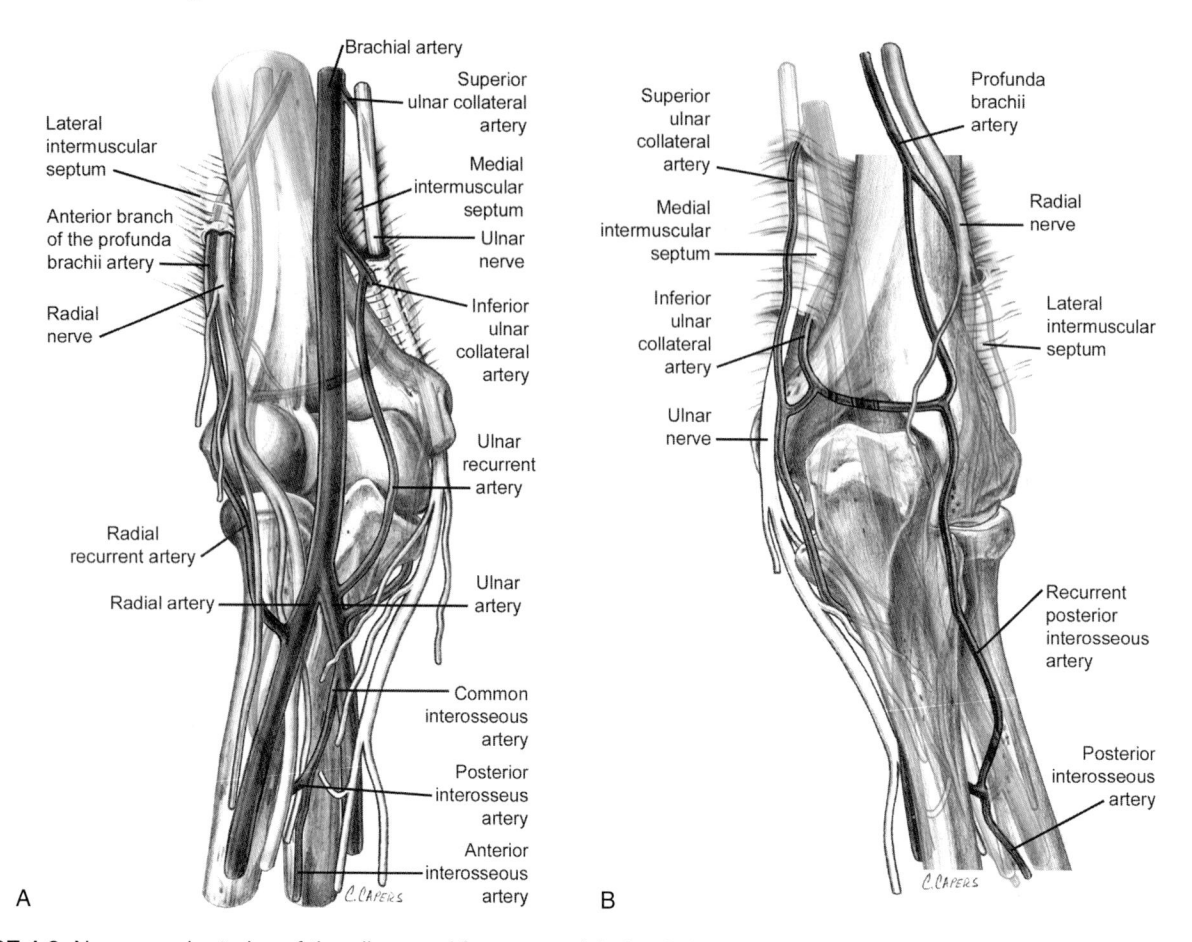

FIGURE 1.3. Nerves and arteries of the elbow and forearm and their relationship to the medial and lateral intermuscular septa of the arm. (A) Anterior aspect. (B) Posterior aspect.

Anconeus Muscle

The anconeus (Fig. 1.7) is the small triangular muscle that covers the lateral aspect of the radiocapitellar joint and is a key landmark for surgical approaches to the elbow. It originates from a small depression on the posterior aspect of the lateral epicondyle[8] and inserts into the lateral dorsal surface of the olecranon and proximal ulna. The second motor branch to the medial head of the triceps (C7, C8) enters the anconeus at its proximal border and innervates the muscle. The anconeus is active in elbow extension, ulnar abduction during pronation, and joint stabilization. This muscle has been used as a local flap for skin coverage over the elbow. We have also used this muscle as a muscular interposition for proximal radioulnar synostosis.

Supinator Muscle

The supinator muscle lies deep to the anconeus muscle and the extensor muscle mass. This muscle is important surgically because of its close proximity to the posterior interosseous nerve.

The deep ulnar head of the supinator originates at the supinator crest and fossa of the ulna and wraps horizon-

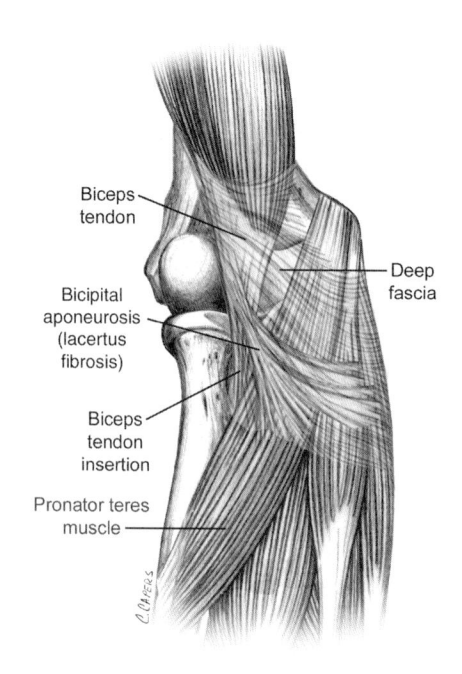

FIGURE 1.4. Relationship of the muscles of the anterior aspect of the elbow to the biceps tendon, deep fascia, and bicipital aponeurosis.

TABLE 1.1. *Muscles of the elbow*

Muscle	Origin	Insertion	Nerve supply	Action
Posterior				
Triceps brachii		Aponeurosis from long and lateral heads blend and insert into olecranon	Radial nerve, C7–C8	Elbow extension
Long head	Infraglenoid tuberosity of scapula			
Lateral head	Humerus above spiral groove			
Medial head	Humerus below spiral groove	Aponeurosis and olecranon		
Anconeus	Posterior lateral epicondyle	Dorsolateral proximal ulna	Motor branch to medial head of triceps, C7–C8	Elbow extension, abduction, and stabilization
Extensor carpi ulnaris	Lateral epicondyle and aponeurosis from subcutaneous border of ulna	Fifth metacarpal	PIN, C6–C7	Wrist extension and ulnar deviation
Extensor digitorum communis	Anterolateral epicondyle	Extensor mechanism of each finger	PIN, C7–C8	Metacarpal phalangeal joint extension
Lateral				
Extensor carpi radialis brevis	Inferolateral lateral epicondyle	Third metacarpal	PIN, C6–C7	Wrist extension
Extensor carpi radialis longus	Lateral supracondylar ridge	Second metacarpal	Radial nerve, C6–C7	Wrist extension
Brachioradialis	Lateral supracondylar ridge	Radial styloid	Radial nerve, C5–C6	Elbow flexion with forearm in neutral rotation
Supinator	Anterolateral lateral epicondyle, lateral collateral ligament, supinator crest of ulna	Proximal and middle third of radius	PIN, C5–C6	Forearm supination
Medial				
Flexor digitorum superficialis	Medial epicondyle, ulnar collateral ligament, medial coronoid and proximal two-thirds of radius	Middle phalanges of fingers	Median nerve, C7–C8	Flexion of PIP joints
Flexor digitorum profundus	Medial olecranon and proximal three-fourths of ulna	Distal phalanges of fingers	Media nerve (index and middle fingers), ulnar nerve (ring and little fingers), C8–T1	Flexion of DIP joints
Anterior				
Biceps brachii		Tendon into bicipital tuberosity of radius	Musculocutaneous nerve, C5–C6	Elbow flexion, supination of flexed
Long head	Supraglenoid tubercle of scapula			
Short head	Coracoid process of scapula	Eponeurosis into forearm fascia and ulna		
Pronator teres	Anterosuperior medial epicondyle, coronoid process of ulna	Pronator tuberosity of radius	Median nerve, C6–C7	Forearm pronation, weak elbow flexion
Humeral head				
Ulnar head				
Flexor carpi radialis	Anteroinferior aspect of medial epicondyle	Second and third metacarpals	Median nerve, C6–C7	Wrist flexion and weak forearm pronation
Palmaris longus	Medial epicondyle	Palmar aponeurosis	Median nerve, C7, C8, T1	Wrist flexion
Flexor carpi ulnaris		Pisiform and fifth metacarpal	Ulnar nerve, C7–C8, T1	Wrist flexion and ulnar deviation
Humeral head	Medial epicondyle			
Ulnar head	Medial olecranon, proximal two-thirds of ulna and aponeurosis from subcutaneous border of ulna			

PIN, posterior interosseous nerve.

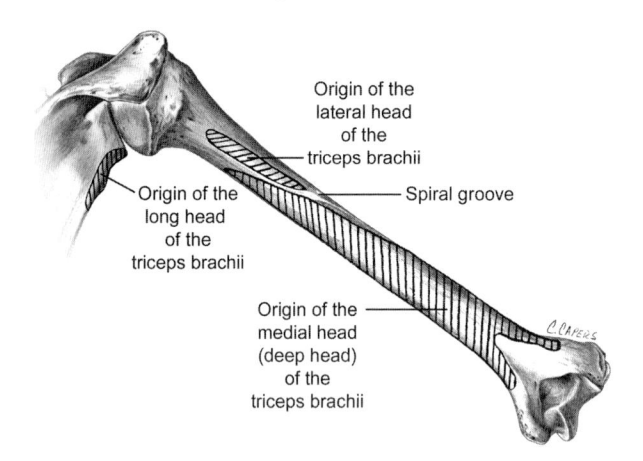

FIGURE 1.5. Origins of the triceps muscle. Note that the medial head also originates from the medial and lateral intermuscular septum.

tally around the radius.[8] The superficial humeral head originates from the distal border of the lateral epicondyle just anterior to the anconeus, the radial collateral ligament, and the proximal ulna just posterior to the supinator crest. The fibers slope downward and overlie the horizontal deep fibers. The arcade of Frohse is the proximal fibrous arch of the superficial head of the supinator muscle.[14] It will be described in more detail when we describe the radial nerve. The muscle is rhomboid in shape. It proceeds distally, obliquely, and radially to wrap around and insert into the proximal and middle thirds of the radius between the anterior and posterior oblique lines.

The posterior interosseous nerve (C5, C6) innervates both heads of the supinator muscle and passes between them into the forearm to supply the extensor muscles of the wrist and digits. Retraction of this nerve when exposing the proximal radius is a common cause of iatrogenic nerve injury.

The supinator muscle assists the biceps muscle with supination of the forearm. The surgeon must be aware of the posterior interosseous nerve's presence in the muscle's substance while dissecting in its vicinity. When exposing the proximal radius, he or she should protect the posterior interosseous nerve by either stripping the supinator muscle subperiosteally from the radius (nerve within the muscle) or by dividing the superficial humeral head (nerve exposed). With pronation of the forearm, the proximal posterior interosseous nerve is translated approximately 1 cm anteromedially. This concept is important to remember when using lateral approaches to the elbow because pronation increases the zone of safety for the posterior interosseous nerve.[15]

Pronator Teres Muscle

The pronator teres muscle is the most proximal of the pronator flexor group and forms the medial border of the cubital fossa. The large humeral head arises from the medial supracondylar ridge and the anterosuperior aspect of the medial epicondyle. The small ulnar head arises from the coronoid process of the ulna and can be absent in 6% of individuals.[16] Before it passes between them into the forearm, the median nerve (C6, C7) supplies a branch to each head. A fibrous arch connects the two heads and may entrap the median nerve that passes beneath it. The common muscle belly proceeds radially and distally under the brachioradialis and inserts into the middle third of the radius.

The pronator teres muscle is the primary pronator of the forearm and is a weak flexor of the elbow. It is an important surgical landmark and is the cause of entrapment of the proximal median nerve.

Cubital Fossa

The cubital fossa is a triangular space on the anterior aspect of the elbow (Fig. 1.8). A line joining the medial

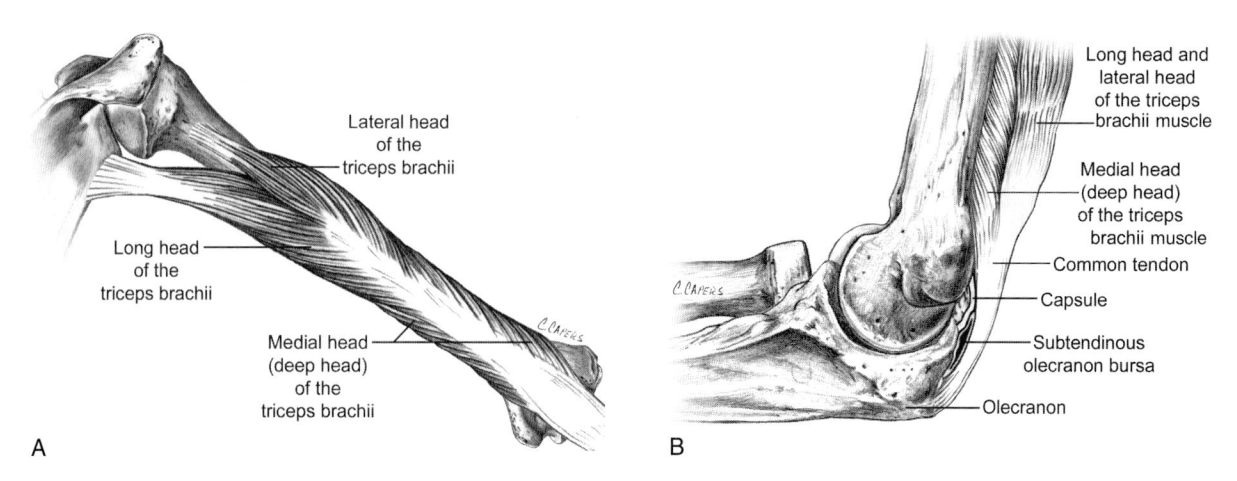

FIGURE 1.6. (A) Triceps muscle on the posterior aspect of the arm. (B) Insertion of the three heads into the capsule. Medial view.

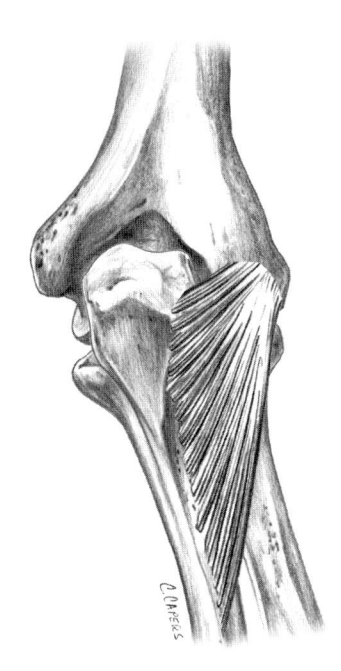

FIGURE 1.7. Anconeus muscle. Posterior aspect.

them to supply the ulnar half of the flexor digitorum profundus muscle, and then supplies the hand.

The ulnar nerve may be entrapped at a number of sites at the level of the elbow: the arcade of Struthers, the cubital tunnel, the arcade of Osborne, and the anconeus epitrochlearis. The **arcade of Struthers** is a band of fas-

and lateral epicondyles of the humerus forms its proximal boundary. The lateral boundary is the medial border of the brachioradialis muscle, and the medial boundary is the lateral border of the pronator teres muscle. Its roof is demarcated by the deep fascia of the forearm and is reinforced by the bicipital aponeurosis. The brachialis and supinator muscles form its floor. The contents of the cubital fossa from medial to lateral are the median nerve, the brachial artery, the biceps tendon, the radial nerve, and the posterior interosseous nerve.

The biceps tendon is flat in the cubital fossa and rotates so that the anterior surface faces laterally to pass between the radius and ulna, inserting into the bicipital tuberosity on the radius. A rough area on the posterior aspect of the tuberosity can be visualized on the dry bone, and a small bursa protects the smooth area anterior to this.[8] The biceps muscle is the primary supinator of the forearm.

The Neural Tunnels Around the Elbow

The **ulnar nerve** is derived from the medial cord of the brachial plexus (C7-C8, T1). It passes posteriorly through the medial intermuscular septum 8 cm above the epicondyle and continues distally along the medial margin of the triceps with the superior ulnar collateral artery. It provides no branches in the arm. The ulnar nerve enters the cubital tunnel (Fig. 1.9) posterior to the medial epicondyle and grooves the posterior portion of the medial collateral ligament. A few small twigs supply the elbow joint.[17] The ulnar nerve supplies motor branches to the heads of the flexor carpi ulnaris muscle, passes between

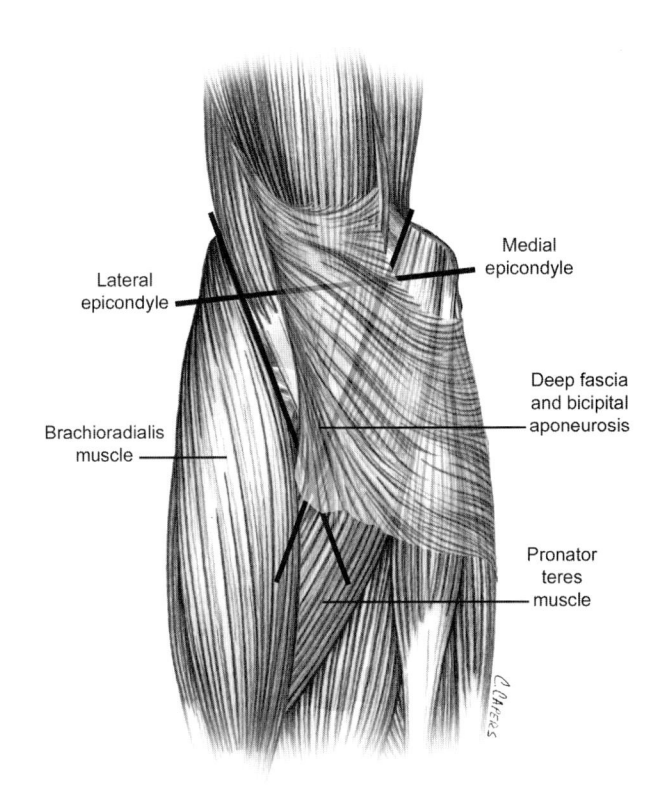

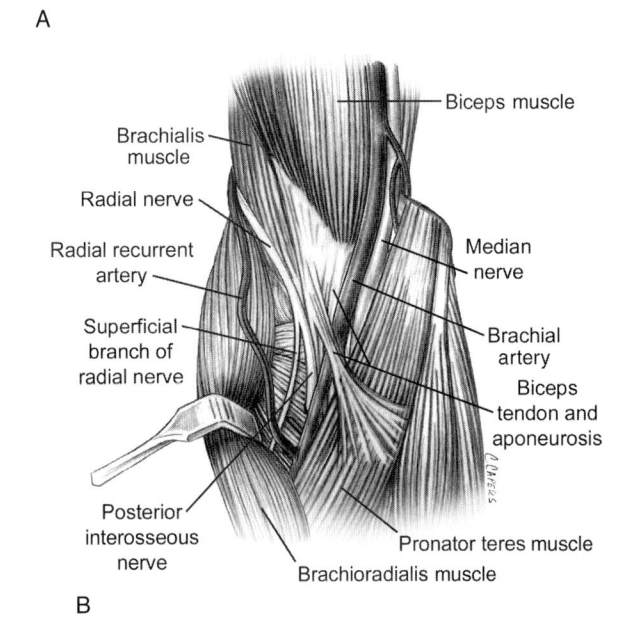

FIGURE 1.8. Cubital fossa. (A) The cubital fossa is the triangular space formed by a line joining the medial and lateral epicondyles and the borders of the brachioradialis and pronator teres muscles. (B) The contents include the nerves, arteries, and biceps tendon.

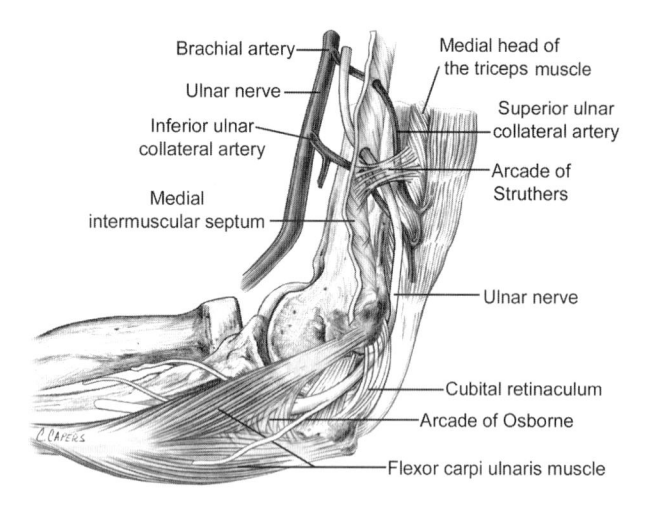

FIGURE 1.9. The ulnar nerve passes through the arcade of Struthers, the cubital tunnel, and the arcade of Osborne.

cia extending from the medial intermuscular septum to the medial head of the triceps and is present in 70% of the population.[18] The ulnar nerve passes under the arcade and is susceptible to compression. This is especially so after anterior transposition of the nerve when adequate release of the arcade is not performed.[18] The **cubital tunnel** is a fibro-osseous tunnel beneath the cubital retinaculum that bridges the medial epicondyle and the olecranon.[18] The boundaries of the cubital tunnel are the ulnar groove of the medial epicondyle anteriorly, the medial collateral ligament laterally, and the cubital retinaculum posteriorly (Fig. 1.10). The sensory and intrinsic motor fibers of the ulnar nerve are superficial and are therefore more predisposed to entrapment neuropathy than the motor fibers to the flexor carpi ulnaris and the flexor digitorum profundus muscles. The cubital retinaculum becomes taut with elbow flexion, thus decreasing the capacity of the cubital tunnel and compressing the ulnar nerve. Absence or redundancy of the cubital retinaculum accounts for developmental subluxation of the ulnar nerve.

The **arcade of Osborne**, which is present in 77% of individuals, is a thickened band of the aponeurosis between the two heads of the flexor carpi ulnaris.[5] It tightens with elbow flexion and can cause nerve compression (see Fig. 1.9). The **anconeus epitrochlearis** is an anomalous muscle that originates at the medial border of the olecranon and inserts into the medial epicondyle. This muscle also can cause ulnar nerve compression.[10]

The **radial nerve** is derived from the posterior cord of the brachial plexus (C5-T1) and courses along the spiral groove to pass through the lateral intermuscular septum 10 cm proximal to the lateral epicondyle. In the anterior compartment, it lies between the brachialis and brachioradialis muscles, supplying motor branches to each (only the lateral portion of the brachialis). The **radial tunnel** is approximately 5 cm long and extends from the level of the radiocapitellar joint to the proximal edge of the superficial head of the supinator muscle.[19] The brachioradialis and extensor carpi radialis longus and brevis form the lateral wall of the radial tunnel. The brachioradialis spirals around and over the nerve from lateral to anterior to form the roof of the tunnel. The anterior capsule of the radiocapitellar joint proximally and the deep head of the supinator distally constitute the floor. The **superficial cutaneous branch** of the radial nerve exits the tunnel proximally, and the **posterior interosseous nerve** diverges posterolaterally to pass beneath the proximal edge of the superficial head of the supinator muscle.

The **arcade of Frohse** is the fibrous proximal aspect of the origin of the superficial head of the supinator. It attaches in a semicircular manner from the tip of the lateral epicondyle, and its fibers arch downward 1 cm and gain attachment to the medial aspect of the lateral epicondyle just lateral to the articular surface of the capitellum.[14] Spinner reported that the lateral half of the arch is fibrous in all individuals and that the medial half is membranous in 70% and fibrous in 30% of individuals.[14] The posterior interosseous nerve passes under this arch and may be compressed when the elbow is in pronation.

The tendinous origin of the **extensor carpi radialis brevis** has a flat, rigid medial edge that may compress the radial nerve. Anterior to the radial head, transverse fibrous bands cross the radial nerve. At the neck of the radius, a fan of vessels including the **recurrent branch of the radial artery** and muscular branches to the mobile wad of three muscles cross the posterior interosseous nerve. These fibrous bands in front of the radial head and the recurrent branch of the radial artery also can cause radial nerve entrapment.

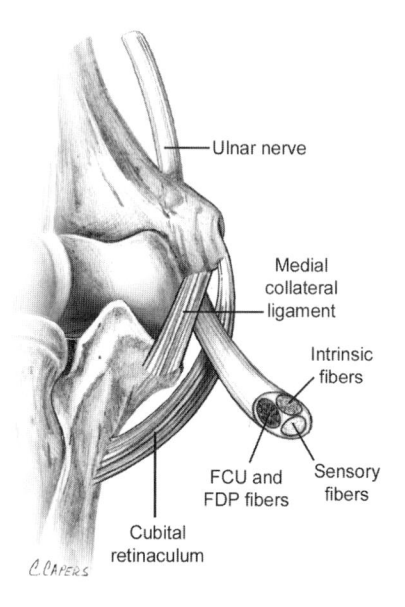

FIGURE 1.10. The ulnar nerve and its components traverse the cubital tunnel (FCU, flexor carpi ulnaris; FDP, flexor digitorum profundus).

The Elbow Capsule and Synovial Membrane

The **synovial membrane** is attached to the articular margins of the joint and lines the capsule and annular ligament. The **capsule** attaches to the articular margin except at the coronoid, radial, and olecranon fossae, where it attaches to the rim of the fossae (Fig. 1.11). The joint capsule does not attach to the radius; it is confluent with the annular ligament that attaches to the anterior and posterior margins of the sigmoid notch and encircles the radius. **Haversian fat pads** are located in each of these fossae between the capsule and synovial membrane. Distention of the joint by hemarthrosis displaces these fat pads out of their respective fossae and produces the characteristic "fat pad sign" seen on lateral radiographs. The anterior capsule is normally a thin transparent structure through which the surgeon can visualize the prominences of the articular condyles. The anterior capsule becomes taut in extension and is an important stabilizer of the extended elbow. The maximum joint capacity is 25 to 30 mL at approximately 80° of flexion.[20]

The ligamentous complexes that stabilize the joint are thickenings of the capsule on its medial and lateral aspects. The **medial collateral ligament complex** consists of three components: the anterior and posterior bundles and the transverse ligament (Fig. 1.12). The **anterior bundle** is structurally and biomechanically the significant component of the medial collateral ligament complex and has three functional bands. The first band arises from the anterior surface of the medial epicondyle and is taut in extreme joint positions. The second band arises below the tip of the epicondyle and is taut in intermediate joint po-

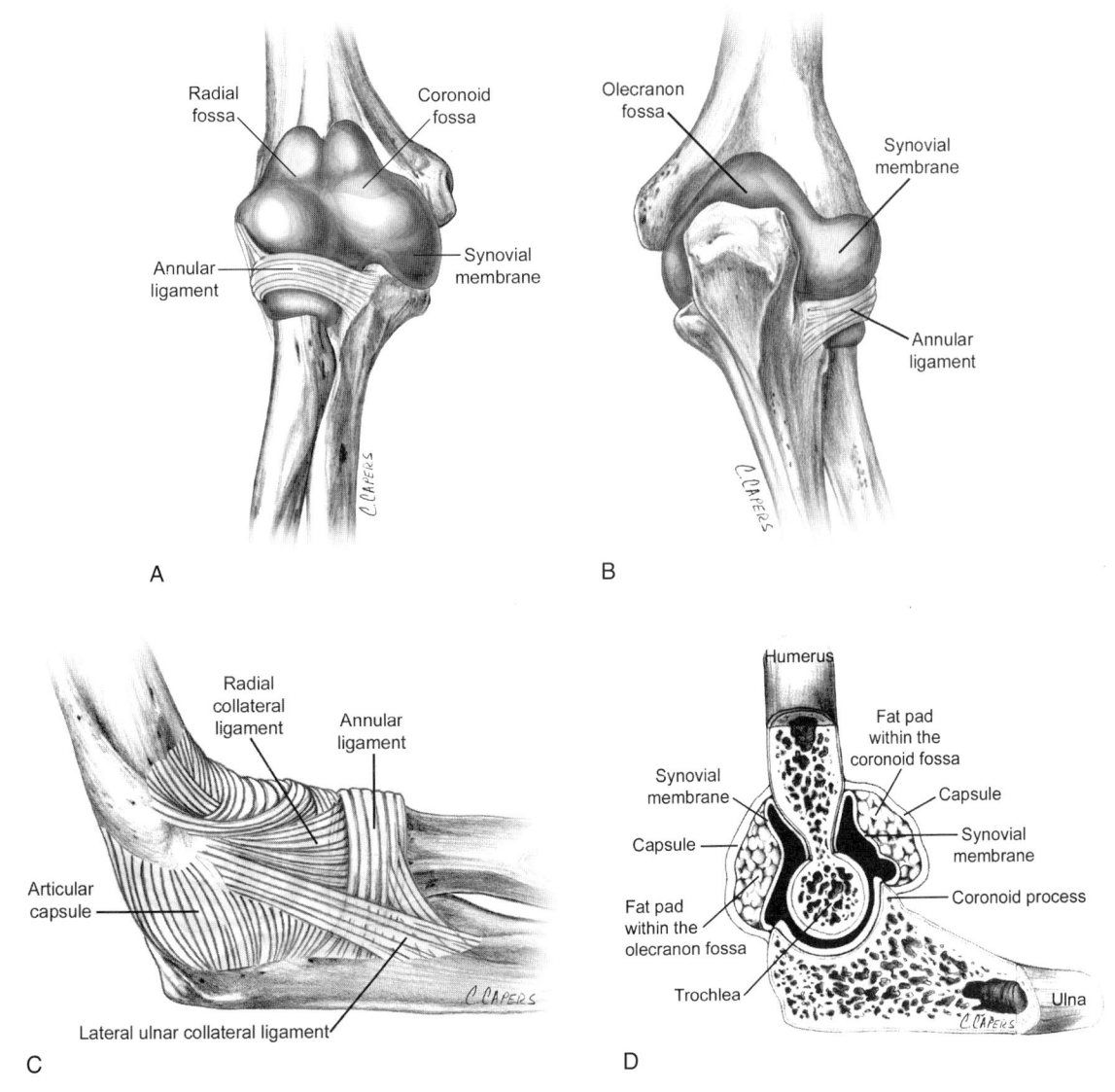

FIGURE 1.11. Elbow capsule and synovial reflections. (A) Anterior view. (B) Posterior view. (C) Lateral view of capsule showing its relationship to annular ligament. (D) Sagittal section of the elbow showing intracapsular extrasynovial Haversian fat pads.

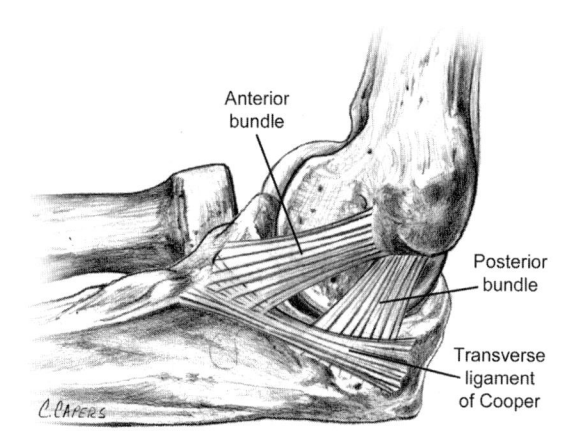

FIGURE 1.12. Medial ligament complex of the elbow.

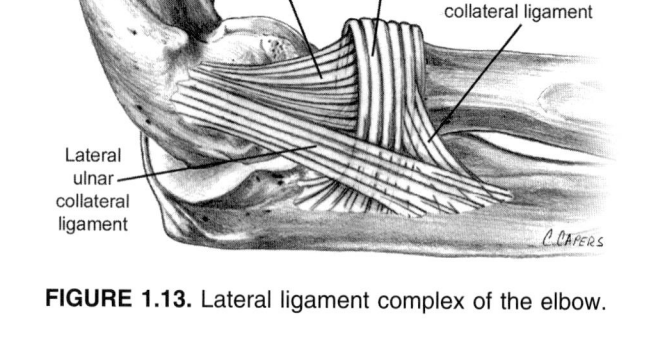

FIGURE 1.13. Lateral ligament complex of the elbow.

sitions. The third band, which arises from the inferior edge of the epicondyle, is taut throughout the full range of joint motion (isometric).[21] The anterior bundle attaches to the sublime tubercle on the medial aspect of the coronoid process. Its mean length and width are 27 mm and 4 to 5 mm, respectively.

The **posterior bundle** (Bardinet's ligament) of the medial collateral ligament complex is fan shaped and attaches inferior and posterior to the axis of rotation on the medial epicondyle.[21] It attaches to the middle of the medial margin of the trochlear notch and is taut during flexion. Its mean length is 24 mm, and its mean width is 5 to 6 mm at the middle portion. This ligament is important because it provides stability to the elbow against pronation. The **transverse ligament of Cooper** (olecranon coronoid ligament) is not always well defined and does not contribute to joint stability because it is limited only to the ulna.

The **medial collateral ligament complex** lies under the prominence of the medial epicondyle. Therefore, when performing a medial epicondylectomy, the surgeon can excise the medial fifth of the width of the epicondyle (1 to 4 mm) without violating the medial collateral ligament.[22] O'Driscoll et al. recommend that the osteotomy should be in a plane between the sagittal and coronal planes, with removal of a greater amount of the posterior portion of the epicondyle.[22]

The **lateral ligament complex** consists of four components: the radial collateral ligament, the annular ligament, the lateral ulnar collateral ligament, and the accessory lateral collateral ligament (Fig. 1.13). The **radial collateral ligament** attaches to the lateral epicondyle and merges indistinguishably with the annular ligament. Its mean length and width are 20 mm and 8 mm, respectively. The **annular ligament** attaches to the anterior and posterior margins of the radial notch of the proximal ulna, encircling the radius but not attaching to it. The most distal aspect of the annular ligament has a smaller diameter that encircles the neck to provide greater stability.

The **lateral ulnar collateral ligament** attaches proximally to the lateral epicondyle and distally to the tubercle of the supinator crest of the ulna. It is the primary lateral stabilizer of the ulnohumeral joint, and its deficiency is the "essential lesion" that produces posterolateral rotatory instability.[23,24] The humeral attachment is at the isometric point on the lateral side of the elbow. In some patients, this ligament cannot be distinguished from the capsule.[25] The capsule posterior to this named ligament is also important because it provides resistance against supination.

The **accessory lateral collateral ligament** blends proximally with the fibers of the annular ligament and distally attaches to the tubercle of the supinator crest. The function of the accessory ligament is to stabilize the annular ligament during varus stress.

The **quadrate ligament** of Denuce is a thin fibrous layer between the inferior margin of the annular ligament and the ulna. It is a stabilizer of the proximal radioulnar joint during full supination.

The **oblique ligament** is a small and inconstant ligament formed by the fascia overlying the deep head of the supinator between the ulna and radius just below the radial tuberosity. It has no known functional importance, but some authors believe this ligament is a cause of rotatory contractures of the forearm.[26]

OSTEOLOGY

The **ossification centers** of the elbow are important because of the prevalence of fractures around the elbow in developing children (Fig. 1.14). At birth, the preosseus form and articular structures constituting the elbow joint are complete. Ossification, however, has only proceeded

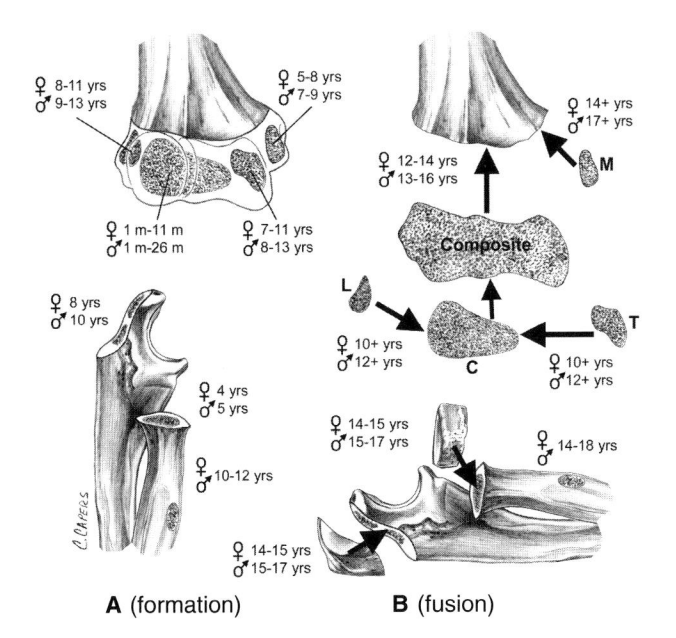

FIGURE 1.14. (A) Appearance of secondary ossification centers about the elbow. (B) Fusion of secondary ossification centers. (M, medial epicondyle; L, lateral epicondyle; C, lateral condyle; T, trochlea.)

to the edges of the joint capsule.[27] The first ossification center to form is the lateral humeral condyle (capitellum); it appears at 6 to 12 months of age and includes the lateral ridge (crista) of the trochlea. The lateral epicondyle, lateral condyle, and trochlear physis (not the medial epicondyle) fuse together at 10 to 12 years of age, and the composite epiphysis fuses to the humeral metaphysis at 12 to 16 years of age. The medial humeral epicondyle fuses to the distal humerus at 14 to 17 years of age.

The **patella cubiti** is an infrequent, separate ossification center that develops in the triceps tendon, is usually unilateral, and can articulate with the trochlea. Wood and Campbell[28] describe it as an accessory sesamoid bone in the triceps muscle. This structure is distinct from the **os supra trochleare dorsale,** which is intra-articular and therefore more anterior. This intra-articular ossicle can grow and fill the olecranon fossa, causing progressive restriction of extension and symptoms. The ossicle could fragment following forced contact with the olecranon, and secondary arthritis of the joint could develop.[28]

The **intraosseous blood supply** of the skeletally mature distal humerus is derived from the central nutrient vessel of the shaft. In the developing distal humerus, the blood supply is more complex and more clinically relevant than in the mature distal humerus. The lateral condylar epiphysis is supplied by two small end vessels that enter the posterior lateral condyle just lateral to the attachment of the capsule near the origin of the anconeus muscle. The trochlea lies within the joint capsule; hence,

the vessels traverse the periphery of the physis to enter the epiphysis. Two end vessels supply the medial crista of the trochlea. The lateral vessel lies on the posterior surface of the humeral metaphysis and penetrates the periphery of the physis to supply the trochlear nucleus. The medial vessel penetrates the nonarticulating portion of the medial crista of the trochlea.[29]

The surgeon must be careful during surgical approaches to the developing lateral condyle so that he or she does not violate the posterior blood supply. The two end vessels to the trochlea are vulnerable to injury, such as a fishtail deformity or a malignant varus deformity.[30]

The bony morphology of the elbow is shown in Figure 1.15. The **trochlea** has anterior, inferior, and posterior articular surfaces. Its obliquity is responsible for the "carrying angle" that exists with the elbow in full extension and supination. The average carrying angle in men is 6.5° (range, 0° to 14°), and in women it is 13° (range, 4° to 20°).[31–33] In extension, the inferoposterior trochlea articulates with the lateral facet of the trochlear notch, and in flexion, the anterior trochlea articulates with the medial facet of the trochlear notch. In relation to the humeral shaft, the distal humeral condyles internally rotate approximately 5°, which may increase following supracondylar fractures.

The **capitellum** is less than half a sphere and has only anterior and inferior articular surfaces. Lateral radiographs show it projecting anteriorly approximately 30° to the shaft of the humerus, which is a useful guide for reducing supracondylar fractures in children.[34] The **coronoid process** is important for stability of the elbow joint, and in type 2 and 3 fractures, the elbow joint is rendered potentially unstable.[35,36]

A **supracondylar process** may project from the medial supracondylar ridge 5 cm proximal to the medial epicondyle and is best seen on an anteroposterior radiograph with the patient's arm in internal rotation. It signifies that a ligament of Struthers is present; this fibrous band spans from the supracondylar process to the medial epicondyle and can entrap the median nerve or the brachial (or ulnar) artery, or both. The pronator teres takes origin from the ligament, if it is present.

THE SURGICAL APPROACHES

The modern historical development of the surgical approaches to the elbow began with the lateral J approach to the elbow that Theodor Kocher described in his book *Textbook of Operative Surgery*[37] published in 1911. Subsequently, many authors, such as Campbell,[38] Van Gorder,[39] Molesworth,[40] Henry,[41] MacAusland,[42] Bryan and Morrey,[43] Morrey and associates,[44–48] and, more recently, Patterson, Bain, and Mehta,[49] have described approaches to the elbow. The surgical approaches to the el-

FIGURE 1.15. Bony morphology of the elbow joint. (A) The joint line is 2 cm distal to the surface markings from the line joining the medial and lateral epicondyles. (B) In extension, the olecranon can be palpated in line with the medial and lateral epicondyles, and (C) in flexion, the three points form an isosceles triangle. (D) Anterior view of the trochlear notch and coronoid process. (E) Anterior view of the capitellum and trochlea. (F) Medial view of trochlear surfaces. (G) Lateral view of trochlear notch and radial notch.

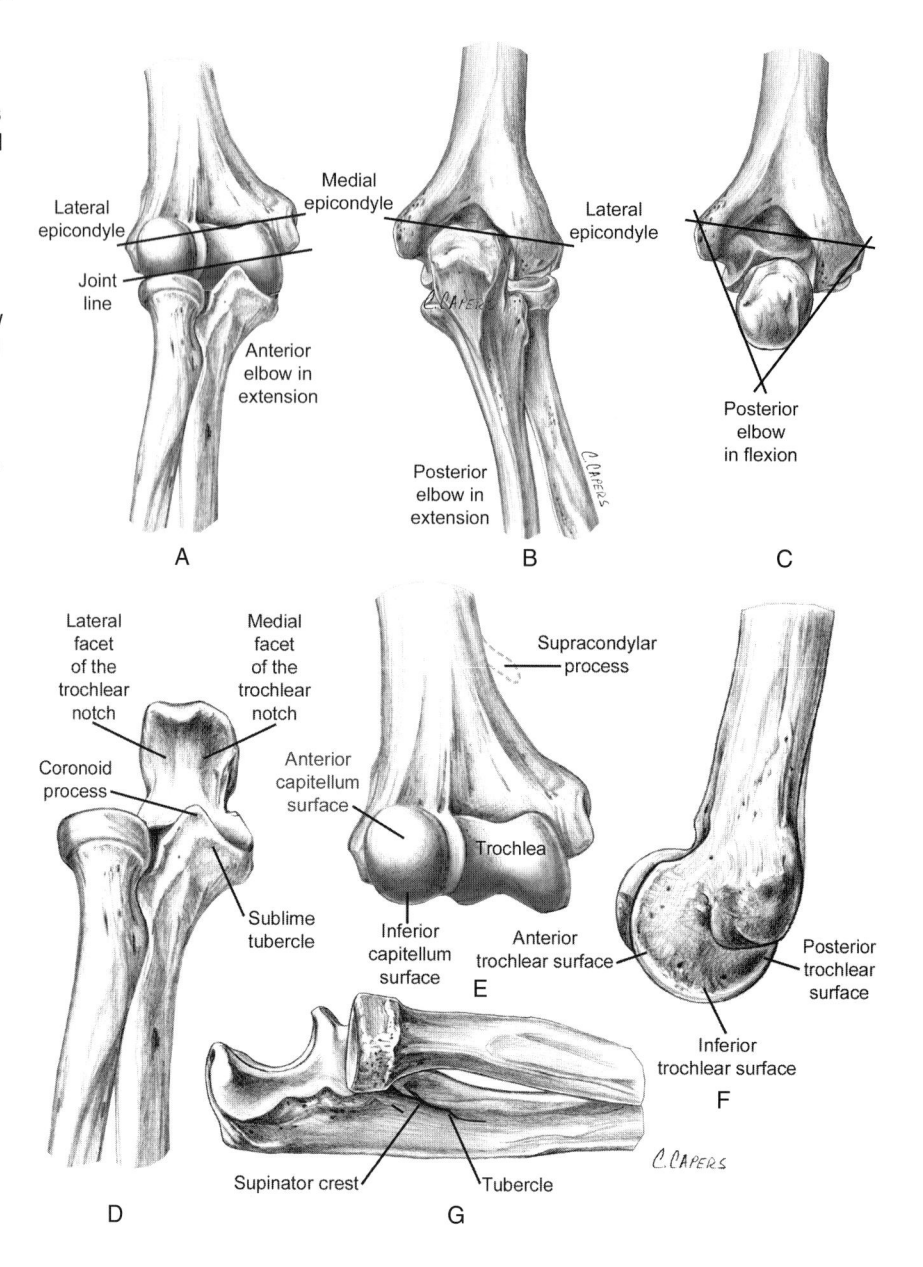

bow can be classified into posterior,[11,12,38,39,42,43,50–53] lateral,[37,54–56] medial,[38,40] combined medial and lateral,[49] and anterior[41] approaches (Table 1.2). Figure 1.16 shows a cross section through the elbow that will help the surgeon to develop an understanding of the named surgical approaches used to treat various disorders. Table 1.3 lists our preferred surgical approaches and their indications.

For major elbow surgery, we place the patient in the lateral decubitus position on a vacuum suction beanbag. We apply an autoclavable, removable tourniquet above the patient's elbow with the arm positioned on a cushioned support. The elbow can be extended easily. With gravity, the elbow flexes to 90°.

Skin Incisions

Surgeons report a high incidence of cutaneous nerve injury with both medial[4,6] and lateral[2,3] incisions. Dowdy et al.[1] reported that a posterior midline skin incision crosses significantly fewer nerves of smaller diameter than either a medial or lateral incision. The cutaneous nerves[1] and the subcutaneous vascular plexus[57,58] lie in the subcutaneous fat and are preserved if full-thickness fasciocutaneous flaps are elevated at the level of the deep fascia.

According to Shawn O'Driscoll, the front of the elbow is at the back. Therefore, we recommend a posterior mid-

TABLE 1.2. *Summary of surgical approaches to the elbow*

Approach	Author	Tissue plane
Posterior	Campbell[38]	Midline triceps split
	Campbell[38]	Triceps aponeurosis tongue, deep head split
	Van Gorder[39]	Triceps tongue (aponeurosis and part of deep head)
	Wadsworth[11]	Triceps tongue (aponeurosis and full-thickness deep head), between ECU and anconeus
	Bryan, Morrey[43]	Elevate triceps mechanism from olecranon and reflect laterally
	Boyd[12]	Lateral border of triceps; anconeus and ECU released from ulna
	Heim, Pfeiffer[53]	Chevron olecranon osteotomy
	Alonso-Llames[50]	Retract triceps medially and laterally
Lateral	Kocher[37]	Between ECU and anconeus
	Cadenat[54]	Between ECRB and ECRL
	Kaplan[55]	Between ECRB and EDC
	Key, Conwell[56]	Between brachioradialis and ECRL
Medial	Molesworth[40]	Medial epicondyle osteotomy and split FCU heads
	Campbell[38]	
Combined	Patterson et al.[49]	Between ECU and anconeus with or without lateral epicondyle osteotomy; FCU elevated from ulna
Anterior	Henry[41]	Between mobile wad and biceps tendon; elevate supinator from radius

ECU, extensor carpi ulnaris; ECRL, extensor carpi radialis longus; ECRB, extensor carpi radialis brevis; EDC, extensor digitorum communis; FCU, flexor carpi ulnaris

line incision for major elbow surgery.[1,49,59] Placement of the incision just lateral to the olecranon takes it away from where the elbow rests on the medial aspect of the olecranon. The entire elbow, including the anterior aspect, can be exposed through this incision, and skin necrosis has not occurred in our patients when we have used this approach. When performing surgical procedures, such as an epicondyle release or an open reduction of simple radial head fractures, we find a more localized approach can be justified, but care for the cutaneous nerves is required.[2–4,6]

For major elbow procedures, we isolate the ulnar nerve and place a tape around it to act as a constant reminder of its location. To avoid inadvertently placing traction on the tape, we do not clamp the tape. Care is taken to preserve the ulnar collateral vessels. We excise the medial intermuscular septum and release the cubital retinaculum to allow the ulnar nerve to be mobilized. At the completion of the procedure, the nerve is placed into its native position. If it is stable throughout the range of motion, it is left in situ. If it dislocates, it is then transposed.

After major elbow surgery, we recommend that the surgeon elevate the patient's elbow in the extended position. We reported the use of the dynamic elbow suspension splint, which is a pediatric Thomas splint suspended from a Balkan frame; it allows the patient to mobilize the extremity while in bed.[59] We now prefer to use a pediatric knee immobilizer because it is more easily applied. Extension facilitates wound closure and healing[46,60] and reduces the risk of fixed flexion deformity.

In the following descriptions of named approaches to the elbow, the details of the skin incision have been omitted unless they have distinct advantages over the posterior midline incision.

Posterior Approaches

The surgeon has a number of options for managing the triceps when approaching the elbow joint (Fig. 1.17). The surgeon can split (Campbell[38]), tongue (Van Gorder[39]), reflect (Kocher[37], Bryan and Morrey[43]), retract (Alonso-Llames,[50] Patterson et al.[49]), or osteotomize the triceps mechanism.

Campbell's Posterolateral Approach

Campbell originally described the triceps splitting approach in 1932[38] (Fig. 1.18). Indications for this posterolateral approach include total elbow arthroplasty and fixation of extra-articular fractures of the distal humerus. After a posterior skin incision is made, a midline incision is made through the triceps fascia and tendon. This incision is continued distally onto the tip of the olecranon and down the ulna. The triceps insertion is released from the olecranon, leaving the extensor mechanism in continuity with the forearm fascia and the medial and lateral muscles. During this approach, the ulnar nerve should be identified and protected.

In the muscular plane, the triceps aponeurosis and the

FIGURE 1.16. (A) Cross section of the elbow at the level of the humeral epicondyles. (B) Location of the named approaches to the elbow. (ECRL, extensor carpi radialis longus; ECRB, extensor carpi radialis brevis; EDC, extensor digitorum communis; ECU, extensor carpi ulnaris.)

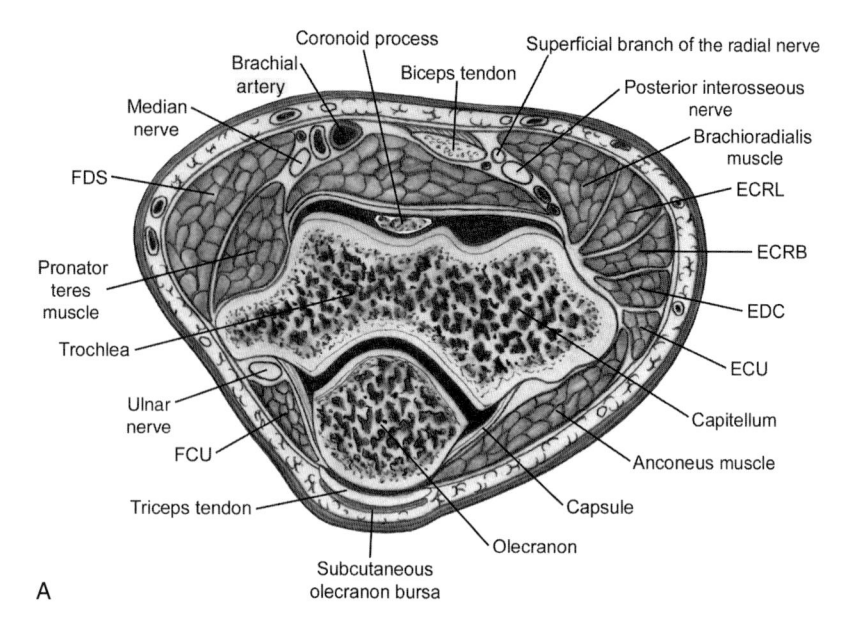

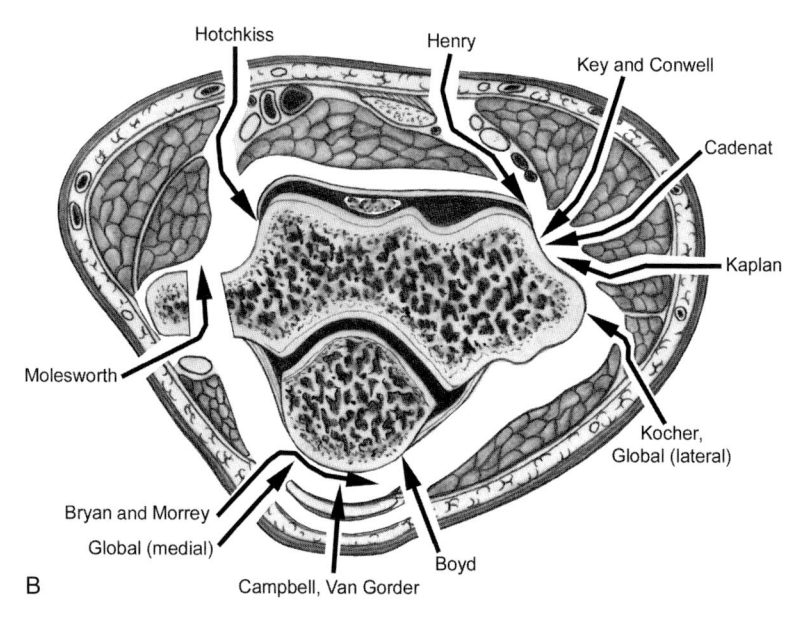

deep medial head are split in the midline. The other muscles around the elbow (anconeus and flexor carpi ulnaris) are released subperiosteally from the humerus and proximal ulna. In the periosteal plane, the joint capsule and the periosteum of the humerus and ulna are divided sharply in the midline to expose the humerus, ulna, and joint.

The soft tissues can be elevated subperiosteally from the distal humerus and olecranon. The surgeon can visualize the posterior distal humerus and elbow joint. The surgeon closes with interrupted sutures to the triceps aponeurosis. We recommend using heavy nonabsorbable transosseous sutures for closure of the triceps mechanism over the point of the olecranon to prevent a boutonnière of the triceps repair.

Wadsworth's Posterolateral Approach

Wadsworth[11] also described a posterolateral approach. Indications for this approach include fixation of distal humeral fractures and total elbow arthroplasty. In the muscular plane, the triceps aponeurosis, along with the underlying deep head of the muscle, is divided in an inverted V with the base attached to the olecranon, leaving a peripheral rim attached to the triceps for later repair. Distally, the surgeon dissects the interval between the extensor carpi ulnaris and the anconeus. The anconeus is reflected medially with the underlying capsule. In the periosteal plane, the lateral exposure can be enhanced by subperiosteal elevation of the common extensor origin and the lateral ligamentous complex.

TABLE 1.3. *Authors' preferred approaches*

Indication	Recommended approach	Alternative approach
Total elbow arthroplasty	Campbell[38] muscle splitting	Bryan and Morrey,[43] Kocher[37]
Soft tissue release	Global (lateral and medial)[49]	Kocher,[37] Bryan and Morrey,[43] Hotchkiss[67]
Supracondylar fracture	Chevron olecranon osteotomy[53]	Wadsworth,[11] Campbell[38]
Radial head, capitellar, or lateral condyle fracture	Global (lateral)[49]	Kocher[37] Chevron olecranon osteotomy[53]
Monteggia fracture	Gordon[63]	—
Coronoid fracture	Global (medial)[49]	Henry[41]
Metaphyseal humeral fracture	Alonso-Llames[50]	Campbell[38] Anterolateral approach to humerus
Radioulnar synostosis	Boyd[12]	Kocher[37]

This exposure extends proximally along the posterior distal humerus and distally along the subcutaneous border of the ulna. The surgeon can visualize the distal humerus and elbow joint. He or she closes the triceps aponeurosis with strong interrupted sutures. Triceps weakness is minimized with secure closure of the aponeurosis.

Modifications. Van Gorder's modification of this technique involves elevating a distally based tongue of approximately 10 cm of triceps aponeurosis (Fig. 1.19).[39] The deep medial head is divided obliquely (posterior proximal to anterior distal) so that no muscle is attached to the proximal tip of the aponeurotic flap, and the entire thickness of the muscle and its insertion are attached to the base of the flap.

Campbell described another modification to this technique.[38] His modified technique involves elevating the tongue of triceps aponeurosis with division of the deep head in the midline. Campbell recommends using the triceps tongue approach only if a triceps contracture is present, and then closure can be performed using a V–Y lengthening. This technique can increase elbow flexion by as much as 40°,[43] but it produces triceps weakness.[44] We believe that the triceps tongue approach should be limited to that originally recommended by Campbell, and, if it is used, we prefer to split the deep medial head in the midline as Campbell described. An advantage of this modification is that it reduces necrosis of the deep head.

Alonso-Llames[50] also reported a modification to the posterolateral technique. Through a midline incision, the surgeon approaches the triceps muscle from the medial and lateral aspects and elevates it from each intermuscular septum. The triceps muscle is simply retracted to expose the distal humerus. He described this approach primarily for the management of supracondylar fractures in children. We have used it successfully to manage extra-articular humeral fractures in adults. When using this approach, the surgeon must protect the ulnar and radial nerves.

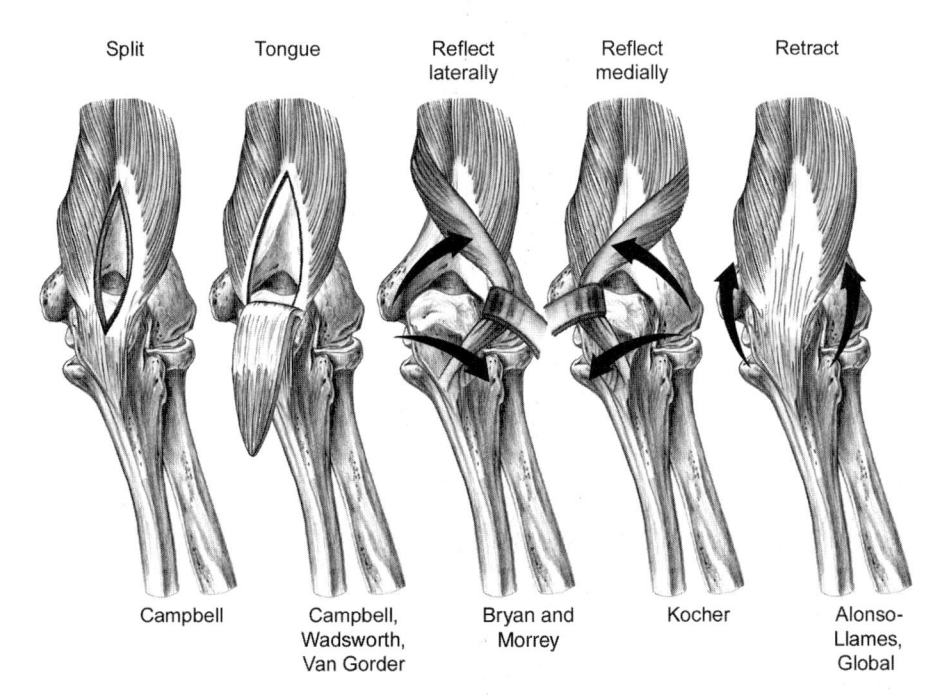

FIGURE 1.17. Surgical options for the triceps mechanism include split, tongue, reflect laterally, reflect medially, or retract techniques. (The surgical option of an osteotomy is not shown here.)

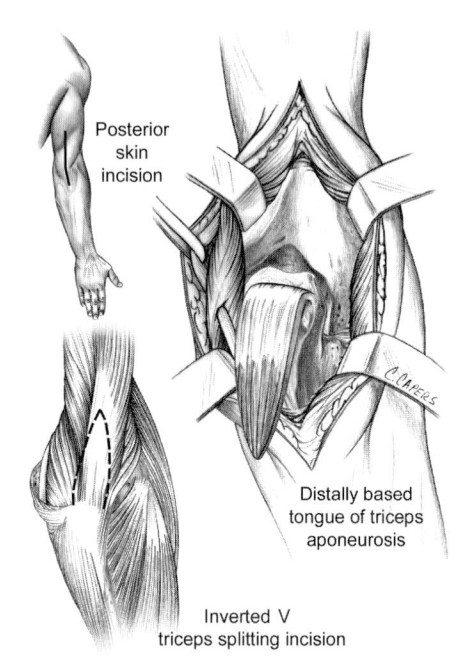

FIGURE 1.18. Campbell's posterolateral approach.

Bryan and Morrey's Extensive Posterior Approach

Bryan and Morrey describe an extensive posterior approach[43] (Fig. 1.20). Indications for this approach include total elbow arthroplasty, fixation of distal humeral fractures, and other cases requiring extensive medial exposure around the elbow.

In the muscular plane, the medial aspect of the triceps is elevated and released from the humerus and the medial intermuscular septum down to the level of the posterior capsule. The fascia of the forearm is incised along the medial aspect of the proximal ulna for approximately 6 cm.

In the periosteal plane, the surgeon elevates and reflects the triceps muscle and its insertion and the fascia and ulnar periosteum as a single unit from medial to lateral. The medial aspect of the junction between the triceps insertion and the ulnar periosteum is the weakest portion of this musculoperiosteal flap, and meticulous care is required during its elevation. Bryan and Morrey[43] recommend that this elevation be accomplished at 20° to 30° of flexion to relieve tension on the flap.

The radial head can be exposed by subperiosteal elevation of the anconeus from the proximal ulna. The posterior capsule usually is reflected with the triceps mechanism, and the tip of the olecranon can be osteotomized to expose the trochlea (see Fig. 1.20B). The medial collateral ligament complex may be reflected by sharp dissection from the humerus to increase the exposure during total elbow arthroplasty.

This exposure extends proximally by subperiosteal dissection of the humerus and distally along the subcutaneous ulna. From this approach, the surgeon can visualize the elbow joint.

For closure, Morrey[48] recommends that the periosteum and triceps insertion be reattached to the proximal ulna with a number 5 crisscrossed transosseous suture (see Fig. 1.20C). An additional transverse suture secures the triceps to the tip of the olecranon. Failure to closely approximate this layer can result in a "sliding" extensor mechanism, with associated pain and weakness. If the medial collateral ligament complex is detached from the humerus, it should be secured with transosseous sutures. The forearm fascia overlying the flexor carpi ulnaris is repaired.

Remember that rupture of the triceps mechanism can occur if care is not taken with elevation of the extensor mechanism from the olecranon. Reattachment should be performed as Morrey[48] recommends.

Modifications. Transosseous exposures require some type of osteotomy. In their modification of Bryan and Morrey's approach, Wolfe and Ranawat recommend that the triceps attachment be released from the ulna by osteotomizing the attachment with a thin wafer of bone and that the entire extensor mechanism with its wafer of bone be reflected laterally.[61]

Boyd's Approach

Boyd[12] describes a posterolateral approach for Monteggia fracture–dislocation, radial head fracture, and reconstruction of the annular ligament (Fig. 1.21). He recommends that a posterolateral incision be made along the lateral border of the triceps muscle and extended distally for 6 cm along the subcutaneous border of the ulna. In

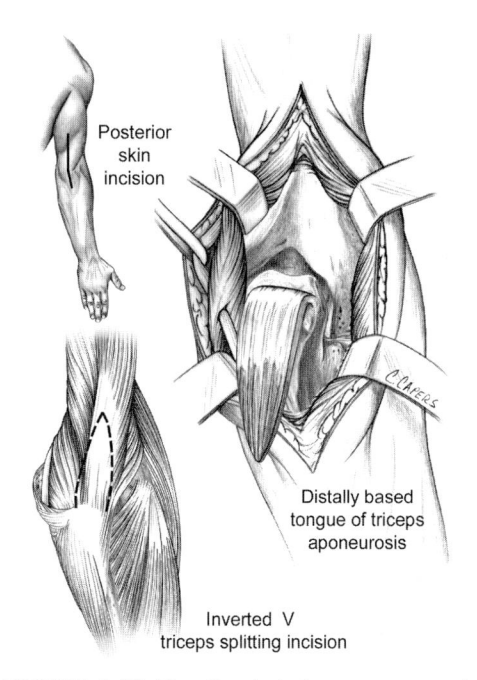

FIGURE 1.19. Van Gorder's tongue approach.

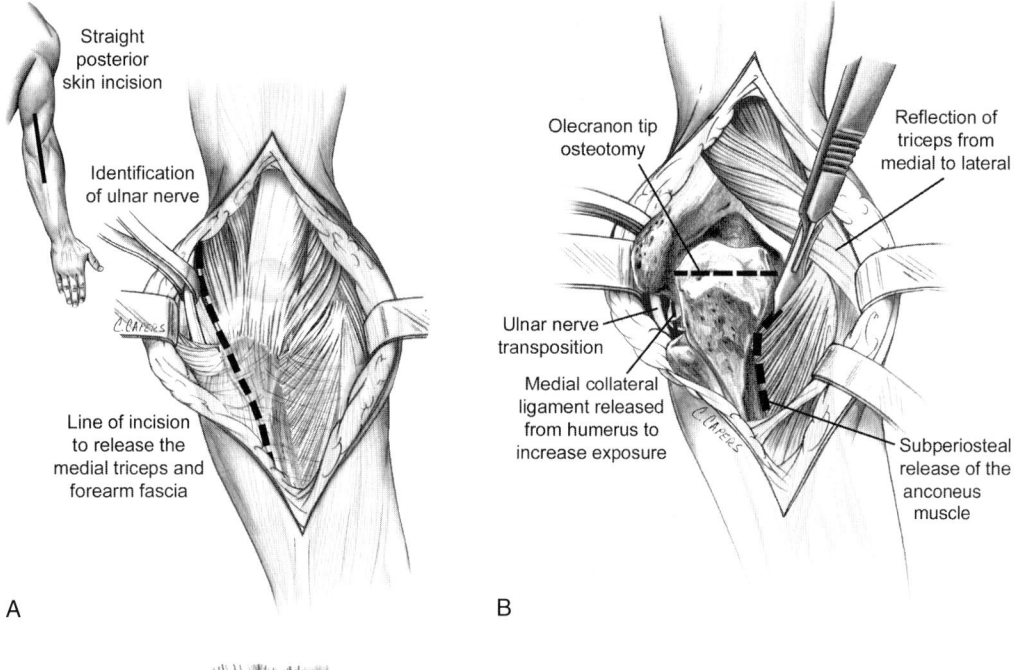

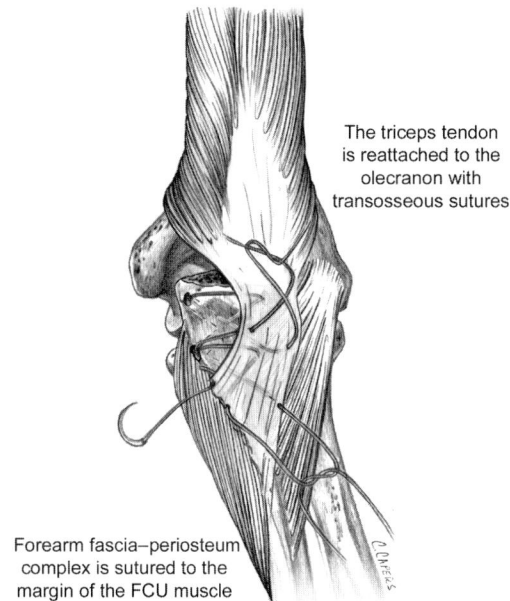

FIGURE 1.20. (A) and (B) Bryan and Morrey's extensive posterior approach. (C) Closure of the extensive posterior approach. (FCU, flexor carpi ulnaris.)

the muscular and periosteal planes, the muscles on the lateral side of the ulna (anconeus and supinator) should be elevated in the subperiosteal plane from the ulna. Retraction of the anconeus and supinator muscles exposes the joint capsule overlying the radial head and neck. This lateral capsule contains the lateral ligamentous complex, and its division can lead to posterolateral rotatory instability. The supinator muscle protects the posterior interosseous nerve.

To expose the radial shaft, the muscles of the lateral aspect of the ulna may be elevated (extensor carpi ulnaris, abductor pollicis longus, and extensor pollicis longus). The muscular flap is retracted at the level of the interosseous membrane. The posterior interosseous and recurrent interosseous arteries may need ligation.

With this approach, the surgeon can view the radiocapitellar joint, proximal quarter of the radius, and the lateral surface of the ulna. For closure, we strongly recommend that the surgeon reattach the lateral ligamentous complex to the supinator crest. The deep fascia is closed.

We have seen posterolateral rotatory instability and radioulnar synostosis result from the Boyd approach and recommend that the surgeon reserve its use for excision or "formation" of radioulnar synostosis (i.e., one-bone forearm). Posterolateral rotatory instability may occur due to detachment of the lateral ligament complex from

FIGURE 1.21. Boyd's approach. (A) Posterior skin incision. (B) Incision is made along the lateral border of the triceps. (ECRL, extensor carpi radialis longus; ECRB, extensor carpi radialis brevis; EDC, extensor digitorum communis; ECU, extensor carpi ulnaris.) (C) The joint capsule is exposed. (D) The supinator muscle overlies the radial head and neck and protects the posterior interosseous nerve. (E) Retraction of the supinator muscle exposes the radial head and neck.

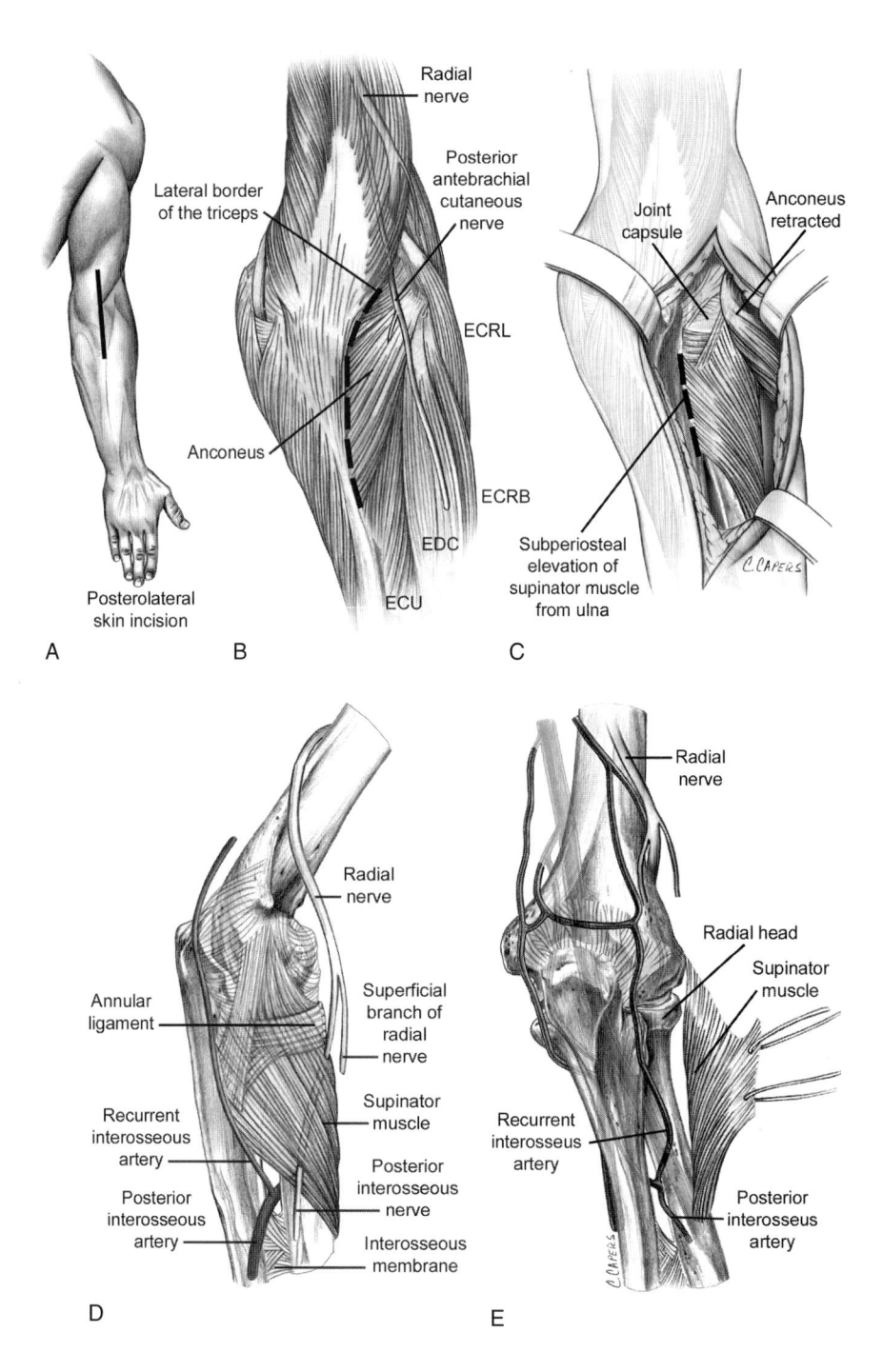

the supinator tubercle. Radioulnar synostosis may occur because the proximal radius and ulna are exposed subperiosteally.[62] The posterior interosseous nerve needs to be protected.

Modifications. For the Monteggia fracture–dislocation, Gordon[63] recommends that the surgeon should expose the ulna with subperiosteal dissection and expose the radial head between the anconeus and the extensor carpi ulnaris (the Kocher interval). Gordon preferred this technique because it preserves the vascularity of the proximal ulnar fragment. We recommend the Gordon modification for the management of Monteggia fracture–dislocation because of the potential complications associated with the Boyd approach.

Olecranon Osteotomy Approach

MacAusland originally described the transolecranon osteotomy approach in 1915[42] (Fig. 1.22). Indications for this approach include fixation of intra-articular fractures of the distal humerus and AO type C3 fractures. In the periosteal plane, the olecranon is exposed and predrilled. The anconeus is elevated from the olecranon, and large

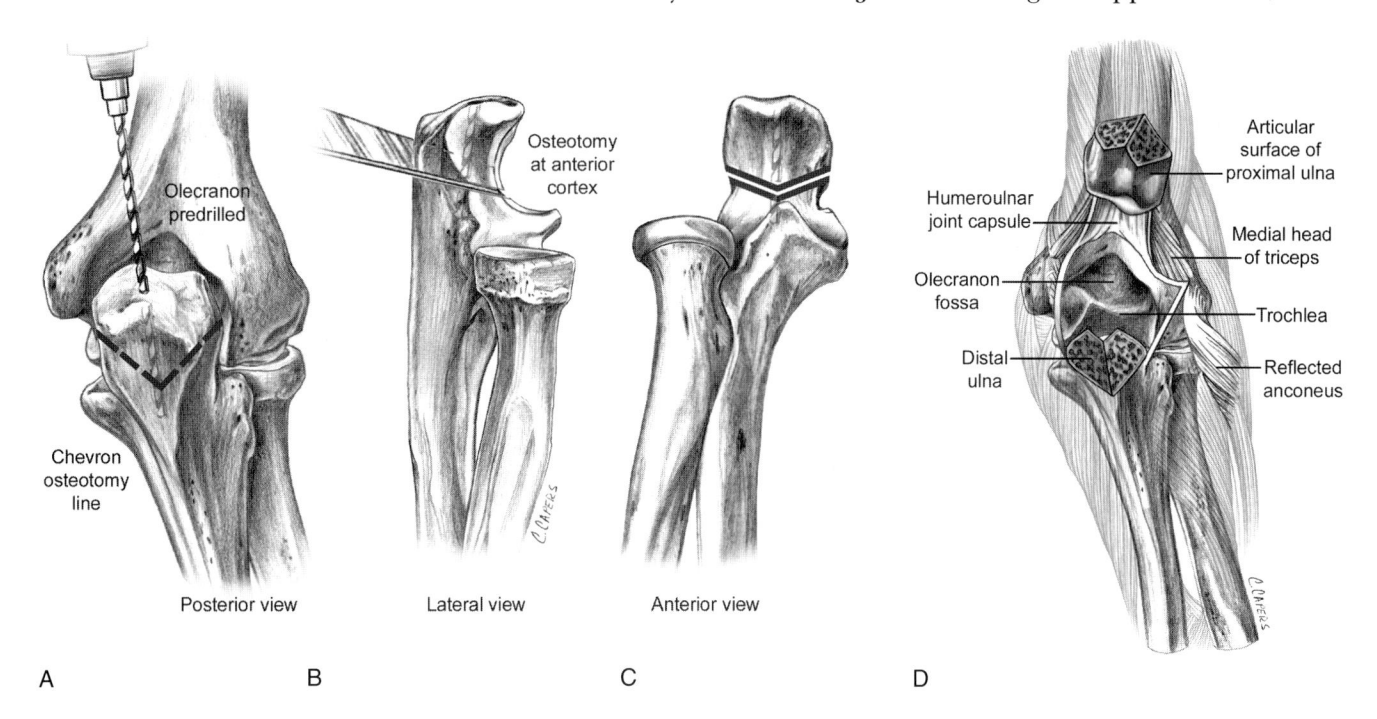

FIGURE 1.22. Chevron olecranon osteotomy. (A) Predrilling of the olecranon. (B) Completion of osteotomy with an osteotome. (C) Point of the osteotomy faces distally. (D) Distal articular surface of the humerus is exposed.

AO bone-holding forceps are used to distract the joint so that the nonarticular area of the olecranon can be identified. The surgeon accomplishes a chevron osteotomy[53] at this site with a thin-bladed oscillating saw up to the anterior cortex and completes it with an osteotome. The olecranon and the triceps mechanism are elevated to expose the distal humerus.[64] The advantage of the chevron osteotomy is that it increases the area for healing and provides some intrinsic rotational control. The point of the chevron osteotomy faces distally so that the collateral ligaments remain attached to the shaft fragment and so that the olecranon fragment is less likely to fracture.

The exposure extends proximally by elevation of the triceps from the humerus and distally by subperiosteal muscular elevation from the proximal ulna. The surgeon can visualize the entire distal articular surface of the humerus.

The olecranon is reattached with a large cancellous screw and tension-band wire. We use a long-threaded, large-fragment AO cannulated screw because it helps to align the olecranon. The guide wire centers the drill and screw into the intramedullary canal. Bone-holding forceps are used to provide rotational control as compression is applied across the osteotomy.

Complications include a 5% incidence of olecranon osteotomy nonunion.[64] Ligamentous instability can occur if the collateral ligaments are violated. Osteoarthritis can occur if the osteotomy is not reduced anatomically. The surgeon needs to avoid malrotation and overtightening of the osteotomy.

Modifications. Müller et al. modified MacAusland's approach and recommend an extra-articular olecranon osteotomy.[51] However, this osteotomy does not provide exposure of the anterior articular surface, which often is comminuted in supracondylar fractures.

Lateral Approaches

Many surgical approaches have been described for the lateral aspect of the joint. The most well-known approach, which Kocher described, involves the interval between the extensor carpi ulnaris and the anconeus.[37] Other lateral approaches have been described.[54–56]

The position of the posterior interosseous nerve is important when using any of the lateral approaches to the elbow. Kaplan stressed the importance of performing the procedure with the forearm in pronation to translate the nerve anteriorly, thus increasing the zone of safety.[55] The posterior interosseous nerve moves approximately 1 cm medially when the forearm is pronated.[15]

Kocher's Lateral Approach

Indications for Kocher's lateral approach (Fig. 1.23)[37] include fixation of distal humeral and radial head fractures, total elbow arthroplasty, radial head arthroplasty, release of soft tissue contractures, removal of loose bodies, and repair or reconstruction of the lateral collateral ligament and associated structures.

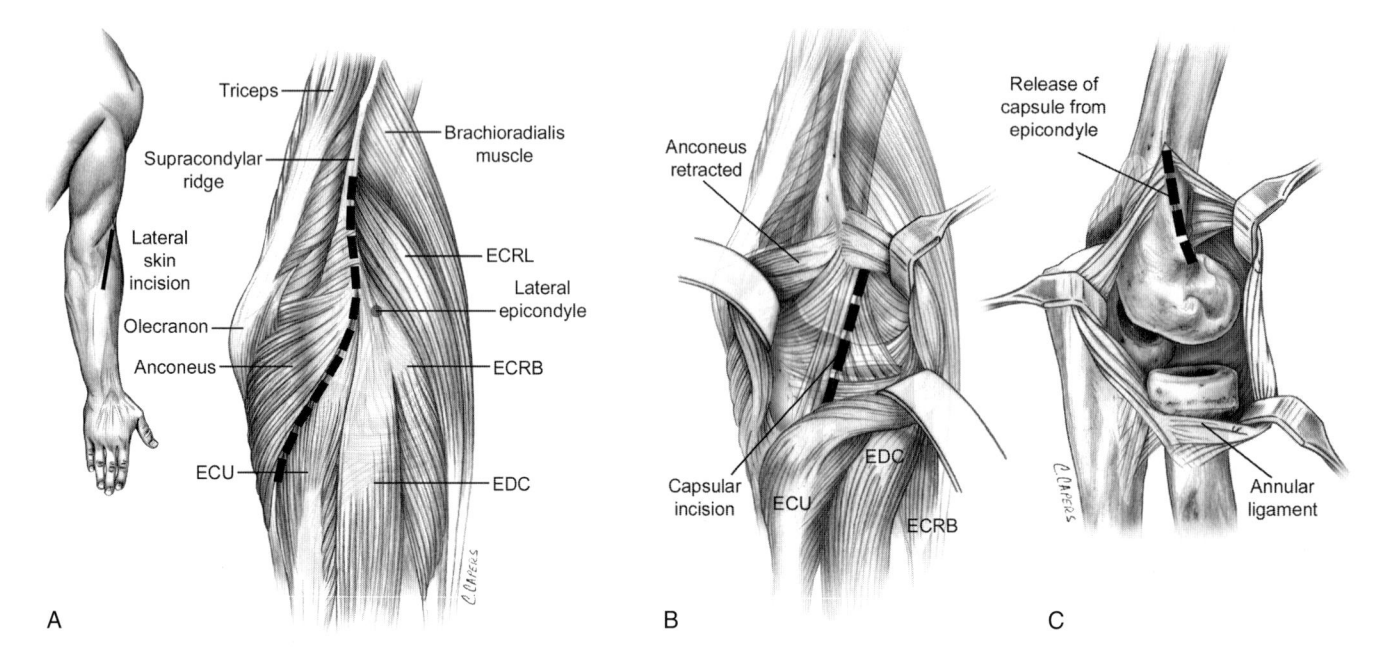

FIGURE 1.23. Modified Kocher's approach. (A) Incision is made from the supracondylar ridge to past the radial head. (B) Lateral capsule is incised anterior to the lateral ulnar collateral ligament. (C) Posterior capsular sleeve released from epicondyle to allow insertion of metallic radial head replacement. (ECRL, extensor carpi radialis longus; ECRB, extensor carpi radialis brevis; EDC, extensor digitorum communis; ECU, extensor carpi ulnaris.)

The surgeon makes a lateral incision from the supracondylar ridge of the humerus distally to 5 cm past the radial head. The interval between the triceps muscle posteriorly and the brachioradialis and extensor carpi radialis longus muscles anteriorly is developed to expose the lateral condyle of the distal humerus and the lateral capsule. Distal to the radial head, the interval between the extensor carpi ulnaris and the anconeus is developed, and the common extensor origin then can be reflected anteriorly to complete the exposure of the lateral capsule and joint. Morrey recommends a modification in which the capsulotomy is performed anterior to the lateral ulnar collateral ligament to prevent posterolateral rotatory instability[47] (see Fig. 1.23B). We have modified this procedure and include a step-cut (Z) incision of the annular ligament anterior to the lateral ulnar collateral ligament. This incision preserves the lateral ulnar collateral ligament and ensures that the annular ligament can be repaired easily without undue tension. This incision is ideal for open reduction of radial head fractures. If a metallic radial head replacement is to be inserted, the posterior capsular sleeve, which includes the lateral ulnar collateral ligament, must be released from the epicondyle and later repaired with transosseous sutures.

The exposure can be extended proximally or distally, as required, to provide greater exposure of the humerus and ulna, respectively.[65] A triceps–anconeus flap can be raised from the olecranon and reflected medially to allow the elbow to dislocate, hinging on the medial collateral ligament. The medial collateral ligament can be released to disengage the humerus and ulna. From this perspective, the surgeon can visualize the entire elbow joint.

We recommend carefully closing the lateral ligamentous complex with transosseous, nonabsorbable, interrupted sutures to prevent posterolateral rotatory instability. The ulnar nerve may be injured during manipulation by a small bony spur, which is commonly present in patients who have rheumatoid arthritis, at the ulnar attachment of the medial collateral ligament.[66] This approach offers more protection to the posterior interosseous nerve and is converted easily to an extensile posterolateral approach if exposure of the entire distal humerus is necessary.

Modifications. The direct lateral approach that Kaplan[55] describes uses the interval between the extensor digitorum communis and the extensor carpi radialis brevis (Fig. 1.24). To move the posterior interosseous nerve as far away from the surgical field as possible, full pronation of the forearm is recommended during this approach. According to Strachan and Ellis, the posterior interosseous nerve moves approximately 1 cm medially with full pronation of the forearm.[15] Even with full pronation of the forearm, the posterior interosseous nerve is still quite close to the surgical field. For this reason, this approach is not used as frequently as that described by Kocher.[37]

In his modification, Cadenat exposes the radial head via

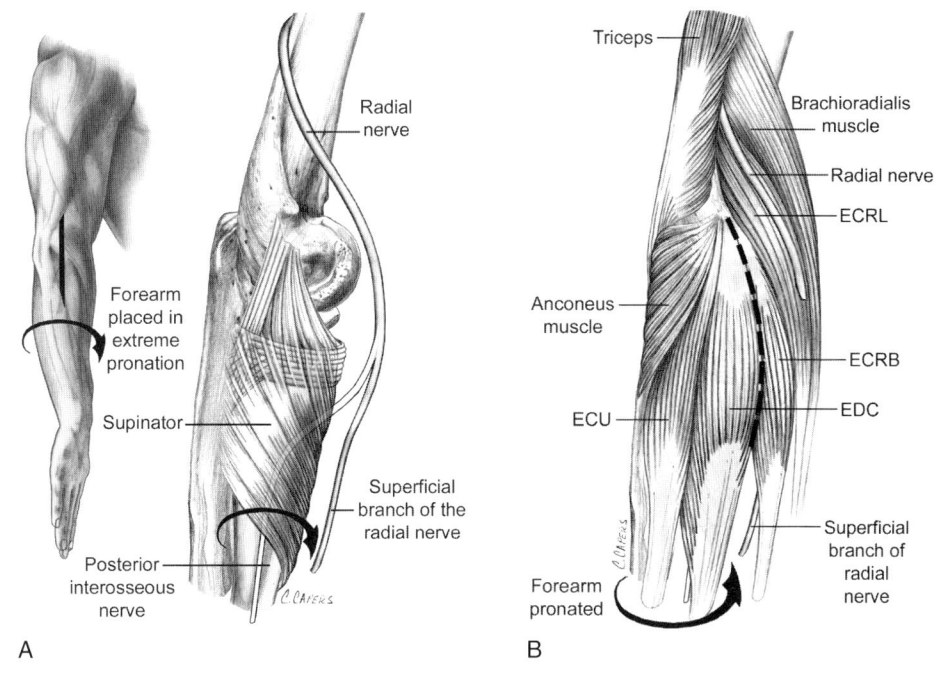

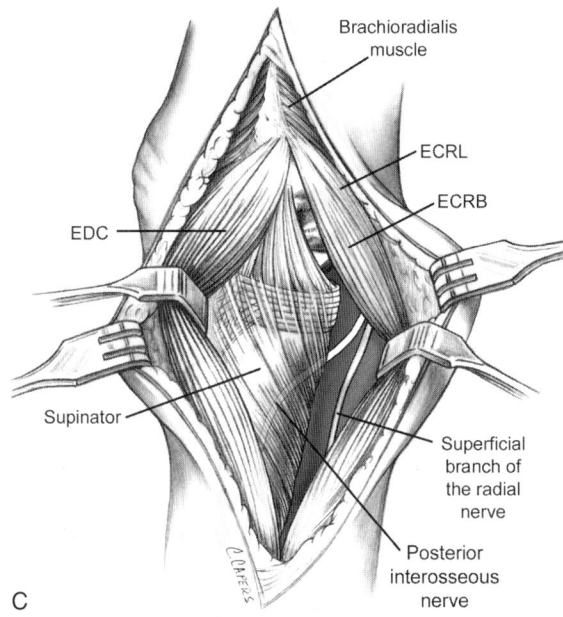

FIGURE 1.24. Kaplan's direct lateral approach. (A) Arm is placed in extreme pronation to protect posterior interosseous nerve. (B) Incision is made between the ECRB and the EDC. (C) Posterior interosseous nerve is at risk. (ECRB, extensor carpi radialis brevis; ECRL, extensor carpi radialis longus; EDC, extensor digitorum communis; ECU, extensor carpi ulnaris.)

the interval between the extensor carpi radialis longus and extensor carpi radialis brevis.[54] This approach can place the nerve to the extensor carpi radialis brevis[55] at risk.

Key and Conwell[56] modified the approach by exposing the radial head between the brachioradialis and the extensor carpi radialis longus. If the exposure is extended proximally, it can place the nerves to the extensor carpi radialis longus and brevis[55] at risk.

In his modified approach, Pankovich exposes the lateral compartment of the elbow by developing the Kocher interval and reflecting the insertion of the anconeus subperiosteally from the ulna[52] (Fig. 1.25). This dissection exposes the supinator muscle, and the dissection can continue in the same fashion as the Boyd approach.

Patterson and associates describe the "global approach" to the elbow with a lateral epicondylar osteotomy to increase exposure of the radial head.[49] The details of this approach are provided in the combined medial and lateral approaches section.

Campbell describes another lateral approach: the transepicondylar approach.[38] The value of this approach is limited and rarely indicated today.

FIGURE 1.25. Pankovich's approach. (A) Incision to release the anconeus from the humerus. (B) Anconeus retracted to expose the lateral joint.

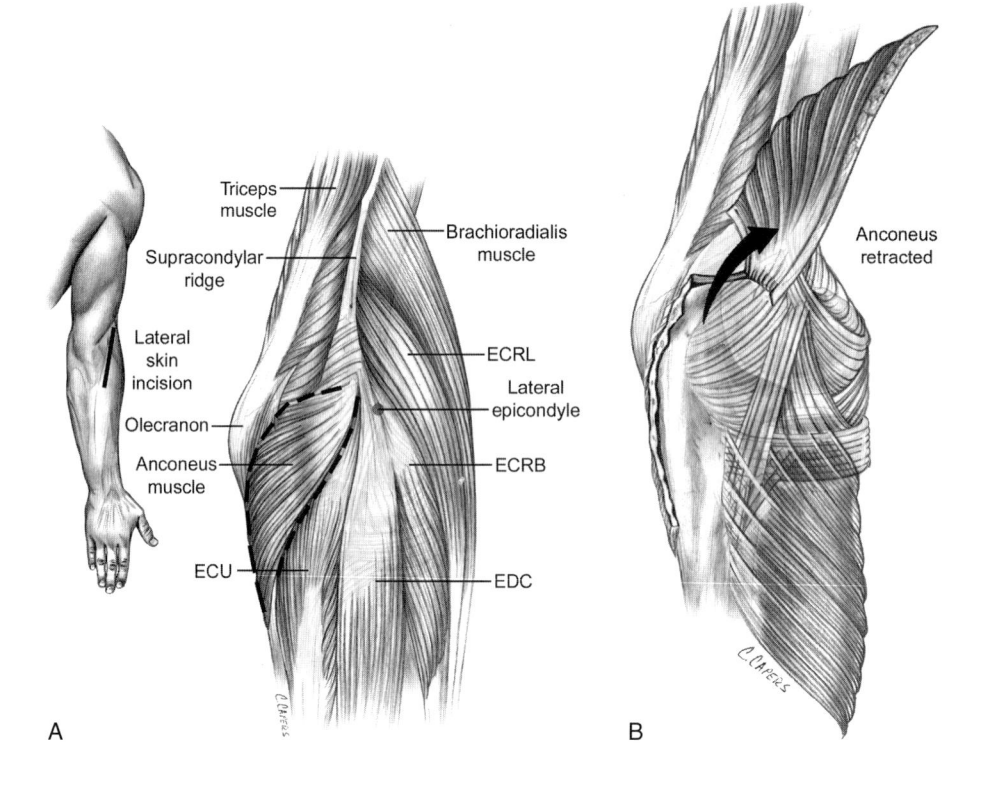

Medial Approach

Molesworth's Medial Approach

Molesworth[40] describes a medial approach. Its indications include fixation of fractures of the medial humeral epicondyle or condyle and fracture–dislocations of the elbow and include removal of loose bodies.

The incision is centered over the medial epicondyle, and the ulnar nerve is isolated and protected. In the muscular plane, the ulnar and humeral heads of the flexor carpi ulnaris are separated, exposing the ulnar nerve in the forearm. The muscular branches are preserved, and the articular branches are sacrificed.

In the subperiosteal planes, the surgeon can see the outline of the trochlea through the capsule. He or she incises the capsule parallel and behind the anterior band of the medial collateral ligament. Through this incision, an osteotome is pressed against the undersurface of the medial epicondyle, adjacent to the medial nonarticular surface of the trochlea after predrilling. The medial epicondyle is osteotomized in an upward direction, and the medial intermuscular septum is detached from this epicondyle after dissecting the pronator teres from the septum. The medial epicondyle with the common flexor origin and the medial collateral ligament are retracted distally. The anterior and posterior portions of the capsule are elevated from the coronoid and olecranon fossae to expose the joint.

Molesworth[40] does not discuss the extensibility of this approach. However, the humerus can be exposed proximally by subperiosteal dissection. Distally, the exposure is limited unless the distal attachment of the collateral ligament is released. Molesworth reported that the entire elbow joint can be visualized with this exposure.

After completing the procedure, the medial epicondyle is reattached with a screw, and the arthrotomy is closed. Molesworth recommends suturing the triceps to the brachialis.

Complications can occur with this approach. The branches of the median nerve to the pronator teres and the common flexor origin must be protected from traction. The ulnar nerve is at risk for injury and must be protected. Secure fixation is important to minimize the risk of nonunion of the osteotomy. Medial collateral instability can occur if the osteotomy is not positioned correctly or if the ligament is violated.

Modifications. Campbell[38] modified the Molesworth approach by performing the osteotomy in an anteroposterior direction.

In his modification, Hotchkiss[67] recommends elevating the pronator teres muscle from the medial supracondylar ridge and retracting it anteriorly to expose the anterior joint capsule. Retraction of the biceps and brachialis provides greater exposure of the anterior capsule. The common flexor origin is left intact. Posteriorly, the triceps is elevated from the distal humerus at the raphe, which is identified distally between the flexor carpi ulnaris and the palmaris longus superficially and between the flexor carpi ulnaris and flexor digitorum superficialis muscles slightly deeper. The ligament complex is exposed, and dissection up to 1 cm distal to the sublime tubercle is permissible. The dissection plane lies in an internervous plane (i.e., median to ulnar), and it has been described extensively for reconstruction of the medial collateral ligament complex.[68]

Jobe describes a medial utility approach for medial collateral ligament reconstruction and for the treatment of medial epicondylitis (Fig. 1.26).[69] A curvilinear incision is made over the anterior aspect of the medial epicondyle, and care is taken to identify and preserve the multiple medial antebrachial cutaneous nerve branches that are encountered. The common flexor tendon can then be divided in line with its fibers or reflected distally to expose the medial capsule and ligaments.

Combined Medial and Lateral Approaches

If required, a combination of the medial and lateral approaches could be used. Indications for this approach include fixation of complex fracture of the radial head, coronoid process, or capitellum and include soft tissue contracture release. Instead of using two separate skin incisions, we recommend that the surgeon use a posterior midline skin incision (Fig. 1.27).

Global Approach

In the muscular and periosteal planes, the muscles of the medial side of the proximal ulna (flexor carpi ulnaris and flexor digitorum profundus) are released subperiosteally, leaving a strip of deep fascia for later repair (Fig. 1.28). The ulnar nerve is released by dividing the cubital retinaculum and releasing the flexor carpi ulnaris fascia. Retraction of the muscles exposes the medial collateral ligament and the anterior joint capsule. Capsulotomy is made anterior to the anterior bundle of the medial collateral ligament. The common flexor origin and medial collateral ligament are left intact. This approach extends proximally along the medial supracondylar ridge and distally by reflecting the flexor carpi ulnaris from the ulna. The medial collateral ligament and the common flexor origin can be released from the medial epicondyle, if required.

Laterally, the interval between the anconeus and the extensor carpi ulnaris is palpated and visualized as a thin strip of fat beneath the deep fascia (Fig. 1.29). It is easily identified distally, and the overlying deep fascia is divided, allowing the anconeus and extensor carpi ulnaris to be retracted to expose the anterolateral joint capsule. The triceps is retracted from the distal humerus to expose the olecranon fossa. The annular ligament is divided with a step-cut incision that allows it to be repaired anatomically. If greater exposure is required for osteosynthesis of the radial head, a lateral capsulotomy is performed as shown in Figure 1.21. Alternatively, a lateral epicondylar osteotomy can be performed. The surgeon predrills the lateral epicondyle and accomplishes a chevron osteotomy that includes the entire extensor origin. The muscles of the supracondylar ridge are elevated subperiosteally. The lateral ulnar collateral ligament is not violated; it remains in continuity with the epicondyle.

On the lateral aspect, the exposure is extensile proximally to where the radial nerve perforates the lateral intermuscular septum. Distally, the exposure extends along the proximal third of the radius. By pronating the forearm, the surgeon translates the posterior interosseous nerve away from the surgical field to increase the zone of safety.[15] The supinator muscle is released from the supinator crest and retracted along with the posterior in-

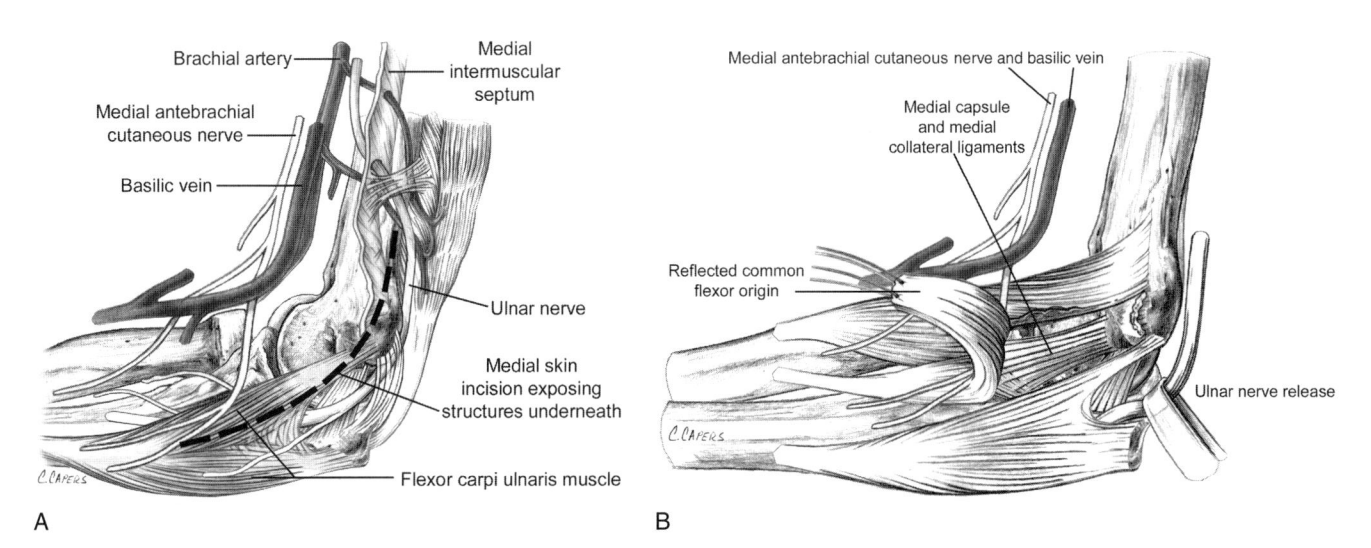

FIGURE 1.26. Jobe's medial utility approach. (A) Skin incision's proximity to branches of medial antebrachial cutaneous nerve. (B) Exposure of capsule and ligaments.

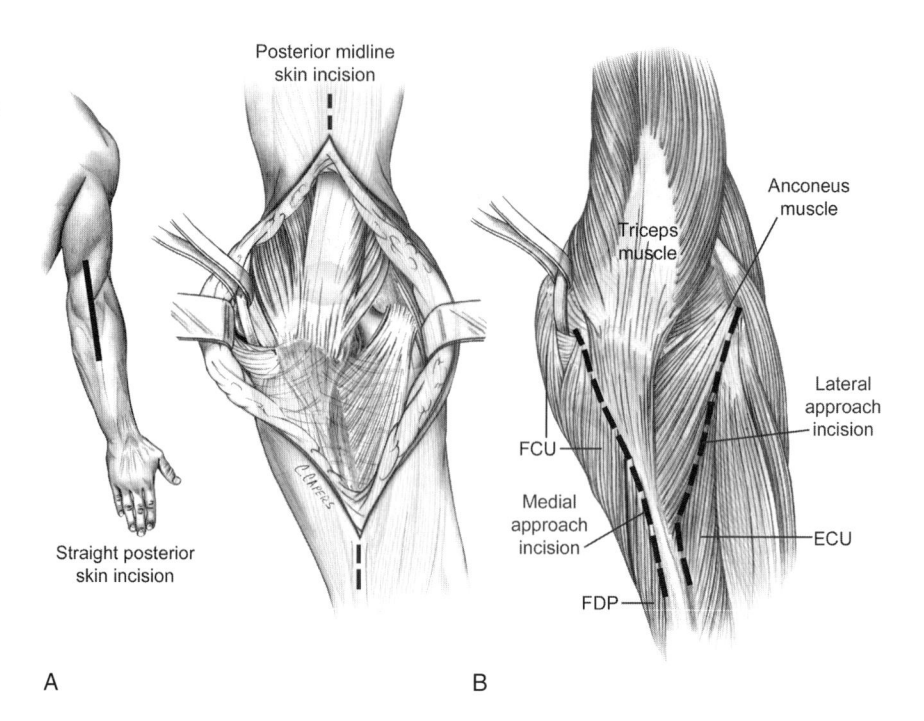

FIGURE 1.27. Global approach. (A) Posterior midline skin incision with full-thickness fasciocutaneous flaps. (B) Medial and lateral muscular and periosteal plane incisions.

terosseous nerve, thereby exposing the radius. The posterior interosseous artery may require ligation.

From this exposure, the surgeon can visualize the elbow joint, distal humerus, proximal radius, and ulna. The medial collateral ligament and the common flexor origin should be repaired with transosseous sutures if they have been elevated. The lateral epicondylar osteotomy is reattached with a screw.

When using this approach, the surgeon must protect the posterior interosseous nerve. We have not witnessed lateral epicondylar osteotomy nonunion and posterolateral rotatory instability or ectopic bone formation with this approach.

Anterior Approach

Henry's Approach

The extensile exposure that Henry[41] describes is the most useful anterior exposure of the elbow joint (Fig. 1.30). Indications for this approach include repair and lengthening of the biceps tendon, anterior release of joint contractures, fixation of proximal radial shaft and coronoid process fractures, decompression of the radial and median nerves, and excision of tumors in the cubital fossa. It also can be used as part of a fasciotomy.

The patient is positioned supine with the upper limb

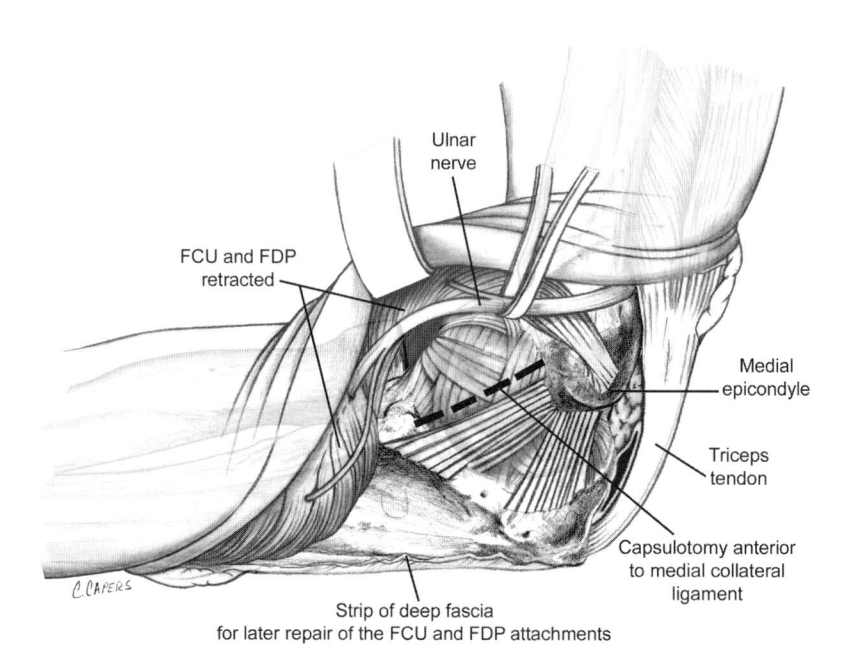

FIGURE 1.28. Global approach. Medial approach is made by reflecting the flexor carpi ulnaris (FCU) from the proximal ulna. (FDP, flexor digitorum profundus.)

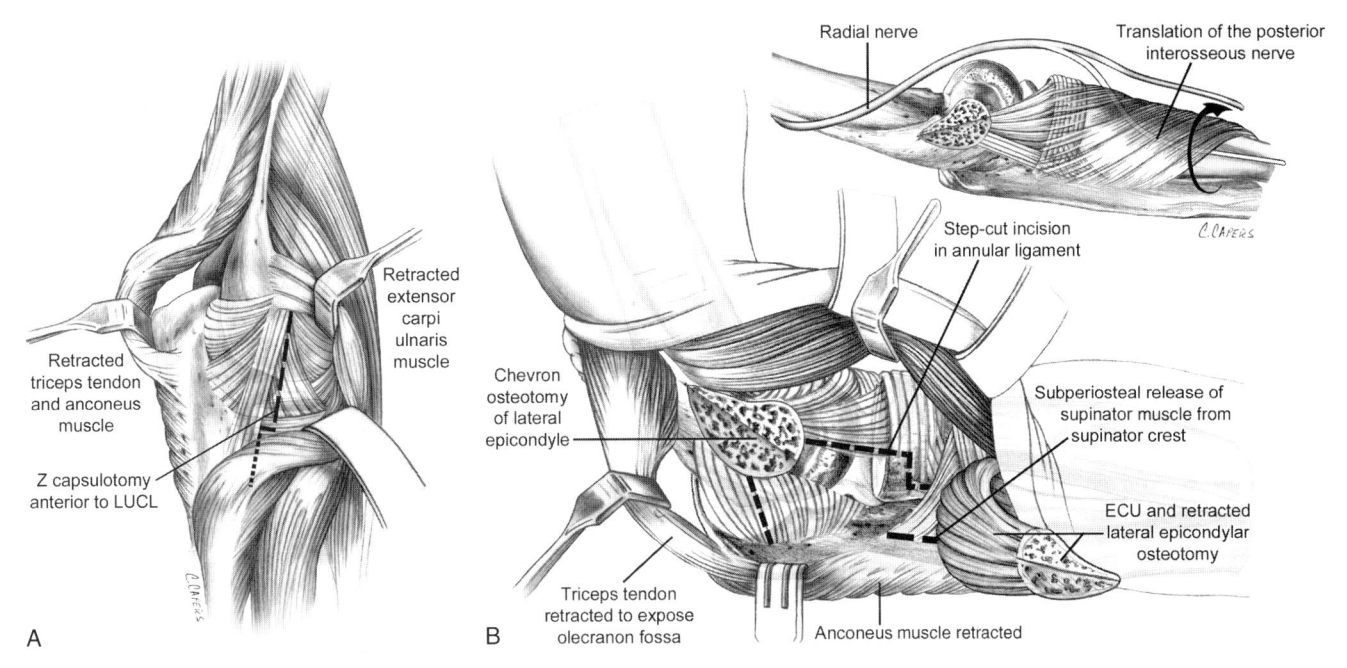

FIGURE 1.29. Global approach. Lateral approach is between the ECU and the anconeus muscle. (A) Olecranon fossa is exposed by retracting the triceps tendon. Z capsulotomy anterior to the LUCL allows simple repair of the annular ligament. (B) Lateral epicondylar osteotomy can be used to increase exposure. With the arm in pronation, the posterior interosseous nerve is moved away from the surgical field (inset). (LUCL, lateral ulnar collateral ligament; ECU, extensor carpi ulnaris.)

on an arm board. The surgeon makes an incision that is a handbreadth proximal to the antecubital flexion crease and a fingerbreadth lateral to the biceps. It curves across the elbow crease and distally along the ulnar border of the mobile wad of three muscles (brachioradialis and extensor carpi radialis longus and brevis). The cephalic vein and the lateral cutaneous nerve of the forearm need to be protected.

In the muscular plane, the biceps tendon is an important landmark and acts as a vertical partition that divides the proximal antecubital fossa into a "dangerous" medial side and a "safe" lateral side[41] (see Fig. 1.8). The deep fascia on the lateral side of the biceps tendon is divided. Henry recommended that the surgeon pass a finger through "the swamp of fat" along the lateral edge of the guiding biceps tendon until the resistance of the "leash

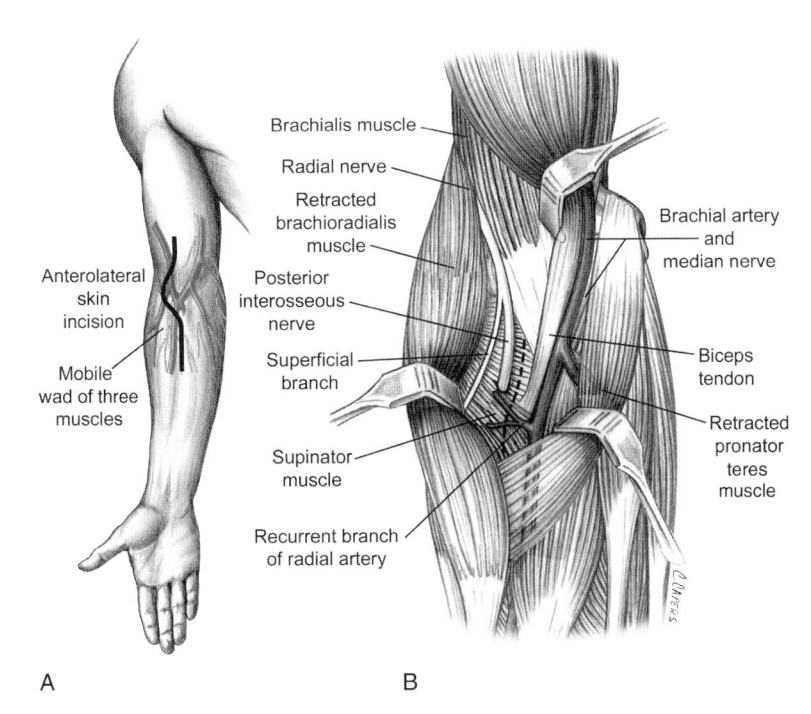

FIGURE 1.30. Henry's anterior approach. (A) Skin incision lateral to biceps tendon curved across the elbow and medial to the mobile wad of three muscles. (B) The deep interval is lateral to the biceps tendon, and the leash of vessels is divided to increase the exposure.

of vessels" in which the recurrent branch of the radial artery is encountered. The recurrent branch is only the proximal rib of a fanlike spread of vessels that lie in several layers, each of which is divided and ligated. If further exposure is required, the muscular branches of the radial artery are divided and ligated. The mobile wad of three muscles is widely mobilized, and the elbow is flexed to 90° to allow exposure of the supinator muscle. The radial nerve branches only laterally; therefore, it can be safely retracted laterally with the brachioradialis.

In the periosteal plane, the dissection then follows the course of the biceps tendon to the radial tuberosity and the bicipital bursa. The bursa is divided, and the supinator muscle is elevated in the subperiosteal plane, sandwiching within its substance the posterior interosseous nerve. The forearm is fully supinated to protect the posterior interosseous nerve, and the supinator muscle is released in a subperiosteal fashion to expose the entire anterior aspect of the elbow joint. This exposure extends distally to the radial styloid. From this approach, the surgeon can visualize the proximal radius, radiocapitellar joint, and the anterolateral humerus.

The muscles are allowed to fall back, and the skin is sutured. Complications can occur with this approach. The posterior interosseous and superficial branch of the radial nerve must be protected. The recurrent branch of the artery should be preserved if possible. Compartment syndrome can occur from bleeding from the recurrent branch of the radial artery.

CONCLUSION

A sound knowledge of the surgical anatomy and approaches to the elbow is critical for the safe and competent execution of elbow surgery. Just as we are sure others do, we prefer certain surgical approaches to others to treat specific elbow injuries or disorders (Table 1.3). We hope that this review of the pertinent surgical anatomy and approaches furthers the practice of the art of elbow surgery.

REFERENCES

1. Dowdy PA, Bain GI, King GJW, et al. The midline posterior elbow incision. An anatomical appraisal. *J Bone Joint Surg* 1995;77B:696–699.
2. Chang CW, Oh SJ. Posterior antebrachial cutaneous neuropathy: Case report. *Electromyogr Clin Neurophysiol* 1990;30: 3–5.
3. Graham B, Adkins P, Scheker LR. Complications and morbidity of the donor and recipient sites in 123 lateral arm flaps. *J Hand Surg* 1992;17B:189–192.
4. Leffert RD. Anterior submuscular transposition of the ulnar nerves by the Learmonth technique. *J Hand Surg* 1982;7A: 147–155.
5. Dellon AL. Techniques for successful management of ulnar nerve entrapment at the elbow. *Neurosurg Clin N Am* 1991; 2:57–73.
6. Dellon AL, MacKinnon SE. Injury to the medial antebrachial cutaneous nerve during cubital tunnel surgery. *J Hand Surg* 1985;10B:33–36.
7. Gray H, Williams PL, Bannister LH, eds. *Gray's anatomy of the human body*, 38th ed. Edinburgh: Churchill Livingstone; 1995.
8. McMinn RMH. *Last's anatomy regional and applied*, 8th ed. Edinburgh: Churchill Livingstone; 1991:13.
9. Romanes GJ. *Cunningham's manual of practical anatomy*, Vol. 1, 14th ed. Oxford: Oxford University Press, 1976.
10. Tountas CP, Bergman RA. *Anatomical variations of the upper extremity*. New York: Churchill Livingstone, 1993.
11. Wadsworth TG. A modified posterolateral approach to the elbow and proximal radioulnar joints. *Clin Orthop* 1979;144: 151–153.
12. Boyd HB. Surgical exposure of the ulna and proximal third of the radius through one incision. *Surg Gyn Obst* 1940;71:86–88.
13. Basmajian JV. *Muscles alive*, 2nd ed. Baltimore: Williams & Wilkins, 1967.
14. Spinner M. The arcade of Frohse and its relationship to posterior interosseous nerve paralysis. *J Bone Joint Surg* 1968; 50B:809–812.
15. Strachan JC, Ellis BW. Vulnerability of the posterior interosseous nerve during radial head resection. *J Bone Joint Surg* 1971;53B:320–323.
16. Dellon AL, Mackinnon SE. Musculoaponeurotic variations along the course of the median nerve in the proximal forearm. *J Hand Surg* (Br) 1987;12:359–363.
17. Bateman JE. Denervation of the elbow joint for the relief of pain. A preliminary report. *J Bone Joint Surg* 1948;30B:635–641.
18. Osterman AL, Kitay GS. Compression neuropathies: Ulnar. In: Peimer CA, ed. *Surgery of the hand and upper extremity*, Vol. 2. New York: McGraw-Hill Book Co, 1995:1339–1362.
19. Lister GD, Belsole RB, Kleinert HE. The radial tunnel syndrome. *J Hand Surg* 1979;4A:52–59.
20. Polonskaja R. Zue frage der arterienanastomosen im gobiete der ellenbagenbeuge des menschen. *Anat Anz* 1932;74:303.
21. Fuss FK. The ulnar collateral ligament of the human elbow joint. Anatomy, function and biomechanics. *J Anat* 1991;175: 203–212.
22. O'Driscoll SW, Jaloszynski R, Morrey BF, et al. Origin of the medial ulnar collateral ligament. *J Hand Surg* 1992;17A:164–168.
23. O'Driscoll SW, Morrey BF, Korinek SL, et al. The patho-anatomy and kinematics of posterolateral rotatory instability (pivot-shift) of the elbow. *Orthop Trans* 1990;14:306.
24. Osborne G, Cotterill P. Recurrent dislocation of the elbow. *J Bone Joint Surg* 1966;48B:340–346.
25. Olsen BS, Vaesel MT, Sojbjerg TO, et al. Lateral collateral ligament of the elbow joint: Anatomy and kinematics. *J Shoulder Elbow Surg* 1996;5:103–112.
26. Bert JM, Linscheid RL, McElfresh EC. Rotatory contracture of the forearm. *J Bone Joint Surg* 1980;62A:1163–1168.
27. Gray DJ, Gardner E. Prenatal development of the human elbow joint. *Am J Anat* 1951;88:429–469.
28. Wood VE, Campbell GS. The supratrochleare dorsale accessory ossicle in the elbow. *J Shoulder Elbow Surg* 1994;3:395–398.

29. Haraldsson S. On osteochondritis deformans juvenilis capituli humeri including investigations of intra osseous vasculature in distal humerus. *Acta Orthop Scand* 1959;38(Suppl).
30. Toniolo RM, Wilkins KE. Avascular necrosis of the trochlea. In: Rockwood CA Jr, Wilkins DE, Beaty JH, eds. *Fractures in children*, 4th ed. Philadelphia: Lippincott-Raven, 1996:822–830.
31. Aebi H. Der ellbowgenwinkel, seine beizehungen zu geschlect. Korperbay und huftbreite. *Acta Anat* 1947;3:228.
32. Beals RK. The normal carrying angle of the elbow. A radiographic study of 422 patients. *Clin Orthop* 1976;119:194–196.
33. Wilkins KE, Beaty JH, Chambers HG, et al. Fractures and dislocations of the elbow region. In: Rockwood CA Jr, Wilkins KE, Beaty JH, eds. *Fractures in children*, 4th ed. Philadelphia: Lippincott-Raven, 1996:653–904.
34. Conwell HE, Reynolds FC. *Key and Conwell's management of fractures, dislocations and sprains*, 7th edition. St. Louis, MO: CV Mosby, 1961.
35. Regan W, Morrey B. Fractures of the coronoid process of the ulna. *J Bone Joint Surg* 1978;71A:1348–1354.
36. Cabanela ME. Fractures of the proximal ulna and olecranon. In: Morrey BF, ed. *The elbow and its disorders*, 2nd ed. Philadelphia: WB Saunders, 1993:382–399.
37. Kocher T. *Textbook of operative surgery*, 3rd ed. London: Adam and Charles Black, 1911:314–319.
38. Campbell WC. Incision for exposure of the elbow joint. *Am J Surg* 1932;15:65–67.
39. Van Gorder GW. Surgical approach in supracondylar "T" fractures of the humerus requiring open reduction. *J Bone Joint Surg* 1940;22:278–292.
40. Molesworth HWL. An operation for the complete exposure of the elbow-joint. *Brit J Surg* 1930;18:303–307.
41. Henry AK. *Extensile exposure*, 3rd ed. Edinburgh: Churchill Livingstone, 1995:95–107.
42. MacAusland WR. Ankylosis of the elbow: with report of four cases treated by arthroplasty. *JAMA* 1915;64:312–318.
43. Bryan RS, Morrey BF. Extensive posterior exposure of the elbow. A triceps-sparing approach. *Clin Orthop* 1982;166:188–192.
44. Morrey BF, Bryan RS, Dobyns JH, et al. Total elbow arthroplasty. A five-year experience at the Mayo Clinic. *J Bone Joint Surg* 1981;63A:1050–1063.
45. Morrey BF, Adams RA. Semiconstrained arthroplasty for the treatment of rheumatoid arthritis of the elbow. *J Bone Joint Surg* 1992;74A:479–490.
46. Morrey BF: Complications of elbow replacement surgery. In: Morrey BF, ed. *The elbow and its disorders*, 3rd ed. Philadelphia: WB Saunders, 2000:667–677.
47. Morrey BF. Surgical exposures of the elbow. In: Morrey BF, ed. *The elbow and its disorders*, 3rd ed. Philadelphia: WB Saunders, 2000:109–134.
48. Morrey BF. Limited and extensile triceps reflecting exposures of the elbow. In: Morrey BF, ed. *The elbow: Master techniques in orthopaedic surgery*. New York: Raven Press, 1994:3–19.
49. Patterson, SD, Bain, GI, Mehta, JA. Surgical approaches to the elbow. *Clin Orthop* 2000;370:19–33.
50. Alonso-Llames M. Bilateraltricipital approach to the elbow. Its application in the osteosynthesis of supracondylar fractures of the humerus in children. *Acta Orthop Scand* 1972;43:479–490.
51. Müller ME, Allgower M, Willenegger H. *Manual of internal fixation: Technique recommended by the AO group*, 2nd ed. New York: Springer-Verlag, 1979.
52. Pankovich AM. Anconeus approach to the elbow joint and the proximal part of the radius and ulna. *J Bone Joint Surg* 1977;59A:124–126.
53. Heim U, Pfieffer KM. *Small fragment set manual: Technique recommended by AO group*, 2nd ed. New York: Springer-Verlag, 1982.
54. Cadenat FM. *Les voies de penetration des membres*. Membre Superieur, p146, Paris Gastoon doin and Cie, 1932.
55. Kaplan EB. Surgical approach to the proximal end of the radius and its use in fractures of the head and neck of the radius. *J Bone Joint Surg* 1941;23:86–92.
56. Key JA, Conwell HE. The management of fractures dislocations and sprains, 2nd ed. St. Louis, MO: CV Mosby, 1937.
57. Pearl RM, Johnson D. The vascular supply to the skin: An anatomical and physiological reappraisal—Part I. *Ann Plast Surg* 1983;11:99–105.
58. Pearl RM, Johnson D. The vascular supply to the skin: An anatomical and physiological reappraisal—Part II. *Ann Plast Surg* 1983;11:196–205.
59. Bain GI, Mehta JA, Heptinstall RJ. The dynamic elbow suspension splint. *J Shoulder Elbow Surg*. 1998;7:419–421.
60. Figgie MP. Elbow arthroplasty. In: Peimer CA, ed. *Surgery of the hand and upper extremity*, Vol. 1. New York: McGraw-Hill Book Co, 1996:535–571.
61. Wolfe SW, Ranawat CS. The osteo-anconeus flap. An approach for total elbow arthroplasty. *J Bone Joint Surg* 1990;72A:684–688.
62. Failla JM, Amadio PC, Morrey BF, et al. Proximal radioulnar synostosis after repair of distal biceps brachii rupture by the two-incision technique. Report of four cases. *Clin Orthop* 1990;253:133–136.
63. Gordon ML. Monteggia fracture. A combined surgical approach employing a single lateral incision. *Clin Orthop* 1967;50:87–93.
64. Jupiter JB. The surgical management of intraarticular fractures of the distal humerus. In: Morrey BF, ed. *The elbow: Master techniques in orthopaedic surgery*. New York: Raven Press, 1994:53–70.
65. Husband JB, Hastings H II. The lateral approach for operative release of posttraumatic contracture of the elbow. *J Bone Joint Surg* 1990;72A:1353–1358.
66. Gschwend N, Simmen BR, Matejovsky Z. Late complications in elbow arthroplasty. *J Shoulder Elbow Surg* 1996;5:86–96.
67. Hotchkiss RN. Compass elbow hinge: Surgical technique. In: *Product manual*. Memphis, TN: Smith & Nephew Richards.
68. Smith GR, Altchek DW, Pagnani MJ, et al. A muscle-splitting approach to the ulnar collateral ligament of the elbow. Neuroanatomy and operative technique. *Am J Sports Med* 1996;24:575–580.
69. Jobe FW. Surgical anatomy of the elbow. In: Jobe FW, ed. *Operative techniques in upper extremity sports injuries*. St. Louis, MO: CV Mosby, 1996:405.

CHAPTER 2

Biomechanics of the Elbow and Throwing Mechanisms

Steven W. Barrentine, Glenn S. Fleisig, Charles J. Dillman, and James R. Andrews

INTRODUCTION

Before treating elbow injuries in the throwing athlete, the surgeon must understand the biomechanics of the elbow joint. Biomechanics is a function of kinematics, kinetics, and electromyography. Kinematics describes how something is moving without stating the causes behind the motion. Specifically, it quantifies linear and angular displacement, velocity, and acceleration—the effects of the motion. Elbow kinematics during throwing includes elbow flexion angles, angular velocities, and angular accelerations. High-speed videography or cinematography often is used to collect kinematic data.

Kinetics explains why an object moves the way it does; it quantifies both the forces and torques that cause the motion. Elbow kinetics includes the forces and torques about the elbow that cause elbow motion to occur. Inverse dynamics equations often are used in conjunction with kinematic and anthropometric data to estimate the net force or torque acting about the elbow.

Electromyography is used to quantify muscle activity. Surface electrodes often are used to detect muscle activity from larger surface muscles, and indwelling electrodes are used to detect muscle activity from smaller deep muscles.

In this chapter, we examine the biomechanics of the elbow, emphasizing the elbow of the throwing athlete. We discuss the overhand and underhand throwing motion, including the baseball pitch, the football pass, the tennis serve, the javelin throw, and the underhand softball pitch. The baseball pitching motion receives the most emphasis because most throwing-related studies have focused on this activity.

BIOMECHANICS OF THE ELBOW

Range of Motion

The elbow complex controls the position of the hand and wrist complex in space and in proximity to the upper body. This control is accomplished primarily with two joints within the elbow complex that have one degree of freedom: flexion and extension at the humeroradial and humeroulnar joints and pronation and supination at the proximal radioulnar joint. Normal range of motion for elbow flexion is 0° to 145°[1,2]; for pronation, 70° to 80°; and for supination, 80° to 85°. Functional range of motion is less than the maximum range because most daily activities (e.g., eating, opening a door, reading, and rising from a chair) are performed within an arc of 100° of flexion (from 30° to 130°) and between 50° of pronation and 50° of supination.[2]

In a study of the passive motion, Morrey and Chao determined that the elbow is not a true hinge joint.[3] They determined that a locus of the instant centers of rotation is present. As Werner and An indicated, further work also has demonstrated that the orientation of the three-dimensional center of rotation varies from person to person.[4] However, Morrey and Chao concluded that, for each individual, the deviation is minimal, and irregularity can be attributed to experimental design.[3] Therefore, it is assumed that the ulnohumeral joint moves as a uniaxial articulation, except for the extreme ranges of flexion and extension.[5]

The axis of rotation for flexion forms a line from the inferior aspect of the medial epicondyle through the center of the lateral epicondyle.[3] This line bisects the longitudinal axis of the humerus, but not the longitudinal axis of the forearm. The longitudinal axis of the humerus and the longitudinal axis of the forearm create a valgus angle (i.e., the carrying angle) because of the configuration of the articulating surfaces. Morrey and Chao[3] found that the carrying angle changes with elbow flexion. London, however, found that the carrying angle remained constant.[6] An et al.[7] concluded that the magnitude of the carrying angle depends on its definition. They also indicated that the change in carrying angle that occurs during flexion and extension has little clinical significance.

Muscle Function

The major flexors across the elbow joint are the brachialis, biceps brachii, brachioradialis, and extensor carpi radialis.[8,9] An et al. determined the physiologic cross-sectional area of each muscle across the elbow joint and concluded that the brachialis had the largest work capacity and potential contractile strength.[8] The brachialis is active regardless of elbow position, type of contraction, or rate of movement, and the position of the shoulder does not affect these factors.

Major elbow extensors are the triceps, extensor carpi ulnaris, and anconeus.[8,9] The triceps has the largest work capacity, and its medial head is the primary force producer.[8] The position of the elbow affects the triceps; however, the position of the shoulder (excluding the long head) does not affect it. The anconeus is active in a variety of motions, so it is considered to be the dynamic stabilizer of the joint.[10]

The muscles involved in pronation include the pronator quadratus and pronator teres. The primary pronator of the forearm is the pronator quadratus.[9] The position of the elbow does not affect the pronator quadratus. The pronator teres functions as a secondary pronator during rapid pronation or during pronation against resistance.

The muscles involved in supination of the forearm are the supinator and the biceps. Supination is achieved primarily by the supinator muscle, with the biceps acting in a secondary role. The supinator acts independently during slow, unrestrained supination. During unrestrained, rapid supination or resisted supination in any position, the biceps assists the supinator muscle. When the biceps assists supination, the extensors must act antagonistically to cancel any flexion that the activity of the biceps creates.

Strength Based on In Vitro Studies

Both the soft tissues and the articulation of the joint afford stability to the elbow. These stabilizers include the medial and lateral collateral ligaments and the articulation of the humeroradial and humeroulnar joints. Morrey and An conducted a cadaveric study investigating the articular and ligamentous contributions to the stability of the elbow joint.[11] Using four cadavers, they analyzed the stability of the joint or the contributions to resisting varus stress, valgus stress, and joint distraction in extended and 90° flexed positions. In the flexed position, the results indicated that the medial collateral ligament, or ulnar collateral ligament, provided 54% of the varus torque needed to resist the valgus stress. The soft tissues and capsule provided 10% of the resistance to valgus stress, and osseous articulation provided approximately 33% of the resistance. In the extended position, the medial collateral ligament provided 31% of the resistance, with the capsule and joint articulation providing 38% and 31%, respectively. The lateral collateral ligament, anconeus, and joint capsule provided stability for resisting varus stress. At 90° of flexion, the lateral collateral ligament contributed 9% of the valgus torque needed to resist varus stress, and the joint articulation and joint capsule provided 75% and 13%, respectively. In the extended position, joint articulation provided 55% of the resistance to varus stress, and the lateral collateral ligament and joint capsule provided 14% and 32%, respectively. Resistance to joint distraction was dependent on the position of the elbow. At 90° of flexion, the medial collateral ligament primarily provided 78% of the resistance to distraction. The lateral collateral ligament contributed 10%, and the joint capsule provided 8%. In the extended position, the contribution to distraction resistance was reversed; the joint capsule provided 85% of the resistance, and the lateral and medial collateral ligaments provided 5% and 6%, respectively.

Dillman et al. measured the ultimate tensile strength of the medial collateral ligament.[12] Using 11 cadaveric elbows, they determined that the ultimate tensile strength of the medial collateral ligament was 642 N before failure. This measurement is equivalent to providing approximately 32 N·m of varus torque to resist valgus stress (using 0.05 m as the moment arm length). Note that the authors of this study investigated the ultimate tensile strength of the ligament. With a large number of loading cycles, the failure load would be less than the ultimate tensile limit. Regan et al. conducted a biomechanical study of ligaments around the elbow, including the lateral collateral ligament and the anterior and posterior bundles of the medial collateral ligament.[13] They determined that the anterior bundle of the medial collateral ligament was the strongest (260-N failure load) and stiffest (1528 N) among these ligaments. The palmaris longus required a 357-N load to achieve failure. The results of this study support the use of the palmaris longus tendon as reconstructive tissue.

The amount of force experienced across the elbow depends on a number of factors including the type of load and the positioning of the hand and elbow. Askew et al. conducted a study measuring the isometric elbow strength in a group of normal individuals (50 men and 54 women) ranging in age from 21 to 79 years.[14] The isometric strength measurements, which were determined by using a custom torque cell dynamometer with the elbow flexed to 90°, included a flexion torque of 71 N·m for men and 33 N·m for women. Supination torque was 9 N·m for men and 4 N·m for women. They generally concluded that the mean extension torque was 61% of flexion torque and that the mean pronation torque was 86% of supination torque. Various models have estimated that forces equal to several times body weight are transmitted across the elbow.[15,16]

Amis et al. developed a three-dimensional model for quantifying joint forces for various activities, including maximal flexion, extension, pulling, abduction, and adduction.[15] During isometric flexion, the model estimated humeroradial and humerocoronoid forces of 3200 N at 30° of flexion. During isometric extension, the peak humeroulnar force was approximately 3200 N at 120° of flexion. According to An and Morrey, the accuracy of these models depends on the number of muscles included and whether antagonistic muscle activity is included.[5] Halls and Travill implanted transducers in cadaveric forearms to measure the distribution of forces across the elbow.[17] They determined that 57% of an applied axial force across the elbow is transferred to the humerus through the radiocapitellar joint and 43% is transferred through the ulnotrochlear joint.

BIOMECHANICS OF THE ELBOW DURING BASEBALL PITCHING

One of the most demanding activities on the elbow in sports is the baseball pitch. The prevalence of overuse injury to the elbow due to pitching is well documented.[12,18–23] Most of these overuse throwing injuries result from repetitive trauma to the elbow. An understanding and application of proper pitching mechanics can help to maximize performance and minimize the potential for injury. Although the baseball pitch is one continuous motion, dividing the motion into phases helps in understanding the elbow biomechanics during pitching. Werner et al. separated the pitch into six phases: windup, stride, arm cocking, arm acceleration, arm deceleration, and follow-through.[24] We provide next a description of the biomechanics of the elbow during each phase.

Windup

The windup phase puts the pitcher in a good starting position (Fig. 2.1). The windup starts when the pitcher initiates the movement (Fig. 2.1A) and ends when the front knee has reached its maximum height and the pitcher is in a balanced position (Fig. 2.1B). This phase typically lasts from 0.5 to 1.0 second. Minimal elbow kinetics and muscle activity are present.[12,24–26] The elbow is flexed throughout the phase, and isometric contractions of the elbow flexors maintain elbow flexion (Table 2.1).[26–28]

Stride

The stride phase begins at the end of the windup when the lead leg begins to fall and move toward the target and the two arms separate from each other (Fig. 2.1C–E). The stride phase ends when the lead foot contacts the mound (Fig. 2.1E). A typical stride lasts from 0.50 to 0.75 second. Moderate activity from the elbow flexors is needed to control elbow flexion and extension. As the hands separate, the elbow flexors first contract eccentrically as the elbow extends and then contract concentrically as the elbow flexes near the completion of the stride. The elbow is flexed from 80° to 100° at lead foot contact.[24,25,29] Minimal elbow kinetics and muscle activity are present during the stride phase (Table 2.1).[20,24–26,28]

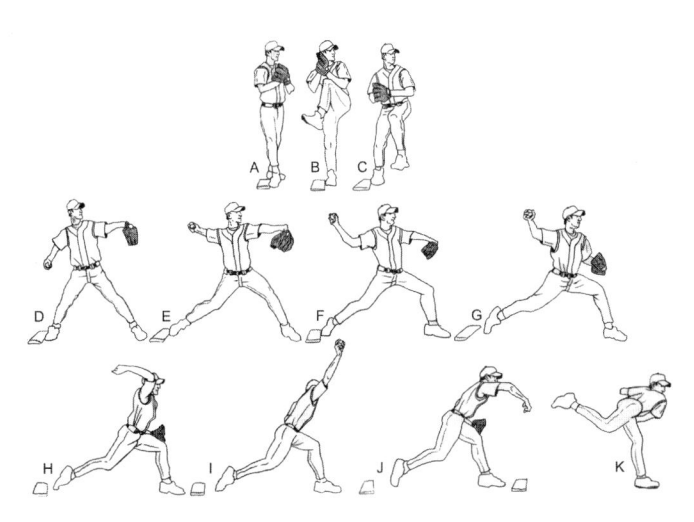

FIGURE 2.1. Sequence of positions during the baseball pitch. (Adapted from Werner et al.[24])

TABLE 2.1. *Muscle activity during pitching, (plus or (minus) standard deviation)**

	n†	Windup	Stride	Arm cocking	Arm acceleration	Arm deceleration	Follow-through
Elbow and forearm muscles							
Triceps	13	4 (6)	17 (17)	37 (32)	89 (40)	54 (23)	22 (18)
Biceps	18	8 (9)	22 (14)	26 (20)	20 (16)	44 (32)	16 (14)
Brachialis	13	8 (5)	17 (13)	18 (26)	20 (22)	49 (29)	13 (17)
Brachioradialis	13	5 (5)	35 (20)	31 (24)	16 (12)	46 (24)	22 (29)
Pronator teres	14	14 (16)	18 (15)	39 (28)	85 (39)	51 (21)	21 (21)
Supinator	13	9 (7)	38 (30)	54 (38)	55 (31)	59 (31)	22 (19)
Wrist and finger muscles							
Extensor carpi radialis longus	13	11 (8)	53 (24)	72 (37)	30 (20)	43 (24)	22 (14)
Extensor carpi radialis brevis	15	17 (17)	47 (26)	75 (41)	55 (35)	43 (28)	24 (19)
Extensor digitorum communis	14	21 (17)	37 (25)	59 (27)	35 (35)	47 (25)	24 (18)
Flexor carpi radialis	12	13 (9)	24 (35)	47 (33)	120 (66)	79 (36)	35 (16)
Flexor digitorum superficialis	11	16 (6)	20 (23)	47 (52)	80 (66)	71 (32)	21 (11)
Flexor carpi ulnaris	10	8 (5)	27 (18)	41 (25)	112 (60)	77 (42)	24 (18)

Adapted from DiGiovine et al.[28]
*Means and standard deviation are expressed as a percentage of the maximal manual muscle test.
†n = number of subjects.

Arm Cocking

The arm-cocking phase, which lasts from 0.10 to 0.15 second, begins at lead foot contact and ends at maximum shoulder external rotation (Fig. 2.1E–H). "Arm cocking" is a more accurate description of this phase than "cocking," because only the arm is cocked during this entire phase.[24] Some parts of the body, such as the pelvis and lower extremities, accelerate or decelerate during this phase. Shortly after the arm-cocking phase begins, the pelvis and upper torso rotate to face the batter.

Elbow joint forces and torques are generated throughout the arm-cocking phase. A low to moderate flexion torque of 0 to 32 N·m is produced at the elbow throughout the arm-cocking phase (Fig. 2.2).[20] Consequently, the elbow flexors demonstrate low to moderate activity, primarily during the middle third of the arm-cocking phase.[24,26,28]

The forearm produces a large valgus torque onto the upper arm at the elbow; the pelvis and upper torso rotation and rapid shoulder external rotation contribute, in part, to this valgus torque. To resist the valgus torque, the upper arm generates a maximum varus torque ranging from 52 to 76 N·m (mean, 64 N·m) onto the forearm shortly before maximum shoulder external rotation (Fig. 2.3).[20] The flexor and pronator muscle mass of the forearm displays moderate to high activity, which helps to contribute to varus torque (Table 2.1).[28] Because these muscles originate at the medial epicondyle, they contract to help to stabilize the elbow. Large tensile forces on the medial aspect of the elbow result from the valgus torque

placed on the arm. Repetitive valgus loading eventually may lead to injury to the ulnar collateral ligament (UCL). Furthermore, inflammation of the medial epicondyle or adjacent tissues may occur (i.e., medial epicondylitis).

As indicated, an in vitro study by Morrey and An showed that the UCL contributes approximately 54% of the resistance to valgus loading in the flexed arm posi-

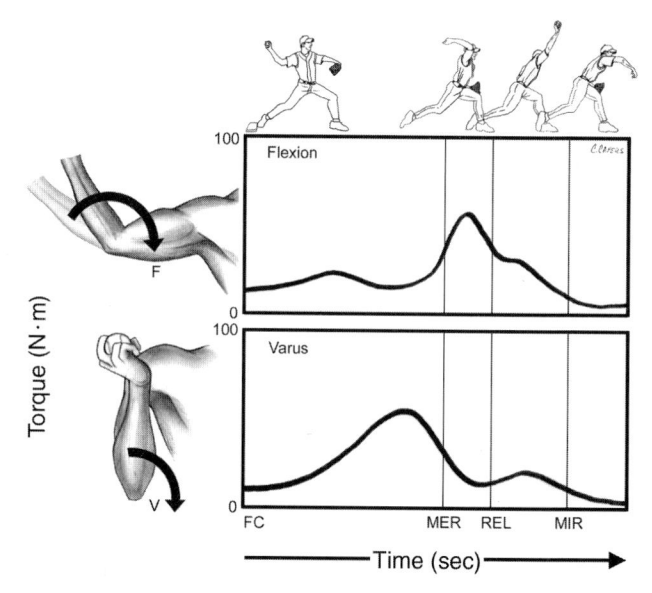

FIGURE 2.2. Torques applied to the forearm at the elbow in the flexion (F) and varus (V) directions. The instants of foot contact (FC), maximum external rotation (MER), ball release (REL), and maximum internal rotation (MIR) are shown. (Adapted from Fleisig et al.[20])

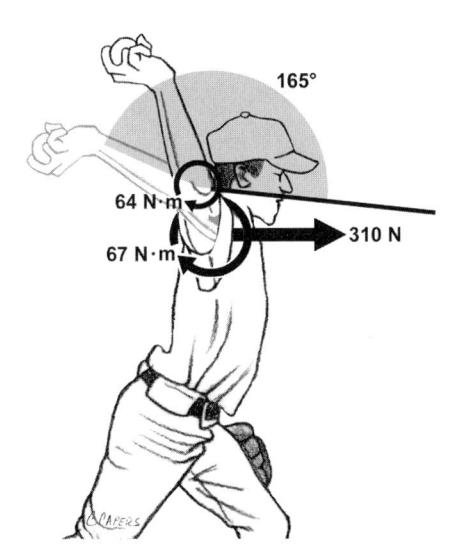

FIGURE 2.3. Shortly before maximum external rotation is achieved, the first critical instant occurs. At this instant, the arm is externally rotated to 165°, and the elbow is flexed to 95°. Among the loads generated at this time are 64 N · m of varus torque at the elbow and 67 N · m of internal rotation torque and 310 N of anterior force at the shoulder. (Adapted from Fleisig et al.[20])

tion.[11] Assuming that the UCL produces 54% of the 52- to 76-N·m maximum varus torque that an elite pitcher generates, the UCL provides approximately 30 to 40 N·m of varus torque. This is similar to the 32-N·m failure load that Dillman et al. reported; thus, during baseball pitching, the UCL appears to be loaded near its maximum capacity.[12,20] However, this result is only an approximation of the UCL's contribution in throwing because the cadaveric research does not account for muscle contributions. Muscle contraction during this phase may reduce the stress seen on the UCL by compressing the joint and adding stability.[24]

Valgus torque also can cause high compressive forces on the lateral elbow, which can lead to lateral elbow compression injury.[20] Specifically, valgus torque can cause compression between the radial head and humeral capitellum.[30] According to the in vitro study by Morrey and An, joint articulation supplies 33% of the varus torque needed to resist the valgus torque that the forearm applies.[11] Thirty-three percent of the 52- to 76-N·m maximum varus torque generated during pitching is 17 to 25 N·m. If the distance from the axis of valgus rotation to the compression point between the radial head and the humeral capitellum is approximately 4 cm, then the compressive force generated between the radius and humerus to produce 17 to 25 N·m of varus torque is approximately 425 to 625 N·m.[20] Muscle contraction about the elbow or loss of joint integrity on the medial side of the elbow can cause this compressive force to increase. Excessive or repetitive compressive force can result in avascular necrosis, osteochondritis dissecans, or osteochondral chip fractures of the radiocapitellar joint.[30]

In addition to a varus torque, the upper arm applies a maximum 240 to 360 N of medial force onto the forearm to resist lateral translation of the forearm at the elbow (Fig. 2.4). This force is significantly greater during a fastball or curveball pitch than during a change-up or slider pitch (Table 2.2).[31] The greater medial force during arm cocking in the curveball pitch compared with other off-speed pitches (e.g., change-up and slider) may be related to medial elbow injuries. Further research is needed to address this issue. The forearm is supinated more during the arm-cocking phase for a curveball pitch than for a fastball pitch, which also may be related to elbow injuries.[32,33]

Other forces also are produced at the elbow during arm cocking. The upper arm applies a maximum anterior force of 80 to 240 N onto the forearm to resist posterior translation of the forearm at the elbow.[20] Similarly, the upper arm applies a maximum compressive force of 150 to 390 N to the forearm to resist elbow distraction.[20]

The elbow achieves a maximum flexion of 85° to 105° approximately 30 ms before maximum shoulder external rotation (Fig. 2.5).[20,24] The triceps muscle appears to control maximum elbow flexion, which shows moderate activity during the last third of the arm-cocking phase.[24,28] This hypothesis is supported by Roberts's data, which

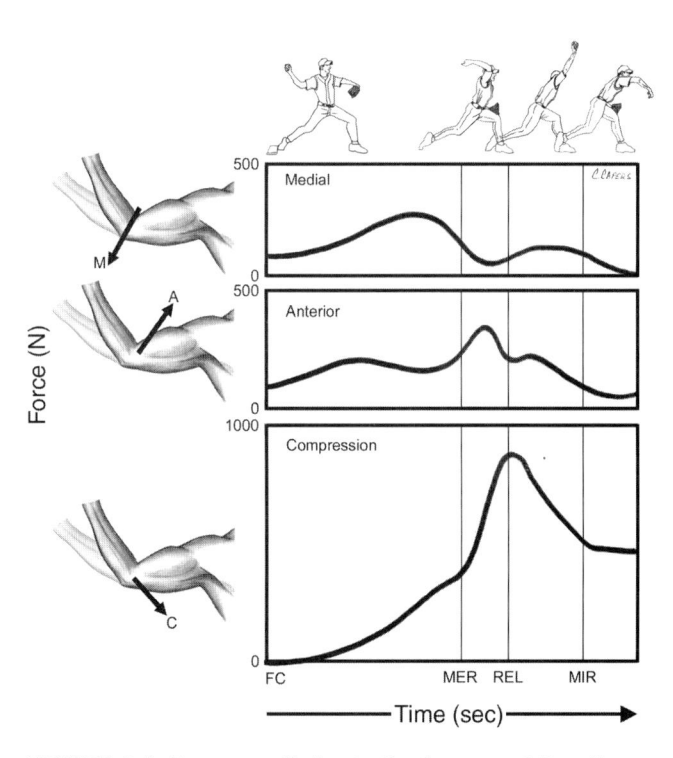

FIGURE 2.4. Forces applied onto the forearm at the elbow in the medial (M), anterior (A), and compressive (C) directions. The instants of foot contact (FC), maximum external rotation (MER), ball release (REL), and maximum internal rotation (MIR) are shown. (Adapted from Fleisig et al.[20])

TABLE 2.2. *Comparison of elbow biomechanics with different pitches*

	Fastball	Curveball	Change-up	Slider
Arm cocking				
Elbow medial force (N)	280	280	240	240
Elbow varus torque (N · m)	55	54	46	47
Arm acceleration				
Elbow extension velocity (degrees/second)	2400	2400	2100	2500
Arm deceleration				
Elbow compressive force (N)	790	730	640	780

Adapted from Escamilla et al.[31] and Escamilla et al.[35]

show that if a radial nerve block paralyzes the triceps muscle the elbow "collapses" and continues flexing near its limit (approximately 145° of elbow flexion).[34] This collapse is caused by a centripetal flexion torque at the elbow that the rapidly rotating upper torso and arm create. The triceps muscle apparently contracts eccentrically and then isometrically in resisting the centripetal elbow flexion torque that occurs during late arm cocking. At approximately the time that the elbow reaches maximum elbow flexion (i.e., approximately 30 ms before maximum shoulder external rotation), the elbow flexors become inactive, and the triceps contracts concentrically to aid in elbow extension.[20,24] Figure 2.5 shows the interactions among muscle activity, elbow joint torque, and elbow extension.

Arm Acceleration

The arm-acceleration phase is the short time from maximum shoulder external rotation to ball release (Fig. 2.1H,I). The entire phase lasts only a few hundredths of a second. A maximum elbow angular velocity of 2100° to 2700° per second occurs approximately halfway through the acceleration phase.[24] Maximum elbow angular velocity is similar for the fastball, curveball, and slider pitches, but is markedly less during the change-up pitch (Table 2.2).[35] This rapid elbow extension may be due primarily to centrifugal force acting on the forearm because of the rotating trunk and arm; the elbow extensors are unlikely to shorten fast enough to generate the high angular velocity measured at the elbow.

Several studies have examined the role of the triceps in extending the elbow during the acceleration phase of throwing.[24,26,28,34,36] Roberts reported that a pitcher with a paralyzed triceps due to a differential nerve block was able to throw a ball at more than 80% of the speed attained before paralyzation.[34] This finding seems to support the concept that the triceps contraction does not generate most of the elbow extension velocity and that centrifugal force is a major factor. Electromyography has shown high triceps and anconeus activity during the arm-acceleration phase, suggesting that the triceps initiates or contributes to some of the angular velocity generated during this phase.[24,26,28,36] However, these muscles may function more as elbow stabilizers than as accelerators.[25]

Toyoshima et al. compared normal throwing using the entire body with throwing using only the forearm to extend the elbow.[37] The latter *forearm throw* involved a maximum voluntary effort to extend the elbow with the upper arm immobilized. Assuming that the triceps muscle shortened as fast as voluntarily possible during the forearm throw, the resulting elbow angular velocity is the maximum that could be generated with maximum triceps contraction alone. The results from this study showed that normal throwing generated approximately twice the elbow angular velocity that could be achieved during the forearm throw. The authors concluded that the elbow was swung open like a whip and that the elbow angular velocity that occurs during throwing is due more to the rotary actions of other parts of the body (e.g., hips, trunk, and shoulder) than to the elbow-extending capabilities of the triceps. They also showed that forearm throwing produced only 43% of the ball velocity generated in normal throwing.

Ahn used computer simulations and optimization techniques in comparing theoretical data with experimental data.[38] The data showed that hand velocity at ball release was approximately 80% of the experimental value when the resultant elbow joint torque was set to zero, approximately 95% of the experimental value when the resultant wrist joint torque was set to zero, and approximately 75% of the experimental value when both the resultant elbow and wrist joint torques were set to zero. Consequently, he concluded that body segments other than the upper extremity (i.e., lower extremities, hips, and trunk) primarily generated ball velocity at release.

During arm acceleration, the need to resist valgus stress at the elbow can result in a wedging of the olecranon against the medial aspect of the trochlear groove and

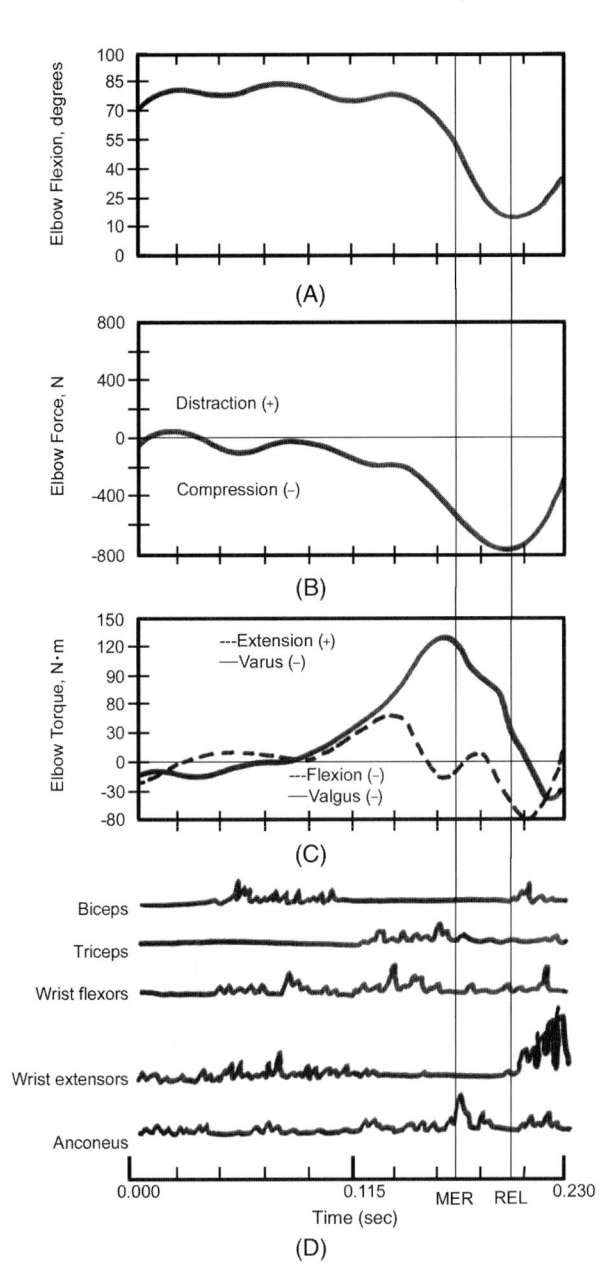

FIGURE 2.5. Time-matched measurements during the baseball pitch: (A) elbow flexion, (B) force applied at the elbow, (C) torque applied at the elbow, and (D) electromyographic muscle activity. (Adapted from Werner et al.[24])

the "valgus extension overload" mechanism that Wilson et al. described.[23] Campbell et al. found greater valgus torque (normalized by body weight times height) in 10-year-old pitchers than in professional pitchers at the instant of ball release. They believed this finding might be related to Little League elbow syndrome in young pitchers.[39]

As the elbow extends and the upper torso continues to rotate, a maximum elbow compressive force of 800 to 1000 N is produced at ball release to prevent elbow distraction due to the centrifugal force acting on the forearm (Fig. 2.4).[20] In addition, low to moderate activity from the elbow flexors generates a maximum elbow flexor torque of 40 to 60 N·m (Fig. 2.2).[20,26,28] Contraction of the elbow flexors in this phase adds compressive force for joint stability and also controls the rate of elbow extension.

Arm Deceleration

The arm-deceleration phase, which only lasts a few hundredths of a second, begins at ball release and ends when the shoulder has reached its maximum internal rotation (Fig. 2.1I,J). An eccentric elbow flexion torque of approximately 10 to 35 N·m is produced throughout the arm-deceleration phase to decelerate elbow extension (Fig. 2.2).[20,24] Moderate to high eccentric contractions of the elbow flexors have been reported during arm deceleration.[24,26,28] Researchers also have shown that the pronator teres is very active in decelerating elbow extension and pronating the forearm.[28,40] The biceps brachii and supinator muscles are responsible for controlling forearm pronation.

A maximum elbow compressive force of 800 to 1000 N occurs just after ball release to prevent elbow distraction (Fig. 2.4).[20] This compressive force is greatest when throwing fastball or slider pitches (Table 2.2).[31] Compressive forces also have been shown to increase as skill level increases.[41] Elbow flexors produce a compressive force, as well as terminate elbow extension, before the olecranon impinges in the olecranon fossa.[24] Elbow extension terminates when the elbow is flexed approximately 20°.[24,25]

the olecranon fossa. This impingement leads to osteophyte production at the posterior and posteromedial aspect of the olecranon tip and can cause chondromalacia and loose body formation.[23] Figure 2.2 shows that substantial varus torque is generated throughout the arm-cocking and arm-acceleration phases in order to resist valgus torque. During these phases, the elbow extends through a range of approximately 65° (from approximately 85° to approximately 20°).[20] This combination of elbow extension and resistance to valgus torque supports

Follow-Through

The follow-through phase begins at maximum shoulder internal rotation and ends when the pitcher attains a balanced fielding position (Fig. 2.1J,K). Motion of the larger body parts, such as the trunk and lower extremities, helps to dissipate energy in the throwing arm during this phase.[1] Forces and torques at the elbow during the follow-through are less than the high levels attained during arm deceleration (Figs. 2.2 and 2.4). During follow-through, the el-

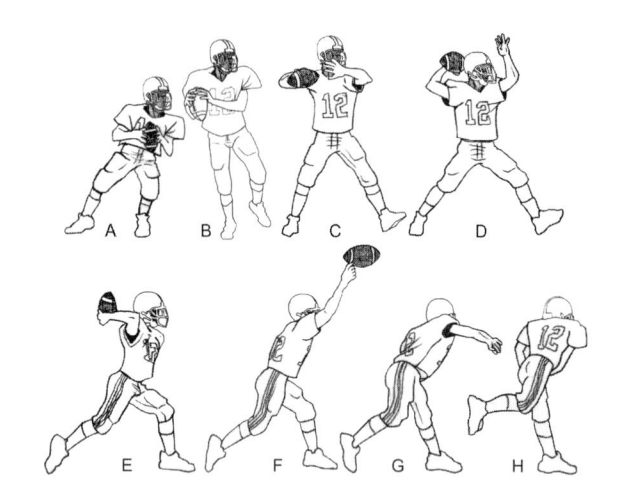

FIGURE 2.6. Sequence of positions during the football pass. (Adapted from Fleisig et al.[42])

bow flexes into a comfortable position as the trunk rotates forward and the arm moves across the body.[25]

BIOMECHANICS OF THE ELBOW DURING OTHER THROWING MOTIONS

Football Passing

The motion of throwing a football is qualitatively similar to throwing a baseball (Fig. 2.6). Quantifying the throwing motion in football and comparing it to baseball pitching have been the emphases of recent studies.[42,43] To compare and contrast baseball pitching and football passing, Fleisig et al.[42] used motion analysis to study 26 baseball pitchers and 26 football quarterbacks. The pitchers threw from a mound to a strike-zone ribbon located 18.4 m away (i.e., regulation distance), and quarterbacks threw drop-back passes an equal distance. The basis for this comparison was the theory that a football could be used as an overload-weighted implement for strengthening the arm of a baseball pitcher. Researchers have documented that overload training can increase ball velocity once pitching with regulation-weight baseballs is resumed.[44–46]

During arm cocking, a quarterback demonstrates greater elbow flexion (range, 100° to 120°) than do pitchers (Fig. 2.6B,C). In addition, during arm cocking, a maximum medial force of 240 to 280 N and a maximum varus torque of 54 N·m are produced at the elbow. During arm acceleration, the elbow reaches a maximum extension velocity of 1760°/sec (Fig. 2.6E). To decelerate the elbow, a quarterback generates a flexion torque of 41 N·m and a compressive force of 620 N. Several kinematic and kinetic differences between baseball pitchers and football passers were found for other joints as well. Rash and Shapiro videotaped 12 collegiate football quarterbacks to quantify the dynamics of the passing motion.[43] They found results similar to those of Fleisig et al., but discrepancies existed between the magnitudes of certain parameters.[43] One explanation for the differences is the sampling rates used for each study.[42] Fleisig et al. collected data at 200 Hz, and Rash and Shapiro collected data at 60 Hz.

Although football passing is qualitatively similar to baseball pitching, it requires markedly less force and torque production to decelerate elbow extension than pitching requires. The lower incidence of elbow injury in quarterbacks who repetitively throw than in baseball pitchers may be attributed to the lower forces and torques generated during the deceleration phase.

In junior high and high school, an athlete with a strong arm often becomes a football quarterback and a baseball pitcher. Because of the kinematic differences between the throwing motions, throwing a baseball and throwing a football during the same season could be detrimental to the development of proper mechanics. However, throwing footballs and baseballs in the off-season may have some positive training benefits. This training may especially benefit the adolescent or prepubescent athlete, whose objective should be to develop general fitness and athletic skills without committing to the specialization of one sport.

Tennis

As with the overhand throw, the tennis serve generates considerable angular velocity at the elbow. Kibler indicated that the angular velocity for elbow extension reaches 982°/sec and forearm pronation reaches 347°/sec.[47] In their investigation of the effectiveness of arm segment rotations in producing racquet-head speed, Sprigings et al.[48] reached conclusions that conflicted with those of Kibler.[47] They found that forearm pronation had the fastest rotation of 1375°/sec; however, it ranked fourth in terms of contribution. They concluded that elbow extension did not contribute significantly to the forward speed of the racquet head. Note that this study analyzed only one player, and the authors indicated that the lack of contribution of elbow extension may be due to technical flaws with this player's particular technique. Cohen et al. investigated relationships among anthropometric data, upper extremity strength, and functional serve velocity and concluded that elbow extension torque production was highly related to serving velocity.[49] Kibler estimated that the elbow joint contributes 15% of the force produced during the tennis serve.[47]

During the serving motion, the elbow moves through a flexion range of approximately 100° (from 116° to 20°), but the range of motion during ground strokes is smaller (11° during the forehand stroke and 18° during the backhand stroke).[47] Electromyographic activity for muscles about the elbow appears to be lower during the ground-stroke motion than during the serving motion.[50] This finding may indicate that during ground-stroke motion, muscle activity stabilizes the elbow and generates velocity during the serve. Morris et al. concluded that high pronator teres and triceps activity (more than 60% manual muscle test) plays a significant role in power production for the serve.[50]

A common interest of researchers and clinicians is the cause of lateral epicondylitis, or tennis elbow, which occurs in 40% to 50% of recreational players.[51] It is often thought to be caused by repeated microtrauma and high wrist extensor activity as soft tissues about the elbow dissipate impact forces. As Roetert et al. and Hatze reported, it is estimated that impact forces during the backhand stroke create torques equal to 17 to 24 N·m.[51,52] Based on studies of the electromyographic activity of muscles about the elbow during the backhand, the cause of injury appears to be related to stroke mechanics and technique, rather than to high muscle activity. Giangarra et al. compared forearm muscle activity during single- and double-hand backhand strokes and found no difference between wrist extensor activity.[53] The authors of this and previous studies concluded that the decreased occurrence of lateral epicondylitis for players using the double-hand technique is attributed to changes in the mechanics of the stroke and the increased ability to absorb the forces created at impact.[53,54] Players with a history of lateral epicondylitis have been shown to have greater wrist extensor and pronator teres activity.[55] The increased activity was attributed to abnormal stroke mechanics observed with cinematography that included leading with the elbow, exaggerated wrist pronation, and off-center ball impact location on the racket head (lower portion). As Roetert et al. indicated, the high involvement of the wrist extensors in all types of strokes increases the chances of overload and the potential for injury for this muscular system.[51] Improper stroke mechanics exacerbate this problem.

Javelin

Some authors have conducted biomechanical analyses of javelin throwing.[56,57] Most of these studies concentrated on kinematic parameters related to performance; consequently, the stress or load experienced at the elbow has not been quantified extensively. Mero et al. investigated the contribution of body segments to the javelin throw during Olympic competition.[56] During the thrust phase (from final foot contact until javelin release), the elbow extends through a flexion range of approximately 40° (from 100° to 57°). Top throwers (i.e., Olympic medal winners) have a 60° range of motion at the elbow (from 96° to 40°), which is comparable with the flexion range for baseball pitchers. This range of motion occurs although the javelin thrower has less elbow flexion than a baseball pitcher or football quarterback at the time of foot contact. The elbow extension angular velocity achieved during the thrust phase is high, reaching a maximum of 1900°/sec.

BIOMECHANICS OF THE ELBOW DURING UNDERHAND THROWING

Although the traditional view is that underhand pitchers have minimal risk for sustaining pitching-related injuries, Loosli et al. found a high incidence of injuries to underhand pitchers.[58] Thirty-one percent of these injuries were at or distal to the elbow. Unfortunately, research investigating the motion involved in underhand throwing is limited.

Barrentine et al. estimated the amount of force experienced at the elbow during underhand softball pitching.[59] During the acceleration phase, a compressive force equivalent to 445 N is exerted to resist elbow distraction. Elbow distraction is caused by the centrifugal force on the forearm resulting from the upper torso rotation of 650°/sec, the arm rotating about the shoulder at 5260°/sec, and the elbow flexing at 880°/sec. A valgus torque of 45 N·m is generated at the elbow to resist varus stress caused by the combination of elbow flexion and shoulder internal rotation. After ball release, a compressive force of 356 N is exerted to resist distraction at the elbow during follow-through. The compressive force exerted on the elbow is smaller during underhand softball pitching than during overhand baseball pitching, and the timings of the maximum loads differ. Peak compressive force loads during underhand pitching occur during the acceleration phase, and peak forces during baseball pitching occur just after ball release during the deceleration phase. Varus torque observed in baseball pitching does not occur in underhand pitching, so fewer elbow injuries result. Elbow injuries often are related to improper mechanics, such as hitting the medial elbow against the hip before ball release. Obvious differences, such as sex, size of the ball, and pitching environment (height of mound), prevent a direct comparison between overhand and underhand pitching; however, based on the results, the elbow in the underhand motion may not be as safe from overuse injuries as previously thought.

CONCLUSION

Common aspects are involved in a variety of throwing motions. During most throwing activities, the elbow is stressed to its biomechanical limits. Through proper coordination with the rest of the body, the muscles about the elbow joint generate the rapid extension, flexion, pronation, and supination needed for sport performance.

Hard and soft joint tissue are loaded to capacity to generate and control these rapid motions. These loads may include large tensile forces on medial soft tissue (e.g., UCL), large compressive forces on lateral hard tissue (e.g., radiocapitellar articulation), soft tissue tensile loads to prevent joint distraction, and hard tissue loads to withstand compression and varus and valgus torques.

REFERENCES

1. Boone DC, Azen SP. Normal range of motion of joints in male subjects. *J Bone Joint Surg* 1979;61A:756–759.
2. Morrey BF, Askew LJ, Chao EY, et al. A biomechanical study of normal functional elbow motion. *J Bone Joint Surg* 1981;63A:872–877.
3. Morrey BF, Chao EY. Passive motion of the elbow joint. *J Bone Joint Surg* 1976;58A:501–508.
4. Werner FW, An KN. Biomechanics of the elbow and forearm. *Hand Clin* 1994;10:357–373.
5. An KN, Morrey BF. Biomechanics of the elbow. In: Morrey BF, ed. *The elbow and its disorders*. Philadelphia: W.B. Saunders, 1985;43–61.
6. London JT. Kinematics of the elbow. *J Bone Joint Surg* 1981;63A:529–535.
7. An KN, Takahashi K, Harrigan TP, et al. Determination of muscle orientations and moment arms. *J Biomech Eng* 1984;106:280–282.
8. An KN, Hui FC, Morrey BF, et al. Muscles across the elbow joint: A biomechanical analysis. *J Biomech* 1981;14:659–669.
9. Basmajian JV. Recent advances in the functional anatomy of the upper limb. *Am J Phys Med* 1969;48:165–177.
10. An KA, Morrey BF. Biomechanics of the elbow. In: Morrey BF, ed. *The elbow and its disorders*, 2nd ed. Philadelphia: W.B. Saunders; 1993:53–72.
11. Morrey BF, An KN. Articular and ligamentous contributions to the stability of the elbow joint. *Am J Sports Med* 1983;11:315–319.
12. Dillman C, Smutz P, Werner S, et al. Valgus extension overload in baseball pitching [abstract]. *Med Sci Sports Exer* 1991;23:S135.
13. Regan WD, Korinek SL, Morrey BF, et al. Biomechanical study of ligaments around the elbow joint. *Clin Orthop* 1991;271:170–179.
14. Askew LJ, An KN, Morrey BF, et al. Isometric elbow strength in normal individuals. *Clin Orthop* 1987;222:261–266.
15. Amis AA, Dowson D, Wright V. Elbow joint force predictions for some strenuous isometric actions. *J Biomech* 1980;13:765–775.
16. Ewald FC, Thomas WH, Sledge CB, et al. Non-constrained metal to plastic total elbow arthroplasty in rheumatoid arthritis. In: *Joint replacement in the upper limb*. London: Institute of Mechanical Engineers; 1977:77–81.
17. Halls AA, Travill A. Transmission of pressures across the elbow joint. *Anat Rec* 1964;150:243–248.
18. Andrews JR, Whiteside JA. Common elbow problems in the athlete. *J Orthop Sports Phys Ther* 1993;17:289–295.
19. DeHaven KE, Evarts CM. Throwing injuries of the elbow in athletes. *Orthop Clin North Am* 1973;4:801–808.
20. Fleisig GS, Andrews JR, Dillman CJ, et al. Kinetics of baseball pitching with implications about injury mechanisms. *Am J Sports Med* 1995;23:233–239.
21. Hang Y-S. Little league elbow: A clinical and biomechanical study. In: Matsui H, Kobayashi K, eds. *Biomechanics VIII-A*. Champaign, IL: Human Kinetics; 1983:70–85.
22. Mirowitz SA, London SL. Ulnar collateral ligament injury in baseball pitchers: MR imaging evaluation. *Radiology* 1992;185:573–576.
23. Wilson FD, Andrews JR, Blackburn TA, et al. Valgus extension overload in the pitching elbow. *Am J Sports Med* 1983;11:83–88.
24. Werner SL, Fleisig GS, Dillman CJ, et al. Biomechanics of the elbow during baseball pitching. *J Orthop Sports Phys Ther* 1993;17:274–278.
25. Feltner M, Dapena J. Dynamics of the shoulder and elbow joints of the throwing arm during a baseball pitch. *Int J Sports Biomech* 1986;2:235–259.
26. Sisto DJ, Jobe FW, Moynes DR, et al. An electromyographic analysis of the elbow in pitching. *Am J Sports Med* 1987;15:260–263.
27. Jacobs P. The overhand baseball pitch: A kinesiological analysis and related strength-conditioning programming. *National Strength and Conditioning Association Journal* 1987;9:5–13.
28. DiGiovine NM, Jobe FW, Pink M, et al. An electromyographic analysis of the upper extremity in pitching. *J Shoulder Elbow Surg* 1992;1:15–25.
29. Fleisig GS. *The biomechanics of baseball pitching* [doctoral dissertation]. Birmingham: University of Alabama; 1994.
30. Atwater AE. Biomechanics of overarm throwing movements and of throwing injuries. *Exerc Sport Sci Rev* 1979;7:43–85.
31. Escamilla RF, Fleisig GS, Alexander E, et al. A kinematic and kinetic comparison while throwing different types of baseball pitches. *Med Sci Sports Exer* 1994;26:S175.
32. Barrentine S, Matsuo T, Escamilla R, et al. Kinematic analysis of the wrist and forearm during baseball pitching. *J Appl Biomech* 1998;14:24–39.
33. Sakurai S, Ikegami Y, Okamoto A, et al. A three-dimensional cinematographic analysis of upper limb movement during fastball and curveball baseball pitches. *J Appl Biomech* 1993;9:47–65.
34. Roberts TW. Cinematography in biomechanical investigation. Selected topics in biomechanics. In: *CIC symposium on biomechanics*. Chicago: The Athletic Institute, 1971:41–50.
35. Escamilla RF, Fleisig GS, Barrentine SW, et al. Kinematic comparisons of throwing different types of baseball pitches. *J Appl Biomech* 1998;14:1–23
36. Jobe FW, Moynes DR, Tibone JE, et al. An EMG analysis of the shoulder in pitching: A second report. *Am J Sports Med* 1984;12:218–220.
37. Toyoshima S, Hoshikawa T, Miyashita M, et al. Contributions of the body parts of throwing performance. In: Nelson RC, Morehouse CA, eds. *Biomechanics IV*. Baltimore: University Park Press, 1974:169–174.
38. Ahn BH. *A model of the human upper extremity and its application to a baseball pitching motion* [dissertation]. East Lansing: Michigan State University; 1991.
39. Campbell KR, Hagood SS, Takagi Y, et al. Kinetic analysis of the elbow and shoulder in professional and Little League pitchers. *Med Sci Sports Exer* 1994;26:S175.

40. Fisk CS. *The dynamic function of selected muscles of the forearm: An electromyographical and cinematographical analysis* [dissertation]. Bloomington: Indiana University; 1976.
41. Fleisig GS, Barrentine SW, Zheng N, et al. Kinematic and kinetic comparison of baseball pitching among various levels of development. *J Biomech* 1999;32:1371–1375.
42. Fleisig GS, Escamilla RF, Andrews JR, et al. Kinematic and kinetic comparison between baseball pitching and football passing. *J Appl Biomech* 1996;12:207–224.
43. Rash GS, Shapiro R. A three-dimensional dynamic analysis of the quarterback's throwing motion in American football. *J Appl Biomech* 1995;11:443–459.
44. DeRenne C, House T. *Power baseball*. New York: West Publishing Co., 1993.
45. Brose DE, Hanson DL. Effects of overload training on velocity and accuracy of throwing. *Res Q* 1967;38:528–533.
46. Litwhiler D, Hamm L. Overload: effect on throwing velocity and accuracy. *Athletic J* 1973;53:64–65, 88.
47. Kibler WB. Clinical biomechanics of the elbow in tennis: Implications for evaluation and diagnosis. *Med Sci Sports Exer* 1994;26:1203–1206.
48. Sprigings E, Marshall R, Elliott B, et al. A three-dimensional kinematic method for determining the effectiveness of arm segment rotations in producing racquet-head speed. *J Biomech* 1994;27:245–254.
49. Cohen DB, Mont MA, Campbell KR, et al. Upper extremity physical factors affecting tennis serve velocity. *Am J Sports Med* 1994;22:746–750.
50. Morris M, Jobe FW, Perry J, et al. Electromyographic analysis of elbow function in tennis players. *Am J Sports Med* 1989;17:241–247.
51. Roetert EP, Brody H, Dillman CJ, et al. The biomechanics of tennis elbow. An integrated approach. *Clin Sports Med* 1995; 14:47–57.
52. Hatze H. Forces and duration of impact, and grip tightness during the tennis stroke. *Med Sci Sports Exer* 1976;8:88–95.
53. Giangarra CE, Conroy B, Jobe FW, et al. Electromyographic and cinematographic analysis of elbow function in tennis players using single- and double-handed backhand strokes. *Am J Sports Med* 1993;21:394–399.
54. Groppel JL, Nirschl RP. A mechanical and electromyographical analysis of the effects of various joint counterforce braces on the tennis player. *Am J Sports Med* 1986;14:195–200.
55. Kelley JD, Lombardo SJ, Pink M, et al. Electromyographic and cinematographic analysis of elbow function in tennis players with lateral epicondylitis. *Am J Sports Med* 1994;22:359–363.
56. Mero A, Komi PV, Korjus T, et al. Body segment contributions to javelin throwing during final thrust phases. *J Appl Biomech* 1994;10:166–177.
57. Bartlett RM, Bent RJ. The biomechanics of javelin throwing. *J Sports Sci* 1988;6:1–38.
58. Loosli AR, Requa RK, Garrick JG, et al. Injuries to pitchers in women's collegiate fast-pitch softball. *Am J Sports Med* 1992;20:35–37.
59. Barrentine SW, Fleisig GS, Whiteside JA, et al. Biomechanics of windmill softball pitching with implications about injury mechanisms. *J Orthop Sports Phys Ther* 1998;28:405–415.

CHAPTER 3

History and Physical Examination of the Elbow

Champ L. Baker and Grant L. Jones

INTRODUCTION

The keys to diagnosing elbow injury are a comprehensive history and a thorough physical examination of not only the elbow but surrounding areas, such as the shoulder, wrist, hand, and cervical spine, to rule out referred pain. In this chapter, we discuss the important components of a complete elbow examination, including history, inspection, palpation, motion, strength testing, reflexes, sensory examination, stability testing, provocative tests, and radiographic evaluation.

HISTORY

Taking a comprehensive history helps the physician to develop a differential diagnosis. The examiner should find out whether a single traumatic event or repetitive traumatic episodes caused the symptoms. Acute injuries include ulnar collateral ligament (UCL) rupture, medial epicondyle avulsion, biceps rupture, loose-body formation, acute musculocutaneous strain or tendon rupture, and acute subluxation of the ulnar nerve. Chronic injuries include UCL strain or rupture, valgus extension overload, musculocutaneous strains, tendonapathies, and osteochondral defects that can progress to degenerative changes.[1]

The examiner should elicit the location of the pain. Dividing the elbow into four anatomic regions (i.e., lateral, medial, anterior, and posterior) helps to narrow the range of differential diagnoses.[1-6] Symptoms in the lateral region of the elbow can indicate radiocapitellar chondromalacia, osteochondral loose bodies, radial head fractures, osteochondritis dissecans (OCD) lesions, or posterior interosseous nerve entrapment. Symptoms in the medial region can indicate UCL strain or rupture, a medial epicondyle avulsion fracture, ulnar neuritis, ulnar nerve subluxation, medial epicondylitis, osteochondral loose bodies, valgus extension overload syndrome, or pronator teres syndrome. The differential diagnoses for symptoms in the anterior region include anterior capsular sprain, distal biceps tendon strain or rupture, brachialis muscle strain, and coronoid osteophyte formation. Finally, symptoms in the posterior region can indicate valgus extension overload, posterior osteophyte with impingement, triceps tendinitis, triceps tendon avulsion, olecranon stress fracture, osteochondral loose bodies, or olecranon bursitis.[1]

The examiner should query the patient about the presence and character of the pain, swelling, and locking and catching episodes. Sharp pain radiating down the medial portion of the forearm with paresthesias in the fifth and the ulnar-innervated half of the fourth digit indicates ulnar neuritis. When these symptoms are associated with a snapping or popping sensation, ulnar nerve subluxation might be the underlying cause. Pain that occurs in the posteromedial portion of the elbow with intense throwing efforts and is associated with localized crepitus might indicate valgus extension overload syndrome.[7,8] Pain localized in the posterior region of the elbow at the triceps tendon insertion can signal triceps tendinitis. Poorly localized, deep, aching pain in the posterior region of the elbow might be associated with an olecranon stress fracture.[1] Sharp pain in the lateral region associated with locking or catching can result from loose bodies in the radiocapitellar joint due to radial head fractures and OCD lesions of the capitellum. Acute, sharp pain in the anterior region of the elbow can result from an acute biceps tendon rupture. Persistent, aching pain in the anterior region can indicate inflammation involving the anterior capsule.[1]

A patient whose symptoms are related to throwing or to an occupational stress should be asked to reproduce the position that causes the symptoms. Pain during the early cocking phase of throwing might result from biceps or triceps tendinitis. Pain during the late cocking phase can result from valgus stresses on the medial region of the elbow and can indicate UCL incompetency or ulnar neuritis. A thrower who reports pain in the posterior region of the elbow during the late cocking and acceleration phases of throwing and reports inability to "let the ball go" might have valgus extension overload syndrome. Pain during the late acceleration or follow-through phases might signal a flexor–pronator tendonapathy due to forceful wrist flexion and forearm pronation during these phases. In the skeletally immature patient, pain in the lateral region of the elbow during the late acceleration and follow-through phases often indicates radiocapitellar joint injuries, such as OCD lesions.

INSPECTION

Careful inspection of the elbow joint and surrounding areas is the next step in evaluating elbow injury. First, the examiner should note atrophy or hypertrophy of muscle groups of the arm or forearm and should obtain girth measurements. Hypertrophy of the forearm musculature often is present in the dominant extremity of the throwing athlete and should be considered a normal variant. Atrophy of arm and forearm musculature, however, might result from an underlying neurologic disorder.

Second, the examiner should measure the carrying angle of the elbow with the arm extended and forearm supinated (Fig. 3.1). The normal carrying angle is 11° in men and 13° in women.[9] An increase in the carrying angle is termed **cubitus valgus**. Often, this angle increases from 10° to 15° in throwing athletes due to adaptive remodeling from repetitive valgus bony stress.[8,10] A progressive cubitus valgus deformity also might result from a nonunited lateral condyle fracture and might lead to a tardy ulnar nerve palsy.[11] A decrease in the carrying angle is termed **cubitus varus**. Cubitus varus might result from a malunited supracondylar humeral fracture or a previous growth plate disturbance due to trauma or inflammation.

Third, the clinician should examine the elbow for swelling. Swelling over the olecranon can indicate olecranon bursitis from trauma or underlying inflammation. Swelling in the area of the lateral soft spot (i.e., an area located in the center of the triangle formed by the lines connecting the olecranon, lateral epicondyle, and radial head) might result from a joint effusion or synovial proliferation due to trauma, infection, or rheumatologic disorder (Fig. 3.2). The clinician should carefully examine the skin in these areas for erythema, which can indicate an infection.

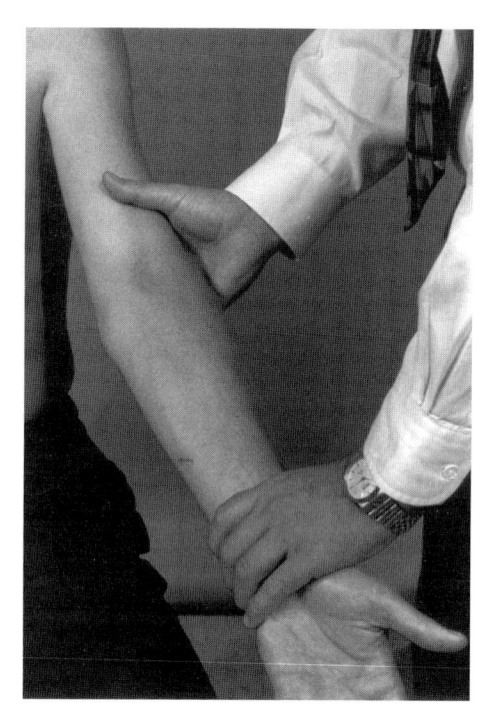

FIGURE 3.1. Observe the carrying angle of the elbow with the arm extended and forearm supinated.

PALPATION

The examiner palpates the medial and lateral epicondyles and olecranon tip and views them from a posterior angle. When the elbow is in full extension, these landmarks normally form a straight line (Fig. 3.3A). With the elbow in

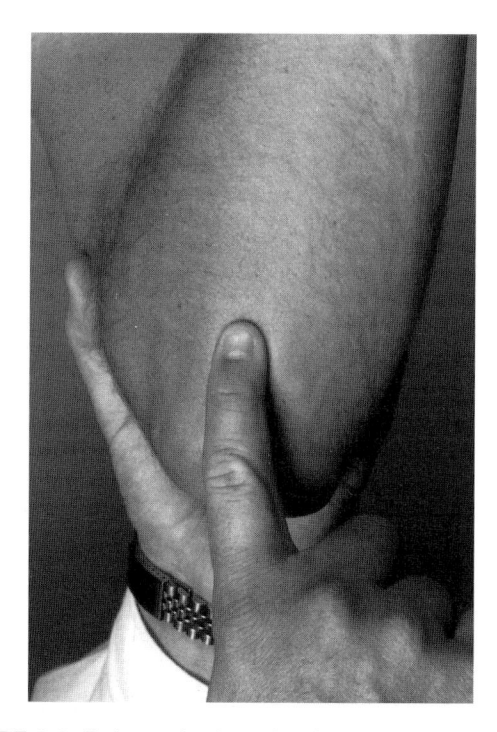

FIGURE 3.2. Palpate the lateral soft spot for swelling from a joint effusion or synovial proliferation.

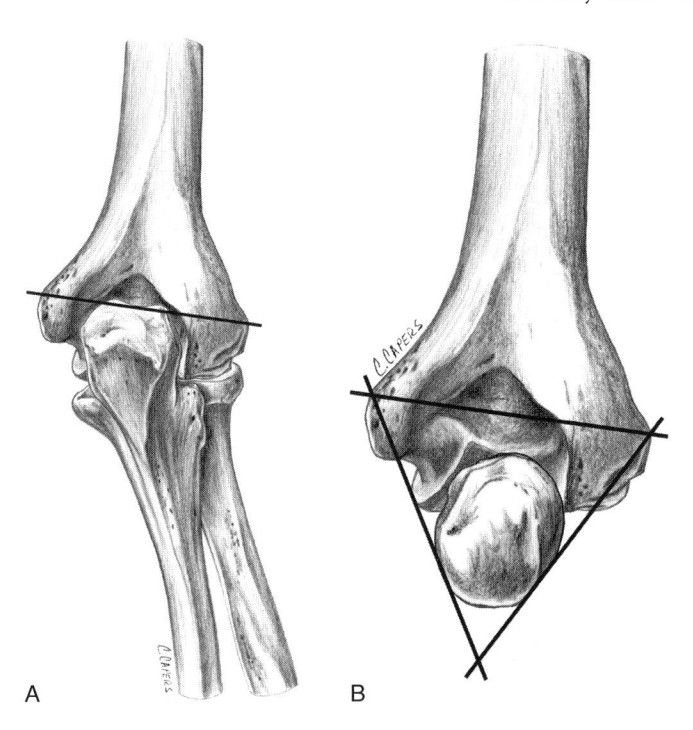

FIGURE 3.3. (A) The medial and lateral epicondyles and olecranon form a straight line with the elbow in full extension. (B) When the elbow is flexed to 90°, these landmarks form an equilateral triangle.

90° of flexion, however, they form an equilateral triangle (Fig. 3.3B). Any abnormalities of these alignments can indicate fracture, malunion, unreduced dislocation, or growth disturbances involving the distal end of the humerus.[12] The examiner should palpate of all four regions of the elbow (i.e., anterior, medial, posterior, and lateral) in an orderly fashion. Beginning with the anterior structures, the cubital fossa is bound laterally by the brachioradialis, the extensor carpi radialis longus, and the extensor carpi radialis brevis muscles; medially by the pronator teres muscle; and superiorly by the biceps muscle. Palpation of the brachioradialis and flexor–pronator muscles might reveal hypertrophy from repetitive use or exercise-induced edema. The examiner can palpate the distal biceps tendon anteromedially in the antecubital fossa with the patient's forearm in supination and elbow in active flexion.[1] Tenderness in this area can indicate biceps tendinitis or a biceps tendon rupture. Deep, poorly localized tenderness can result from anterior capsulitis or coronoid hypertrophy due to hyperextension injuries or repetitive hyperextension stress.[5] Next, the examiner should feel the brachial artery pulse deep to the lacertus fibrosus, which is just medial to the biceps tendon. Finally, he or she should conduct a Tinel's test in the area of the lacertus fibrosus, which is a common site of median nerve compression.[13] A positive Tinel's sign might indicate pronator syndrome.

Next, the clinician should palpate the structures in the medial region of the elbow, beginning with the supracondylar ridge. A congenital medial supracondylar process might be present in this area, which gives rise to a fibrous band (known as the **ligament of Struthers**) that inserts on the medial epicondyle. This band can compress the brachial artery and median nerve and result in neurovascular symptoms with strenuous use of the extremity. The examiner should palpate the medial epicondyle and flexor pronator mass. Tenderness at the origin of the flexor pronator mass on the epicondyle can reflect an avulsion fracture in adolescents or medial epicondylitis (i.e., golfer's elbow) in adults. Flexor pronator strains produce pain anterior and distal to the medial epicondyle. The UCL also is present in this area as it courses from the anteroinferior surface of the medial epicondyle to insert on the medial aspect of the coronoid process at the sublime tubercle.[14] Flexing the patient's elbow to 100° facilitates palpation of the UCL and uncovers the distal insertion of the anterior oblique portion of the UCL[1] (Fig. 3.4).

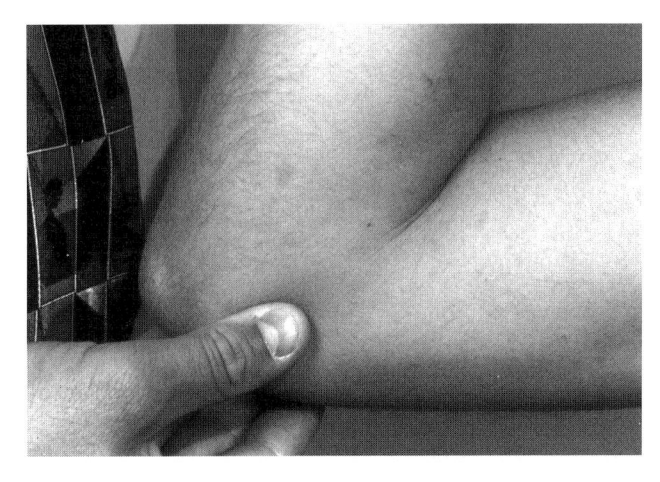

FIGURE 3.4. The examiner flexes the patient's elbow to 100° to facilitate palpation of the ulnar collateral ligament (UCL) and to uncover the distal insertion of the anterior oblique portion of the UCL.

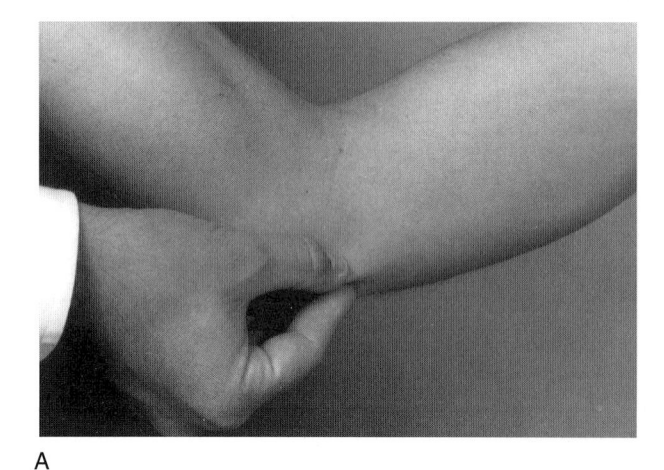

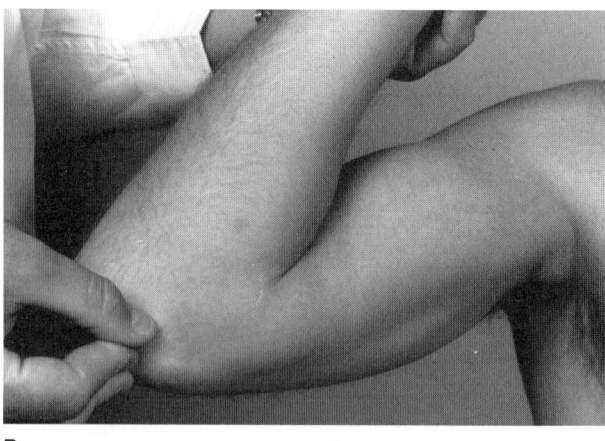

FIGURE 3.5. As the patient's elbow is brought from extension to flexion, the examiner might feel the ulnar nerve subluxate or dislocate anteriorly over the medial epicondyle, as in this subject who has a hypermobile nerve.

In the posteromedial area of the elbow, the ulnar nerve is easily palpable in the ulnar groove. An inflamed ulnar nerve is tender and can have a doughy consistency. The examiner should conduct Tinel's testing in three areas: proximal to the cubital tunnel (zone I), at the level of the cubital tunnel where the fascial aponeurosis joining the two heads of the flexor carpi ulnaris muscle forms (zone II), and distal to the cubital tunnel where the ulnar nerve descends to the forearm through the muscle bellies of the flexor carpi ulnaris (zone III).[15] A positive test produces paresthesias in the fifth digit and ulnar-innervated half of the fourth digit and indicates ulnar neuritis due to entrapment, trauma, or subluxation. The clinician also should test the nerve for hypermobility. The clinician brings the patient's elbow from extension to terminal flexion as he or she palpates the nerve to determine if it subluxates or completely dislocates over the medial epicondyle[16] (Fig. 3.5).

In the posterior region of the elbow, the examiner evaluates the olecranon bursa for swelling and fluctuation that indicate olecranon bursitis. He or she also examines this area for palpable osteophytes along the subcutaneous border of the olecranon that might contribute to an overlying bursitis. The examiner palpates the proximal one-third medial subcutaneous border of the olecranon because tenderness in this area can indicate a stress fracture. Next, he or she evaluates the insertion of the triceps tendon (Fig. 3.6). The three heads of the triceps converge to form an aponeurosis that attaches to the tip of the olecranon. Tenderness in this area can indicate triceps tendinitis or triceps avulsion injury if a palpable defect also is found. Finally, the clinician palpates the posterior, medial, and lateral aspects of the olecranon in varying degrees of flexion to detect osteophytes and loose bodies. Palpation of the posteromedial olecranon can reveal an osteophyte and swelling, which are present in the valgus extension overload syndrome of the throwing athlete.[7]

Examination of the lateral region of the elbow begins with the lateral epicondyle, which is readily palpable by tracing the lateral supracondylar ridge distally and with the mobile wad of Henry, which originates at the lateral region. Tenderness over the lateral epicondyle is typical of lateral epicondylitis (i.e., tennis elbow) (Fig. 3.7); however, tenderness approximately 4 cm distal to the lateral epicondyle and over the extensor muscle mass is present with radial tunnel syndrome, which is a compression neuropathy of the radial nerve as it travels from the radial head to the supinator muscle.[15] Finally, tenderness distal

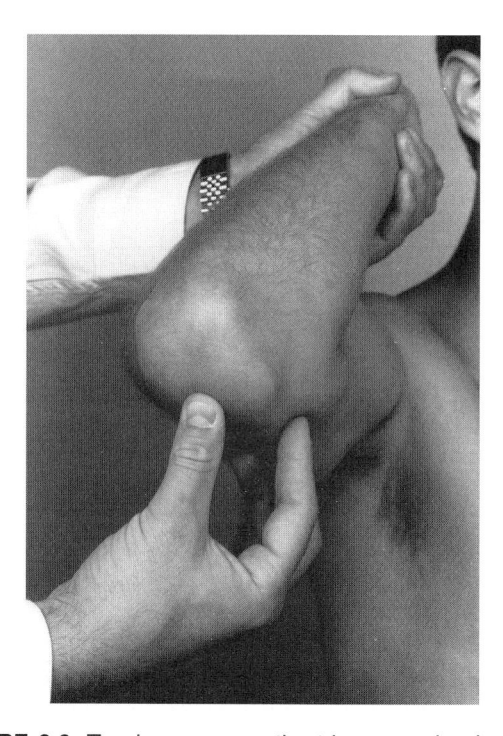

FIGURE 3.6. Tenderness over the triceps tendon insertion on the olecranon might indicate triceps tendinitis or triceps avulsion injury.

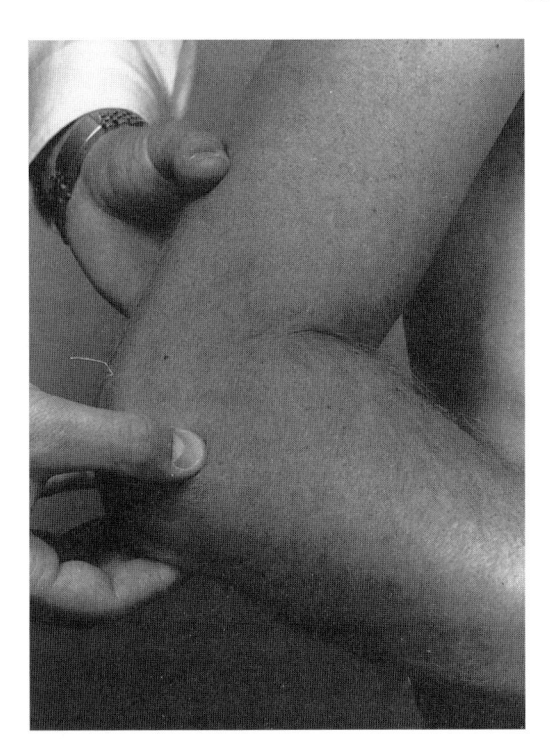

FIGURE 3.7. Lateral epicondylitis causes tenderness over the lateral epicondyle.

might demonstrate hyperextension of the elbow due to hypermobility. Injuries that cause loss of extension include capsular strain, flexor muscle strain, and intra-articular loose bodies. Injuries that cause abnormal lack of full flexion include loose bodies, capsular tightness, triceps strain, anterior osteophytes, and coronoid hypertrophy.

To measure pronation and supination, the examiner has the patient flex the elbows to 90° while holding pencils in each hand (Fig. 3.9). The examiner must immobilize the humerus in a vertical position when evaluating forearm rotation, because patients tend to adduct or abduct the shoulder to compensate for loss of forearm pronation or supination. Acceptable norms for full pronation and supination are 70° and 85°, respectively.[12] The functional arc of motion is 50° for both pronation and

to the location of the radial tunnel might be due to compression of the posterior interosseous nerve as it descends beneath the arcade of Frohse and the supinator muscle.

Next, the examiner palpates the radial head and radiocapitellar joint distal to the lateral epicondyle. Pronation and supination of the forearm enhance evaluation. Tenderness in this area might indicate fracture or dislocation of the radial head, osteochondrosis or Panner's disease in the adolescent athlete, or articular fragmentation and bony overgrowth with possible progression to loose-body formation in the young adult athlete.[1] Finally, palpation of the lateral recess, or soft spot, easily identifies an elbow effusion.

MOTION

Range of motion of the elbow occurs about two axes: (1) flexion and extension and (2) pronation and supination. The normal arc of flexion and extension ranges from 0° of extension to 140° of flexion (±10°),[17] but the functional arc about which most activities of daily living are performed ranges from 30° to 130° [18,19] (Fig. 3.8). The examiner must compare the range of motion of the contralateral extremity to account for normal individual variance. An athlete who has pitched many innings may have a flexion contracture on the dominant side that can increase as the season progresses and can decrease between seasons. However, a younger, less experienced pitcher

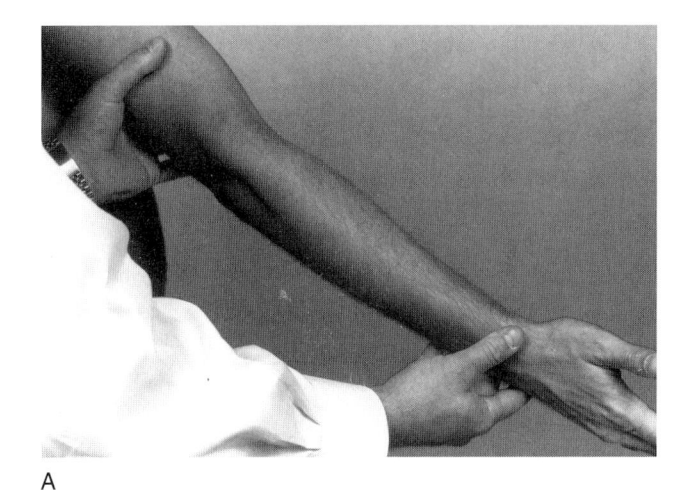

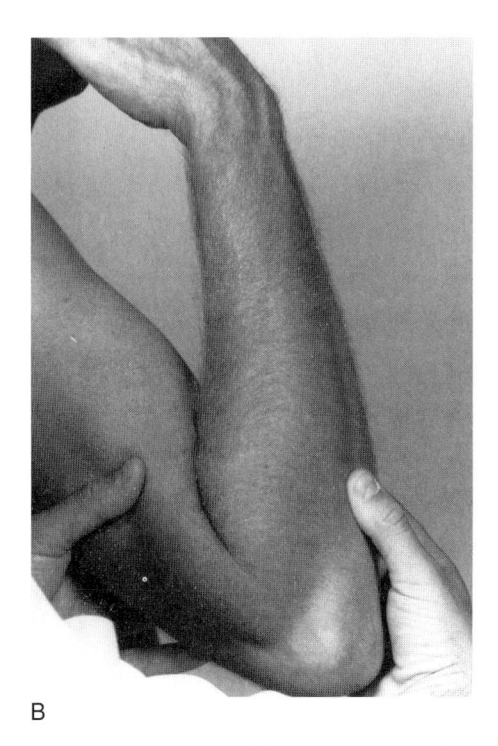

FIGURE 3.8. Normal arc of (A) extension and (B) flexion.

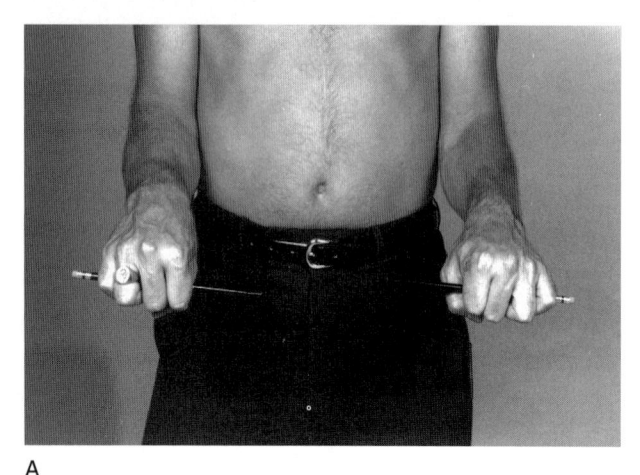

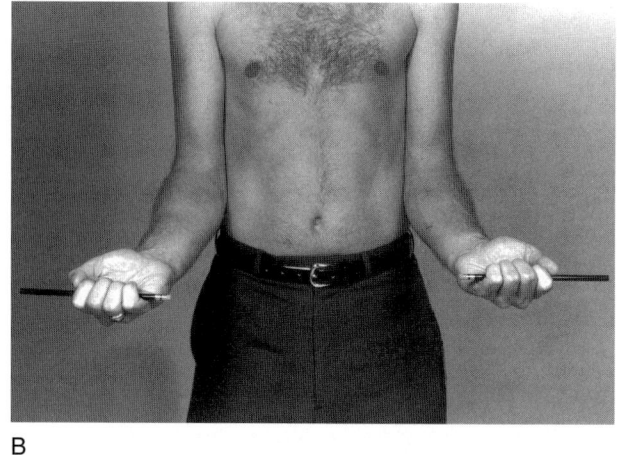

FIGURE 3.9. While the patient holds pencils in each hand and flexes the elbows to 90°, measure (A) pronation and (B) supination. Due to a previous fracture in the distal radius, this patient demonstrates a slight loss of pronation in the left extremity compared with the right extremity.

supination.[12] Pronation is the primary arc of motion on the dominant side for eating and writing, and patients compensate for loss of pronation by abducting the shoulder to perform these tasks. Loss of supination can cause difficulty in performing personal hygiene tasks, taking change in the palm, and turning door handles. Shoulder and wrist motion, however, poorly compensate for the lack of supination required in performing these tasks. Loss of pronation or supination can be caused by loose bodies, radiocapitellar osteochondritis, radial head subluxation, or motor nerve entrapment resulting in weakness of the biceps, pronator teres, pronator quadratus, or supinator muscles.[1] The examiner also should assess the wrist, because wrist injury can cause loss of forearm rotation.

When testing range of motion, the examiner also should note the presence or absence of crepitus. He or she must test both active and passive range of motion, because crepitus might not be present on passive motion and might be unveiled only through active range of motion. In addition, the clinician should assess active and passive limitation of motion; if motion is full on passive testing but limited on active testing, pain or paresis might be the limiting factor, rather than a mechanical block. Finally, the quality of the endpoint of motion should be noted. Firm endpoints often point to bony blocks, such as loose bodies, osteophytes, or other joint incongruities, as the cause of limited motion. Conversely, soft endpoints most likely result from soft-tissue contractures, such as flexion contractures seen in baseball pitchers and weight lifters.

STRENGTH TESTING

Although only gross estimates of strength are attainable in the clinical setting, the clinician must examine the strength of the elbow, wrist, and hand motors, particularly when assessing for a neurologic problem or a tendonapathy. Biceps brachii muscle strength testing is best conducted against resistance with the forearm supinated and the shoulder flexed from 45° to 50°[1] (Fig. 3.10). Triceps strength testing, however, is best conducted with the shoulder flexed to 90° and the elbow flexed from 45° to 90°[1] (Fig. 3.11). Elbow extension strength is normally 70% of flexion strength.[17] Pronation, supination, and grip strength then are studied with the elbow in 90° of flex-

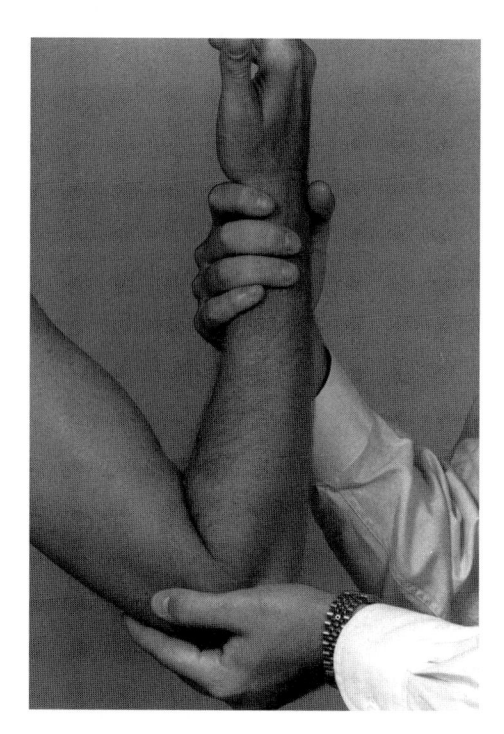

FIGURE 3.10. Biceps muscle strength is assessed with the forearm supinated and the shoulder flexed from 45° to 50°. The examiner applies resistance to flexion.

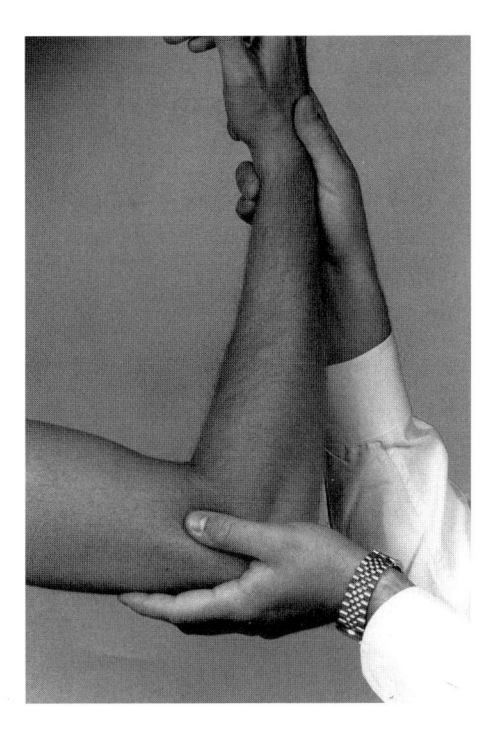

FIGURE 3.11. Triceps muscle strength is best tested with the shoulder flexed to 90° and the elbow flexed from 45° to 90°.

ion and the forearm in neutral rotation. Supination strength is approximately 15% greater than pronation strength, and the dominant extremity is from 5% to 10% stronger than the nondominant extremity.[17]

Finally, the examiner tests the forearm musculature and hand intrinsic strength. The extensor carpi radialis longus musculotendinous unit is best studied with the elbow flexed to 30° and resistance applied to wrist extension.[1] However, the extensor carpi radialis brevis musculotendinous unit is best isolated by providing resistance to wrist extension with the elbow in full flexion. The examiner studies the extensor carpi ulnaris muscle by resisted ulnar deviation of the wrist. Weakness in the wrist, finger, and thumb extensor might indicate a posterior interosseous nerve palsy. Similarly, the examiner should test the wrist, finger, and thumb flexors. Weakness of the flexor pollicis longus and flexor digitorum profundus muscles of the index finger is present in an entrapment palsy of the anterior interosseous nerve, which branches from the median nerve approximately 5 cm distal to the medial epicondyle.[20] Finally, weakness in the hand intrinsics can indicate ulnar nerve entrapment at the cubital tunnel.

REFLEXES

Reflexes are evaluated to rule out potential sources of referred pain, such as a cervical radiculopathy. An increased response to stimulation can indicate an upper motor neuron lesion, whereas a decreased response can sig-nify a lower motor neuron lesion. The examiner tests the C5 nerve root by the biceps reflex, the C6 nerve root by the brachioradialis reflex, and the C7 nerve root by the triceps reflex.

SENSORY EXAMINATION

The clinician conducts a comprehensive sensory examination to assess for a cervical radiculopathy or a peripheral neuropathy. This examination depends on the patient's subjective response to light touch or pinprick. As discussed earlier, diminished sensation in the fifth and ulnar-innervated half of the fourth digits can signify an ulnar neuropathy. Unfortunately, however, many entrapment neuropathies of the elbow and forearm, such as anterior interosseous neuropathy, pronator syndrome, posterior interosseous neuropathy, and radial tunnel syndrome, do not demonstrate abnormal objective sensory examinations.

STABILITY TESTING

Either an acute traumatic event or a chronic overload syndrome can result in valgus instability of the elbow. Attenuation or rupture of the anterior oblique bundle of the UCL causes this pattern of instability.[1,21,22] Medial elbow stability is tested with the patient sitting, the patient's elbow flexed from 20° to 30° to unlock the olecranon from its fossa, and the patient's forearm secured between the examiner's arm and trunk[1] (Fig. 3.12). While apply-

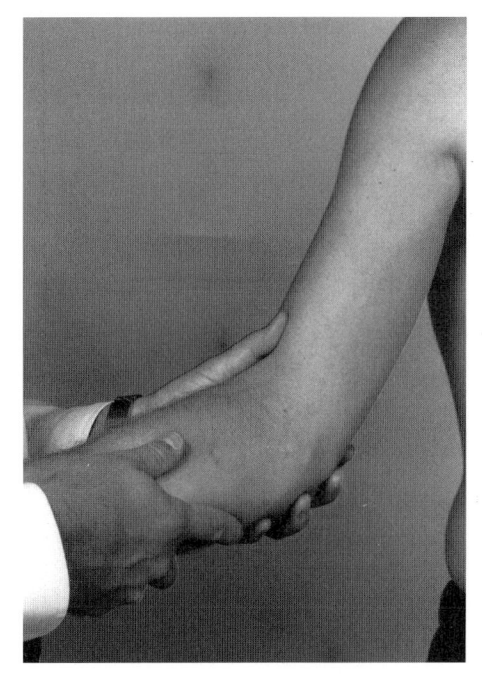

FIGURE 3.12. Valgus stress testing is accomplished with the patient's elbow flexed from 20° to 30° and his or her arm secured between the examiner's arm and trunk.

ing a valgus stress, the examiner notes the presence of pain and increased medial opening and evaluates the quality of the endpoint. Another method for examining the UCL is to have the patient lie supine with the shoulder abducted to 90° and the elbow flexed from 20° to 30°.[1] The examiner applies a valgus force against the supinated forearm and uses the opposite thumb to palpate the medial portion of the joint line to determine the amount of opening. O'Driscoll[22] tested for stability with the forearm fully pronated so that he would not mistake posterolateral instability for valgus instability. Posterolateral instability due to lateral collateral ligament disruption is present when the ulna and radius as a unit rotate away from the humerus in response to a valgus stress. Calloway et al.[23] described another variation of the standard technique for evaluating valgus instability. They suggested performing the test at 90° of flexion. In their medial collateral ligament selective cutting study in cadavers, they found valgus opening to be the greatest at this degree of flexion.

Varus instability is caused by disruption of the lateral collateral ligament complex and is present acutely when the elbow dislocates and chronically when the ligament fails to heal.[22] This pattern of instability is not as apparent as posterolateral rotatory instability, which is always present when the lateral collateral ligament is disrupted. The examiner conducts a varus stress test with the patient's shoulder internally rotated and the elbow flexed from 20° to 30° to unlock the olecranon. He or she palpates the radiocapitellar joint to detect the degree of opening in the lateral joint line.

Posterolateral rotatory instability is essentially a rotational displacement of the ulna and radius on the humerus that causes the ulna to supinate away from the trochlea.[22] In almost all patients, the ulnar part of the lateral collateral ligament is attenuated or disrupted with this pattern of instability.[24–26] The examiner can diagnose posterolateral rotatory instability using the lateral pivot-shift test.[26] With the patient placed in the supine position and the affected extremity placed overhead, the examiner grasps the wrist and elbow. (This grasping is similar to the way that the examiner would hold the knee and ankle when conducting a pivot-shift test on the knee.) The elbow is supinated, and a valgus moment and axial compression are applied as the elbow slowly is moved from full extension to flexion (Fig. 3.13). In a patient who has posterolateral rotatory instability, this movement produces an apprehensive response, because it reproduces the patient's symptoms and a sense that the elbow is about to dislocate. Reproduction of the actual subluxation and reduction is difficult to accomplish in a patient who has not had either local or general anesthesia, because the patient tends to tighten the muscles to guard the joint. The pivot-shift maneuver causes posterolateral subluxation or dislocation of the radius and ulna off the humerus that reaches a maximum at 40° of flexion, creating a posterolateral prominence over the dislocated radial head and a dimple between the radius and capitellum. As the elbow is flexed past 40°, reduction of the ulna and radius together on the humerus occurs suddenly and produces a palpable and visible snap (Fig. 3.14).

PROVOCATIVE TESTS

Lateral

Stress to the extensor carpi radialis longus and brevis muscles reproduces the discomfort associated with lateral epicondylitis. To create this stress, the patient fully extends the elbow and resists active wrist and finger extension (Fig. 3.15). This maneuver elicits pain at the lateral epicondyle and is the most sensitive provocative maneuver for lateral epicondylitis. Passive flexion of the wrist with the elbow

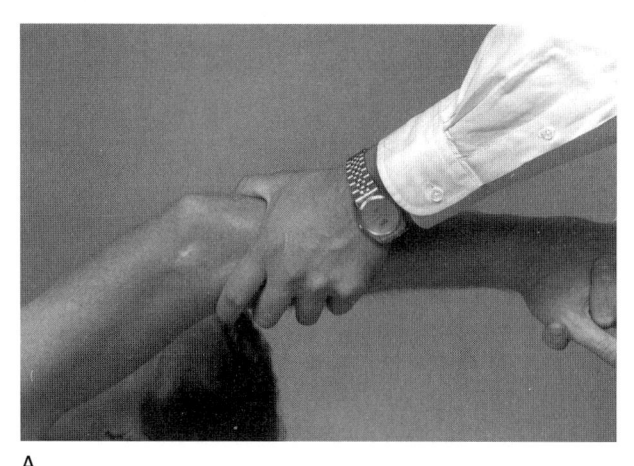

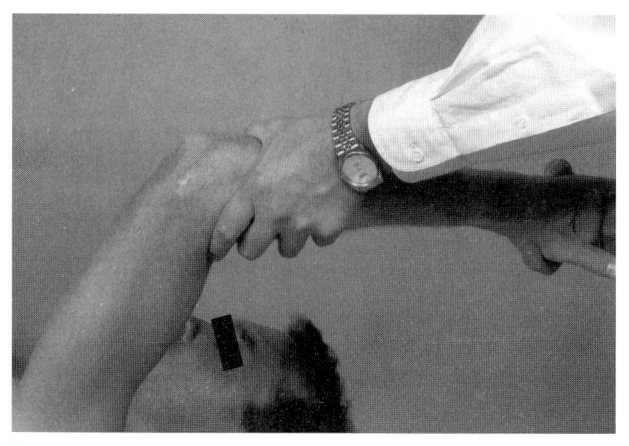

FIGURE 3.13. Lateral pivot-shift test. The examiner supinates the elbow, applies a valgus moment and axial compression, and moves the elbow from full extension (A) to flexion (B).

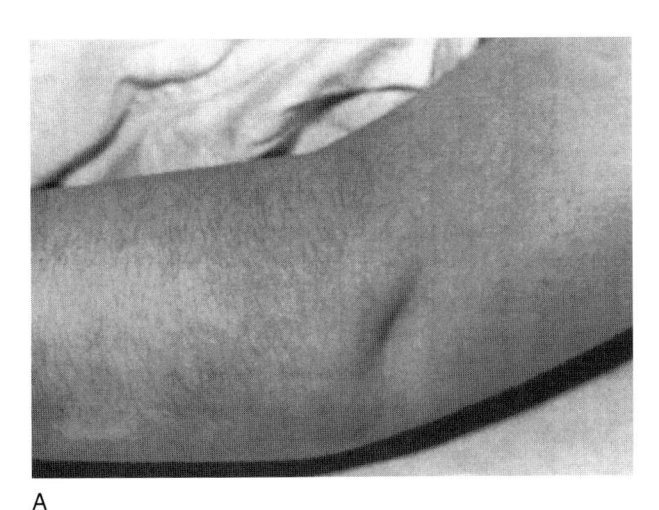

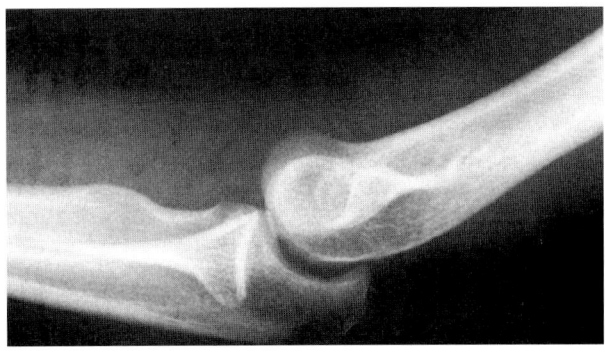

FIGURE 3.14. (A) Positive test for posterolateral rotatory subluxation of the elbow. The posterolateral dislocation of the radiohumeral joint produces an osseous prominence and an obvious dimple in the skin just proximal to the dislocated radial head. (B) Lateral radiograph made simultaneously with the photograph. The radiohumeral joint is dislocated posterolaterally, and there is rotatory subluxation of the ulnohumeral joint. The semilunar notch of the ulna is rotated away from the trochlea. (Reprinted with permission.[24])

extended also can cause discomfort because it stretches the extensor tendons. Finally, the *chair test* can help the examiner diagnose lateral epicondylitis.[27,28] In this test, the patient raises the back of a chair with the elbow in full extension, the forearm pronated, and the wrist dorsiflexed (Fig. 3.16). Before he or she raises the chair, a patient who has lateral epicondylitis often exhibits apprehension.

When resisted supination produces pain approximately 4 to 5 cm distal to the lateral epicondyle, it is the most sensitive test for radial tunnel syndrome. However, when the maneuver produces pain on resisted third-digit extension, it is not specific for radial tunnel syndrome, because the maneuver causes similar pain in patients who have lateral epicondylitis. Another indicator of radial tun-

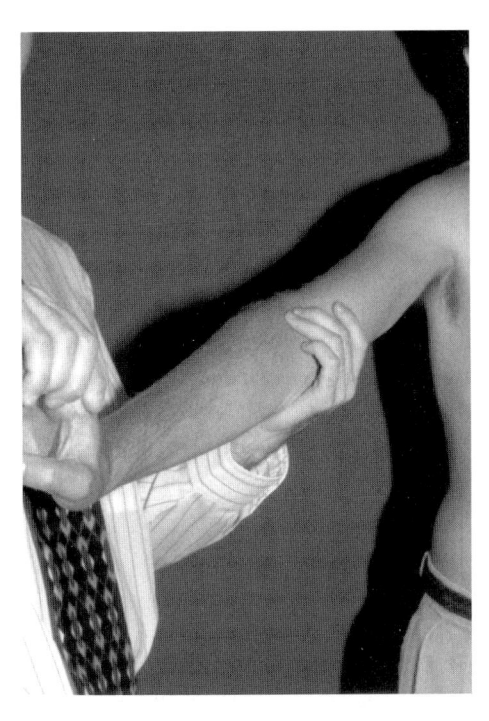

FIGURE 3.15. Test for lateral epicondylitis. Stress to the origin of extensor carpi radialis brevis and longus tendons, which is created by resisting active wrist extension with the elbow fully extended, elicits pain at the lateral epicondyle.

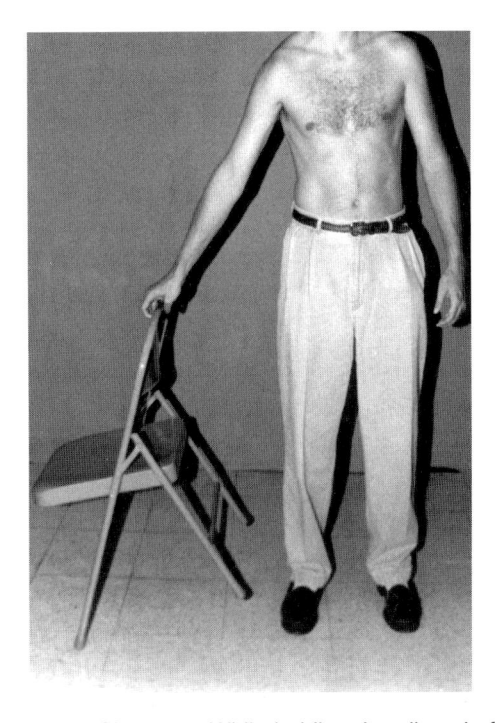

FIGURE 3.16. Chair test. While holding the elbow in full extension, pronating the forearm, and dorsiflexing the wrist, the patient lifts the back of a chair. The test elicits apprehension in patients with lateral epicondylitis.

nel syndrome is the pronation–supination sign.[29] This test is positive if direct tenderness over the radius at 5 cm distal to the lateral epicondyle is markedly greater in full supination than in pronation; the radial nerve is located in this position in full supination, but moves medially and distally with pronation.

Finally, the examiner tests damage to the articular surface of the radiocapitellar joint. With the patient's elbow extended, the examiner applies an axial load to the joint while supinating and pronating the forearm repeatedly. A positive radiocapitellar compression test elicits pain.[1]

Medial

The most sensitive indirect maneuver for the diagnosis of medial epicondylitis is resisted forearm pronation, which is positive in 90% of patients who have this disorder[29] (Fig. 3.17). A positive test elicits pain at the flexor–pronator muscle mass origin on the medial epicondyle. The second most sensitive maneuver is resisted palmar flexion, which is positive in 70% of patients.[29] Passive extension of the wrist and fingers also can elicit pain at the medial epicondyle in these patients.

The most sensitive and specific provocative test maneuver for locating the site of ulnar nerve compression is the elbow flexion test conducted with direct pressure over the cubital tunnel.[20] With the patient's wrist neutral and forearm supinated, the examiner flexes the elbow to 135° and applies digital pressure over the cubital tunnel for a

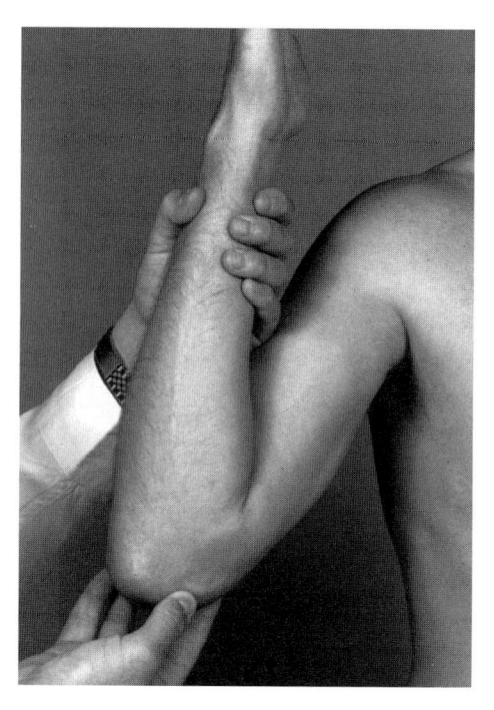

FIGURE 3.18. Elbow flexion test for ulnar nerve compression. With the patient's wrist neutral and forearm supinated, the examiner flexes the patient's elbow to 135° as he or she applies digital pressure over the cubital tunnel.

period of 3 min[30] (Fig. 3.18). A positive test results in paresthesias or dysesthesias in the fifth and ulnar-innervated half of the fourth digits. A simple nerve compression test (e.g., digital compression of the nerve at the inferior medial epicondyle) and Tinel's test also are used to aid in the diagnosis.

Anterior

Vague anterior elbow or proximal forearm pain can result from entrapment of the median nerve at many sites. First, as discussed earlier, the median nerve can become compressed under the ligament of Struthers. In this case, resisted flexion of the elbow between 120° and 135° of flexion aggravates the symptoms.[15] Active elbow flexion with the forearm in pronation, which tightens the lacertus fibrosus, elicits symptoms resulting from compression of the nerve by the lacertus fibrosus.[15] If resisted pronation of the forearm combined with flexion of the wrist reproduces the symptoms, the nerve can become compressed as it passes through the pronator teres muscle.[15,20] Finally, if resisted flexion of the superficialis muscle of the third digit aggravates the pain, the nerve can become entrapped in the superficialis arch.[15]

Anterior elbow pain also can be due to biceps or brachialis tendinitis. These diagnoses are suggested when re-

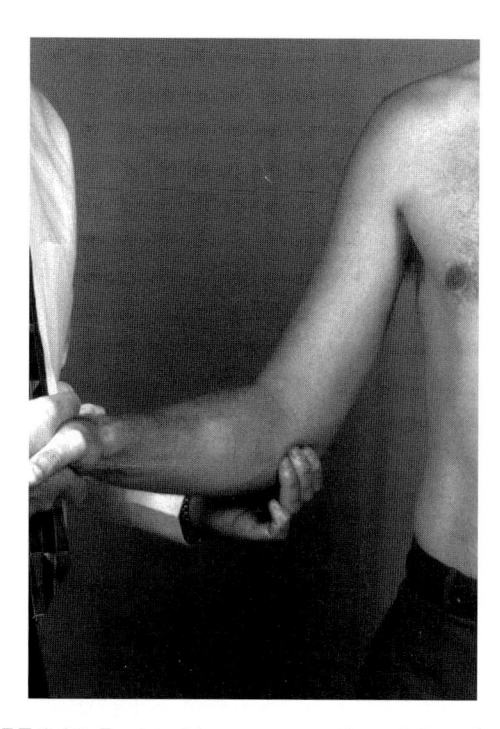

FIGURE 3.17. Resisted forearm pronation elicits pain at the medial epicondyle in patients who have medial epicondylitis.

sisted forearm supination and elbow flexion produce increased pain.

Posterior

The throwing athlete subjects the elbow to a tremendous amount of valgus stress and extension. As a result, the olecranon becomes impinged in the posteromedial portion of the olecranon fossa of the distal humerus.[7] Eventually, degenerative changes develop with resultant articular cartilage damage and osteophyte formation. This problem is known as the valgus extension overload syndrome, and it can lead to significant pain that limits throwing ability. The valgus extension overload test and valgus extension snap maneuver consistently produce discomfort in patients who have this disorder.[1] With the patient in the seated position, the examiner applies a moderate amount of valgus stress to the elbow as he or she moves the elbow from 30° of flexion to full extension. This maneuver simulates posteromedial olecranon impingement and re-creates the pain that the athlete experiences during the late acceleration phase of throwing.

RADIOGRAPHIC EVALUATION

Routine Views

After taking a history and making a physical examination of the patient, the examining physician may need to make ancillary tests. Routine radiographs remain a very cost efficient initial approach to elbow imaging. They enable the physician to gather formative information on bone, on joint positioning, and on the presence or absence of soft-tissue swelling, loose bodies, ectopic ossification, and foreign bodies. If more information is required, specialized studies, including fluoroscopy, computerized tomography, and arthrography, can be valuable. Initial routine radiographic views include anteroposterior (AP) and lateral views. An AP view is taken with the arm in full extension and the forearm supinated (Fig. 3.19). This position allows good visualization of the medial and lateral epicondyles and of the radiocapitellar joints and the trochlear articulation with the medial epicondyle. A portion of the olecranon fossa also can be visualized. A lateral view completes the initial examination with two tangential views (see Fig. 3.20). The lateral radiographic view should be taken with the elbow flexed to 90° and the beam reflected distally approximately 70° to account for the normal valgus position of the elbow. The lateral view demonstrates the distal humerus, the elbow joint, and the proximal forearm. It gives an excellent view of the coronoid process anteriorly and the olecranon tip posteriorly. If the examiner suspects that the patient has a fracture of the radial head, he or she can obtain an additional view in the lateral position, or the radial head view (Fig. 3.21). This radiograph usually allows for visualization of the head without a view of the overlapping coronoid process. The tube is angled 45° toward the shoulder, the elbow is flexed to 90°, and the

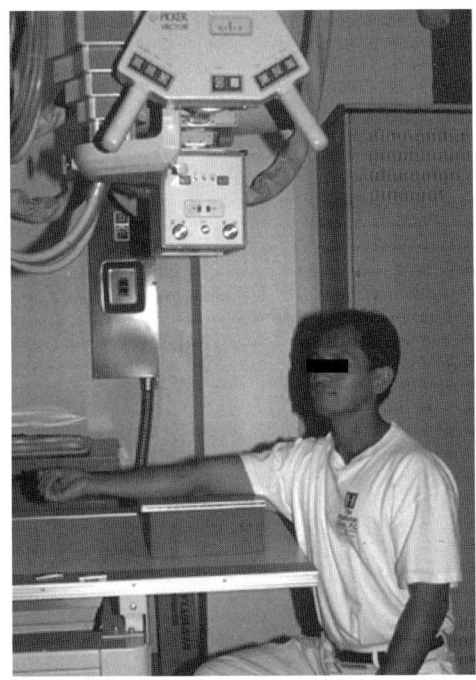

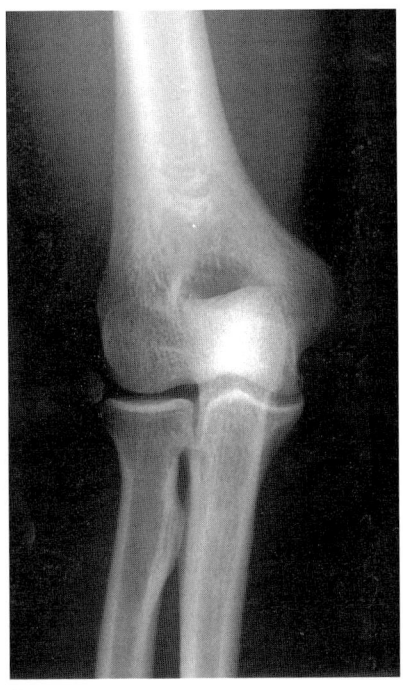

FIGURE 3.19. (A) Patient positioned for anteroposterior (AP) radiographic view. (B) AP radiographic view.

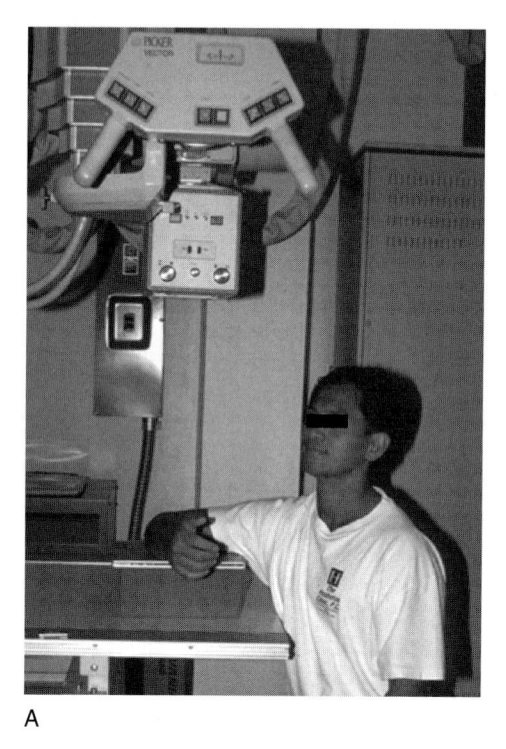

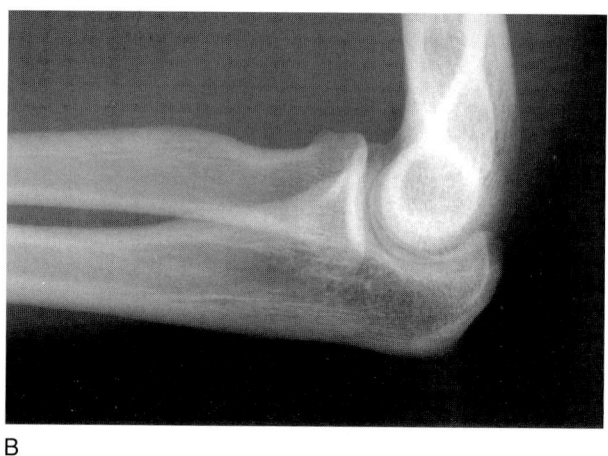

FIGURE 3.20. (A) Patient positioned for lateral radiographic view. (B) Lateral radiographic view.

thumb is placed in a vertical position. This special view may be indicated if a radial head fracture is suspected after the examiner views the fat pad sign on a plain radiograph.

The elbow joint has both anterior and posterior fat pads that are intercapsular but extrasynovial. Trauma to the joint and increased fluid in the joint push these fat pads away from the bony surface. The appearance of the anterior fat pad on a radiograph sometimes is normal. However, if the posterior fat pad is seen on the lateral radiographic view, it is always abnormal. The appearance of the posterior fat pad, particularly after trauma, may suggest an intra-articular fracture, and additional radiographs or studies may be indicated.

The axial view is another routine radiograph that may be indicated, particularly in throwers. This flexed elbow view (Fig. 3.22) is taken to allow visualization of the posterior compartment, specifically visualization of the articulation of the posterior olecranon and the humerus. The view helps the examiner to evaluate the thrower's elbow

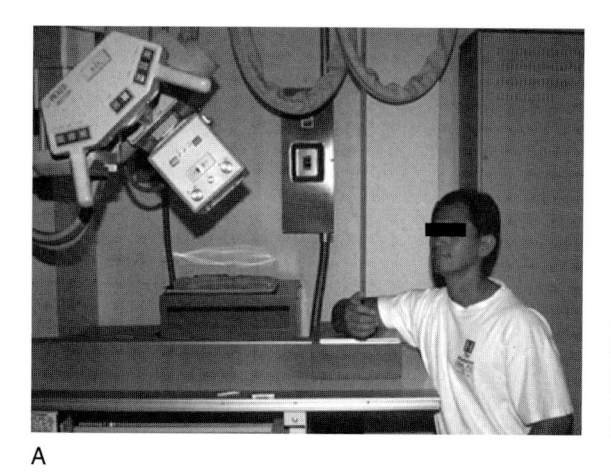

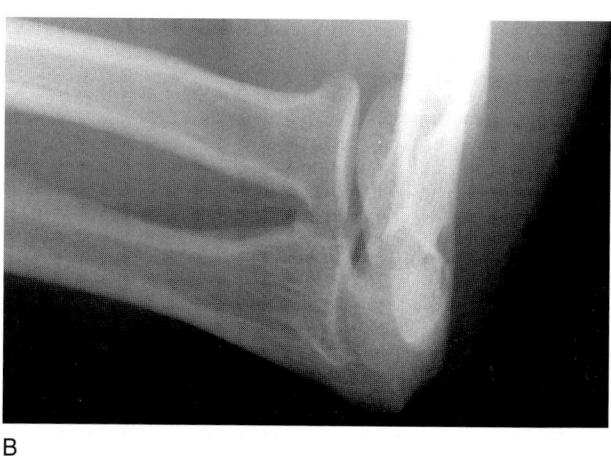

FIGURE 3.21. (A) Patient positioned for radial head radiographic view. (B) Radial head radiographic view.

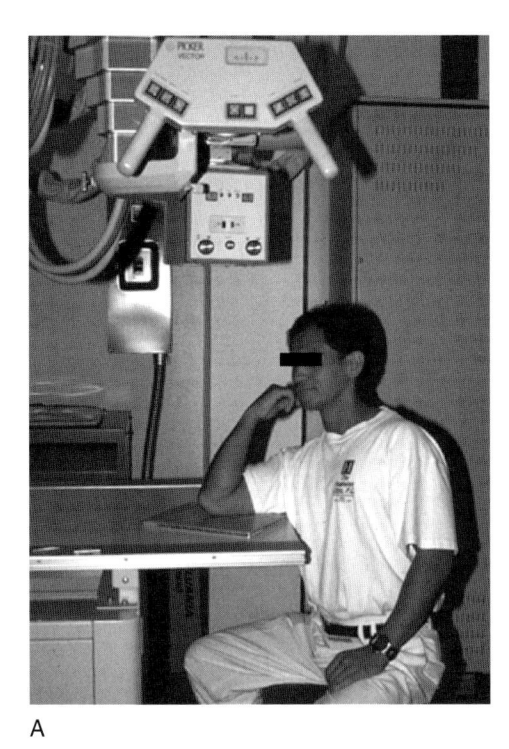

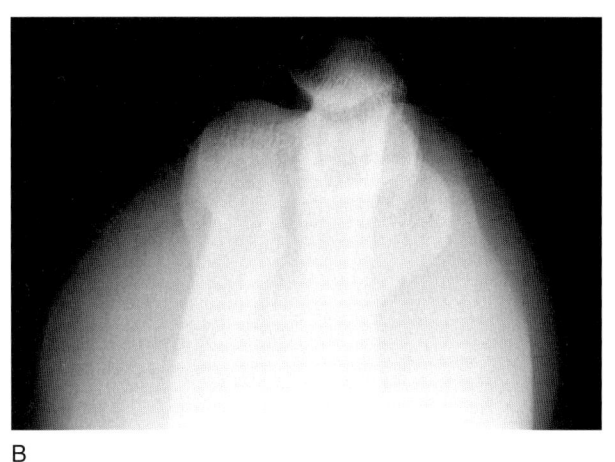

FIGURE 3.22. (A) Patient positioned for axial radiographic view. (B) Axial radiographic view.

for a posteromedial spur, which is seen in valgus extension overload.

Direct Views

The valgus gravity radiograph is often described as a means of demonstrating medial laxity of the elbow. In reality, this view is seldom taken. When addressing suspected medial collateral laxity of the elbow, fluoroscopy may be helpful, particularly in looking for loose bodies or evulsion fractures of the epicondyle or medial epicondyle. The predetermination of instability, however, is not well visualized on a dynamic basis and is best seen on a static film, such as an arthrogram or magnetic resonance imaging.

Arthrography can provide useful information about the capsule, the thick subarticular surface, and capsular tears and ligament disruptions. Contrast arthrography is best used for delineating loose bodies and capsular tears. The T sign, as Timmerman and coworkers[31] described, may indicate a ligament tear without complete rupture; if the contrast material easily flows from a lateral injection out of the medial compartment, then complete rupture is present. However, other studies, specifically magnetic resonance imaging, have largely replaced invasive arthrography as a means of detecting ligament disruption.

Tomography

In the elbow, computed tomography largely has replaced tomography, which allows thin sections of both AP and lateral projections to show the bony contours. Computed tomography allows the surgeon to view bony detail in many different planes, and it can be extremely helpful in assessing complex fractures as a means of planning before fixation. Contrast can be beneficial as an adjunct to computed tomography for defining both articular and subchondral abnormalities. It can be helpful in assessing osteochondritis dissecans and determining whether loose bodies or a spur is present in or about the elbow.

CONCLUSION

A comprehensive history and physical examination of the elbow and surrounding joints is the most important part of the evaluation of elbow disorders. The examiner can use further diagnostic studies, such as radiographs and magnetic resonance imaging (if necessary), to confirm the diagnosis or further narrow the scope of potential diagnoses. The elbow joint is a complex and difficult joint to examine; therefore, evaluating it in a thorough and orderly fashion is important. Every portion of the examination should be conducted because a wide variety of disorders has similar signs and symptoms.

REFERENCES

1. Andrews JR, Whiteside JN, Buettner CM. Clinical evaluation of the elbow in throwers. *Oper Tech Sports Med* 1996;4(2):77–83.
2. Slocum DB. Classification of elbow injuries from baseball pitching. *Tex Med* 1968;64:48–53.
3. Jobe FW, Nuber GN. Throwing injuries of the elbow. *Clin Sports Med* 1986;5:621–635.
4. Dehaven KE, Evarts CM. Throwing injuries of the elbow in athletes. *Orthop Clin North Am* 1973;4:801–808.
5. Barnes DA, Tullos HS. An analysis of 100 symptomatic baseball players. *Am J Sports Med* 1978;6:62–67.
6. Bennett GE. Elbow and shoulder lesions of baseball players. *Am J Surg* 1959;98:484–492.
7. Wilson FD, Andrews JR, Blackburn TA, et al. Vaglus extension overload in the pitching elbow. *Am J Sports Med* 1983;11:83–87.
8. King JW, Brelsford HJ, Tullos HS. Analysis of the pitching arm of the professional baseball pitcher. *Clin Orthop* 1969;67:116–123.
9. Beals RK. The normal carrying angle of the elbow. A radiographic study of 22 patients. *Clin Orthop* 1976;19:194–196.
10. Andrews JR, Wilk KE, Satterwhite YE, et al. Physical examination of the thrower's elbow. *J Orthop Sports Phys Ther* 1993;17:296–304.
11. Flynn JC, Richards JF, Saltzman RI. Prevention and treatment of non-union of slightly displaced fractures of the lateral humeral condyle in children. An end-result study. *J Bone Joint Surg* 1975;57A:1087–1092.
12. Volz RE, Morrey BF. The physical examination of the elbow. In: Morrey BF, ed. *The elbow and its disorders*. Philadelphia: WB Saunders, 1985:62–72.
13. Gessini L, Jandolo B, Pietrangeli A. Entrapment neuropathies of the median nerve at and above the elbow. *Surg Neurol* 1983;19:112.
14. O'Driscoll SW, Jaloszynski R, Morrey BF, et al. Origin of the medial ulnar collateral ligament. *J Hand Surg* 1992;17A:164–168.
15. Eversmann WW. Entrapment and compressive neuropathies. In: Green DP, ed. *Operative hand surgery*. New York: Churchill Livingstone; 1993:1341–1385.
16. Childress HM. Recurrent ulnar-nerve dislocation at the elbow. *Clin Orthop* 1975;108:168–173.
17. Boone DC, Azen SP. Normal range of motion of joints in male subjects. *J Bone Joint Surg* 1979;61A:756–759.
18. Morrey BF, Askew LJ, An K-N, et al. A biomechanical study of normal functional elbow motion. *J Bone Joint Surg* 1981;63A:872–877.
19. Askew LJ, An K-N, Morrey BF, et al. Functional evaluation of the elbow: normal motion requirements and strength determinations. *Orthop Trans* 1981;5:304–305.
20. Wright TW. Nerve injuries and neuropathies about the elbow. In: Norris TR, ed. *Orthopaedic knowledge update: Shoulder and elbow*. Rosemont, IL: American Association of Orthopedic Surgeons; 1997:369–377.
21. Jobe FW, Stark H, Lombardo SJ. Reconstruction of the ulnar collateral ligament in athletes. *J Bone Joint Surg* 1986;68A:1158–1163.
22. O'Driscoll SW. Elbow instability. In: Norris TR, ed. *Orthopaedic knowledge update: Shoulder and elbow*. Rosemont, IL: American Association of Orthopedic Surgeons; 1997:345–354.
23. Calloway GH, Field LD, Deng XH, et al. Biomechanical evaluation of the medial collateral ligament of the elbow. *J Bone Joint Surg* 1997;79A:1223–1231.
24. O'Driscoll SW, Bell DF, Morrey BF. Posterolateral rotatory instability of the elbow. *J Bone Joint Surg* 1991;73A:440–446.
25. O'Driscoll SW, Horii E, Morrey BF, et al. Anatomy of the ulnar part of the lateral collateral ligament of the elbow. *Clin Anat* 1992;5:296–303.
26. O'Driscoll SW, Morrey BF, Korinek S, et al. Elbow subluxation and dislocation. A spectrum of instability. *Clin Orthop* 1992;280:186–197.
27. Plancher KD, Halbrecht J, Lourie GM. Medial and lateral epicondylitis in the athlete. *Clin Sports Med* 1996;15:283–305.
28. Gardner RC. Tennis elbow: diagnosis, pathology and treatment: nine severe cases treated by a new reconstructive operation. *Clin Orthop* 1970;72:248–253.
29. Gabel GT, Morrey BF. Tennis elbow. *Instructional Course Lect*. 1998;47:165–172.
30. Buehler MJ, Thayer DT. The elbow flexion test. A clinical test for cubital tunnel syndrome. *Clin Orthop* 1988;233:213–216.
31. Timmerman LA, Schwartz ML, Andrews JR. Preoperative evaluation of the ulnar collateral ligament by magnetic resonance imaging and computed tomography arthrography. Evaluation in 25 baseball players with surgical confirmation. *Am J Sports Med* 1994;22:26–31.

CHAPTER 4

Magnetic Resonance Imaging of the Elbow

Russell C. Fritz

INTRODUCTION

An accurate diagnosis is the essential first step toward a successful treatment plan in patients who present with elbow pain. The diagnostic approach to elbow pain always begins with a thorough history and physical examination. Imaging plays an important role in confirming the initial clinical diagnosis so that a rational plan of treatment can be selected. Diagnostic imaging is especially important when there is significant uncertainty regarding the cause of elbow pain, and the outcome can be improved by timely treatment.

Magnetic resonance imaging (MRI) is the imaging procedure of choice for evaluating the ligaments, tendons, and muscles of the elbow. Direct visualization of the bone marrow makes MRI useful and accurate for evaluating osteomyelitis, tumor extension, and radiographically occult fractures. Direct visualization of unossified cartilage makes MRI useful for evaluating fractures of the growth plate and epiphysis in children. MRI is also the imaging procedure of choice for evaluating soft-tissue masses and nerve entrapment about the elbow. It provides clinically useful information in assessing the elbow joint. Superior depiction of muscles, ligaments, and tendons and the ability to directly visualize nerves, bone marrow, and hyaline cartilage are advantages of MRI relative to conventional imaging techniques. These features of MRI may help to establish the cause of elbow pain by accurately depicting the presence and extent of bone and soft-tissue pathology. Ongoing improvements in surface coil design and newer pulse sequences have resulted in higher-quality MR images of the elbow that can be obtained more rapidly. Recent clinical experience has shown the utility of MRI in detecting and characterizing disorders of the elbow in a noninvasive fashion.

MRI TECHNIQUE

The elbow typically is scanned with the patient in a supine position with the arm at the side. A surface coil is essential for obtaining high-quality images. Depending on the size of the patient and the size of the surface coil relative to the bore of the magnet, it may be necessary to scan the patient in a prone position with the arm extended overhead. In general, the prone position is less well tolerated and results in a greater number of motion-degraded studies. When the patient's elbow is scanned, it should be in a comfortable position to avoid motion artifact. The elbow typically is extended and the wrist is placed in a neutral position. Technologists have more difficulty positioning patients who cannot extend the elbow; therefore, they must take more time and skill to obtain optimal images. Taping a vitamin E capsule or other marker to the skin at the site of tenderness or at the site of a palpable mass helps to ensure that the area of interest has been included in the study, especially when no abnormalities are identified on the images.

Excellent images may be obtained with both midfield and high-field MR systems. Proton-density and T2-weighted images typically are obtained in the axial and sagittal planes using the spin-echo or fast spin-echo technique. T1-weighted and short TI inversion recovery (STIR) sequences usually are obtained in the coronal plane. Although the STIR sequence has a relatively poor signal-to-noise ratio because of the suppression of signal from fat, abnormalities are often more conspicuous due to the effects of additive T1 and T2 contrast.

The axial images, in general, should extend from the distal humeral metaphysis to the radial tuberosity. The common flexor and extensor origins from the medial and lateral humeral epicondyles and the biceps insertion on the radial tuberosity are routinely imaged with this coverage. This coverage usually is obtained with 3- or 4-mm-thick slices using a long time of repetition (TR) sequence. The coronal images are angled parallel to a line through the humeral epicondyles on the axial images. The sagittal images are angled perpendicular to a line through the humeral epicondyles on the axial images.

The field of view on the axial images should be as small as the signal of the surface coil and the size of the patient's elbow allow. To include more of the anatomy about the elbow, the field of view selected on the coronal and sagittal sequences is usually larger than the field of view on the axial images. This guideline is especially true when imaging a ruptured biceps tendon that may retract to the normal superior margin of coverage. The slice thickness, interslice gap, and TR may be increased on the axial sequences just as the field of view is increased on the coronal and sagittal sequences as long as the surface coil provides adequate signal to image the entire length of the abnormality.

Additional sequences may be added or substituted depending on the clinical problem that must be solved. T2*-weighted gradient-echo sequences provide useful supplemental information for identifying loose bodies within the elbow. In general, gradient-echo sequences should be avoided after elbow surgery because magnetic susceptibility artifacts associated with micrometallic debris may obscure the images and also may be mistaken for loose bodies. Fast spin-echo and fast STIR sequences may be substituted for conventional T2-weighted spin-echo and conventional STIR sequences if available; these newer sequences allow greater flexibility in imaging the elbow while continuing to provide information that is comparable with that of the conventional spin-echo and conventional STIR sequences. The speed of fast spin-echo sequences may be used to obtain higher-resolution T2-weighted images in the same amount of time as the conventional spin-echo sequences, or it simply may be used to increase the speed of the examination. The ability to shorten the examination with fast spin-echo has been useful when scanning claustrophobic patients or patients who become uncomfortable in the prone position with the arm overhead.

Fat suppression may be added to various pulse sequences to improve visualization of the hyaline articular cartilage. Avoidance of chemical shift artifact at the interface of cortical bone and fat-containing marrow permits a more accurate depiction of the overlying hyaline cartilage. T1-weighted images with fat suppression are useful whenever gadolinium is administered, either intravenously or directly into the elbow joint. Intravenous gadolinium may provide additional information in the assessment of neoplastic or inflammatory processes about the elbow. Articular injection of saline or dilute gadolinium may be useful in patients without a joint effusion to detect loose bodies, to determine if the capsule is disrupted, or to determine if an osteochondral fracture fragment is stable.

ELBOW PATHOLOGY

Medial Collateral Ligament Injury

Degeneration and tearing of the medial collateral ligament (MCL) with or without concomitant injury of the common flexor tendon commonly occurs in throwing athletes. Injury of these medial stabilizing structures is due to chronic microtrauma from repetitive valgus stress during the acceleration phase of throwing.

Acute injury of the MCL can be detected, localized, and graded with MRI. The status of the functionally important anterior bundle of the MCL complex may be determined by assessing the coronal and axial images. Acute ruptures of the MCL are well seen with standard MRI (Fig. 4.1). Partial detachment of the deep undersurface fibers of the anterior bundle also may occur in pitchers with medial elbow pain and are more difficult to diagnose with standard MRI. These partial tears of the MCL characteristically spare the superficial fibers of the anterior bundle and, therefore, are not visible from an open surgical approach unless the ligament is incised to inspect the torn capsular fibers. As a result, MRI is important to localize these partial tears, which are treated with repair or reconstruction. Detection of these undersurface partial tears is improved when intra-articular contrast is administered and computed tomography (CT) arthrography or MR arthrography is performed. The capsular fibers of the anterior bundle of the MCL normally insert on the medial margin of the coronoid process. Undersurface partial tears of the anterior bundle are characterized by distal extension of fluid or contrast along the medial margin of the coronoid process (Fig. 4.1).

Midsubstance MCL ruptures can be differentiated from proximal avulsions or distal avulsions with MRI. Midsubstance ruptures of the MCL accounted for 87%, whereas distal and proximal avulsions were found in 10% and 3%, respectively, in a large series of surgically treated throwing athletes.[1] Other authors have found a lesser percentage of midsubstance ruptures. The fibers of the flexor digitorum superficialis muscle blend with the anterior bundle of the MCL.[2-4] A strain of the flexor digitorum superficialis muscle commonly is seen when the MCL is injured (Fig. 4.1). Chronic degeneration of the MCL is characterized by thickening of the ligament secondary to scarring, often accompanied by foci of calcification or

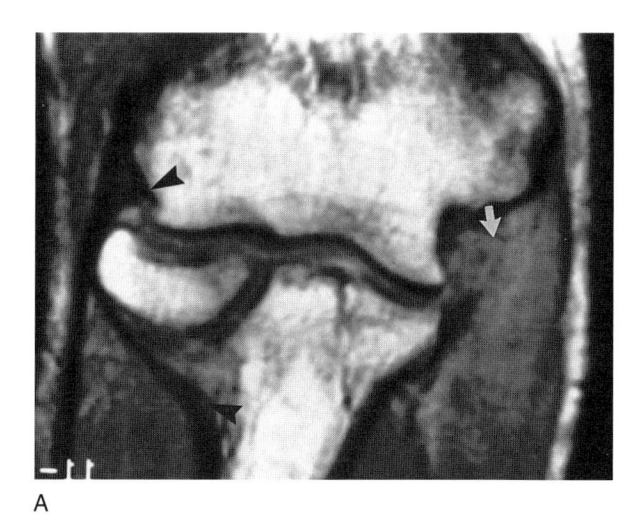

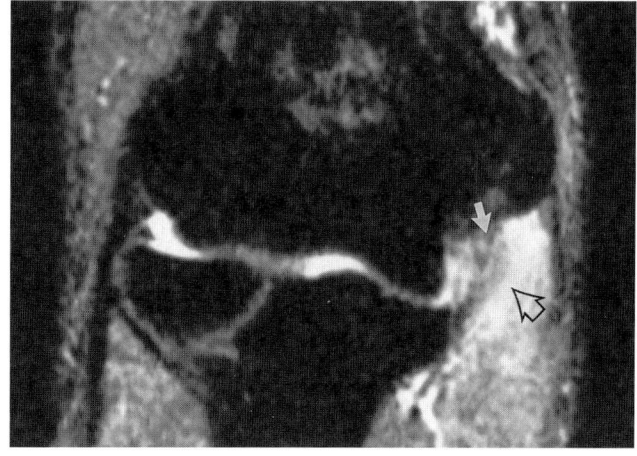

FIGURE 4.1. Rupture of the medial collateral ligament in a 24-year-old pitcher. T1-weighted (A) and STIR (B) coronal images reveal increased signal and poor definition of the fibers of the anterior bundle of the medial collateral ligament (white arrows). A strain of the adjacent flexor muscles is also noted (open arrow). The normal LUCL is also well seen (arrowheads).

heterotopic bone. Patients with symptomatic MCL insufficiency usually are treated with reconstruction using a palmaris tendon graft. Graft failure is unusual, but it may be evaluated with MRI (Fig. 4.2). Lateral compartment bone contusions may be seen in association with acute MCL tears and may provide useful confirmation of recent lateral compartment impaction secondary to valgus instability.

A number of different conditions may occur secondary to the repeated valgus stress to the elbow that occurs with throwing. Medial tension overload typically produces extra-articular injury, such as flexor–pronator strain, MCL sprain, ulnar traction spurring, and ulnar neuropathy. Lateral compression overload typically produces intra-articular injury, such as osteochondritis dissecans of the capitellum or radial head, degenerative arthritis, and loose-body formation. MRI can assess for each of these related pathologic processes associated with repeated valgus stress.[5,6] The additional information that MRI provides can be helpful in formulating a logical treatment plan, especially when surgery is being considered.

Rupture of the MCL also is encountered commonly as a result of posterior dislocation of the elbow. The extent of injury secondary to elbow dislocation is well delineated with MRI.

Medial Epicondylitis

Medial epicondylitis, also known as golfer's elbow, pitcher's elbow, or medial tennis elbow, is caused by degeneration of the common flexor tendon secondary to overload of the flexor–pronator muscle group that arises from the medial epicondyle.[7–9] The spectrum of damage to the muscle–tendon unit that may be characterized with MRI includes muscle strain injury, tendon degeneration (tendinosis), and tendon disruption (Fig. 4.3).

MRI is useful for detecting and characterizing acute muscle injury and for following its resolution.[10] The STIR sequence is the most sensitive for detecting muscle abnormalities. The common flexor tendon and MCL should be evaluated carefully for associated tearing when there is evidence of medial muscle strain injury on MRI. Alternatively, increased signal intensity on STIR and T2-weighted sequences may be seen after an intramuscular injection and may persist for as long as one month.[11] Abnormal signal intensity within a muscle may simply be

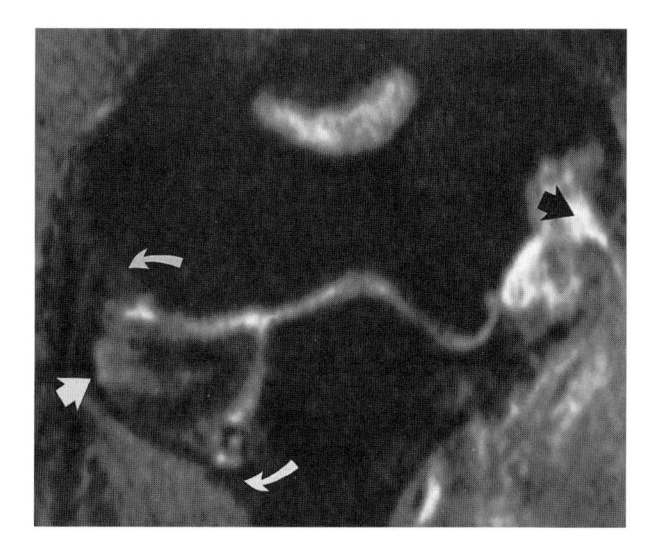

FIGURE 4.2. MCL graft rupture and contusion of the radial head in a professional baseball player. A STIR coronal image reveals increased signal at the site of a ruptured MCL graft (black arrow). Increased signal is also seen within the lateral portion of the radial head secondary to impaction from valgus insufficiency (white arrow). The normal LUCL is also well seen (curved white arrows).

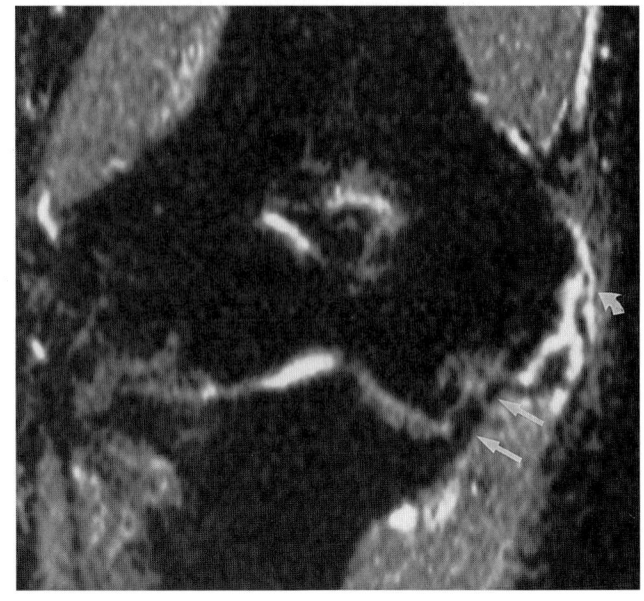

FIGURE 4.3. A 42-year-old golfer with persistent symptoms of medial epicondylitis after a steroid injection. T1-weighted (A) and STIR (B) coronal images reveal detachment of the common flexor tendon from the medial epicondyle (curved arrows). The underlying anterior bundle of the MCL (straight arrows) appears normal.

due to the effect of a therapeutic injection for epicondylitis rather than an indication of muscle strain. Steroid injections ideally should be done after MRI to avoid the confounding appearance of the injection on the structures about the elbow.

A normal muscle–tendon unit tears at the myotendinous junction.[12] A much more common clinical entity, however, is failure of a muscle–tendon unit through an area of tendinosis.[13] Degenerative tendinosis is common about the elbow.[9,14] MRI can determine if tendinosis is present, rather than partial tearing or complete rupture. This distinction is primarily made on the T2-weighted images by evaluating the morphology of the tendon adjacent to the epicondyle. The tendon fibers are normal or thickened in cases of degenerative tendinosis, thin in cases of partial tears, or absent in cases of complete tears. The coronal, sagittal, and axial sequences are all useful for assessing the degree of tendon injury.

The appearance of medial and lateral epicondylitis about the elbow is similar to the appearance of other common degenerative tendinopathies that involve the attachment of tendons to bone. Similar criteria can be used to evaluate the common flexor and common extensor tendons in the elbow, the supraspinatus tendon in the shoulder, the patellar tendon in the knee, and the plantar fascia in the foot on MRI. In each of these conditions, degenerative tendinosis and a failed healing response precede rupture.[13,15–17]

MRI facilitates surgical planning by delineating and grading tears of the common flexor tendon and by evaluating the underlying MCL and adjacent ulnar nerve. Ulnar neuritis commonly accompanies common flexor tendinosis and may be difficult to identify clinically. Patients who have a concomitant ulnar neuropathy have a significantly poorer prognosis after surgery compared with patients who have isolated medial epicondylitis.[18,19] Patients who have coexisting ulnar neuritis and common flexor tendinosis (25% to 50% of patients who undergo surgery for medial epicondylitis) need transposition or decompression of the ulnar nerve in addition to debridement and repair of the abnormal flexor tendon.[7,8,18,19]

In skeletally immature individuals, the flexor muscle–tendon unit may fail at the unfused apophysis of the medial epicondyle. Stress fracture, avulsion, or delayed closure of the medial epicondylar apophysis may occur in young baseball players secondary to overuse (Little League elbow).[20] MRI may detect these injuries before complete avulsion and displacement by revealing soft tissue or marrow edema about the medial epicondylar apophysis on the STIR images.[21]

Lateral Epicondylitis and Lateral Collateral Ligament Injury

Lateral epicondylitis, also called tennis elbow, is caused by degeneration and tearing of the common extensor tendon.[22] This condition often occurs as a result of repetitive sports-related trauma to the tendon, although it is seen far more commonly in nonathletes.[9] In the typical patient, the degenerated extensor carpi radialis brevis tendon is partially avulsed from the lateral epicondyle.[22] Scar tissue

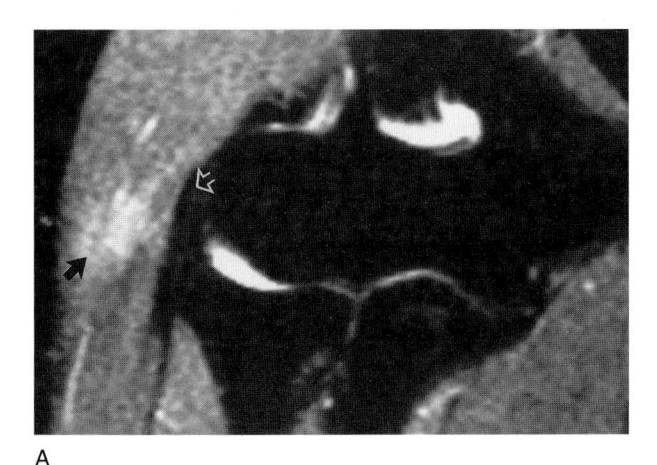

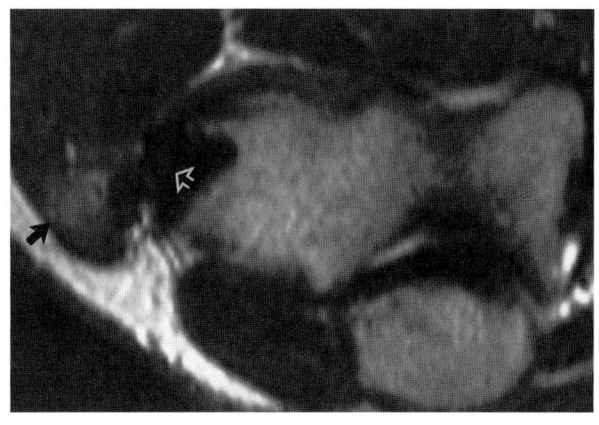

FIGURE 4.4. Clinically suspected tennis elbow in a patient who did not respond to a local steriod injection. A STIR coronal image (A) and a T2-weighted axial image (B) reveal a completely normal common extensor tendon (open arrows) and increased signal within the adjacent extensor carpi radialis longus muscle (solid arrows) secondary to a recent steroid injection. Abnormal signal may persist for weeks after an injection and be mistaken for primary muscle pathology on MRI.

forms in response to this partial avulsion, which then is susceptible to further tearing with repeated trauma. Recent histologic studies have shown angiofibroblastic tendinosis with a lack of inflammation in the surgical specimens of patients who have lateral epicondylitis; this suggests that the abnormal signal seen on MR images is secondary to tendon degeneration and repair rather than tendinitis.[14,17] Local steroid injections commonly are used to treat lateral epicondylitis and may increase the risk of tendon rupture.[23,24] Signal alteration in the region of a local steroid injection should not be confused for primary muscle abnormality on MRI (Fig. 4.4).

Overall, 4% to 10% of cases of lateral epicondylitis are resistant to nonoperative therapy[14,25]; MRI is useful in assessing the degree of tendon damage in such cases. Tendinosis and tearing typically involve the extensor carpi radialis brevis portion of the common extensor tendon anteriorly. Degenerative tendinosis is manifested by normal to increased tendon thickness, with increased signal intensity on T1-weighted images that is not as bright as fluid on properly windowed T2-weighted images. Partial tears are characterized by thinning of the tendon that is outlined by adjacent fluid on the T2-weighted images (Fig. 4.5). Complete tears may be diagnosed on MRI by identifying a fluid-filled gap separating the tendon from its adjacent bony attachment site.

At surgery for lateral epicondylitis, 97% of the tendons appear scarred and edematous and 35% have macroscopic tears.[22] MRI is useful in identifying high-grade partial tears and complete tears that are unlikely to improve with rest and repeated steroid injections. In addition to determining the degree of tendon damage, MRI also provides a more global assessment of the elbow and is therefore able to detect additional abnormal conditions that may explain the lack of a therapeutic response. For example, unsuspected ruptures of the lateral collateral ligament complex may occur in association with tears of the common extensor tendon (Fig. 4.6). Morrey recently reported on a series of 13 patients who underwent reoperation for failed lateral epicondylitis surgery; stabilization procedures were required in 4 patients with either iatrogenic or unrecognized lateral ligament insufficiency.[26] Iatrogenic tears of the lateral ulnar collateral ligament (LUCL) may occur secondary to an overly aggressive release of the common extensor tendon.[27] Operative release of the extensor tendon may further destabilize the elbow

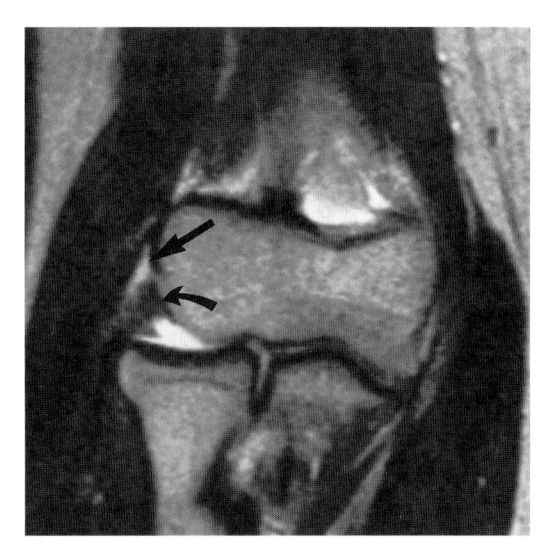

FIGURE 4.5. Lateral epicondylitis in a 30-year-old tennis player. A T2-weighted coronal image reveals increased signal and attenuation of the common extensor tendon (large arrow) compatible with a partial tear. The underlying LUCL (curved arrow) is thickened and mildly increased in signal compatible with degeneration.

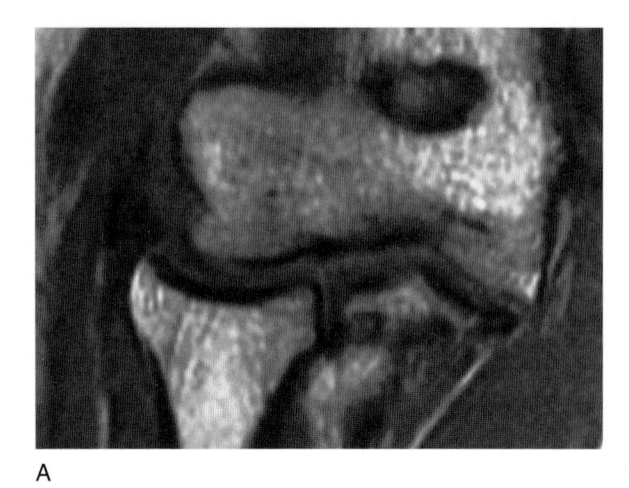

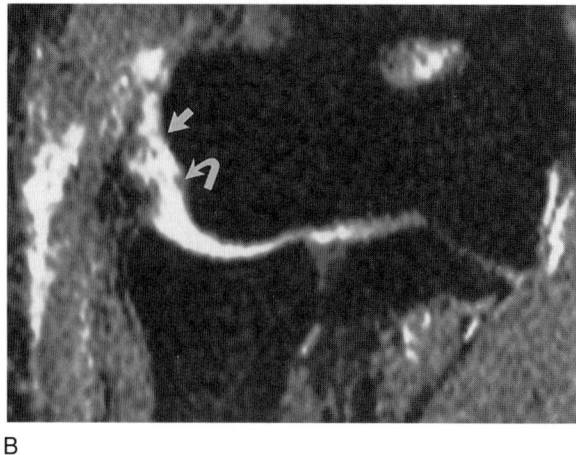

FIGURE 4.6. A 50-year-old tennis player with symptoms of lateral epicondylitis. T1-weighted (A) and STIR (B) coronal images reveal detachment of the common extensor tendon from the lateral epicondyle (straight arrow). The underlying LUCL is also torn from its attachment site on the humerus (curved arrow).

when rupture of the LUCL and subtle associated instability are not recognized clinically. MRI can reveal concurrent tears of the LUCL and common extensor tendon in patients who have lateral epicondylitis and isolated LUCL tears in patients who have posterolateral rotatory instability. Moreover, the lack of a significant abnormality involving the common extensor tendon on MRI may prompt consideration of an alternative diagnosis, such as radial nerve entrapment that can mimic or accompany lateral epicondylitis.[28,29]

Posterior Dislocation Injury and Instability

Posterior dislocation of the elbow is an unusual event; however, it is the second most common major joint dislocation (after the shoulder) in adults, and it is the most common dislocation in children less than 10 years of age.[30] Many of the dislocations that occur in children go unrecognized because of spontaneous reduction, with swollen, tender elbow as the only finding.[31] MRI in such cases usually shows both an effusion and a contusion or strain of the brachialis muscle (Fig. 4.7). Bone contusions may be seen at the posterior margin of the capitellum and at the radial head and coronoid process.

We have found MRI to be very reliable in detecting rupture of the LUCL. This ligament usually tears proximally at the lateral margin of the capitellum and is best evaluated on coronal and axial images.[5,32] The LUCL may tear as an isolated finding on MRI in patients who have posterolateral rotatory instability in stage 1. Tears of the LUCL also may be detected in association with rupture of the MCL in stage 3B. Disruption of the LUCL is commonly seen in patients who have severe tennis elbow and tears of the common extensor tendon on MRI.

Fractures

Radiographically occult or equivocal fractures may be assessed with MRI. In general, the findings of bone injury may be subtle on proton-density, T2-weighted, and T2*-weighted sequences and are more conspicuous on T1-weighted, fat-suppressed T2-weighted, or STIR sequences.

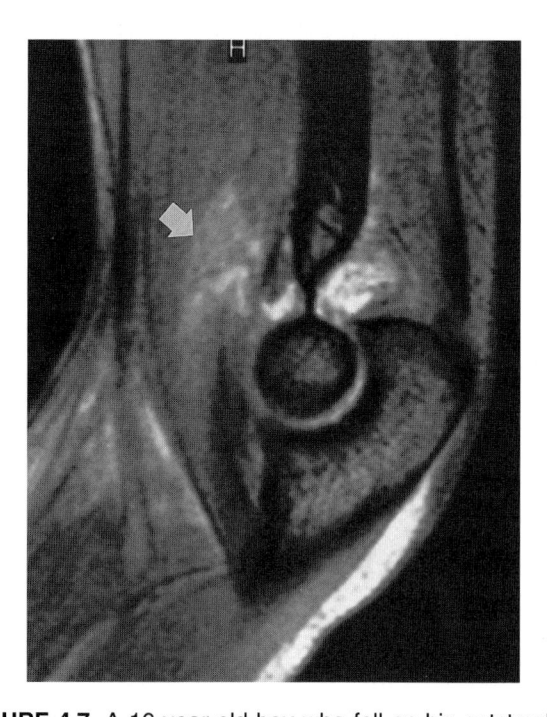

FIGURE 4.7. A 16-year-old boy who fell on his outstreched arm now complains of painful limitation of elbow extension. A T2*-weighted gradient-echo sagittal image reveals increased signal (arrow) compatible with a strain of the brachialis muscle. Brachialis muscle injury is commonly seen after posterior subluxation or dislocation of the elbow.

Approximately 10% of elbow dislocations result in fractures of the radial head; conversely, about 10% of patients with a radial head fracture have an elbow dislocation.[33] Displaced fractures of the radial head are best treated with internal fixation when there is ligamentous disruption and instability.[34] CT is the technique of choice when additional information about the fracture morphology or degree of comminution is needed. MRI may detect and characterize radial head fractures and is useful for excluding associated collateral ligament injury that may contribute to instability. The integrity of the MCL is especially important if excision of the radial head is being considered.

MRI may identify or exclude supracondylar fractures in children when radiographic evidence of a joint effusion is present and a fracture is not visualized. In children, supracondylar fractures that do not involve the physis are more common than all physeal injuries about the elbow combined.[35,36] However, the elbow is a relatively common site of physeal injury, occurring most frequently after distal radial and distal tibial physeal fractures are considered.[37] Fractures of the lateral humeral condyle are the most common specific type of physeal injury about the elbow. Injury to the physis and the unossified epiphyseal cartilage may be assessed with arthrography or MRI in these cases (Fig. 4.8).[37–39] This information is important as Salter–Harris type IV fractures of the lateral humeral condyle tend to be unstable and require surgical intervention, whereas Salter–Harris type II fractures can be treated successfully with closed reduction.

Osteochondritis Dissecans

MRI can reliably detect and stage osteochondritis dissecans; however, the accuracy of staging is improved by performing MR arthrography using dilute gadolinium.[40] Unstable lesions are characterized by fluid or contrast encircling the osteochondral fragment on T2-weighted images. Loose in situ lesions also may be diagnosed by identifying a cystlike lesion beneath the osteochondral fragment.[41] These cystlike lesions typically contain loose granulation tissue at surgery, which explains why they may enhance after intravenous administration of gadolinium (Fig. 4.9). Few authors have reported their experience with intravenous gadolinium-enhanced scans to evaluate osteonecrosis and osteochondritis dissecans in the elbow.[42]

Osteochondritis dissecans should be distinguished from osteochondrosis of the capitellum, which is known as Panner's disease. Panner's disease is characterized by fragmentation and abnormally decreased signal intensity within the ossifying capitellar epiphysis on the T1-weighted images similar in appearance to Legg–Calve–Perthes disease in the hip. Panner's disease is believed to represent avascular necrosis of the capitellar ossification center that occurs secondary to trauma. Subsequent scans reveal normalization of these changes with little or no residual deformity of the capitellar articular surface. The articular surface typically remains intact and does not undergo fragmentation or loose-body formation.

Loose Bodies

Large loose bodies are well seen with MRI, especially when an effusion is present (Fig. 4.10).[43] Small loose bodies may be more difficult to detect and differentiate from other foci of signal void on MRI, such as thickened synovium (Fig. 4.11). Air bubbles also may mimic loose bodies on MRI.[44] Small air bubbles may arise naturally from vacuum phenomenon or may be introduced iatrogenically during aspiration or injection of fluid. Vacuum phenomenon is unusual in the elbow joint, whereas small bubbles are commonly seen with MR arthrography. Even with good arthrographic technique, it is not uncommon to inject several small air bubbles into the joint that may mimic loose bodies on MRI. These air bubbles can be recognized by a characteristic margin of high signal adjacent to the signal void, which is due to a magnetic susceptibility artifact and is not found along the margins of a real loose body. A similar appearance of multiple foci of magnetic susceptibility artifact also may be seen at the site of micrometallic deposition associated with previous

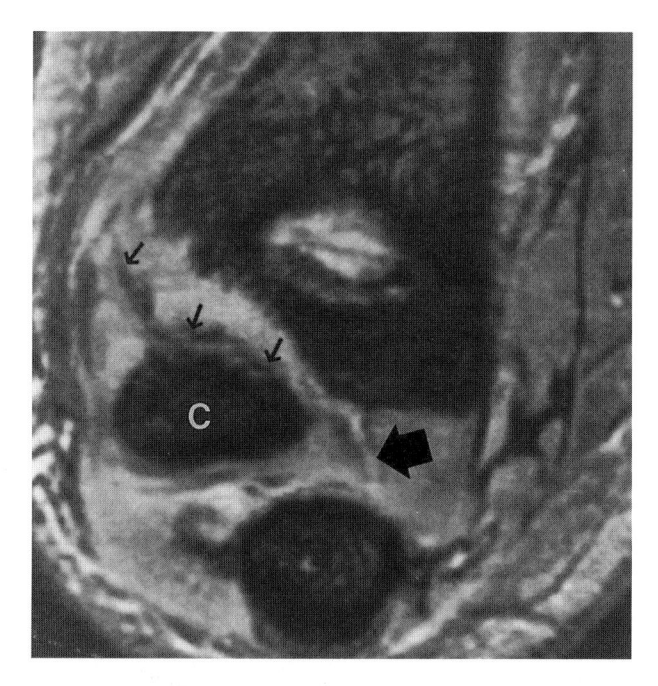

FIGURE 4.8. Salter–Harris type IV fracture of the lateral humeral condyle. A T2*-weighted gradient-echo coronal image of a partially flexed elbow reveals the thin metaphyseal fracture fragment (small arrows) and extension of the fracture through the unossified trochlear epiphysis (large arrow). These fractures may require open reduction and internal fixation. C, capitellum. (Courtesy of Phoebe Kaplan, MD)

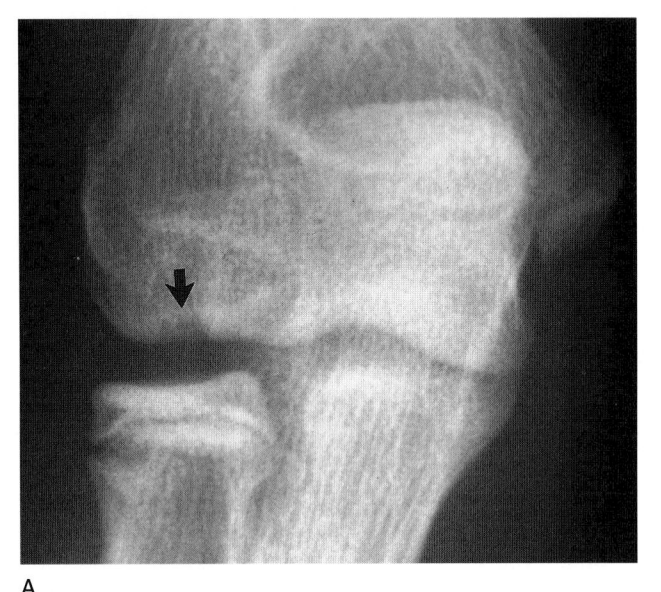

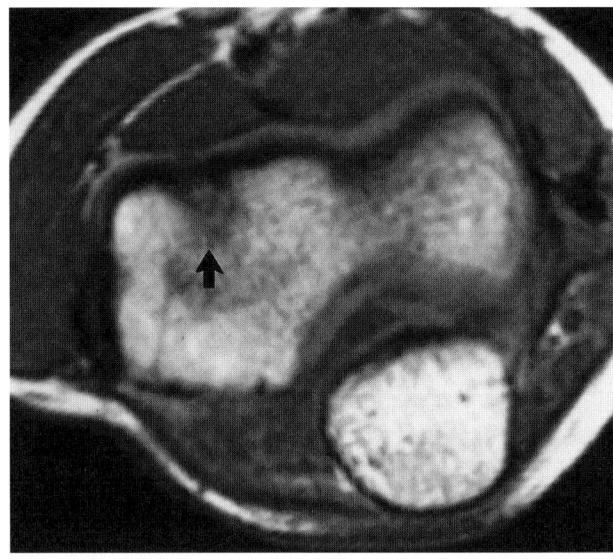

FIGURE 4.9. Osteochondritis dissecans (OCD) in an 11-year-old female gymnast. (A) Plain X-ray reveals a small lucency in the capitellum (arrow). (B) T1-weighted axial image reveals a small focus of OCD in the anterior aspect of the capitellum (arrow). (C) T1-weighted axial image obtained after IV administration of gadolinium reveals enhancement of thickened irregular synovium (curved arrows) compatible with synovitis. Enhancing granulation tissue is seen highlighting the overlying osteochondral defect (arrow).

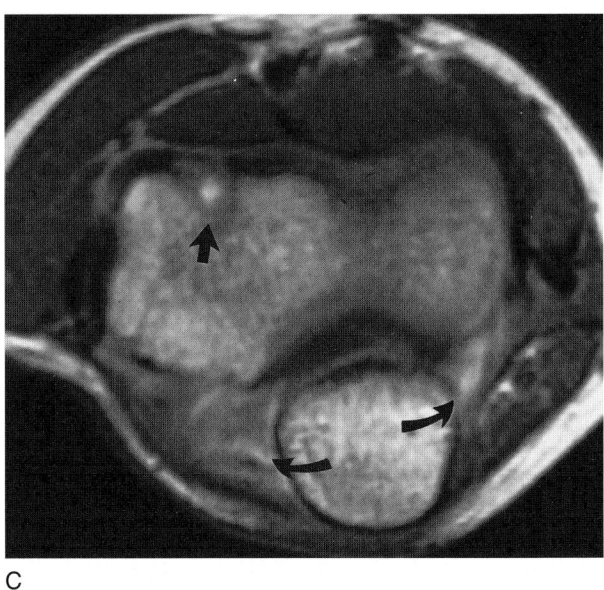

surgery. These foci of magnetic susceptibility artifact are most prominent on gradient-echo T2*-weighted images.

Noncalcified chondral loose bodies cannot be visualized on CT or radiographs; however, they can be identified with MRI. Calcified loose bodies are very conspicuous on MRI, especially with gradient-echo T2*-weighted sequences. Calcified loose bodies may appear slightly larger than their actual size on gradient-echo T2*-weighted images as a result of magnetic susceptibility effects that are normally dampened by the 180° refocusing pulse on spin-echo images.

Biceps Tendon Injury

Complete tears of the distal biceps are thought to be much more common than partial tears.[45,46] MRI is useful in evaluating these injuries because degenerative tendinosis, partial tears, and complete ruptures may be distinguished.[6,47,48]

Distal biceps tendinosis is common and has been shown to precede spontaneous tendon rupture.[13] Tendinosis of the distal biceps is probably a multifactorial process that involves repetitive mechanical impingement of a poorly vascularized distal segment of the tendon. Irregularity of the radial tuberosity and chronic inflammation of the adjacent radial bicipital bursa also may contribute.[49,50] A zone of relatively poor blood supply exists within the distal biceps tendon approximately 10 mm from its insertion on the radial tuberosity.[51] In addition, this hypovascular zone may be impinged between the radius and the ulna during pronation. The space between the radius and ulna progressively narrows by 50% during pronation, with average measurements of approxi-

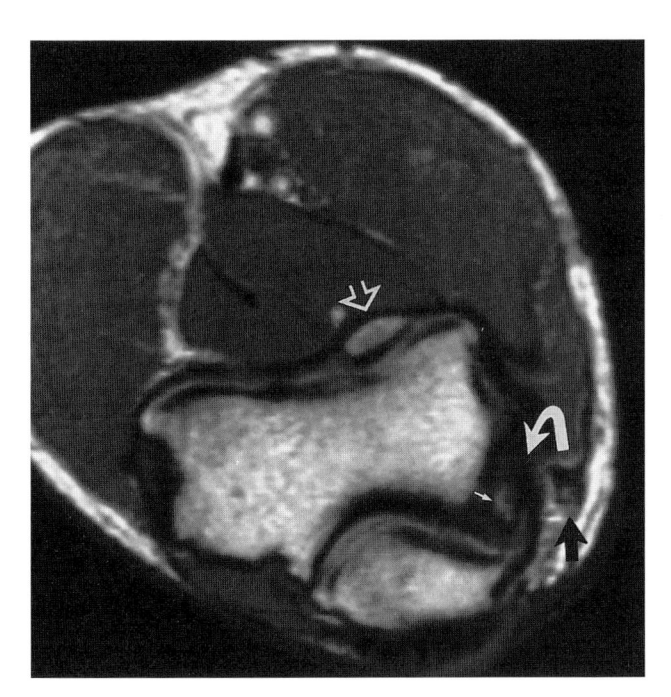

FIGURE 4.10. Loose bodies in a professional pitcher with ulnar neuritis. A T1-weighted axial image distal to the medial epicondyle reveals an anterior compartment loose body (open arrow) and a posteromedial loose body (small white arrow) and thickened medial collateral ligament (curved arrow) that undermine the floor of the cubital tunnel adjacent to the ulnar nerve (black arrow).

mately 8 mm in supination, 6 mm in neutral position, and 4 mm in pronation recorded in asymptomatic volunteers with CT and MRI.[51] Repetitive impingement during pronation coupled with an intrinsically poor blood supply of the distal biceps tendon may result in a failed healing response and degenerative tendinosis. Enlargement of the degenerated tendon and irregularity and hypertrophy of the radial tuberosity may lead to inflammation of the adjacent bursa. Each of these factors may contribute to worsening impingement between the radial tuberosity and the ulna, leading to further degeneration of the distal biceps tendon. Ultimately, this process may result in complete tendon rupture or, less commonly, partial tendon rupture or bursitis.

The distal biceps tendon is covered by an extrasynovial paratenon and is separated from the radial tuberosity by the bicipital radial bursa. Inflammation of this cubital bursa may accompany tendinosis and tearing of the distal biceps (Fig. 4.12). Enlargement of the bicipital radial bursa may occasionally present as a nonspecific antecubital fossa mass as large as 5 cm in diameter.[50,52] Intravenous administration of gadolinium may aid in recognition of this enlarged bursa on MRI and may allow differentiation of this benign entity from a solid neoplasm.[52] Cubital bursitis, tendinosis, and partial tendon rupture may coexist to differing degrees and may be impossible to distinguish clinically.[45,50] Cubital bursitis and partial tendon rupture may both cause irritation of the adjacent median nerve, further complicating the clinical findings.[50,53]

The T2-weighted axial images are most useful for determining the degree of tendon tearing. These images also are useful for evaluating the lacertus fibrosus (Fig. 4.13). The axial images should extend from the musculotendinous junction to the insertion of the tendon on the radial tuberosity. MRI provides useful information regarding the degree of tearing, the size of the gap, and the location of the tear for preoperative planning. The tendon typically tears from its attachment on the radial tuberosity as a result of attempted elbow flexion against resistance.[9] Rupture of the distal biceps tendon generally is treated with prompt surgical repair and reattachment to the radial tuberosity to restore flexion and supination strength. Early diagnosis of biceps tendon rupture is important because surgical outcome is improved in patients treated during the first several weeks after injury.[54] After several months, the tendon retracts into the substance of the biceps muscle, making retrieval and reattachment more complicated. MRI may be useful in such cases to confirm the clinical diagnosis and to plan reconstructive surgery.

Triceps Tendon Injury

Rupture of the distal triceps tendon has been considered one of the least common tendon injuries, with approximately 60 cases reported in the literature to date. Partial tears may occur, but they generally have been consid-

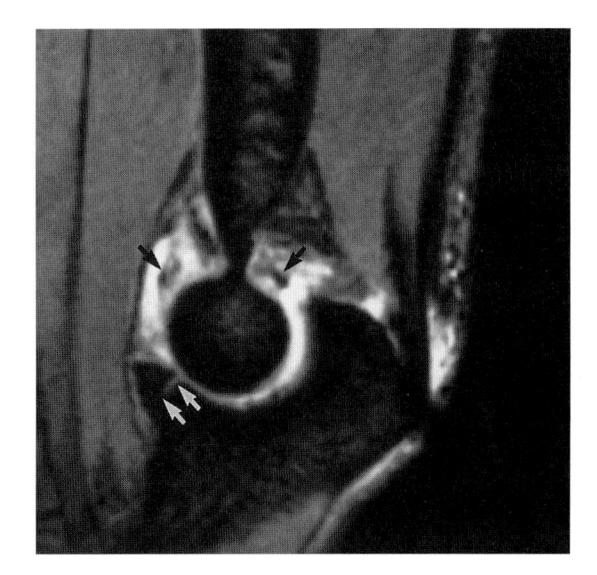

FIGURE 4.11. Radiographically occult type I fracture of the coronoid process in a patient with pain and loss of motion after a fall. A T2*-weighted gradient-echo sagittal image reveals a nondisplaced sheer fracture of the coronoid process (white arrows). An effusion and foci of thickened synovium (black arrows) are also noted. The synovial thickening should not be mistaken for small loose bodies on these images.

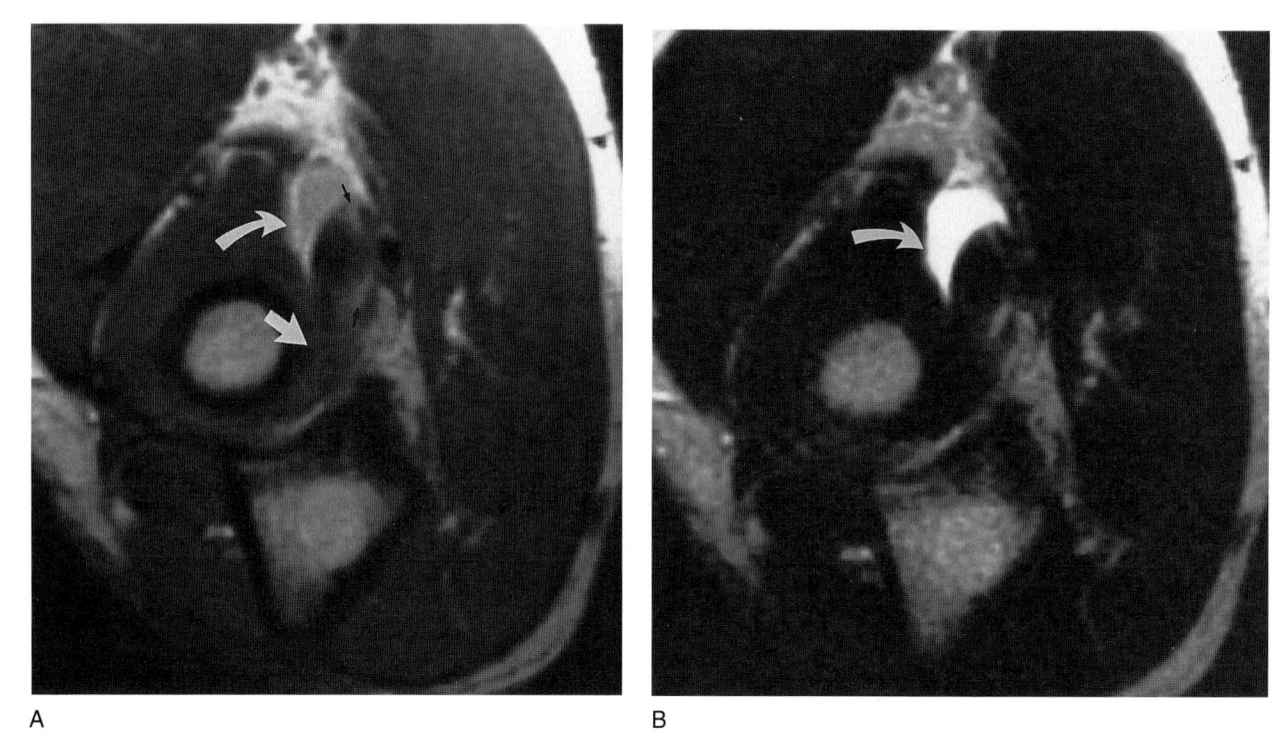

FIGURE 4.12. Cubital bursitis, tendinosis, and intrasubstance partial tearing of the distal biceps tendon. Proton-density (A) and T2-weighted (B) axial images reveal prominent distention of the bicipital radial bursa (curved arrows). The bursa separates the biceps tendon from the radial tuberosity further distally. Moderate increased signal is seen in the biceps tendon on the proton-density image (straight white arrow) consistent with degenerative tendinosis. A small longitudinal split (small black arrows) is seen in the medial aspect of the thickened tendon. Partial rupture of the distal biceps and bursitis may be difficult to distinguish clinically and may also coexist.

ered less common than complete ruptures of the triceps tendon.[55–57]

The consequences of overloading the extensor mechanism of the elbow depend largely on the age of the patient and the presence of pre-existing tendon degeneration. Most often, the tendon ruptures at the site of degenerative tendinosis. In skeletally immature individuals, separation of the olecranon growth plate may occur and require internal fixation. Acute overload of the extensor mechanism in an adolescent with a partially closed olecranon growth plate may result in a Salter–Harris type II fracture that may be radiographically subtle. MRI may be useful in this setting to evaluate the extensor mechanism and detect occult injury to the growth plate.

Injuries of the triceps tendon and muscle are well seen with MRI.[6,58,59] The normal triceps tendon often appears lax and redundant when the elbow is imaged in full extension or mild hyperextension. This appearance resolves when the elbow is imaged in mild degrees of flexion and should not be mistaken for an abnormality. Degenerative tendinosis is characterized by thickening and signal alteration of the distal tendon fibers. Acute rupture is well seen on T2-weighted or STIR images due to surrounding fluid. Partial tears are much less common than complete rupture and are more difficult to diagnose clinically.[60]

MRI can distinguish between complete tears that require surgery and partial tears that may do well with protection and rehabilitation. MRI also can help delineate the degree of tendon retraction and muscular atrophy that is present when rupture of the triceps has been missed and a more extensive reconstruction of the defect is required.

Entrapment Neuropathies

The ulnar nerve is well seen on axial MR images as it passes through the cubital tunnel.[61,62] Anatomic variations of the cubital tunnel retinaculum may contribute to ulnar neuropathy.[63] These variations in the cubital tunnel retinaculum and the appearance of the ulnar nerve itself can be identified with MRI. The retinaculum may be thickened in 22% of the population, resulting in dynamic compression of the ulnar nerve during elbow flexion. In 11% of the population, the cubital tunnel retinaculum may be replaced by an anomalous muscle, the anconeus epitrochlearis, resulting in static compression of the ulnar nerve (Fig. 4.14).[63] The cubital tunnel retinaculum may be absent in 10% of the population, allowing anterior dislocation of the ulnar nerve over the medial epicondyle during flexion with subsequent friction neuritis

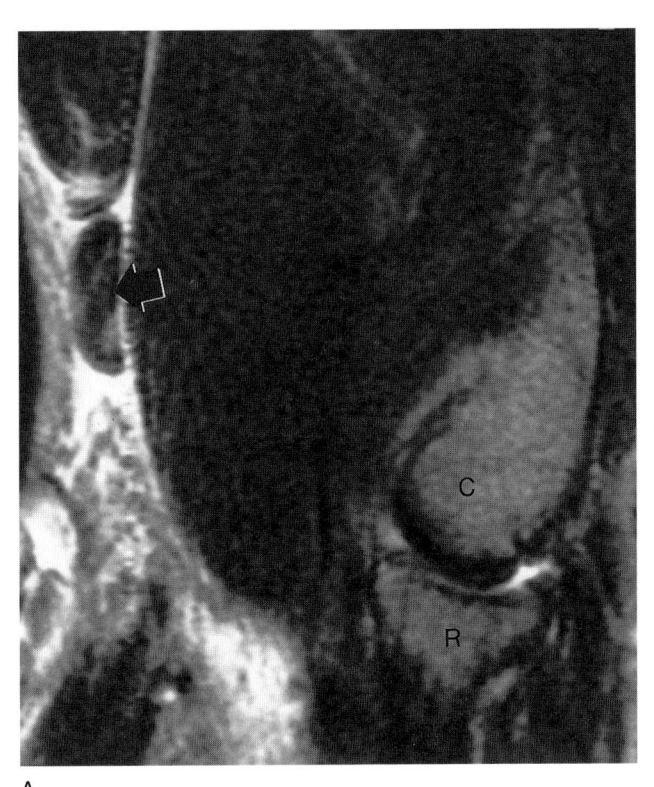

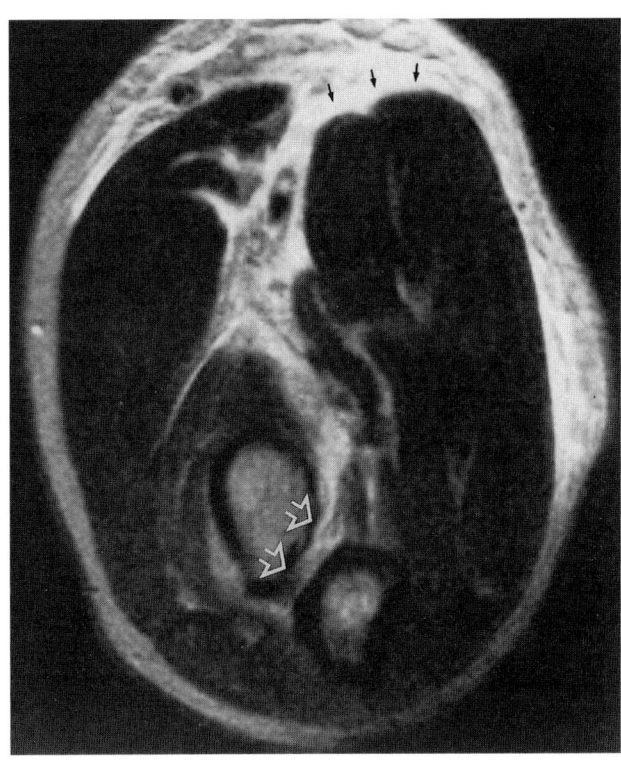

FIGURE 4.13. Rupture of the biceps tendon and bicipital aponeurosis (lacertus fibrosus). **(A)** T2-weighted sagittal image reveals the retracted biceps tendon (arrow) within the antecubital fossa. **(B)** There is increased signal and poor definition of the lacertus fibrosus (small black arrows) on this T2-weighted axial image. There is increased signal at the expected attachment site of the distal biceps tendon to the radial tuberosity (open arrows). Hypertrophy of the radial tuberosity is seen contributing to narrowing of the space between the ulna and radius where the torn distal biceps tendon was previously impinged. (C, capitellum, R, radius)

(Fig. 4.15).[64] This subluxation of the ulnar nerve, as well as subluxation of the medial head of the triceps in cases of snapping elbow syndrome, may be depicted with MR images of the elbow in flexion.[65]

MRI signs of ulnar neuritis and entrapment include displacement and flattening of the nerve adjacent to a mass, swelling and enlargement of the nerve proximal or distal to a mass, infiltration of the perineural fat, and increased signal intensity within the nerve on T2-weighted images.[62,66] Peripheral nerves are normally intermediate in signal intensity on T2-weighted images. The ulnar nerve must be followed carefully to avoid mistaking it for enlargement of the adjacent veins. The posterior ulnar recurrent artery and the deep veins that accompany it are normally small structures that course with the ulnar nerve through the cubital tunnel. Enlargement of a deep vein may appear as a bright tubular structure on T2-weighted, gradient-echo, or STIR sequences and may mimic an edematous ulnar nerve.[66]

Entrapment of the median nerve and radial nerve also may be evaluated with MRI. Median nerve entrapment may be due to a variety of uncommon anatomic variations about the elbow including the presence of a supracondyloid process with a ligament of Struthers, anomalous muscles, an accessory bicipital aponeurosis, and hypertrophy of the ulnar head of the pronator teres.[67] These anatomic variants and abnormal mass lesions, such as an enlarged radial bicipital bursa, may entrap the median nerve and may be identified with MRI. Radial nerve entrapment may occur due to thickening of the arcade of Frohse along the proximal edge of the supinator muscle. Ganglion cysts may arise from the anterior margin of the elbow joint and compress the radial nerve.[68]

MRI may be complementary to electromyography and nerve conduction studies in cases of nerve entrapment about the elbow.[61] In subacute denervation, the affected muscles have prolongation of T1 and T2 relaxation times secondary to muscle fiber shrinkage and associated increases in extracellular water.[69] Entrapment of a nerve about the elbow may therefore cause increased signal within the muscles innervated by that nerve on T2-weighted or STIR images. These changes may be followed to resolution or progressive atrophy and fatty infiltration.[70,71] Moreover, the site and cause of entrapment may be discovered with MRI by following the nerve implicated from the distribution of abnormal muscles on MRI.[72]

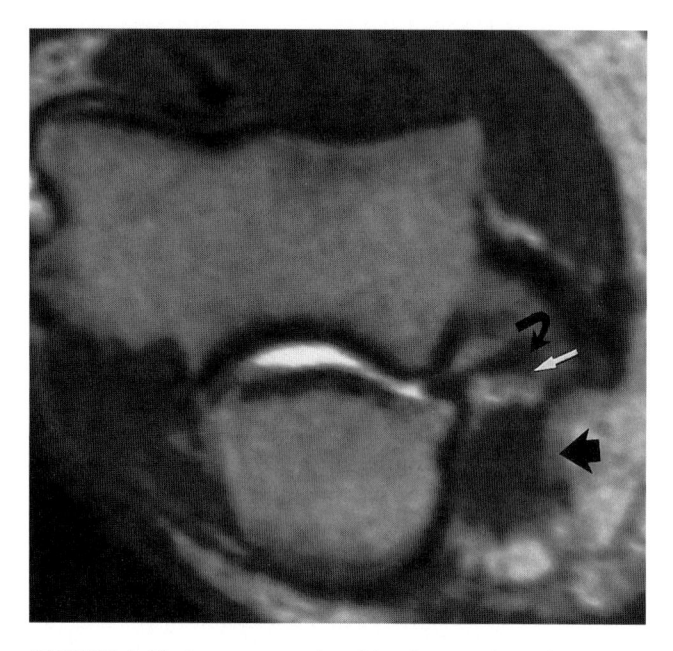

FIGURE 4.14. Anconeus epitrochlearis muscle replacing the cubital tunnel retinaculum. A T2-weighted axial image reveals the ulnar nerve (white arrow) deep to an anomalous anconeus epitrochlearis muscle (black arrow) and superficial to the posterior bundle of the medial collateral ligament (curved arrow).

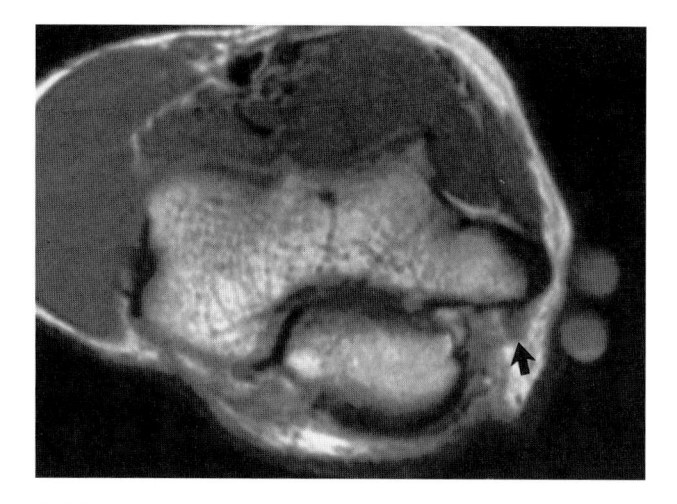

FIGURE 4.15. Ulnar neuritis in a patient with questionable ulnar nerve subluxation on physical examination. A T1-weighted axial image reveals prominent enlargement and medial subluxation of the ulnar nerve (arrow). The overlying cubital tunnel retinaculum is developmentally absent, allowing anterior dislocation of the ulnar nerve during elbow flexion with subsequent friction neuritis. The nerve was increased in signal intensity on the T2-weighted images (not shown).

SUMMARY

MRI imaging provides clinically useful information in assessing the elbow joint. Superior depiction of muscles, ligaments, and tendons and the ability to directly visualize nerves, bone marrow, and hyaline cartilage are advantages of MRI relative to conventional imaging techniques. Ongoing improvements in surface coil design and newer pulse sequences have resulted in higher-quality MRI of the elbow. Traumatic and degenerative disorders of the elbow are well seen with MRI. The sequelae of medial traction and lateral compression from valgus stress include medial collateral ligament injury, common flexor tendon abnormalities, medial traction spurs, ulnar neuropathy, and osteochondritis dissecans. These conditions, as well as lateral collateral ligament injury and lateral epicondylitis, may be characterized with MRI. Post-traumatic osseous abnormalities well seen with MRI include radiographically occult fractures, stress fractures, bone contusions, and apophyseal avulsions. MRI also can be used to assess cartilaginous extension of fractures in children. Intra-articular loose bodies can be identified with MRI, especially if fluid or contrast material is present within the elbow joint. Biceps and triceps tendon injuries can be diagnosed and characterized. MRI also can provide additional information regarding entrapment neuropathies about the elbow. MRI perhaps is most useful when patients have not responded to nonoperative therapy, and surgery, as well as additional diagnoses, is being considered.

REFERENCES

1. Conway JE, Jobe FW, Glousman RE, et al. Medial instability of the elbow in throwing athletes. Treatment by repair or reconstruction of the ulnar collateral ligament. *J Bone Joint Surg* 1992;74A:67–83.
2. Jordan SE. Surgical anatomy of the elbow. In: Jobe FW, ed. *Operative techniques in upper extremity sports injuries.* St. Louis, MO: CV Mosby; 1996:402–410.
3. Morrey BF. Anatomy of the elbow joint. In: Morrey BF, ed. *The elbow and its disorders.* 2nd ed. Philadelphia: WB Saunders; 1993:56–52.
4. Timmerman LA, Andrews JR. Histology and arthroscopic anatomy of the ulnar collateral ligament of the elbow. *Am J Sports Med* 1994;22:667–673.
5. Fritz RC. Magnetic resonance imaging of the elbow. *Semin Roentgenol* 1995;30:241–264.
6. Murphy BJ. MR imaging of the elbow. *Radiology* 1992;184:525–529.
7. Ollivierre CO, Nirschl RP, Pettrone FA. Resection and repair for medial tennis elbow. A prospective analysis. *Am J Sports Med* 1995;23:214–221.
8. Vangsness CT Jr, Jobe FW. Surgical treatment of medial epicondylitis. Results in 35 elbows. *J Bone Joint Surg* 1991;73B:409–411.

9. Wilkins KE, Morrey BF, Jobe FW, et al. The elbow. *Instructional Course Lect* 1991;40:1–87.
10. Fleckenstein JL, Weatherall PT, Parkey RW, et al. Sports-related muscle injuries: Evaluation with MR imaging. *Radiology* 1989;172:793–798.
11. Resendes M, Helms CA, Fritz RC, et al. MR appearance of intramuscular injections. *AJR Am J Roentgenol* 1992;158:1293–1294.
12. Garrett WE Jr. Injuries to the muscle–tendon unit. *Instructional Course Lect* 1988;37:275–282.
13. Kannus P, Jozsa L. Histopathological changes preceding spontaneous rupture of a tendon. A controlled study of 891 patients. *J Bone Joint Surg* 1991;73A:1507–1525.
14. Nirschl RP. Elbow tendinosis/tennis elbow. *Clin Sports Med* 1992;11:851–870.
15. Doran A, Gresham GA, Rushton N, et al. Tennis elbow. A clinicopathologic study of 22 cases followed for 2 years. *Acta Orthop Scand* 1990;61:535–538.
16. Jozsa L, Lehto M, Kvist M, et al. Alterations in dry mass content of collagen fibers in degenerative tendinopathy and tendon-rupture. *Matrix* 1989;9:140–146.
17. Regan W, Wold LE, Coonrad R, et al. Microscopic histopathology of chronic refractory lateral epicondylitis. *Am J Sports Med* 1992;20:746–749.
18. Gabel G, Morrey BF. Operative treatment of medial epicondylitis. Influence of concomitant ulnar neuropathy at the elbow. *J Bone Joint Surg* 1995;77A:1065–1069.
19. Kurvers H, Verhaar J. The results of operative treatment of medial epicondylitis. *J Bone Joint Surg* 1995;77A:1374–1379.
20. Brogdon BG, Crow NE. Little Leaguer's elbow. *AJR Am J Roentgenol* 1960;83:671–675.
21. Patten RM. Overuse syndromes and injuries involving the elbow: MR imaging findings. *AJR Am J Roentgenol* 1995;164:1205–1211.
22. Nirschl RP, Pettrone FA. Tennis elbow: The surgical treatment of lateral epicondylitis. *J Bone Joint Surg* 1979;61A:832–839.
23. Halpern AA, Horowitz BG, Nagel DA. Tendon ruptures associated with corticosteroid therapy. *West J Med* 1977;127:378–382.
24. Unverferth LJ, Olix ML. The effect of local steroid injections on tendon. *J Sports Med* 1973;1:31–37.
25. Coonrad RW, Hooper WR. Tennis elbow: Its course, natural history, conservative and surgical management. *J Bone Joint Surg* 1973;55A:1177–1182.
26. Morrey BF. Reoperation for failed surgical treatment of refractory lateral epicondylitis. *J Shoulder Elbow Surg* 1992;1:47–55.
27. Morrey BF. Surgical failure of the tennis elbow. In: Morrey BF, ed. *The elbow and its disorders*, 2nd ed. Philadelphia: WB Saunders; 1993:553–559.
28. Verhaar J, Spaans F. Radial tunnel syndrome. An investigation of compression neuropathy as a possible cause. *J Bone Joint Surg* 1991;73A:539–544.
29. Werner CO. Lateral elbow pain and posterior interosseous nerve entrapment. *Acta Orthop Scand Suppl* 1979;174:1–62.
30. Linscheid RL, O'Driscoll SW. Elbow dislocations. In: Morrey BF, ed. *The elbow and its disorders*, 2nd ed. Philadelphia: WB Saunders; 1993:441–452.
31. Letts M. Dislocations of the child's elbow. In: Morrey BF, ed. *The elbow and its disorders*, 2nd ed. Philadelphia: WB Saunders; 1993:288–315.
32. Potter HG, Weiland AJ, Schatz JA, et al. Posterolateral rotatory instability of the elbow: Usefulness of MR imaging in diagnosis. *Radiology* 1997;204:185–189.
33. Morrey BF. Radial head fracture. In: Morrey BF, ed. *The elbow and its disorders*, 2nd ed. Philadelphia: WB Saunders; 1993:383–404.
34. O'Driscoll SW. Elbow instability. *Hand Clinics* 1994;10:405–415.
35. Peterson HA. Physeal fractures of the elbow. In: Morrey BF, ed. *The elbow and its disorders*, 2nd ed. Philadelphia: WB Saunders; 1993:248–265.
36. Klassen RA. Supracondylar fractures of the elbow in children. In: Morrey BF, ed. *The elbow and its disorders*. 2nd ed. Philadelphia: WB Saunders; 1993:206–247.
37. Beltran J, Rosenberg ZS, Kawelblum M, et al. Pediatric elbow fractures: MRI evaluation. *Skeletal Radiol* 1994;23:277–281.
38. Jaramillo D, Hoffer FA. Cartilaginous epiphysis and growth plate: Normal and abnormal MR imaging findings. *AJR Am J Roentgenol* 1992;158:1105–1110.
39. Jaramillo D, Waters PM. Abnormalities of the pediatric elbow: Evaluation with MR imaging. *Radiology* 1992;185(P):137.
40. Kramer J, Stiglbauer R, Engel A, et al. MR contrast arthrography (MRA) in osteochondrosis dissecans. *J Comput Assist Tomogr* 1992;16:254–260.
41. De Smet AA, Fisher DR, Burnstein MI, et al. Value of MR imaging in staging osteochondral lesions of the talus (osteochondritis dissecans): Results in 14 patients. *AJR Am J Roentgenol* 1990;154:555–558.
42. Peiss J, Adam G, Casser R, et al. Gadopentetate-dimeglumine-enhanced MR imaging of osteonecrosis and osteochondritis dissecans of the elbow: Initial experience. *Skeletal Radiol* 1995;24:17–20.
43. Quinn SF, Haberman JJ, Fitzgerald SW, et al. Evaluation of loose bodies in the elbow with MR imaging. *J Magn Reson Imaging* 1994;4:169–172.
44. Patten RM. Vacuum phenomenon: A potential pitfall in the interpretation of gradient-recalled-echo MR images of the shoulder. *AJR Am J Roentgenol* 1994;162:1383–1386.
45. Bourne MH, Morrey BF. Partial rupture of the distal biceps tendon. *Clin Orthop* 1991;271:143–148.
46. Nielsen K. Partial rupture of the distal biceps brachii tendon. A case report. *Acta Orthop Scand* 1987;58:287–288.
47. Fitzgerald SW, Curry DR, Erickson SJ, et al. Distal biceps tendon injury: MR imaging diagnosis. *Radiology* 1994;191:203–206.
48. Falchook FS, Zlatkin MB, Erbacher GE, et al. Rupture of the distal biceps tendon: Evaluation with MR imaging. *Radiology* 1994;190:659–663.
49. Davis WM, Yassine Z. An etiological factor in tear of the distal tendon of the biceps brachii. *J Bone Joint Surg* 1956;38A:1365–1368.
50. Karanjia ND, Stiles PJ. Cubital bursitis. *J Bone Joint Surg* 1988;70B:832–833.
51. Seiler JG III, Parker LM, Chamberland PD, et al. The distal biceps tendon. Two potential mechanisms involved in its rupture: Arterial supply and mechanical impingement. *J Shoulder Elbow Surg* 1995;4:149–156.

52. Kosarek FJ, Hoffman CJ, Martinez S. Distal bicipital bursitis: MR imaging characteristics. *Radiology* 1995;197(P):398.
53. Foxworthy M, Kinninmonth AW. Median nerve compression in the proximal forearm as a complication of partial rupture of the distal biceps brachii tendon. *J Hand Surg* 1992;17B:515–517.
54. Agins HJ, Chess JL, Hoekstra DV, et al. Rupture of the distal insertion of the biceps brachii tendon. *Clin Orthop* 1988;234:34–38.
55. D'Alessandro DF, Shields CL. Biceps rupture and triceps avulsion. In: Jobe FW, ed. *Operative techniques in upper extremity sports injuries*. St. Louis, MO: CV Mosby; 1996:506–517.
56. Tarsney FF. Rupture and avulsion of the triceps. *Clin Orthop* 1972;83:177–183.
57. Farrar EL III, Lippert FG III. Avulsion of the triceps tendon. *Clin Orthop* 1981;161:242–246.
58. Tiger E, Mayer DP, Glazer R. Complete avulsion of the triceps tendon: MRI diagnosis. *Comput Med Imaging Graph* 1993;17:51–54.
59. Bos CF, Nelissen RG, Bloem JL. Incomplete rupture of the tendon of triceps brachii. A case report. *Int Orthop* 1994;18:273–275.
60. Morrey BF, Regan WD. Tendinopathies about the elbow. In: DeLee JC, Drez D Jr., eds. *Orthopaedic sports medicine: Principles and practice*. Philadelphia: WB Saunders; 1994:860–881.
61. Rosenberg ZS, Beltran J, Cheung YY, et al. The elbow: MR features of nerve disorders. *Radiology* 1993;188:235–240.
62. Britz GW, Haynor DR, Kuntz C, et al. Ulnar nerve entrapment at the elbow: Correlation of magnetic resonance imaging, clinical, electrodiagnostic, and intraoperative findings. *Neurosurgery* 1996;38:458–465.
63. O'Driscoll SW, Horii E, Carmichael SW, et al. The cubital tunnel and ulnar neuropathy. *J Bone Joint Surg* 1991;73B:613–617.
64. Morrey BF. Applied anatomy and biomechanics of the elbow joint. *Instructional Course Lect* 1986;35:59–68.
65. Spinner RJ, Hayden FR Jr, Hipps CT, et al. Imaging the snapping triceps. *AJR Am J Roentgenol* 1996;167:1550–1551.
66. Rosenberg ZS, Beltran J, Cheung Y, et al. MR imaging of the elbow: Normal variant and potential diagnostic pitfalls of the trochlear groove and cubital tunnel. *AJR Am J Roentgenol* 1995;164:415–418.
67. Spinner M, Linscheid RL. Nerve entrapment syndromes. In: Morrey BF, ed. *The elbow and its disorders*, 2nd ed. Philadelphia: WB Saunders, 1993:813–832.
68. Ogino T, Minami A, Kato H. Diagnosis of radial nerve palsy caused by ganglion with use of different imaging techniques. *J Hand Surg (Am)* 1991;16:230–235.
69. Polak JF, Jolesz FA, Adams DF. Magnetic resonance imaging of skeletal muscle. Prolongation of T1 and T2 subsequent to denervation. *Invest Radiol* 1988;23:365–369.
70. Fleckenstein JL, Watumull D, Conner KE, et al. Denervated human skeletal muscle: MR imaging evaluation. *Radiology* 1993;187:213–218.
71. Shabas D, Gerard G, Rossi D. Magnetic resonance imaging examination of denervated muscle. *Comput Radiol* 1987;11:9–13.
72. Uetani M, Hayashi K, Matsunaga N, et al. Denervated skeletal muscle: MR imaging. Work in progress. *Radiology* 1993;189:511–515.

CHAPTER 5

Little League Elbow

Stephen J. Augustine, George M. McCluskey III,
and Luis Miranda-Torres

INTRODUCTION

The sports medicine community has become increasingly aware of injuries in the elbows of child and adolescent athletes. The elbow is one of the most common sites of injury in children and adolescent baseball players.[1,2] In 1965, Adams reported elbow pain in 45% of sixty 9- to 14-year-old pitchers studied.[3] On radiographs, all the pitchers had some degree of accelerated joint separation and fragmentation of the medial epicondylar epiphysis of their throwing arm. Larson and coworkers reported that 20% of one hundred and twenty 11- to 12-year-old pitchers had elbow tenderness.[4] Gugenheim and associates found elbow symptoms in 17% of 595 Little League pitchers ages 9 to 12 years old.[1] The high demands of repetitive throwing can cause injuries to the immature elbow that not only limit performance immediately, but can also lead to significant long-term sequelae.

The term **Little League elbow** is attributed to Brogdon and Crow, who described the most common radiographic changes and clinical features of osteochondrosis of the medial epicondyle in young pitchers.[5] Later, Adams expanded the definition to include all the elbow problems associated with skeletally immature baseball players.[3]

Currently, the term is used to describe a constellation of elbow problems in immature throwers that are secondary to repetitive medial tension, extension overload, and lateral compression forces. Disorders termed Little League elbow include the following: medial epicondylar fragmentation and avulsion, delayed or accelerated apophyseal growth of the medial epicondyle, delayed closure of the medial epicondylar growth plate, osteochondrosis and osteochondritis of the capitellum, osteochondrosis and osteochondritis of the radial head, hypertrophy of the ulna, olecranon apophysitis, and delayed closure of the olecranon apophysis.

Pathogenesis of Injury

Skeletal maturation of the elbow centers on the primary ossification centers of the humerus, ulna, and radius and on six distinct secondary centers of ossification. The chronological appearance and closure of these centers has been well documented[6,7,8] (Fig. 5.1). Childhood terminates with the appearance of all secondary centers of ossification, adolescence terminates with the fusion of all secondary centers of ossification, and young adulthood terminates with the completion of all bone growth and the achievement of final muscular form. These events usually occur 6 months to 1 year earlier in girls than in boys.

Immature athletes are different anatomically, biomechanically, and biochemically from adult athletes. These differences give rise to unique injury patterns in the young throwing athlete's elbow. The most common sites of injury in the young athlete's elbow are the epiphyseal plate, the joint surface, and the apophyseal insertion of the major tendon units. The growing athlete has unique injury risk factors due to the growth process itself. Longitudinal bone growth may cause injury to the muscle–tendon units, bone, and joints from a relative strength and flexibility imbalance, especially during growth spurts. The increase in muscle–tendon tightness about the elbow joint enhances the susceptibility to overuse injury. The presence of physeal cartilage at the plate, at joint surfaces, and at all sites of major tendinous insertions creates a special type of overuse and traumatic injuries. Growth cartilage, including the articular cartilage, is more susceptible to injury from repetitive microtrauma than is adult cartilage. The zone of hypertrophy is the structurally weakest portion of the epiphyseal plate, especially between the layers of degeneration and partial calcification. During adolescent growth spurts, this area of the physeal plate is weaker than the surrounding ligaments. As the

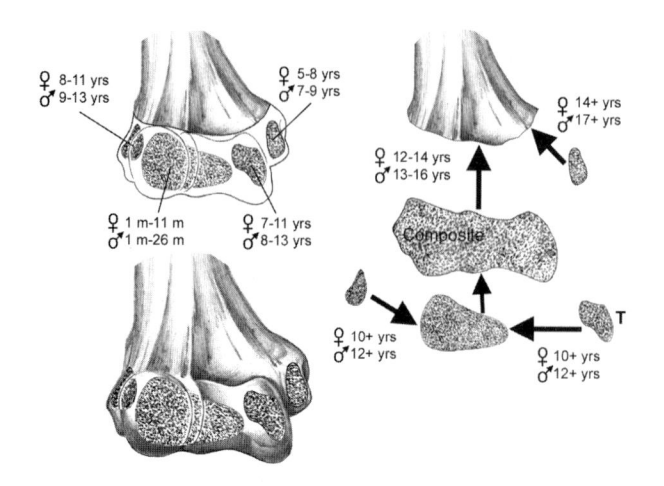

FIGURE 5.1. Ages of appearance and fusion for secondary ossification centers about the elbow (m, months).

plate matures and becomes stronger than the surrounding ligaments, the area of potential injury changes. Therefore, adolescents tend to sustain physeal plate injuries, whereas the prepubescent child or skeletally mature athlete is more likely to sustain tendinous or ligamentous injuries.

Throwing imparts significant stresses on the developing elbow. To understand the mechanism of injury, it is important to understand the biomechanics of the overhead throwing motion, which is discussed in detail in Chapter 2 (Fig. 5.2). Certain stresses on the elbow occur during different phases of the throwing motion.[9] Most injuries occur during the late cocking and acceleration phases. During these phases, the forces placed on the elbow result in valgus stress and hyperextension creating medial tension (distraction) overload on the medial restraints, lateral compression overload on the capitellar and radial head articular surfaces, posterior medial shear forces on the posterior articular surfaces and structures, and distraction anteriorly on the capsule (Fig. 5.3). All the manifestations of Little League elbow result from these forces.

Little League elbow is predominately an overuse syndrome of immature baseball pitchers but its manifestations are also seen in all positions of baseball and in other overhead activities, such as tennis, volleyball, javelin, and the quarterback position in football.[10] Passing a football, serving a tennis ball, and spiking a volleyball place similar forces on the elbow as the pitching motion does. These overuse problems also occur in young gymnasts who place similar forces on the elbow by using it as a weight-bearing joint during maneuvers.[11,12]

The most common risk factor for developing Little League elbow is overuse. Poor throwing technique may also be a cause, and sometimes it is a combination of the two. The two can be cumulative as well, with overuse leading to fatigue, which contributes to poor technique and, conversely, poor technique leading to fatigue and overuse. Either way the end result is loss of the balanced interaction between muscle, ligament, and bone, creating an environment that places the elbow at risk of injury. There is a positive correlation between pitching frequency and repetitive trauma injuries.[13] Overuse injuries result from repetitive submaximal loads that cause an accumulation of microtrauma that damages tissues quicker than the bodies ability to repair them. These injuries include stress fractures (bone and physeal), tendon breakdown, joint cartilage impaction injuries, and progressive ligament and capsular stretching. Overuse injuries can be insidious and chronic in nature or sudden, with an acute event superimposed on already weakened and damaged tissues or structures.

Often young athletes are subjected to the misguided "too much, too soon" training phenomenon.[14] Many factors contribute to this phenomenon. Sport-specific summer camps have become popular during which the young athlete is required to participate suddenly in intensive training, often without preconditioning. Many young athletes now participate on multiple teams and throughout the entire year. Particularly at risk are those young athletes who demonstrate above-average skills. These outstanding young players are called on to perform too often. Coaches and parents are often guilty of trying to create an all-star athlete or to have a winning team while not understanding the potential risk of injury to a talented young player. All these factors contribute to potential overuse problems from excessive throwing and too little time for recovery.

Poor throwing techniques increase the stresses on the elbow beyond normal limits, making it it more susceptible to injury. In contrast, proper throwing techniques have been shown to reduce the incidence of injury in pitchers.[15] Analysis of the overhand pitching mechanism and the sidearm pitching mechanism has demonstrated that the sidearm motion is three times more likely to lead to elbow problems.[15] The type of pitch thrown can also increase the stresses on the elbow and focus these stresses in certain locations about the joint. At the end of the follow-through, the fastball pitch places more stress on the radiocapitellar joint because of terminal pronation, whereas the curveball creates more stress on the medial joint line because of terminal supination. Electromyographic and high-speed film analysis has shown that the forearm supination required to throw a curveball pitch creates higher stresses on the elbow than a fastball pitch.[13]

PHYSICAL EXAMINATION AND TREATMENT

The condition known as Little League elbow comprises a large group of injuries or disorders about the elbow joint

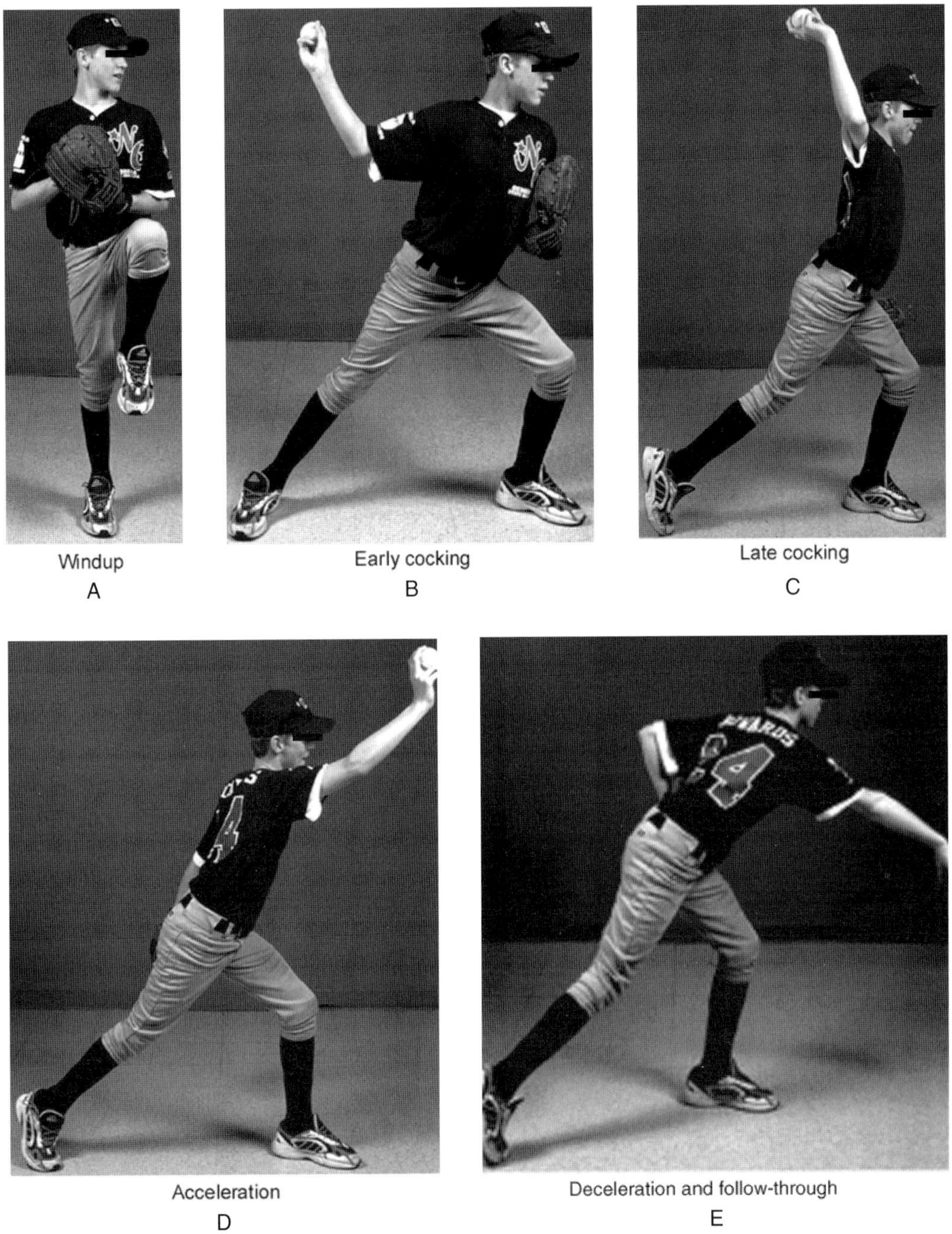

FIGURE 5.2. The five phases of the throwing motion: (A) windup; (B) early cocking; (C) late cocking; (D) acceleration; and (E) deceleration and follow-through.

in young throwing athletes. These entities are divided into three main groups based on anatomic location and mechanism of injury: medial tension injuries, lateral compression injuries, and posterior extension injuries. Comparative anteroposterior, lateral, axial, and oblique radiographic views are needed to evaluate elbow complaints in the young thrower.

Medial Tension Injuries (True Little League Elbow)

Medial tension injuries are the most common entities associated with Little League elbow. Young throwers typically present with the classic history triad of medial elbow pain, decreased throwing effectiveness, and de-

FIGURE 5.3. (A) Anterior view of the elbow demonstrating medial and lateral forces placed on the elbow structures during the throwing motion. (B) Posterior view of the elbow showing forces typically placed on the elbow structures during the late cocking and acceleration phases. The valgus load can cause impingement at the posteromedial ulnohumeral articulation and lead to osteophyte formation.

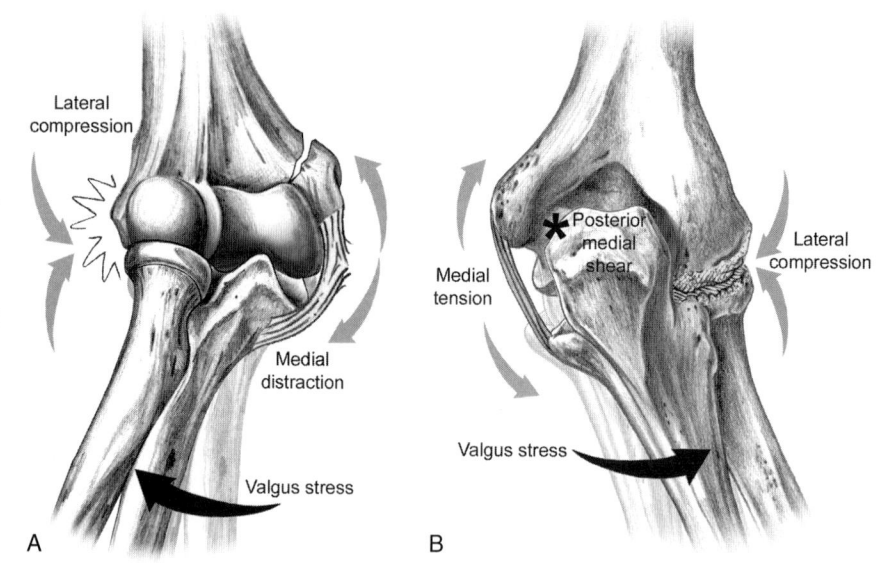

creased throwing distance. The physical examination includes a complete evaluation of the upper extremity from the neck down to the hand.

Medial Epicondylar Osteochondrosis (Stress Injury)

The physical examination reveals point tenderness at the medial epicondyle and pain with resisted flexion and pronation, as well as with valgus stress at 25° of elbow flexion. Often there is a flexion contracture of less than 15°. The radiographs show fragmentation and widening of the medial epicondylar physis. If uncertainty exists, a bone scan or magnetic resonance imaging (MRI) may be helpful in identifying an injury.

The treatment is always nonoperative and includes 4 to 6 weeks of relative rest (wrist and elbow range of motion are maintained), ice massage, and nonsteroidal anti-inflammatory medication or acetaminophen until tenderness of the medial epicondyle subsides. After the symptoms resolve, a gradual return to throwing is begun using a supervised interval-throwing program. Anytime a young thrower is seen for elbow complaints, a proper evaluation of throwing technique by a trained throwing coach or therapist is mandatory to assure that he or she is using proper mechanics.

Medial Epicondylar Avulsion

Examination demonstrates point tenderness at the medial epicondyle and exacerbation of pain with resisted wrist flexion and pronation; valgus stress at 25° is frequently found. In patients with a complete medial epicondylar avulsion, a medial aspect hematoma can be seen on inspection, and grating can be noted with range of motion if the fragment is in the joint.

Radiographs may show widening of the medial epicondyle and, in the case of complete avulsion, there will be displacement of the medial epicondyle from its actual posteromedial position in the humerus. Avulsion fractures are commonly displaced into the normal position of the trochlear ossification center. Because the medial epicondylar nucleus appears before the trochlear center, any radiograph showing the presence of a trochlear center and no medial epicondylar center indicates a dislocated avulsion fracture of the medial epicondyle. The medial epicondyle is extra-articular, and no fat pad sign will be visible. If there is any question concerning the presence or position of an apophyseal or epiphyseal growth center in any of these entities, a contralateral elbow series should be obtained for comparison. Tomograms, computed tomography (CT) scans, and MRI are rarely needed for evaluation of medial epicondylar avulsions. If injury to the ligament is of concern, a CT arthrogram or contrast-enhanced MRI may be used to diagnose undersurface medial collateral ligament (MCL) tears, and MRI is the study of choice for suspected complete MCL tears.[16–18]

The treatment of medial epicondylar avulsion is based on the amount of fragment displacement. This treatment guideline is used for young throwing athletes who continue to place high demands on their elbows through future sports participation, and greater amounts of displacement may be acceptable for nonoperative treatment in a nonathletic child. For minimal displacement (<2 mm), a posterior splint is applied with the elbow flexed slightly less than 90° to relax the flexor–pronator group for 2 to 3 weeks. After 2 weeks, range of motion exercises are begun and are advanced as tolerated by the patient. At 6 weeks, radiographs are taken to assess healing. The athlete can start an interval-throwing program at 8 weeks if the fracture has healed and is painless. A full return to competition is permitted at 12 weeks.

When there is significant displacement (>2mm), open reduction and internal fixation are recommended. In addition, a relative indication for open reduction and internal fixation is the presence of ulnar nerve dysfunction.[19,20]

The operation is performed through a medial incision centered over the medial epicondyle. The fragment is usually displaced anterior and distally and is reduced to its posteromedial location by holding it with a towel clip while flexing and pronating the forearm. The fixation is achieved with one or more cannulated 3.0-mm AO screws, depending on the fragment size (Fig. 5.4). The ulnar nerve is identified and protected throughout the procedure. It is important to preserve the medial antebrachial cutaneous nerve during the superficial dissection to avoid bothersome neuromas. After the completion of the procedure, the elbow is splinted for 2 weeks. Range of motion is started after 2 weeks and rehabilitation continues as described above for minimally displaced avulsion fractures.

Other Associated Entities

Ulnar neuritis is less common in young throwers than in adult throwers. Subluxation of the nerve can contribute to the problem, but be aware that 30% of the adolescent population has asymptomatic subluxation.[21] Players often relay a history of numbness and tingling in the ring and long fingers, weakness and clumsiness of the hand after throwing, and a snapping sensation in the elbow during the acceleration phase. Examination may demonstrate sensory changes in the ulnar distribution, possible muscle atrophy, and a positive Tinel's sign at the cubital tunnel. An electromyographic (EMG) study confirms the diagnosis. Treatment of ulnar neuritis is nonoperative, consisting of rest, nonsteroindal anti-inflammatory medication, immobilization in a sling or splint for 2 to 3 weeks, if necessary, followed by a gradual return to a throwing program. Recurrence is common and is usually due to underlying medial collateral ligament laxity or poor throwing mechanics, both of which increase valgus stresses that place the nerve on stretch. Symptomatic subluxation without underlying laxity in young players can be treated with ulnar nerve transposition with good results.[22]

Other manifestations of medial tension stresses are medial prominence overgrowth, which is a cosmesis problem, and delayed closure of the medial epicondylar growth plate, which is more of a radiological finding than a functional problem.[19]

Medial collateral ligament injuries in young players are rare but, when present, they should be treated with repair or reconstruction based on the tear sites.[5] If the injury is treated surgically, the postoperative splint is removed at 2 weeks and a valgus-stress-preventing brace is applied for 4 weeks. At this time, rehabilitation begins.

Complications associated with the medial tension injuries are loss of motion, specifically the final 5° to 10° of extension, ligament ossification, and valgus instability. In medial epicondylar avulsions that have been treated surgically, painful retained hardware should be removed after the fracture has healed.

Lateral Compression Injuries

The entities associated with lateral compression injuries are osteochondritis dissecans, osteochondrosis of the capitellum, and osteochondrosis or deformation of the radial head.

Osteochondritis Dissecans (OCD) of the Capitellum

The repetitive lateral compression forces placed on the elbow with throwing result in microfractures of the capitellar cartilage surface and subsequent edema of the underlying bone. This edema produces avascular necrosis because of the precarious circulation in the epiphyseal vessels of the developing capitellum. In advanced cases, this process can result in loose-body formation.

The patient is usually older than 13 years of age and presents with an insidious onset of poorly localized lateral elbow pain while throwing. The physical examination reveals radiocapitellar tenderness and possible joint effusion. In a series by Gill and Micheli, 79% of the cases revealed effusion and radiocapitellar tenderness.[8] The patient's range of motion is diminished. There can be a progressive flexion contracture (>15°) and, sometimes, locking or catching from loose bodies.[5,23]

In these patients, radiographs show mottling at an early stage. Radiographic changes seen in later stages of the process are opacification, a focal area of involvement in the capitellum with well-defined sclerotic borders (Fig. 5.5), loose bodies, and an enlarged radial head in advanced cases. Tomograms are very sensitive for this condition.[13] CT arthrography is useful for identifying loose bodies without calcification. Magnetic resonance imag-

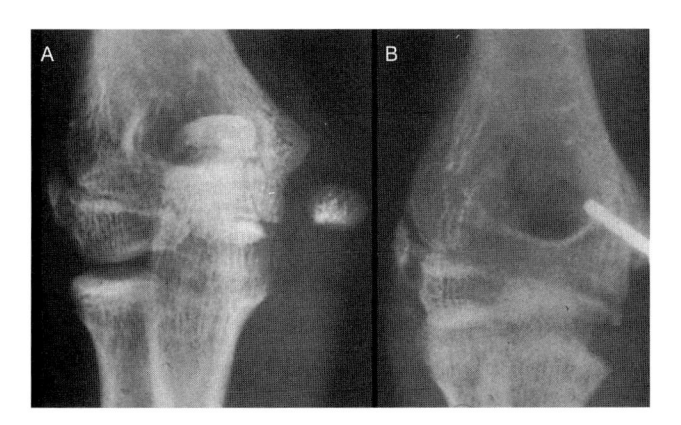

FIGURE 5.4. (A) Anteroposterior radiograph of a displaced medial epicondyle fracture. (B) Postoperative radiograph shows fracture fixation with a single screw after open reduction and internal fixation.

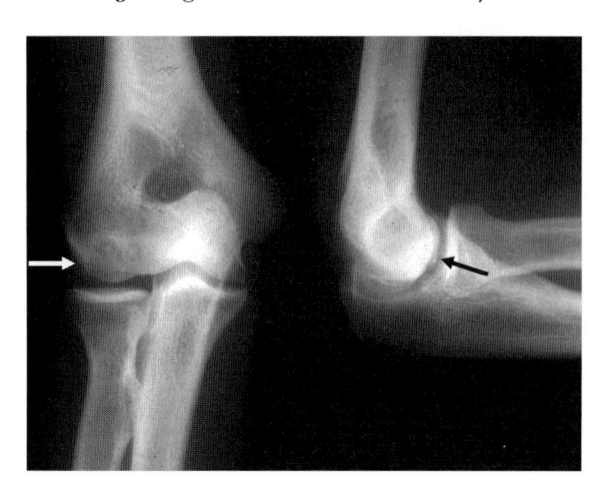

FIGURE 5.5. Anteroposterior and lateral radiographs show osteochondritis dissecans of the capitellum. Arrow indicates area of lesion.

ing is not only helpful in confirming the diagnosis of OCD lesions, but in preoperative staging of the lesion and assessment of the status of overlying cartilage[10,16] (Fig. 5.6).

The lesions are grouped into three stages based on the characteristics of the articular cartilage. This classification is used to direct treatment. In stage I, the articular surface is intact, and there is no subchondral displacement or fracture. Stage II lesions have articular surface fractures and fissuring. There may be partial detachment of a fragment. In stage III, the chondral or osteochondral fragments have become unstable and detached, producing intra-articular loose bodies.

The treatment for a stage I lesion is splinting for 4 weeks, followed by rest and range of motion for another 4 weeks. After 8 weeks, a follow-up radiograph is taken to assess evidence of revascularization and healing. If the patient is still symptomatic after 8 weeks, arthroscopic retrograde drilling is recommended.

The treatment for a stage II lesion is open drilling of the subchondral bed and stabilization of the partially detached lesion with one or more compression screws. Consideration should be given to the use of bioabsorbable screws. If the surgeon is unable to stabilize the lesion, it is treated as a stage III lesion. The stage III treatment involves arthroscopic or open removal of the loose bodies and microfracture or drilling of the lesion. Occasionally, the loose fragment is large enough and its quality is good enough to consider reduction and fixation. The use of osteochondral autografts or allografts is still experimental.

Immediately after surgery, the patient begins gentle passive range-of-motion exercises. The patient progresses to active-assisted range-of-motion exercises, as tolerated, during the first week. After the second week, emphasis is placed on improving strength and endurance. The preparation of the athlete to return to functional activities begins when he or she achieves full, nonpainful range of motion and strength, usually after the sixth week. The athlete starts a supervised interval-throwing program at approximately the eighth week and progresses to full activity, as tolerated.

The ability to return to throwing sports depends on the age of the patient (the likelihood of healing is better for younger patients), the stage of the lesion, and the presence or absence of symptoms.[24,25] Although OCD is the leading cause of permanent elbow disability in throwing athletes, 85% of those treated with the excision and drilling return to throwing competitively in 6 to 12 months.[26]

A common complication of this condition and its treatment is an elbow flexion contracture. Flexion contracture is caused by the intimate congruency of the elbow complex, the tightness of its capsule, and a tendency of the anterior capsule to scar and form adhesions. Emphasis on early range of motion, elbow mobilization, and low-load, long-duration stretching is instituted in nonoperatively and operatively treated patients to avoid capsular restrictions. Radiological arthritic changes can occur in up to half of these patients regardless of treatment. Early detection and prevention are the best way to avoid these complications.

Osteochondrosis of the Capitellum (Panner's Disease)

Panner's disease is a condition of the growing elbow that is often compared with Legg–Calvé–Perthes disease in the hip. It most often occurs in children between 7 and 12 years of age and is usually atraumatic and self-limiting (3-year period). The process begins with resorption followed by fragmentation, regeneration, and, finally, recalcification. The patient presents with a dull lateral ache,

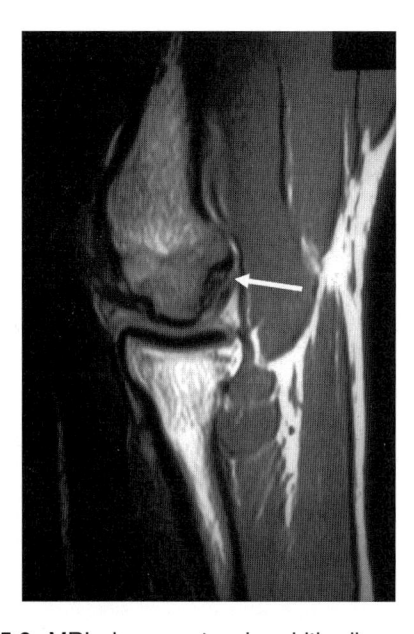

FIGURE 5.6. MRI shows osteochondritis dissecans of the capitellum. Arrow indicates area of lesion.

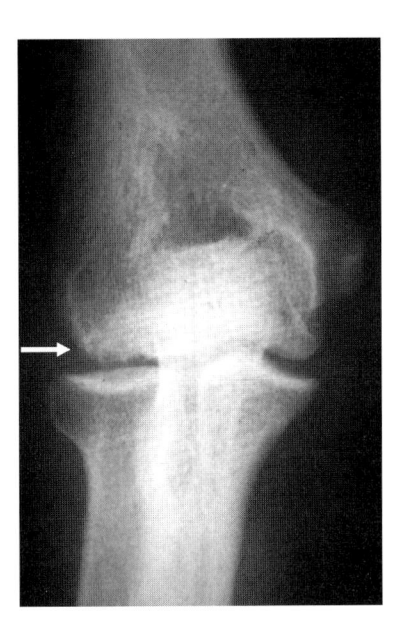

FIGURE 5.7. Anteroposterior radiograph shows typical lesion of the capitellum (arrow) in a patient with Panner's disease.

a swollen elbow, and lack of extension. Radiographs show capitellar epiphyseal fragmentation and patchy rarefaction[5,25,26] (Fig. 5.7). After ruling out OCD, treatment is always nonoperative and consists of rest until symptoms subside, followed by range-of-motion exercises and a supervised throwing program when the patient achieves pain-free motion and healing is evident on radiographs. The prognosis is favorable for relief of symptoms and return to play with excellent functional results.

Radial Head Osteochondrosis or Deformation

Injury to the radial head results from the lateral compressive forces, as well. These changes can occur in association with OCD lesions of the capitellum. The ossific nucleus of the radial head appears later than the ossific nucleus of the humeral capitellum.[5] Moreover, the surface area of the capitellum is greater than that of the radial head.[27] These factors concentrate lateral compression stresses on the epiphyseal plate of the radial head, leading to growth disturbances and angulation.[11] The plasticity of the immature skeleton allows greater deformation of the articular surface when subjected to the chronic repetitive stress, which in turn results in more pronounced damage.[11]

The patient presents with diffuse dull pain and some joint stiffness. There is limitation of extension that increases with time and eventually interferes with sport participation. Some may show spontaneous locking and joint effusion.

When the radial head is ossified in a juvenile baseball player, radiographs show anterior angulation of the radial head.[27] In these patients, OCD and even formation of loose bodies can occur later in life.

The treatment is nonoperative with rest until symptoms resolve, and an interval-throwing program is begun when the patient achieves a normal range of motion and strength. In patients in whom loose bodies or OCD lesions are present, the treatment is arthroscopic removal and drilling of the lesion.

Although this condition has excellent functional results after treatment, the patient might have loss of motion secondary to residual radial head spurring and anterior angulation.

Posterior Extension Injuries

Olecranon Apophysitis and Triceps Strain

This entity is the result of repetitive posterior tension and shear forces applied to the developing olecranon apophysis through the pull of the triceps in children younger than 13 years of age. Excessive force during the late cocking and acceleration phases of throwing can lead to failure at the olecranon apophysis or triceps tendon insertion.[5] This condition is similar to Osgood–Schlatter's disease of the tibial tubercle.[3]

The patient presents with vague posterior elbow pain and an inability to fully extend the elbow. The physical examination reveals tenderness at the olecranon or triceps insertion, or both, and pain with elbow extension against resistance. The radiographs show an irregular pattern of olecranon apophysis ossification (sclerosis, widening, or fragmentation) compared with the uninvolved side. An MRI shows apophyseal edema or physeal separation, triceps tendon edema (tendinosis), and degeneration or detachment.

This condition responds well to rest while preserving wrist and elbow motion, ice, nonsteroidal anti-inflammatory medication, and a carefully monitored rehabilitation that includes a return-to-throwing program. Treatment for olecranon avulsion consists of cast immobilization for 3 to 4 weeks. If the displacement is greater than 4 to 5 mm or if the elbow fails to heal despite cast immobilization, surgery is warranted.

Open reduction and internal fixation are performed using either a compression screw or the tension-band technique (use of suture is acceptable). In chronic cases, bone grafting is indicated. This treatment does not affect longitudinal growth because the proximal ulnar physis growth contribution is minimal. When the triceps tendon is avulsed or partially detached, debridement or reattachment may be necessary. Postoperatively, a splint is used for 10 days, after which protected range of motion is begun. Radiographs are taken at 8 weeks to document healing. An interval-throwing program is started at 10 weeks with progression to full activity. Return to play is allowed if there is full and painless range of motion and 90% strength in the injured extremity when compared with the uninjured extremity.

Olecranon Oblique Fracture

These fractures most commonly occur in adolescents (>13 years). They are caused by impaction of the posteromedial olecranon on the medial wall of the olecranon fossa and by impingement of the lateral aspect of the coronoid on the intercondylar notch during resistance to valgus stress.[28]

The patient presents with pain that is worse during the acceleration phase of the pitching motion and an inability to perform at his or her previous level. The physical examination reveals tenderness over the olecranon and sometimes along the anterior band of the medial collateral ligament. Radiographs show an oblique-type fracture with sclerotic changes along the fracture line. If the radiographs fail to show the fracture, a tomogram should be obtained to make the diagnosis.

Although the initial treatment is nonoperative with a combination of rest, stretching, and anti-inflammatory medication for 4 weeks, Suzuki and associates suggest early surgical treatment.[28] If the fracture fails to heal, it is bone grafted and fixed internally with a compression screw across the fracture line. If present, partial injuries to the medial collateral ligament heal spontaneously with the treatment of the fracture and therefore do not require specific treatment.[28]

Complications from these lesions are the result of the operative treatment itself. As with any other surgery requiring hardware placement around the elbow, pain from hardware is the most common complication. This is treated by removal after the fracture has healed, as determined on radiographs. Spur formation secondary to overgrowth of the olecranon epiphysis can occur.[19] In some patients, it becomes symptomatic and may have to be excised. Apophyseal arrest rarely occurs and does not have a significant effect on elbow function.

SUMMARY

Immature throwers are different anatomically, biomechanically, and biochemically from adult throwers. Consequently, the growing child is vulnerable to many different and unique musculoskeletal lesions about the elbow as a result of the medial tension, lateral compression, and posterior shear forces repetitively encountered during the throwing motion. An understanding of the biomechanics of the throwing motion and an in-depth knowledge of the developing anatomy of the elbow and how it relates to the temporal radiographic findings are combined to delineate how various musculotendinous, ulnar nerve, medial epicondylar, lateral compression, and olecranon injuries can occur. This understanding and knowledge are paramount to the physician who evaluates and treats the young thrower's elbow. Such knowledge also reinforces the importance of proper overhand throwing technique in reducing potential injury in immature athletes.

Early recognition and treatment are vital because most entities of Little League elbow respond to nonoperative treatment. Early treatment can also reduce long-term sequelae, such as ulnar neuritis, valgus instability, valgus deformity, loose bodies, osteophyte formation, flexion contracture, flexor–pronator musculotendinous problems, residual pain, and loss of supination and pronation, that cause functional disability and permanent deformity. Although early recognition and treatment of Little League elbow entities is important, prevention is really the answer to reducing the risk of developing the associated problems.

Overuse and improper throwing mechanics are the most common risk factors for developing elbow problems and, because they are preventable, certain guidelines and recommendations are necessary. Children usually have less coordination and slower reaction times and therefore a decreased ability to throw accurately and use proper mechanics. Because most young pitchers throw with more enthusiasm than skill, supervised coaching should emphasize proper basic overhand throwing mechanics and concentrate on accuracy. Young players should be advised to avoid sidearm and curveball pitches. They should focus on fastball and change-up (off-speed) pitches. Presently, the American Little League guidelines limit a pitcher to six innings of pitching per week, which is equal to 18 to 200 pitches. This does not account for warm-up pitches, hard throws from other positions, pitches or hard throws in practice, or pitches thrown while participating in another league. The Japanese recommend counting both pitches and hard throws as a total number (not to exceed 300 per week) and, because of this, it may be a better guideline. Rest periods between pitching appearances are mandatory. Training should not increase throwing by more than 10% per week, and conditioning should be done before intensive summer camp participation or competitive league play.

Enforcing these guidelines is very difficult, and it is up to local program directors, parents, and coaches to adhere to it. As physicians, we must educate those who are responsible for young athletes about the possibility of overuse injuries that result from excessive pitching and throwing and poor throwing mechanics.

REFERENCES

1. Gugenheim JJ, Stanley RF, Woods GW, Tullow HS. Little League survey: the Houston study. *Am J Sports Med* 1976;4: 189–200.

2. Torg JS, Pollack H, Sweterlitsch P. The effects of competitive pitching on the shoulders and elbows of preadolescent baseball players. *Pediatrics* 1972;49:267.
3. Adams JR. Injury of the throwing arm: a study of traumatic changes in the elbow joint of boy baseball players. *Calif Med* 1965:102–127.
4. Larson RL, Singer KLM, Bergstrom R, Thomas S. Little League survey: the Eugene study. *Am J Sports Med.* 1976;4: 201–209.
5. Brogdon BE, Crow WF. Little Leaguer's elbow. *Am J Roentgenol* 1960;63:671–675.
6. Gray DJ, Gardner E. Prenatal development of the human elbow joint. *Am J Anat* 1951;88:429–469.
7. Haraldsson S. On osteochondrosis deformans juvenilis capituli humeri including investigation of intraosseous vasculature. *Acta Orthop Scand (Suppl.)* 1946;38:1–232.
8. Gill TJ, Micheli LJ. The immature athlete. *Clin Sports Med* 1996;15:401–423.
9. DiGiovine NM, Jobe PW. An electromylographic analysis of the upper extremity on pitching. *J Shoulder Elbow Surg* 1992; 1:15–25.
10. Caldwell GL Jr., Safran MR. Elbow problems in the athlete. *Orthop Clin North Am* 1995;26:465–485.
11. Maffulli N, Chan D, Aldridge MJ. Derangement of the articular surfaces or the elbow in young gymnasts. *J Pediatr Orthop* 1992;12:344–350.
12. Priest JD. Elbow injuries in gymnastics. *Clin Sports Med* 1985;4:73–81.
13. DaSilva MF, Williams JS, Fadale PD, Hulstyn MJ, Ehrlich MG. Pediatric throwing injuries about the elbow. *Am J Orthop* 1998;27:90–96.
14. Micheli LJ. Overuse injuries in children's sports: The growth factor. *Orthop Clin North Am* 1983;14:337–360.
15. Albright IA, et al. Clinical study of baseball pitchers. *Am J Sports Med* 1978;6:15–21.
16. Patten RM. Overuse syndromes and injuries involving the elbow: MR imaging findings. *Am J Roentgenol* 1995;164:1205–1211.
17. Sugimoto H, Ohsawa T. Ulnar collateral ligament in the growing elbow: MR imaging of normal development and throwing injuries. *Radiol* 1994;1992:417–422.
18. Timmerman LA, Schwartz ML, Andrews JR. Preoperative evaluation of the ulnar collateral ligament by magnetic resonance imaging and computed tomography arthrography. *Am J Sports Med* 1994;22:26–32.
19. Rockwood CA, Wilkins KE. *Fractures in children,* 4th ed. Philadelphia: Lippincott-Raven; 1996: p. 814.
20. Schwab GH, Bennett JB, Woods GW, Tullos HS. Biomechanics of elbow instability: the role of the medial collateral ligament. *Clin Orthop* 1980;146:42–52.
21. Gerbino PG, Waters PM. Elbow injuries in young athletes. *Op Tech Sports Med* 1998;6(4):259–267.
22. Jobe FW, Fanton GS. Nerve injuries. In Morrey BF, ed. *The elbow and its disorders*, 1st ed. Philadelphia: WB Saunders; 1985:497–501.
23. Brown R, Blazina ME, Kerlan RK, et al. Osteochondritis of the capitellum. *J Sports Med* 1974;2:27–46.
24. Renstrom P. Swedish research in sports traumatology. *Clin Orthop* 1984;191:144–158.
25. Tivnon MC, Anzel SH, Waugh TR. Surgical management of osteochondritis dissecans of the capitellum. *Am J Sports Med* 1976;4:121–128.
26. McManama GB, Micheli LJ, Berry MV, Sohn RS. The surgical treatment of osteochondritis of the capitellum. *Am J Sports Med* 1985;13:11–21.
27. Morrey BF, An KN. Stability of the elbow joint: a biomechanical assessment. *Am J Sports Med* 1983;11:315–319.
28. Suzuki K, Minami A, Suenaga N, Kondoh M. Oblique stress fracture of the olecranon in baseball pitchers. *J Shoulder Elbow Surg* 1997;6:491–494.

CHAPTER 6

Lateral and Medial Epicondylitis

George M. McCluskey III and Michael S. Merkley

INTRODUCTION

Lateral and medial epicondylitis are diagnostic terms that describe the constellation of pain and localized tenderness at the epicondyles of the distal humerus. Major originally coined the term **tennis elbow** in 1883.[1] This eponym remains despite the fact that 95% of affected people are not tennis players.[2] However, 10% to 50% of persons who regularly play tennis will, at some time, experience symptoms characteristic of this disorder.[3]

Lateral epicondylitis is far more common than medial epicondylitis, with ratios of reported incidences ranging from 4:1 to 7:1.[4-6] The incidence is equal among men and women, with male tennis players affected more often than female players. The average peak age distribution is 42 years (range, 30 to 50 years). A bimodal distribution is present: acute onset of symptoms is much more common in young athletes, and the chronic, recalcitrant pattern most often occurs in older individuals.

The cause of the disorder seems to be repetitive eccentric or concentric overloading of the flexor or extensor muscle masses. It affects the dominant extremity twice as often as the nondominant extremity. Most cases are related to occupational exposure and cause subacute or chronic symptoms. Only 10% to 20% of patients, usually young tennis players (lateral) or throwing athletes (medial),[4] have an acute injury.

In athletes, the occurrence of lateral epicondylitis is almost exclusively limited to tennis players. The pain commonly is felt on the backhand stroke when the wrist extensors are actively stabilizing the racquet to absorb the impact from the ball. If medial epicondylitis is present in a tennis player, the pain can be reproduced on the forehand, serve, or overhead stroke.[5]

Medial epicondylitis can affect golfers or throwing athletes. Baseball pitchers and javelin hurlers are particularly susceptible, because their specialized throwing styles place considerable strain on the flexor–pronator origin. The valgus overload that these throwing motions produce also predisposes athletes to acute or chronic medial ligamentous insufficiency.

In 1969, Nirschl reported his observation of "mesenchymal syndrome."[7] This term described a subset of patients who seemed predisposed to tendinitis. Repetitive overuse of the affected extremities commonly was not present. This unique group of patients constituted about 15% of cases. The involved patient typically was a woman between 35 and 55 years of age. In these patients, Nirschl identified varying combinations of disorders, including rotator cuff tendinopathy, medial epicondylitis, ulnar neuropathy, lateral epicondylitis, carpal tunnel syndrome, DeQuervain's tenosynovitis, and trigger finger. Almost invariably, the rheumatologic evaluation was negative. This finding led to the postulation that constitutional factors, such as estrogen deficiency or a hereditary predisposition to tendon degeneration, predisposed a patient to generalized tendinitis.

In this chapter, we discuss the pathology, clinical presentation, and treatment of lateral and medial epicondylitis. After briefly describing nonoperative treatment, we focus on the operative techniques for treating these disorders and touch on postoperative care, results, and failures.

PATHOLOGY

Although the term **epicondylitis** implies the presence of an inflammatory condition, inflammation is present only in the earliest stages of the disease process. In 1936, Cyriax postulated that microscopic or macroscopic tears of the common extensor origin were involved in the disease process.[8] However, he made this report without studying any diseased or surgical specimens. Goldie,[9] Coonrad and

Hooper,[2] and Nirschl and Pettrone[10] demonstrated that the condition is actually a degenerative tendinopathy. Goldie[9] described granulation tissue found at the extensor carpi radialis brevis (ECRB) origin, but did not describe any tearing of the tissue. Coonrad and Hooper first described macroscopic tearing in association with the histologic findings in 1973.[2] Nirschl termed this histologic process "angiofibroblastic tendinosis." It is characterized by disorganized, immature collagen formation with immature fibroblastic and vascular elements.[3] This gray, friable tissue is found in association with varying degrees of tearing in the involved tendinous origins. The most common anatomic locations of the tendinosis are the ECRB tendon laterally and the pronator teres and flexor carpi radialis medially. Universally, the ECRB tendon is involved in lateral epicondylitis.[11] A bony exostosis, or traction spur, can be identified at the lateral epicondyle in 20% of patients.

CLINICAL PRESENTATION OF LATERAL EPICONDYLITIS

Clinically, a patient who has lateral epicondylitis presents with pain localized to the lateral epicondyle. Wrist extensor activity provokes pain. A subjective feeling of wrist weakness may be present and may or may not correlate with strength testing. The pain may radiate into the extensor mass or proximally to the elbow. On physical examination, localized tenderness at the ECRB origin must be present to make the diagnosis. This origin is located just distal and slightly anterior to the lateral epicondyle. Resisted wrist extension with the forearm in pronation and elbow extended (Thomsen maneuver) should reproduce the patient's pain. If this does not reproduce the patient's symptoms, the examining physician should reconsider the diagnosis of lateral epicondylitis. Resisted supination commonly reproduces the pain as well. In chronic cases, a mild flexion contracture may be present at the elbow. Coonrad[12] believed that the "coffee cup" test was pathognomonic. He described this test as lateral epicondylar pain aggravated by lifting a full coffee cup.

The radiocapitellar joint should be examined to rule out intra-articular abnormalities. If tenderness is present over the course of the radial nerve or is more than 1 to 2 cm distal to the epicondyle, radial nerve entrapment may be present. Pain on resisted supination or with resisted long-finger extension suggests this disorder. The coincidence of radial nerve entrapment with lateral epicondylitis has been reported as 5%.[4] In our experience, pain on resisted long-finger extension often accompanies pain on resisted wrist extension and may represent involvement of the common extensor tendon. Common extensor tendon involvement is present in 35% of surgical patients.[3]

The differential diagnosis of lateral elbow pain is extensive. A thorough history and physical examination are necessary to localize the cause. In patients who have lateral ligamentous instability, an initial traumatic event is usually present. Intra-articular abnormalities, such as osteochondritis dissecans, loose bodies, degenerative arthritis, or radiocapitellar chondromalacia can present with mechanical symptoms. Cervical radiculopathy rarely can mimic the pain of lateral epicondylitis. Provocative maneuvers for lateral epicondylitis typically do not reproduce the patient's pain. Local nerve entrapment syndromes, such as those involving the posterior interosseous, radial, or lateral antebrachial cutaneous nerves, may occur concomitantly and be discerned by careful examination.

CLINICAL PRESENTATION OF MEDIAL EPICONDYLITIS

Medial epicondylitis is also known as **golfer's elbow**. It is far less common than lateral epicondylitis. Typically, the patient profile is similar to that for lateral epicondylitis. The exception is the young (i.e., 15 to 25 years of age) throwing athlete who presents with either acute or subacute onset of symptoms.

Tenderness is present at the origin of the common flexor tendon at the medial epicondyle. Resisted wrist flexion with the forearm supinated or resisted pronation reproduces the patient's pain. The examining physician should carefully evaluate the ulnar nerve for signs of neuritis because these conditions commonly coexist. Nirschl reported a 60% incidence of ulnar nerve entrapment in association with medial epicondylitis.[11] Most commonly, the site of entrapment was distal to the medial epicondyle (Nirschl's zone III) where the nerve passes between the heads of the flexor carpi ulnaris. In throwing athletes, assessing the integrity of the ulnar collateral ligament is imperative. With the wrist in flexion and the forearm in pronation, the physician applies a valgus force to the slightly flexed elbow. In patients who have medial ligamentous insufficiency, opening of the joint and pain is evidenced. This test should not cause pain in isolated medial epicondylitis.

NONOPERATIVE TREATMENT

Almost all cases of epicondylitis initially should be managed nonoperatively. Exceptions may be made for elite or upper-level athletes who have acute ruptures. With appropriate nonoperative treatment, a success rate of more than 90% can be expected. A combination of patient education, anti-inflammatory agents, orthoses, and physical therapy exercises and modalities can be used. Most importantly, the patient must avoid provocative activities. The patient should be counseled regarding the expected course and duration of the disorder. Primarily, the goal of treatment is relief of pain. For mild or moderate symptoms, treatment includes rest, ice, and anti-inflammatory medications. A counterforce brace or wrist extension splint may be added at the physician's discretion. If pain is severe or symptoms persist after 3 months of appropriate treatment, then a corticosteroid injection is recommended. Subcutaneous deposition of the injection must be avoided to prevent hypopigmentation (Fig. 6.1) and fat atrophy. An increase in pain is expected after the injection, but should resolve by 8 to 12 hours. The patient should be counseled appropriately.

Improved throwing mechanics and endurance exercises are stressed for throwers. The importance of a proper warm-up and stretching cannot be overemphasized. For tennis players, alterations in grip size, racquet weight, and string tension are significant for the treatment and prevention of lateral epicondylitis.

Once pain and tenderness have been reduced, a regimented physical therapy program is initiated. As part of the program, the patient begins muscle stretching and gradual strengthening exercises. Counterforce bracing (Fig. 6.2) is employed during rehabilitation. A combination of isotonic and isometric exercises is used. Initially, the patient's opposite hand should provide resistance. As strength increases, a program involving dumbbell weights in 1-lb increments can be implemented. Repetitions are increased as the patient can tolerate them. If pain returns at any time, a return to a lower level of exercise is indicated. If pain persists despite the decreased activity level,

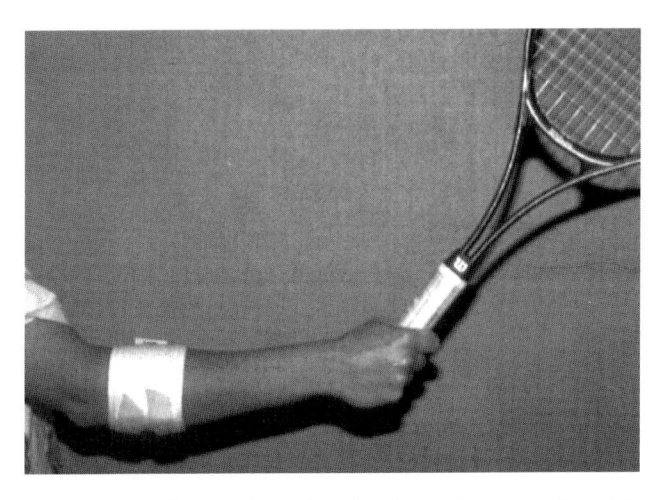

FIGURE 6.2. Counterforce bracing is used as an adjunct to rest and rehabilitation in treating tendinosis of the elbow.

the physician should consider administering another corticosteroid injection. Therapeutic modalities are added at the physician's discretion.

OPERATIVE TREATMENT

Indications

Pain that persists despite an adequate period of nonoperative treatment is the main indication for surgical intervention. The pain must limit activity and function to the point where the patient's activity level and thus quality of life are unacceptable. The duration of what constitutes an adequate period of nonoperative treatment typically is at least 6 months. Patient compliance with activity modification and therapy exercises is mandatory. Failure to gain relief after corticosteroid injection is no longer considered an absolute indication for surgery.[4] Patients who have an acute onset of symptoms often do not respond to nonoperative treatment and may be considered candidates for earlier surgical intervention.

Contraindications to surgical treatment are a noncompliant patient who will not modify his or her activities or who has not completed an adequate nonoperative treatment program. Many individuals who have epicondylitis are involved in workers' compensation claims; therefore, secondary gain issues must be considered. Before considering surgical intervention in these patients, the surgeon should examine them many times and should closely monitor their nonoperative treatment program.

Procedures

Before considering surgery, the surgeon should re-examine the patient to confirm the exact location of the tenderness and to assess the results of provocative maneu-

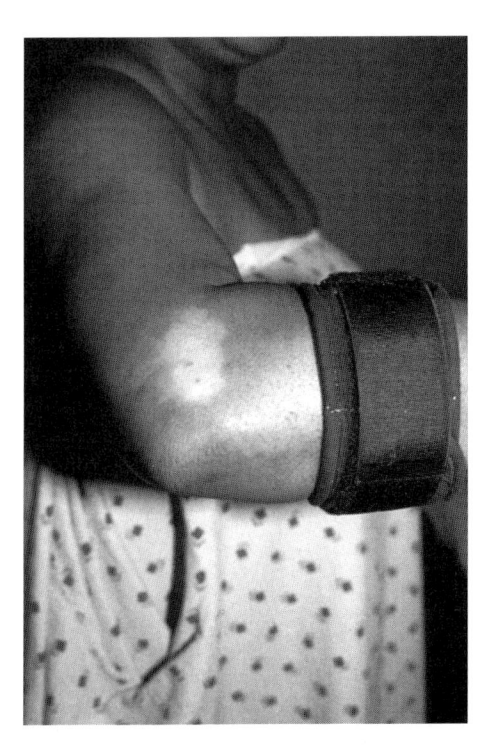

FIGURE 6.1. After an injection of the elbow for tendinopathy, subcutaneous deposition of the steroid can cause hypopigmentation of the skin in the area.

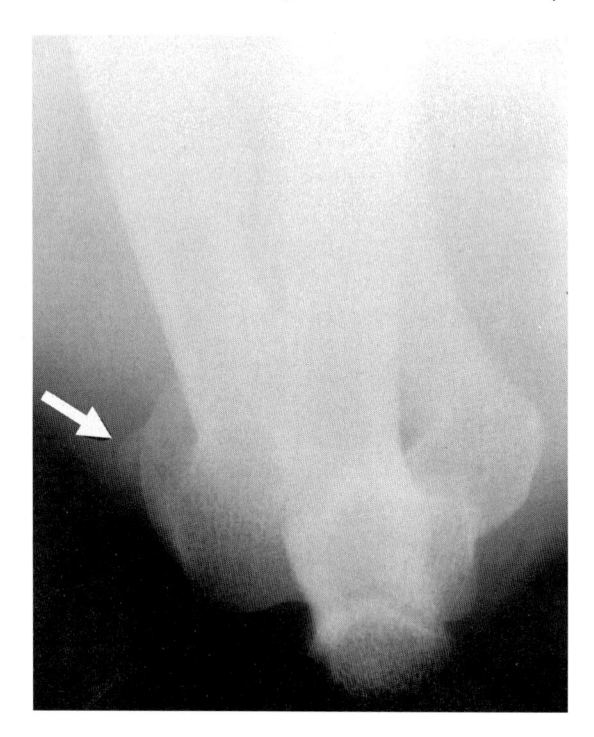

FIGURE 6.3. Axial view of the elbow reveals calcification at the lateral epicondylar extensor tendon attachment site. This finding suggests a chronic and advanced pathologic process.

vers to ensure that he or she has made the correct diagnosis. For patients who have medial epicondylitis, the presence of ulnar nerve symptoms and signs is important to note so that, if indicated, the nerve can be released appropriately. Quality anteroposterior, lateral, and oblique radiographic views should be assessed for the presence of calcification or a bony exostosis (Fig. 6.3). In patients who have medial epicondylitis, a cubital tunnel, or posteroanterior axial, view can be substituted for the oblique view.

Surgical treatment of lateral epicondylitis has been directed toward the structures that the surgeon believes are abnormal elements. Bosworth initially described excision of the orbicular ligament in 1955; he later modified his procedure to include release of the ECRB.[13] Other procedures involve removal of a radiohumeral bursa or excision of the radiohumeral synovial fringe.[4] Procedures to address possible neurologic causes include denervation by neurotomy of articular branches of the radial nerve[14] and radial tunnel release.[15]

Researchers widely accept that the ECRB is the location of the disease process, and current surgical approaches to lateral epicondylitis are directed at either complete removal of what is believed to be the diseased tissue, release of tension in the ECRB, or a combination of these techniques. Release of the ECRB or common extensor origin has been reported to give excellent pain relief, but concerns exist over possible weakening.[16] In Germany, Hohmann originally described lateral release of the common extensor origin in 1926.[17] Several authors have reported on variations of this procedure, with success rates generally around 90%. Percutaneous extensor tenotomy recently has been reported and can be performed as an office procedure. The authors reported a 93.5% success rate with at least 1-year follow-up in 109 patients.[18] Initially, authors reported that proximal extensor fasciotomy and distal ECRB lengthening gave good results.[19,20] However, further studies have been unable to reproduce these findings.[21]

The senior author (GMM) favors a surgical technique similar to the technique that Nirschl and Pettrone or Coonrad described.[10,12] Abnormal portions of the tendon are excised and, if the common extensor origin is violated, it is reattached. The goal is removal of all abnormal material and prevention of postoperative extensor weakness due to release of the common extensor tendon. Using this described technique, Nirschl and Pettrone reported 97% good to excellent results in a series of 88 patients.[10]

Lateral Epicondylitis Technique

The patient is placed in the supine position. A nonsterile tourniquet is used, and the arm is draped free on a hand table. The extremity is exsanguinated, and the tourniquet is inflated to 250 mm Hg. The lateral incision begins just anterior to the epicondyle and extends distally 3 to 4 cm (Fig. 6.4). Dissection is carried down through the subcutaneous tissue until the superficial fascia is identified. The superficial fascia is incised in line with the skin incision, and the interval between the extensor carpi radialis longus (ECRL) and the common extensor tendon is identified (Fig. 6.5). The ECRB tendon is under the ECRL at this point. The interval between the longus and the common extensor tendon is incised, extending from just anterior to the epicondyle to the level of the joint. The depth of this incision should be limited to 2 to 3 mm because the

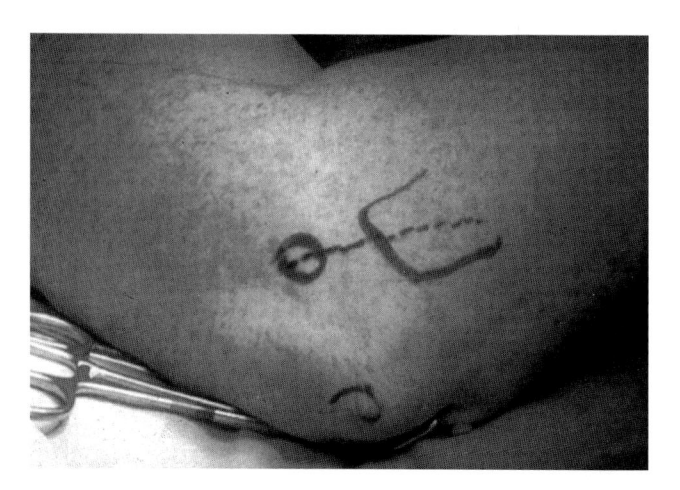

FIGURE 6.4. The lateral incision begins just anterior to the epicondyle and extends distally for about 4 cm.

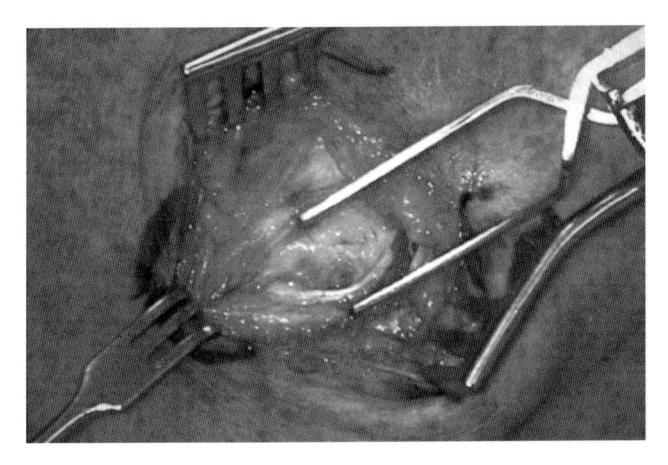

FIGURE 6.5. The interval between the common extensor aponeurosis and the extensor carpi radialis longus is incised.

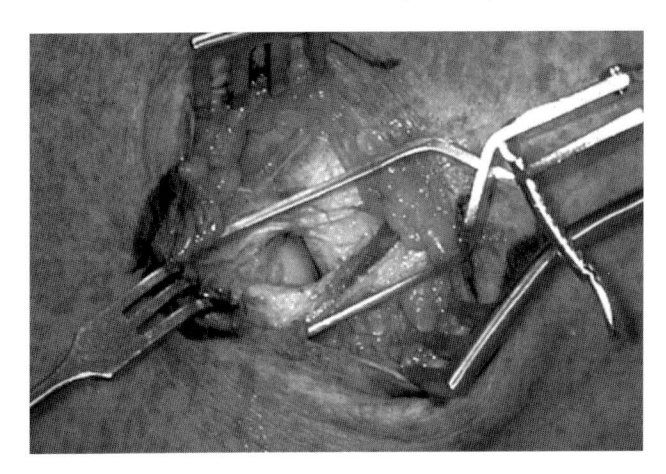

FIGURE 6.7. Pathologic tissue involving the extensor carpi radialis brevis tendon and occasionally the common extensor tendon should be excised. The lateral intra-articular compartment of the elbow joint should also be inspected following incision of the capsule.

ECRL is very thin at this point. Next, the ECRL is elevated sharply and retracted anteriorly to expose the ECRB tendon (Fig. 6.6).

The entire origin of the brevis tendon should be exposed. At this point, abnormal tissue should be identified (Fig. 6.7). Universally, the ECRB is involved, and in 35% of patients the anterior edge of the common extensor aponeurosis concurrently is affected.[11] Abnormal tissue is identified by its dull gray hue and edematous, friable consistency.[3] Typically, this tissue is easily distinguished from the surrounding normal tendon. The affected tendon is excised completely. This excision usually involves releasing the tendon origin from the epicondyle and the anterior edge of the extensor aponeurosis. If the aponeurosis is involved, this abnormal tissue is also excised.

In about 20% of patients, an exostosis is present at the lateral epicondyle. In this case, the leading edge of the aponeurosis is elevated sharply from the epicondyle, and the prominence is removed by rongeur and smoothed with a rasp. The aponeurosis is reattached later through drill holes or using suture anchors into the epicondyle.

Resection of the diseased tissue leaves a defect at the origin of the ECRB tendon. The tendon does not shorten because of its attachments to the orbicular ligament, extensor aponeurosis, and ECRL. At this time, the surgeon usually makes a small synovial opening and inspects the radiocapitellar joint. Intra-articular abnormalities rarely are identified; however, this arthrotomy does not add morbidity to the procedure, and it may prevent overlooking a concomitant loose body or other abnormality.

Next, the lateral epicondyle is drilled with a $\frac{5}{64}$-in. bit (Fig. 6.8). By encouraging revascularization, drilling is believed to promote healing of the defect that resection of the abnormal tendon leaves.[11] Watertight closure of the interval between the ECRL and extensor aponeurosis is accomplished with no. 1 absorbable sutures in an interrupted, or running, fashion (Fig. 6.9). The subcutaneous layer is closed, and skin closure is obtained through a running subcuticular stitch using 3-0 nonabsorbable sutures and Steri-Strips.

The extremity is dressed and immobilized in a posterior splint at 90° of flexion and neutral rotation. At the patient's first postoperative visit, the splint is removed and range of motion is initiated.

Arthroscopic Lateral Epicondylitis Technique

Baker and coworkers presented an arthroscopic technique to address lateral epicondylitis (Fig. 6.10).[22–24] They retrospectively reviewed the results in 40 patients (42 elbows) who had arthroscopic treatment of recalcitrant lateral epicondylitis.[23] Three types of lesions were identified through the arthroscope. Arthroscopically, type I lesions

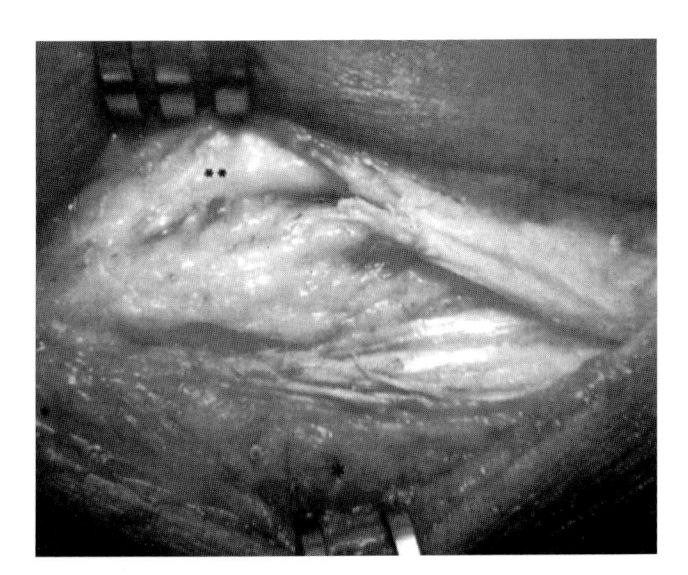

FIGURE 6.6. Anterior retraction of the extensor carpi radialis longus exposes the underlying extensor carpi radialis brevis tendon origin.

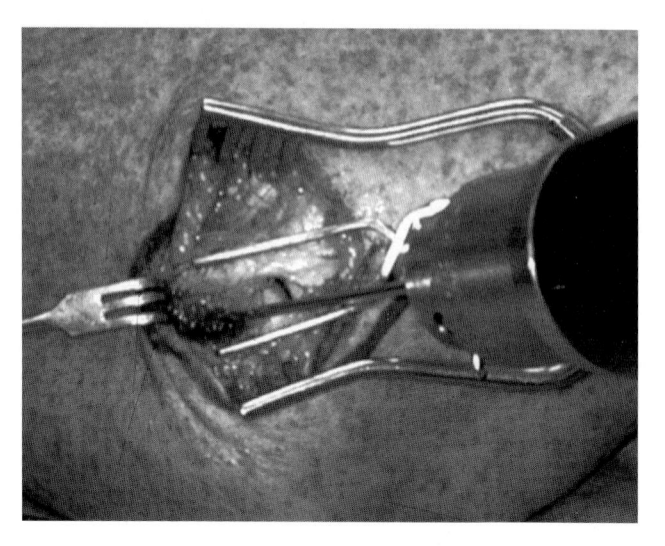

FIGURE 6.8. Drilling of the lateral epicondyle promotes vascularization and healing of soft tissues to bone.

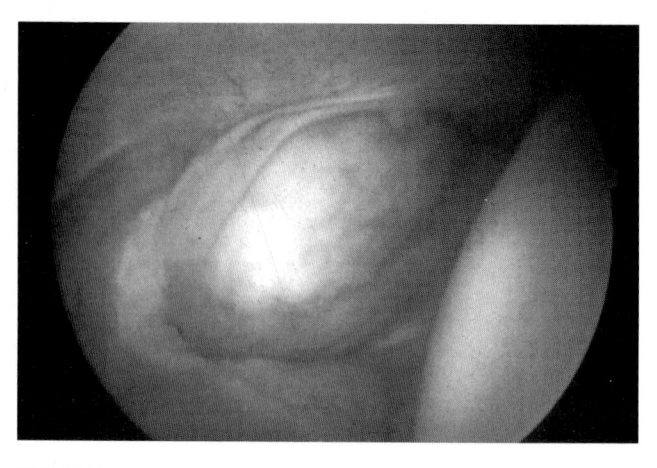

FIGURE 6.10. Arthroscopic visualization of the lateral compartment reveals the capsular and extensor carpi radialis brevis tendon injury. Debridement of pathologic tissue can be performed arthroscopically.

appeared as an intact capsule (15 elbows). Type II changes appeared as linear capsular tears (15 elbows). Type III lesions appeared as complete ruptures and retraction of the capsule with a frayed extensor carpi radialis brevis tendon (12 elbows). Of the 39 elbows in the 37 patients who were available for follow-up, 37 were improved. These results compared favorably with results that Nirschl and Pettrone found (i.e., 97.7% improvement rate).[10] Patients returned to work in an average of 2.2 weeks. No correlation could be found between the type of lesion and clinical outcome.[23]

The surgical indications for endoscopic intervention are the same as for open procedures. Taking a thorough history and physical examination is essential. Previous surgery, especially an ulnar nerve transposition, may al-

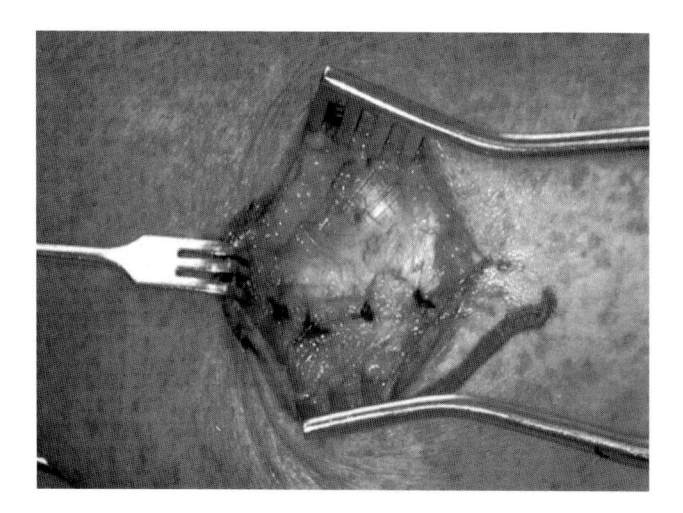

FIGURE 6.9. Anatomic repair of the interval between the posterior edge of the extensor carpi radialis longus and the common extensor aponeurosis allows early postoperative range of motion.

ter portal placement. In addition, the surgeon should note any instability of the nerve in the epicondylar groove on flexion and extension of the elbow. A complete neurovascular examination should be documented in the medical record.

A general anesthetic is administered to the patient, then he or she is positioned prone. Rolled towels are placed under the thorax. Bony prominences are padded and checked to make sure that no undue pressure is placed on them. The extremity is positioned with the shoulder abducted to 90° and the arm supported in a precut foam holder. The forearm hangs freely over the edge of the table with the elbow flexed to 90°. A tourniquet is applied proximally to the arm.

After preparing and draping the extremity in a sterile fashion, the surgeon identifies and outlines landmarks, including the medial and lateral epicondyles, radial head, ulnar nerve, and olecranon. Next, potential portal sites are located and marked.

The joint is distended with 30 mL of saline injected through the direct lateral portal using an 18-gauge needle. Distention of the joint increases the distance between the portals and neurovascular structures. The tubing is removed from the spinal needle, and backflow is confirmed to ensure adequate distention.

The proximal medial or superomedial portal is located approximately 2 cm proximal to the medial epicondyle and 1 cm anterior to the intermuscular septum. The portal is created using a no. 11 blade to incise the skin, followed by blunt, hemostat dissection to spread the underlying tissue. A blunt trocar is passed into the joint capsule through the proximal flexor muscle mass near the brachialis muscle. The trocar is advanced toward the radial head, maintaining contact with the anterior humerus at all times. A 2.7-mm 30° arthroscope is placed into the joint, and diagnostic arthroscopy is initiated.

Abnormal changes are present at the lateral capsule and undersurface of the ECRB tendon. After identifying abnormal tissue, the surgeon establishes the proximal lateral portal. If the lateral capsule has remained intact, it is debrided with a motorized shaver to expose the undersurface of the ECRB tendon. The tendon is removed using a motorized shaver or radiofrequency ablator. The lateral epicondyle is decorticated using a curette or motorized shaver.

Care must be taken to limit epicondylar resection to protect the lateral collateral ligament. Resecting too far posteriorly on the epicondyle places the ligament at risk for injury. After the ECRB tendon has been debrided and released, the fibers of the overlying extensor musculature should be visible.

Postoperatively, the patient's arm is placed in a sling, and gentle range-of-motion exercises are initiated. Gradual progression to wrist extension strengthening and upper extremity conditioning are added as indicated.

Medial Epicondylitis Technique

Little has been published regarding operative techniques for medial epicondylitis. Vangsness and Jobe reported good to excellent results in 88% of patients following excision of the diseased tendon and reattachment of the pronator teres and flexor carpi radialis origin.[25] The association of medial epicondylitis and ulnar neuropathy has been well documented.[26,27] Gabel and Morrey elucidated the influence of associated ulnar neuropathy.[26] They developed a classification system that they showed to be prognostically significant.

Before proceeding with surgery for medial epicondylitis, examination of the ulnar nerve is necessary. Ulnar nerve involvement is found in 40% to 60% of patients.[26,27] Electromyography and nerve conduction velocity testing can be useful when ulnar nerve symptoms are present. Progressive ulnar neuritis is an indication for surgical intervention regardless of the response of the epicondylitis to nonoperative treatment. The surgeon should suspect damage to the ulnar collateral ligament in patients who present with acute symptoms or in throwing athletes who apply a significant valgus load to the elbow (e.g., baseball and javelin throwers). Valgus stability of the elbow should be examined, and stress radiographs or magnetic resonance imaging should be obtained if indicated. If damage to the ulnar collateral ligament is suspected, the surgeon should be prepared to explore the anterior bundle of the ligament and, if indicated, to reconstruct it.

To treat medial epicondylitis, we favor a technique similar to the technique that Ollivierre, Nirschl, and Pettrone described[28] (Fig. 6.11). The incision begins about 2 cm proximal to the medial epicondyle and parallels the epicondylar groove to a point 5 cm distal to the epicondyle (Fig. 6.11A). Straying anterior to the epicondyle places the medial antebrachial cutaneous nerve at risk for injury. A bothersome neuroma can result from transection of the nerve. Dissection through the subcutaneous tissue exposes the deep fascia overlying the ulnar head of the flexor carpi ulnaris. Dissection should proceed anterolaterally over the epicondyle to expose the common flexor tendon. Normally, at this point, disease is not evident because the degeneration is deep. A longitudinal incision is made in the tendon overlying the area of maximal point tenderness. This incision is usually at the origin of the pronator teres and flexor carpi radialis. Gabel and Morrey described the "accessory anterior oblique ligament" (Fig. 6.11B); this structure defines the interval between the flexor carpi ulnaris and flexor carpi radialis and serves as a critical landmark in medial epicondylitis surgery.[4] Because involvement of the flexor carpi ulnaris in medial epicondylitis is rare, dissection should remain anterior to the accessory anterior oblique ligament. The anterior oblique ligament is immediately posterior to the accessory anterior oblique ligament. Dissection of the flexor–pronator origin posterior to the accessory anterior oblique ligament may result in iatrogenic valgus instability secondary to injury of the anterior oblique ligament.

If abnormal tissue is present, it is readily apparent after incision of the pronator teres–flexor carpi radialis origin. As in lateral epicondylitis surgery, all diseased tendon is excised, usually leaving an elliptical defect (Fig. 6.11C).

Preoperative and intraoperative findings dictate ulnar nerve management. The typical site of ulnar nerve compression is at the cubital tunnel; in rare cases, the compression may be proximal to the epicondyle.[27] Nirschl et al. described three possible zones of median nerve compression: zone 1 is proximal to the epicondyle (medial intramuscular septum), zone 2 is at the level of the epicondyle, and zone 3 is distal to the epicondyle where the nerve passes between the heads of the flexor carpi ulnaris.[11] In more than 90% of cases, the compression is found in zone 3.

If ulnar neuropathy is mild, the nerve can simply be decompressed at the cubital tunnel. However, if the neuropathy is moderate to severe with more than a single site of compression, a subcutaneous transposition is performed. Other indications for transposition include instability of the nerve in the epicondylar groove as the elbow is placed through range of motion, epicondylitis associated with ulnar neuropathy, and the need for ulnar collateral ligament reconstruction.[11] We do not favor a submuscular transposition because it is technically more difficult, adds morbidity to the procedure, and has not been shown to affect functional results.

After addressing the ulnar nerve if needed, the surgeon addresses the tendon defect. The epicondyle is drilled with a $\frac{5}{64}$-in. bit to produce a bleeding surface. The defect is closed with no. 1 absorbable sutures, and the subcutaneous layer is closed (Fig. 6.11D). The skin is closed with a running, subcuticular stitch using 3-0 nonabsorbable sutures.

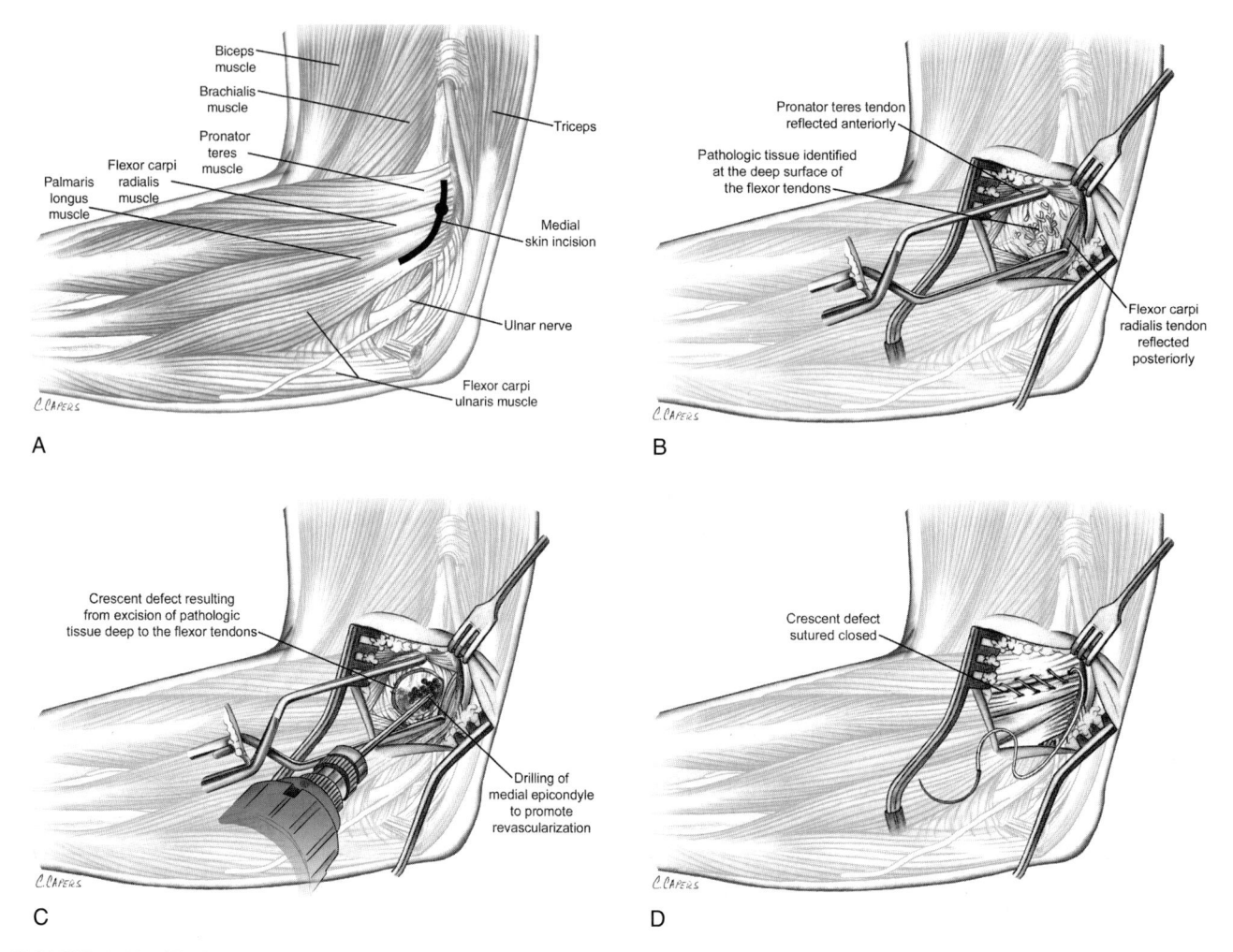

FIGURE 6.11. (A) The medial skin incision begins about 2 cm proximal to the medial epicondyle, parallels the epicondylar groove, and ends at a point 5 cm distal to the epicondyle. (B) The pronator teres and flexor carpi radialis are identified and incised. Pathologic tissue generally is located on the undersurface of these flexor tendons. (C) The pathologic soft tissue is excised, and the medial epicondyle is drilled to promote vascularization and healing. (D) The flexor–pronator tendons are reattached anatomically to the medial epicondyle if they were detached from bone, or they are repaired side to side if the bony attachment was not disturbed.

POSTOPERATIVE MANAGEMENT

Initially, patients wear a posterior splint for 1 week after surgery. When the splint is removed, the patient begins range-of-motion exercises of the wrist and elbow. Once motion is regained, a gradual program of strengthening that concentrates on endurance is undertaken from week 4 to week 6 after surgery. A counterforce brace is employed during the rehabilitation phase. Return to competitive athletics or the workplace is restricted until full strength has returned to the extremity. Patients need to be counseled against the temptation to return too quickly. The usual return to activities is 4 months after surgery for lateral epicondylitis. After surgery for medial epicondylitis, the patient should expect to return after 5 or 6 months; the return will take longer if the patient had a concomitant ligament reconstruction.

SURGICAL RESULTS

In patients who have undergone resection and repair for recalcitrant lateral epicondylitis, a success rate of more than 90% can be expected.[4,10,12,16] Nirschl reported a total of 97% good to excellent results in his series.[10] Eighty-five percent of the patients had a full return to activity and complete absence of pain, and 12% had pain only with aggressive activities.[10] Glousman reported similar results in 1991, with 94% of the 60 patients in his series experiencing significant improvement in their symptoms.[29]

Medial epicondylitis results need to be assessed carefully because concomitant ulnar neuropathy affects the outcome. Gabel and Morrey reported less than 50% good to excellent results in patients who had moderate or severe ulnar neuropathy compared with more than 90% in patients who had mild or no neuropathy.[26] Vangsness and Jobe reported that 86% of patients had no limitations of elbow function in their series.[25] However, the incidence of ulnar nerve abnormalities in their series was 23%, which is about half of what other authors have reported.[4,11]

SURGICAL FAILURE

The surgical procedures to address tennis elbow are extremely reliable. Success rates of approximately 90% can be expected. Typically, the most common cause of perceived surgical failure is a return to activity that is too aggressive. In the absence of secondary gain issues (i.e., workers' compensation claims), pain from 6 to 9 months after surgery is unusual in a compliant patient.

Morrey differentiated surgical failures into two types: type I, patients whose symptom complex is similar to their preoperative state; and type II, patients whose symptom complex is different.[30] The most common cause of type I failure is incomplete resection of all abnormal tissue.[27,30] When identical symptoms persist, the initial diagnosis must be questioned. Other causes of pain at the lateral aspect of the elbow need to be considered. These include intra-articular pathologic conditions, posterior interosseous nerve entrapment at the arcade of Frohse, extensor compartment syndrome,[4] and instability. Especially in workers' compensation patients, the issues of patient motivation, job satisfaction, and secondary gain all deserve attention.

Type II failures are usually iatrogenic. Ligamentous instability, synovial fistula, and adventitial bursa formation are the typical culprits. Synovial fistula formation is associated with percutaneous techniques.[18] Posterolateral instability results from incompetency of the ulnar band of the lateral collateral ligament. Medial instability usually is caused by dissection posterior to the accessory anterior oblique ligament, with subsequent disruption of the anterior oblique ligament.

Diagnostic injections can be very useful in the evaluation of failed tennis elbow surgery. Morrey presented a logical algorithm for the evaluation of failed procedures (Fig. 6.12).[30] Injections can be used at the epicondyle or at the arcade of Frohse to differentiate posterior interosseous nerve compression from persistent lateral epicondylitis. Fluoroscopy or arthrography can be used to evaluate potential instability. The arthrogram also demonstrates bursal or capsular defects. If a definitive diagnosis can be made with the use of the algorithm, surgical treatment can be recommended.

The results of surgical procedures for failed epicondylitis surgery cannot be expected to approach the 90% reported with primary procedures. The surgeon must remember that these are salvage procedures. Organ et al. reported 83% good to excellent results in patients who underwent excision and repair after failed procedures.[27] Morrey reported satisfactory results in 11 of 13 (85%) patients following secondary procedures in a select group of patients.[30]

CONCLUSION

Surgical intervention for medial or lateral epicondylitis is only indicated when the physician is sure that the correct diagnosis has been made and the patient has not improved after an adequate nonoperative treatment program. Following the previously outlined surgical techniques gives the best likelihood of successful operative results. However, we cannot overemphasize the point that, with a proper course of rest, immobilization, medication, and physical therapy exercises and modalities, only 10% of patients, or fewer, should require surgical intervention.

REFERENCES

1. Major HP. Lawn-tennis elbow. *Br Med J* 1883;2:557.
2. Coonrad RW, Hooper WR. Tennis elbow: Its courses, natural history, conservative and surgical management. *J Bone Joint Surg* 1973;55A:1177–1182.
3. Nirschl RP. Elbow tendinosis/tennis elbow. *Clin Sports Med* 1992;11:851–870.
4. Gabel GT, Morrey BF. Tennis elbow. *Instr Course Lect* 1998;47:165–172.
5. Leach RE, Miller JK. Lateral and medial epicondylitis of the elbow. *Clin Sports Med* 1987;6:259–272.
6. Nirschl RP. Soft-tissue injuries about the elbow. *Clin Sports Med* 1986;5:637–652.

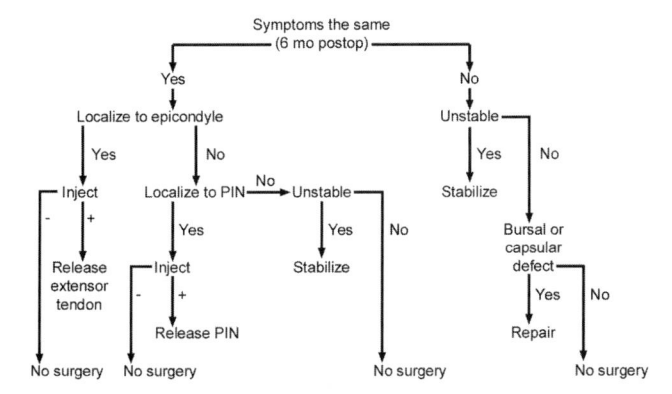

FIGURE 6.12. A logical sequence of assessment for patients with surgical failure for lateral epicondylitis. Notice that the majority of categories indicates that no surgical intervention is necessary. Also note the major distinction between symptoms that are the same (type I) and those that are different (type II). (From Morrey BF.[30])

7. Nirschl RP. Mesenchymal syndrome. *Va Med Monthly* 1969; 96:659–662.
8. Cyriax JH. The pathology and treatment of tennis elbow. *J Bone Joint Surg* 1936;18:921–940.
9. Goldie I. Epicondylitis lateralis humeri (epicondylagia or tennis elbow): A pathologic study. *Acta Chir Scand Suppl* 1964: 339.
10. Nirschl RP, Pettrone FA. Tennis elbow: The surgical treatment of lateral epicondylitis. *J Bone Joint Surg* 1979;61A:832–839.
11. Nirschl RP. Muscle and tendon trauma: Tennis elbow. In: Morrey BF, ed. *The elbow and its disorders*, 1st ed. Philadelphia: WB Saunders; 1985:537–552.
12. Coonrad RW. Tennis elbow. *Instructional Course Lect* 1986; 35:94–101.
13. Bosworth DM. Surgical treatment of tennis elbow. A follow-up study. *J Bone Joint Surg* 1965;47A:1533–1536.
14. Kaplan EB. Treatment of tennis elbow (epicondylitis) by denervation. *J Bone Joint Surg* 1959;41A:147–151.
15. Moss SH, Switzer HE. Radial tunnel syndrome: A spectrum of clinical presentations. *J Hand Surg* 1983;8:414–420.
16. Jobe FW, Ciccotti MG. Lateral and medial epicondylitis of the elbow. *J Am Acad Orthop Surg* 1994;2:1–8.
17. Hohmann G. Über den Tennisellenbogen. *Verhandlungen der Deutschen Orthopädischen Gesellschaft*. 1926;21:349.
18. Yerger B, Turner T. Percutaneous extensor tenotomy for chronic tennis elbow: An office procedure. *Orthopedics* 1985; 8:1261–1263.
19. Garden RS. Tennis elbow. *J Bone Joint Surg* 1961;43B:100–106.
20. Michele AA, Krueger FJ. Lateral epicondylitis of the elbow treated by fasciotomy. *Surgery* 1956;39:277–284.
21. Carroll RE, Jorgensen EC. Evaluation of the Garden procedure for lateral epicondylitis. *Clin Orthop* 1968;60:201–204.
22. Baker CL Jr, Cummings PD. Arthroscopic management of miscellaneous elbow disorders. *Oper Tech Sports Med* 1998;6: 16–21.
23. Baker CL Jr, Murphy KP, Gottlob CA, Curd DT. Arthroscopic classification and treatment of lateral epicondylitis: two-year clinical results. *J Shoulder Elbow Surg* 2000;9:475–482.
24. Brooks AA, Baker CL. Arthroscopy of the elbow. In: Stanley D, Kay N, eds. *Surgery of the elbow: Scientific and practical aspects*. London: Edward Arnold; 1998:71–81.
25. Vangsness CT Jr, Jobe FW. Surgical treatment of medial epicondylitis. Results in 35 elbows. *J Bone Joint Surg* 1991;73B: 409–411.
26. Gabel GT, Morrey BF. Operative treatment of medial epicondylitis: Influence of concomitant ulnar neuropathy of the elbow. *J Bone Joint Surg* 1995;77A:1065–1069.
27. Organ SW, Nirschl RP, Kraushaar BS, et al. Salvage surgery for lateral tennis elbow. *Am J Sports Med* 1997;25:746–750.
28. Ollivierre CO, Nirschl RP, Pettrone FA. Resection and repair for medial tennis elbow. A prospective analysis. *Am J Sports Med* 1995;23:214–221.
29. Glousman RE. Surgical treatment of lateral epicondylitis (tennis elbow). *Techniques Orthop* 1991;6:33–38.
30. Morrey BF. Sports—and overuse injuries to the elbow. In: Morrey BF, ed. *The elbow and its disorders*, 2nd ed. Philadelphia: WB Saunders; 1993:558.

CHAPTER 7

Ulnar Collateral Ligament Injuries

Nathan M. Breazeale and David W. Altcheck

INTRODUCTION

The ulnar (medial) collateral ligament (UCL) of the elbow consists of three bundles: anterior, posterior, and transverse. Researchers have shown that the anterior bundle is the primary restraint to valgus stress at the elbow.[1-8] Ligament injury rarely leads to symptomatic instability.[3,9] An exception is UCL injury in an athlete who participates in a sport involving overhead throwing motions, such as javelin or baseball throwing or tennis serving. The extreme valgus loads that the throwing motion generates place tremendous stress across the medial portion of the joint. Subtle injury to the UCL can lead to disabling valgus instability in the throwing athlete who places repetitive valgus stress on the elbow.[2,9-15] Instability that prevents the athlete from returning to competition often indicates the need for surgical reconstruction.

CLINICAL ANATOMY

A thorough understanding of the anatomy and biomechanics of the elbow is essential to diagnosing and treating injuries of the UCL. The anterior bundle of the UCL is the most discrete of the three portions of the ligament complex (i.e., anterior, posterior, and transverse bundles) (Fig. 7.1). Its margins are readily distinguishable from the surrounding joint capsule, and its fibers often are associated intimately with the deep surface of the flexor mass.[16] The posterior bundle consists of a less distinct fan-shaped thickening of the posterior capsule.[4] The transverse fibers originate and insert on the ulna, covering a bony depression on the medial portion of the trochlear notch, and they contribute little or nothing to the stability of the elbow.[4,16]

The anterior bundle is the most important portion of the complex when treating valgus instability of the elbow. The ligament originates from the anteroinferior surface of the medial epicondyle. The width of the origin varies but, in most cases, occupies the middle two-thirds to three-quarters of the epicondyle in the coronal plane (Fig. 7.2).[17] A small space remains between the lateral edge of the ligament and the medial crista of the trochlea. This space allows for a synovial reflection in the joint, which the surgeon readily can visualize with magnetic resonance imaging (MRI). In their study, Morrey and An found that the mean length of the anterior bundle is 27.1 ± 4.3 mm and the mean width is 4.7 ± 1.2 mm.[4] The anterior bundle inserts on the medial border of the coronoid at the sublime tubercle.[4,16]

Timmerman and Andrews defined the histology and arthroscopic anatomy of the anterior bundle.[16] The medial capsule consists of a synovial lining with two distinct capsular layers between which the anterior and posterior bundles pass (Fig. 7.3).[16] The anterior bundle consists of well-defined collagen bundles in parallel arrangement, which is typical of ligaments. In cross section, the bundle consists of two portions: one layer within the two synovial layers of the joint capsule and one layer that is superficial to the capsule and that blends with the deep surface of the flexor muscle mass. The posterior bundle consists of a smaller area of collagen within the capsular layers.

Understanding the functional anatomy of the UCL requires a synthesis of the kinematics of elbow motion with the biomechanics of the throwing mechanism. The ulnohumeral joint is a hinge, or ginglymus, joint that permits flexion and extension. The articulation between the greater sigmoid notch of the olecranon and the trochlea of the humerus is one of the most congruous and constrained joints in the body. With loading, the elbow flexors and extensors tend to seat the olecranon in the trochlea of the humerus, contributing valgus stability under dynamic conditions. Biomechanical studies of the loaded

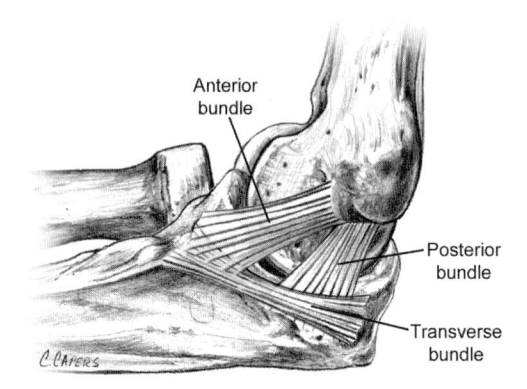

FIGURE 7.1. The anterior, posterior, and transverse bundles compose the ulnar collateral ligament. The anterior bundle is the primary stabilizer of the elbow when it resists valgus stress.

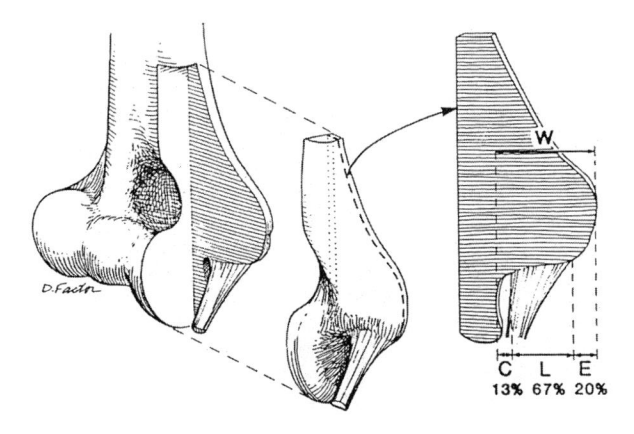

FIGURE 7.2. The anterior part of the medial epicondyle removed by orthogonal osteotomies. On the right, a 2-mm-thick slice through the widest portion of the origin of the anterior bundle of the ulnar collateral ligament. (Mean values are shown.) W, width of medial epicondyle; C, distance from lateral edge of anterior medial collateral ligament origin to medial side of condyle (trochlea); L, width of origin of anterior medial collateral ligament; E, distance from tip of epicondyle to medial edge of anterior band of the medial collateral ligament origin. (From O'Driscoll SW, et al.[17])

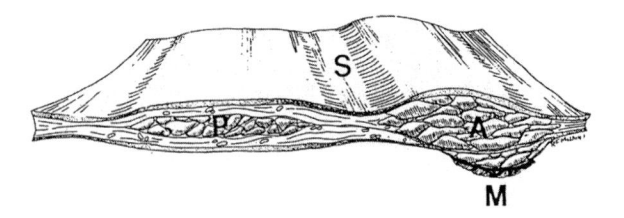

FIGURE 7.3. Cross-sectional anatomy of the medial capsule of the elbow at the level of the joint line. A, anterior bundle; M, muscle; P, posterior bundle; S, synovium. (From Timmerman LA, Andrews JR[16])

and unloaded cadaveric elbow by Morrey et al. demonstrated decreased valgus laxity against a gravity valgus stress in the loaded specimens compared with the unloaded specimens both before and after sectioning the anterior bundle of the UCL.[8]

Researchers have shown that the anterior bundle of the UCL is the primary restraint to valgus stress and that the radial head is a secondary restraint.[1,6,8] With anterior bundle sectioning, the resultant instability is greatest between 60° and 70° and is least at full extension and full flexion.[6] True lateral radiographs show that the flexion–extension axis, or center of rotation, of the elbow lies in the center of the trochlea and capitellum.[18,19] The origin of the anterior bundle of the UCL lies slightly posterior to the rotational center of the elbow (Fig. 7.4). The anterior bundle is further divided into an anterior band and a posterior band.[20] The eccentric origin of these anterior bundle components in relation to the rotational center through the trochlea creates a cam effect during flexion and extension. The anterior band tightens during extension, and the posterior band tightens during flexion. This reciprocal tightening of the two functional components of the anterior bundle allows the ligament to remain taut throughout the full range of flexion (Fig. 7.5).[20]

Researchers have documented the rupture of the UCL in athletes in many sports; however, most ruptures occur in athletes participating in throwing sports.[12,21–23] An understanding of the throwing mechanism and its relationship to injury is essential when treating UCL tears.

The throwing motion is one of the most violent athletic activities. The transition from the late cocking phase to early acceleration places extreme valgus stress on the medial structures of the elbow. Researchers have estimated that between 100 and 120 N · m of varus torque are required to resist the valgus stress that the throwing motion produces in elite-level pitchers.[24,25] After comparing the electromyographic data in throwing athletes who had healthy elbows with the data in throwing athletes who had UCL instability, researchers found that the muscles (specifically, the flexor carpi radialis, pronator teres, and flexor carpi ulnaris muscles) that were positioned to function as dynamic stabilizers of the medial elbow did not appear to compensate for UCL laxity. In

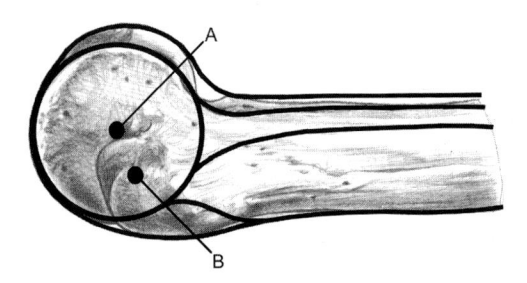

FIGURE 7.4. Lateral projection of the distal humerus showing the axis of rotation of the elbow through the center of the humeral trochlea (A) and the origin of the ulnar collateral ligament (B).

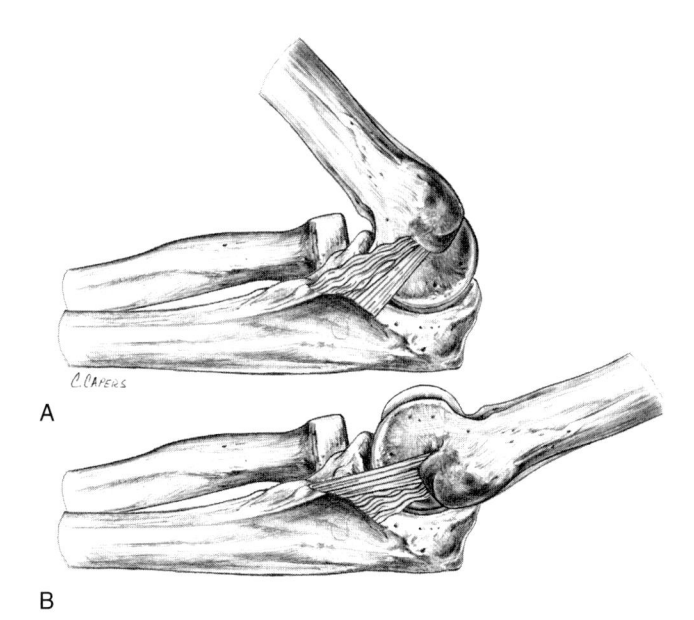

FIGURE 7.5. Lateral projections of the elbow demonstrating the reciprocal tightening of the anterior and posterior bands of the anterior bundle of the ulnar collateral ligament. (A) The posterior band tightens during flexion. (B) The anterior band tightens during extension.

fact, they found slightly decreased activity in these muscles in the UCL-insufficient pitchers during throwing.[26,27] This finding suggests that the flexor–pronator muscles have limited ability for dynamic stabilization of the elbow in high-demand throwers who have valgus instability.

HISTORY AND PHYSICAL EXAMINATION

History

A detailed history and physical examination is essential in evaluating the elbow for UCL insufficiency. Most athletes who present for evaluation participate in activities involving repetitive overhead throwing motions. Knowledge of previous elbow injuries and treatments aids the examiner in the initial examination. The chronology of the development of elbow pain can give clues to the underlying problems and can indicate where the injury lies on the spectrum of UCL injury.

A history of mild pain following a return to activities involving overhead throwing motions or a significant increase in activity intensity or duration indicates an overuse syndrome. This syndrome generally responds to nonoperative treatment directed at inflammation after overuse. Athletes who have this problem often are able to continue throwing at 100% of their maximal effort, but develop pain with progression to heavy throwing or with alteration in throwing mechanics.[21,22,28]

Pain in the medial portion of the elbow with throwing beyond 60% to 75% of maximal effort can indicate ligament attenuation. Athletes who have ligament attenuation often have a history of recurrent medial elbow injury and might sense movement in the elbow when attempting to throw beyond 75% of maximal effort. In a chronic case of UCL insufficiency, the athlete might experience mechanical symptoms, such as locking and catching, or crepitation, that suggest the presence of loose bodies or early degenerative changes in the joint.

In contrast to this gradual development of UCL insufficiency, an acute rupture of the ligament can occur in athletes who might or might not have had previous symptoms. They often report developing a sudden, sharp pain over the medial portion of the elbow. They can identify the exact moment that symptoms developed and might feel or sense a pop at the moment of ligament rupture. Medial elbow opening with valgus stress can cause ulnar nerve stretching with paresthesia radiating into the medial forearm, hand, and fourth and fifth digits. A pitcher might not be able to continue throwing or to exceed 75% of maximal effort.

Physical Examination

Physical examination of the elbow for UCL injury entails assessing the integrity of the ligament and evaluating the joint and surrounding structures for associated injuries.

Inspection of the upper extremity in overhead athletes often reveals hemihypertrophy of the dominant extremity.[23] In acute cases of UCL injury, pain or guarding might limit elbow range of motion. In chronic cases and especially in throwers, motion might be limited at terminal extension due to bony changes in the posterior compartment, anterior capsular contracture, or loose bodies in the olecranon fossa. Crepitation with motion suggests the presence of loose bodies or degenerative changes in the joint.

Palpation over the ligament usually elicits tenderness along its course when the athlete has an acute injury. The anterior bundle of the UCL originates at the anteroinferior portion of the medial epicondyle of the humerus and inserts on the medial border of the coronoid process at the sublime tubercle.[16,17] Pain at the ligament's origin can mimic medial epicondylitis or, in extreme injury, rupture of the flexor–pronator muscle mass origin.[12,22,23] Pain elicited at the origin of the tendon with resisted wrist flexion, resisted forearm pronation, or firm fist clench differentiates the isolated UCL injury from these other injuries.

Injury to the insertion of the UCL occurs distal to the medial epicondyle, and the location of the point of tenderness differentiates it from injury to the origin. The examiner uses the "milking maneuver" to facilitate identification and palpation of the ligament underneath the mass of the flexor–pronator muscle origin.[27] During examination, the patient places the opposite hand under the elbow and grasps the thumb of the injured arm. With the injured elbow flexed to more than 90°, the patient applies a valgus stress to the elbow by pulling the thumb with the opposite hand. Hyperflexion isolates the anterior bundle of the UCL, and valgus stress stretches it. Positioning the elbow in this fashion facilitates location and palpation of the tensioned ligament beneath the mass of the flexor–pronator origin. Positioning for the maneuver alone can elicit pain over the medial elbow as the anterior bundle is placed on stretch.

Valgus stability of the elbow is best examined with the elbow positioned in approximately 30° of flexion, which frees the olecranon tip from the fossa posteriorly. Forearm pronation and wrist flexion relax the flexor–pronator mass and allow isolation of the UCL. While holding the pronated hand either in one of his or her hands or between his or her trunk and arm, the examiner places his or her other hand on the lateral side of the elbow and applies a valgus stress to the arm. While applying the valgus stress, the examiner palpates the ligament for tenderness. The examiner also assesses the extent of joint opening and quality of the ligament's endpoint with this maneuver and compares the findings with the findings in the contralateral elbow. Even with complete ligament rupture, the side to side difference in joint opening might be only 3 to 4 mm, and the difference in endpoint quality can be subtle, making the maneuver difficult to master.

We recommend a variation of the stress test to aid the examiner in sensing the amount or extent of medial joint opening. After applying the valgus stress and palpating the endpoint, the examiner places a varus stress on the elbow. It often is easier to sense the amount of joint opening by the extent of joint-line closure when moving from the valgus to varus stress. As the ulnohumeral articulation closes, the endpoint palpated during varus stress is firm and discrete and can assist the examiner in determining the amount of medial joint laxity.

Complete examination of the elbow that might have a UCL injury requires assessment of other structures in the medial portion of the elbow. Ulnar nerve irritation can be mistaken for ligament injury or can occur in conjunction with it. Bony hypertrophy, medial joint spurring, or inflammation associated with UCL injury can compress the ulnar nerve in the cubital tunnel. Nerve subluxation, especially during the late cocking phase of throwing, can lead to pain in the medial portion of the elbow. Careful examination of the nerve is essential for ruling out isolated or associated ulnar nerve injury. The examination should focus on nerve sensitivity and tenderness, presence of Tinel's sign, and distal sensory and motor function. The examiner can assess nerve stability by looking for hypermobility or anterior subluxation. Nerve involvement associated with UCL incompetence might require nerve transposition in conjunction with ligament reconstruction.

Valgus extension overload associated with throwing can lead to several well-recognized bony changes across the posteromedial portion of the elbow.[15] Olecranon tip spurring and osteophyte formation along with bony hypertrophy of the olecranon fossa and loose-body formation can lead to impingement of the olecranon tip in the fossa at terminal extension, especially in throwing athletes. Snapping extension of the elbow can elicit pain.

Chondral injury and degenerative changes in the posterior portion of the joint also can cause pain in the medial portion similar to the pain that UCL tears cause. Applying a valgus stress with the elbow in extension can reproduce pain in cases of posteromedial instability due to a UCL tear. The examiner must explore all sources of pain in the medial portion of the elbow and address any concurrent injury at surgery for a successful outcome in UCL reconstruction.

Radiographs are helpful in evaluating the elbow for UCL injury. Using plain radiographs, the examiner can identify degenerative changes in the elbow and loose bodies (Fig. 7.6). Chronic UCL injury can cause calcification along the course of the ligament and medial joint-line spurring (see Fig. 7.6B). Osteophytes in the posteromedial portion of the elbow are seen easily on the anteroposterior and the hyperflexion lateral views as the tip of the olecranon is advanced out of the fossa (Fig. 7.6C). Secondary degenerative changes also can be seen at the radiocapitellar joint, and at the ulnohumeral joint in chronic cases of UCL insufficiency. Stress radiographs can be useful in the examination; however, we have found that they can be negative in known cases of UCL rupture. Use of computed tomography and arthrography can help in diagnosing an undersurface tear of the ligament.[14,29]

MRI has become the study of choice in evaluating the elbow that might have a UCL injury. It shows the integrity of the ligament and associated injuries (Fig. 7.7). By placing the patient's elbow in extension, the examiner can well visualize the anterior bundle on coronal section and can differentiate among proximal, distal, and mid-substance ligament tears. MRI also allows the examiner to view the articular surfaces and adjacent neuromuscular structures for evaluation of any abnormalities identified on physical examination or radiographic evaluation (Fig. 7.8). The examiner can use MRI after surgery to evaluate graft integrity, placement, or reinjury (Fig. 7.9). Because of the small size of the ligament, technical considerations (e.g., arm positioning, signal-to-noise ratio, and signal sequencing) are important in producing an optimal image.[30]

NONOPERATIVE TREATMENT

Treatment options for UCL injuries vary according to the severity of the injury and the patient's athletic requirements. For ligament strains, the basic treatment princi-

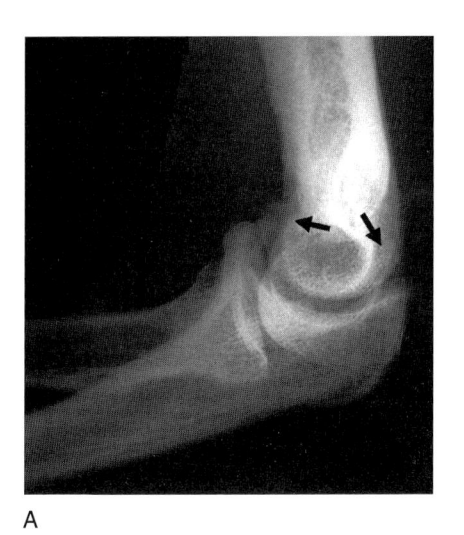

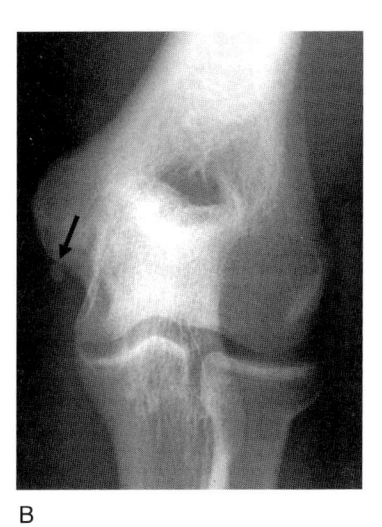

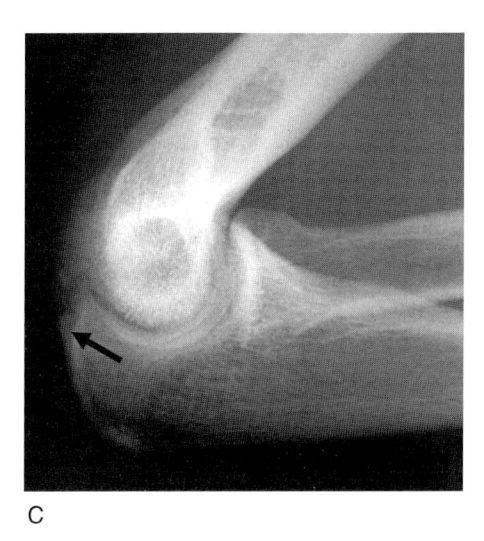

FIGURE 7.6. (A) Lateral radiograph shows degenerative osteophyte formation at the anterior ulnohumeral joint (left arrow) and a loose body in the posterior fossa (right arrow). (B) Anteroposterior radiograph shows calcification at the origin of the ulnar collateral ligament. (C) Hyperflexion lateral radiograph demonstrates improved visualization of the spurring at the tip of the olecranon process.

ples for any ligament injury apply: cold and heat therapy, rest, nonsteroidal anti-inflammatory medications, range-of-motion and strengthening exercises, therapeutic modalities, and a gradual return to sport participation. For overhead athletes, a multidisciplinary approach to recovery (including the athletic trainer, physical therapist, coach, and physician) is used. These sport and medical professionals should pay special attention to sport technique, especially with pitchers, to help the athlete to avoid technical errors that place excessive valgus stress on the medial portion of the elbow.[28] Temporarily moving the athlete to a playing position that involves less throwing

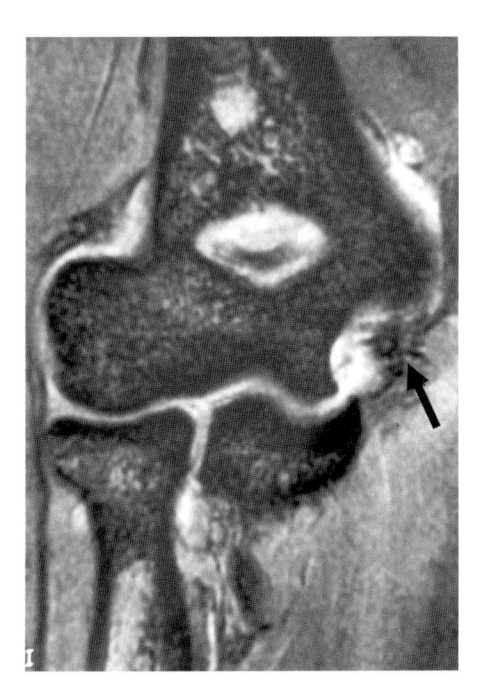

FIGURE 7.7. Coronal gradient-recalled magnetic resonance imaging of the right elbow of a 20-year-old lacrosse player who had sustained a valgus load to the elbow 12 hours earlier. The ulnar collateral ligament (arrow) is disrupted completely off the humeral insertion. A large joint effusion is evident. Note the increased signal intensity in the flexor–pronator muscle mass inferior to the ligament due to associated contusion. (Courtesy of Hollis G. Potter, MD)

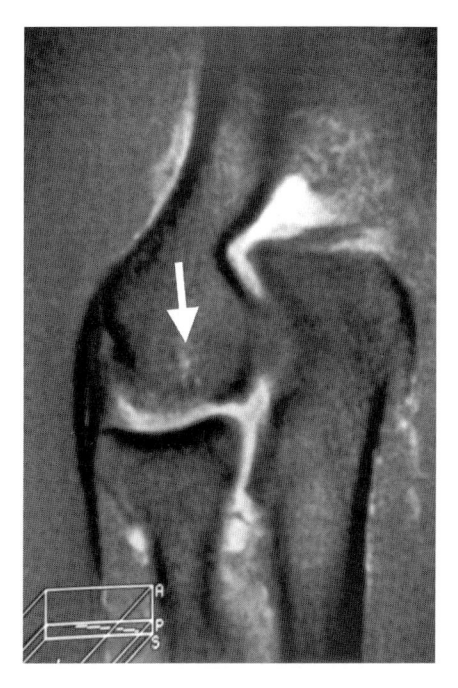

FIGURE 7.8. Coronal fat-suppressed, fast-spin, echo magnetic resonance imaging demonstrating osteochondral impaction of the capitellum with marrow edema (arrow) secondary to a valgus load. (Courtesy of Hollis G. Potter, MD)

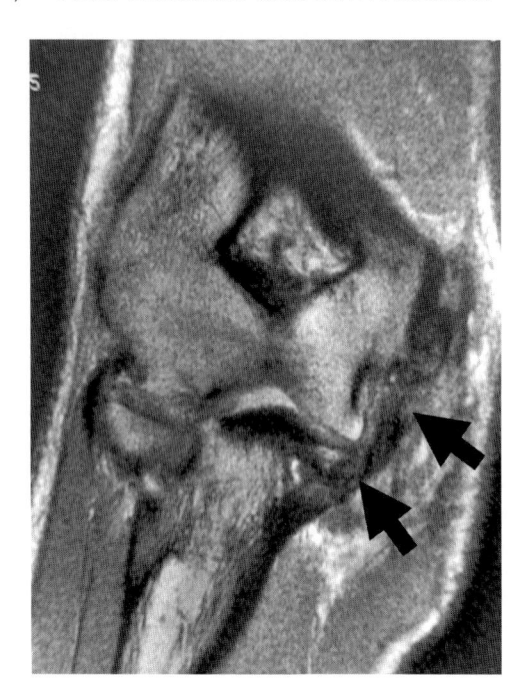

FIGURE 7.9. Coronal fast-spin, echo magnetic resonance imaging through the right elbow of a 30-year-old professional baseball player who had had an ulnar collateral ligament reconstruction using a palmaris longus tendon graft (arrows). Magnetic resonance imaging obtained after reinjury demonstrates partial-thickness disruption of the proximal aspect of the graft (superior arrow), but no evidence of full-thickness discontinuity. Using appropriate pulse sequences, previous surgery, or orthopedic instrumentation does not preclude diagnostic imaging. (Courtesy of Hollis G. Potter, MD)

can aid the recovery process. Many athletes who do not pitch but have chronic UCL laxity can adapt their throwing technique to minimize valgus stress and can remain active. However, pitchers who have laxity tend to develop symptoms with repetitive attempts at throwing beyond 75% of their maximal effort.

As with chronic UCL laxity, acute ligament rupture in most athletes can be managed nonoperatively. Patients rarely have significant pain or dysfunction after the initial inflammatory phase resolves, and they can return gradually to most sports. Athletes who participate in sports that involve valgus-loading upper-extremity maneuvers, such as javelin and baseball throwing and volleyball and tennis serving, do not respond as well to nonoperative treatment. They often need surgical treatment in order to return to their preinjury level of function. Rehabilitation programs for athletes who have symptomatic UCL laxity or complete ligament rupture have yielded poor results in returning these high-demand athletes to their previous level of function.

Electromyographic analysis in UCL-deficient throwers shows a paradoxical inhibition of muscle recruitment of the flexor–pronator mass during throwing compared with the results in uninjured throwers.[26,31] This inhibition might imply that, despite this muscle group's ideal orientation to compensate for the deficient UCL, it might not be able to overcome the tremendous valgus stress occurring across the medial portion of the elbow during the throwing mechanism. This problem, in part, might account for the poor results that rehabilitation alone in these athletes produces.

OPERATIVE TREATMENT

Indications

In most overhead athletes who do not throw, the spectrum of UCL injuries can be managed nonoperatively, allowing even elite-level participation in most sports. However, reconstruction is indicated for athletes participating in sports that place high demand on the upper extremity, such as baseball pitching, javelin throwing, and serving. If nonoperative treatment fails, ligament reconstruction is a treatment option for overhead-throwing athletes who have pain in the medial aspect of the elbow or have a sense of movement in the elbow with the application of valgus loads during sports participation and have UCL laxity or rupture diagnosed on physical examination and confirmed by imaging studies. The surgeon should forewarn the patient that the recovery period following surgery is lengthy and that their sports requirements and aspirations should be consistent with this significant investment in attempting to restore a highly specific elbow function.

Contraindications

Athletes who do not place high demands on their elbow and do not subject it to extreme valgus loads and who are able to return to their sport after injury and rehabilitation usually are not candidates for reconstruction despite objective evidence of ligament rupture.[11] Athletes who have UCL deficiency and who do not plan to continue participation in throwing or other high-demand activities also are not candidates for reconstruction.

Technique

Treatment options for UCL insufficiency include repair of the acute ligament disruption and reconstruction using a free autogenous tendon graft. Results of surgical repair have not been as encouraging as reconstruction.[11] Indications for repair remain narrow and include an acute proximal avulsion in which the tissue is of good quality and no calcification is present in the ligament. This presentation is rare, and reconstruction generally is recommended because the success rate in returning an athlete to competition is higher with reconstruction and because the recovery time is nearly the same for the two procedures.[11]

The graft of choice in UCL reconstruction is the palmaris longus tendon.[5,11] Minimal morbidity is associated with its removal; however, the surgeon must take care to avoid damaging the adjacent median nerve. In our clinical experience, harvest of the ipsilateral palmaris longus tendon does not lead to marked postoperative morbidity and has been used successfully at other institutions.[11] The strength characteristics of the graft are excellent; the ultimate strength is four times that of the anterior bundle of the UCL.[5] Other graft options include the contralateral palmaris longus tendon, the plantaris tendon, the lesser toe extensor tendons, or a 3- to 5-mm strip of the Achilles or hamstring tendon.

Authors' Preferred Method

The preoperative examination in the throwing athlete who has a UCL injury often reveals an intra-articular injury that needs to be evaluated and addressed at the time of ligament reconstruction. In addition, some athletes who have suspected ligament laxity might have equivocal opening on valgus stress examination. For these reasons, we often evaluate the elbow using arthroscopic surgery in conjunction with the ligament reconstruction procedure.

The arthroscopic evaluation permits visualization of the anterior and posterior compartments. The surgeon evaluates the anterior compartment for loose bodies and spur formation and examines the capitellum surface for reciprocal chondral lesions, which occur in acute or chronic UCL deficiency, and for osteochondritis dissecans lesions (Fig. 7.8). Application of a valgus stress produces from 2 to 3 mm of opening between the medial ulnohumeral joint in patients who have UCL insufficiency and serves as a useful diagnostic confirmation when ligament instability is uncertain.[18] Although only 20% to 30% of the anterior bundle is visible from the anterior portal,[16] medial elbow stability can be assessed during arthroscopic surgery.

We use arthroscopic surgery to evaluate the posterior compartment for loose bodies as well. Overhead-throwing athletes often develop a medial olecranon spur in association with the valgus extension overload that occurs during throwing.[15] The surgeon easily can debride the spur at this time. We also evaluate the chondral surfaces of the posterior compartment. We have seen a characteristic reciprocal chondral lesion of the medial crista of the posterior humeral trochlea occur in association with the olecranon spurring in throwers who have UCL insufficiency. For these reasons, we have found arthroscopy to be a valuable adjunct to the evaluation and treatment of UCL injuries.

For arthroscopy alone, we prefer prone positioning of the patient. However, to prepare for both the arthroscopic surgery and the reconstruction, the patient is positioned supine. The arm is placed in the over-the-chest position, and an assistant either holds the hand or secures it with an arm holder, such as the McConnell® device. A pneumatic tourniquet is used for hemostasis. Routine arthroscopy portals are used to evaluate the elbow. After completion of the arthroscopic surgery, the arm is abducted and externally rotated and is placed on an arm board for the reconstruction procedure.

The surgeon makes a 10-cm curvilinear incision that is centered over the medial epicondyle. The fascia and aponeurosis of the flexor–pronator muscle group are carefully exposed, and the medial antebrachial cutaneous nerve is isolated and protected (Fig. 7.10). The nerve crosses the field anywhere from 3 to 60 mm distal to the epicondyle.[32] If the patient has had a previous ulnar nerve transposition, the surgeon should isolate and protect this nerve. This possibility emphasizes the need for taking a thorough preoperative history.

After exposing the flexor pronator, the surgeon has two options for exposing the ligament. The standard approach, as Jobe et al. described, involves transecting the conjoined tendon of the flexor–pronator muscle mass 1 cm distal to the medial epicondyle and reflecting it distally to gain exposure to the medial capsule (Fig. 7.11).[12] Although this technique is reliable for ligament exposure, we prefer the less traumatic, potentially less time consuming muscle-splitting approach.[32]

The interval for the muscle split is the fascial raphe between the ulnar-innervated flexor carpi ulnaris muscle and the median-innervated common flexor muscle mass. This raphe usually is identified easily at the posterior one-third of the flexor–pronator muscle group (Fig. 7.10). The

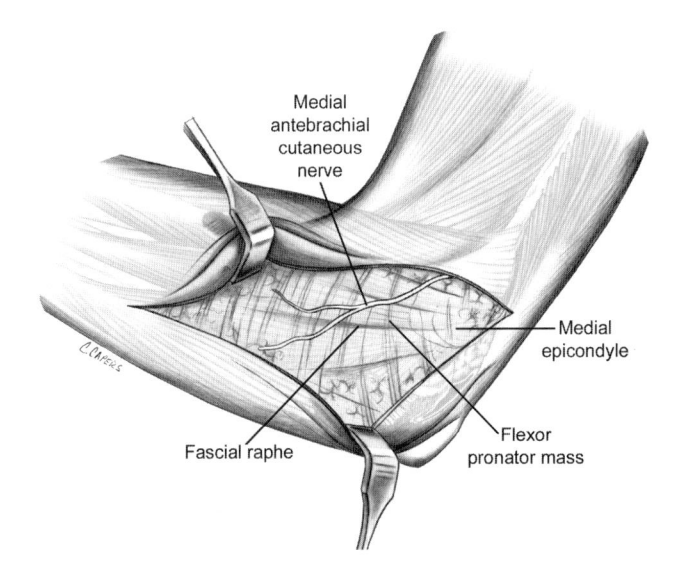

FIGURE 7.10. Exposure of the fascia and aponeurosis of the flexor–pronator muscle mass. Branches of the medial antebrachial cutaneous nerve cross the surgical field. The raphe separating the common flexor muscle origin and the flexor carpi ulnaris muscle marks the line for the fascial incision for the muscle-splitting approach.

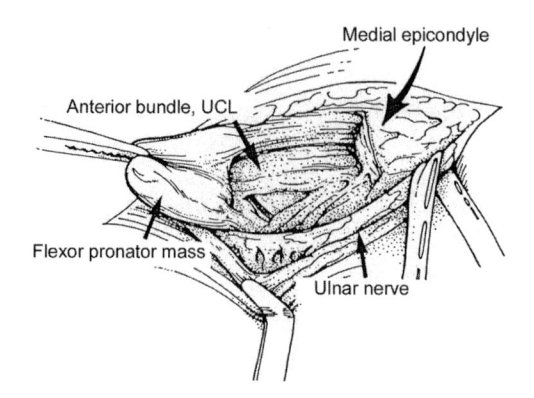

FIGURE 7.11. The conjoined tendon of the flexor–pronator muscle mass is cut approximately 1 cm distal to the medial epicondyle and retracted to expose the ulnar collateral ligament and capsule. UCL, ulnar collateral ligament. (From Jobe FW, et al.[12])

surgeon incises the fascia longitudinally along the raphe from the medial epicondyle to 1 cm distal to the sublime tubercle of the ulna, which he or she identifies using deep fingertip palpation through the flexor mass. The ulnar nerve lies just posterior to this interval, and the surgeon should identify and protect it before completing the muscle split. To expose the medial joint capsule, the surgeon uses blunt dissection to split the muscle fibers longitudinally in line with the fibers (Fig. 7.12). This interval separates the flexor carpi ulnaris muscle (medial) from the palmaris longus muscle (lateral) in the superficial dissection and separates the flexor carpi ulnaris muscle from the flexor digitorum superficialis muscle in the deeper dissection.[32] After exposing the capsule, the surgeon exposes the medial ulna distal to the sublime tubercle using subperiosteal dissection to avoid transecting the motor branches of the flexor carpi ulnaris muscle. When developing the approach, Smith and associates used anatomic dissection data that identified the points of motor branch innervation from both the median and ulnar nerves to avoid denervation of the surrounding muscle.[32]

Next, blunt retractors are used to retract the anterior and posterior muscle masses, giving access to the capsule and ligament. A valgus stress is applied with the elbow flexed to 30° to assess the ligament. If the ligament is insufficient, the joint opens at least 3 to 4 mm when the surgeon applies a valgus stress.

By incising the ligament longitudinally, the surgeon gains access to the medial portion of the joint and can assess it for intra-articular injury. He or she should preserve as much as possible of the ligament's origin and insertion. The ligament and capsule can be closed before graft tensioning in a pant-over-vest imbrication to add support to the reconstruction. The entire anterior bundle is exposed from its origin to the insertion on the ulna. The subperiosteal dissection is continued distally for approximately 1 cm on the ulna to allow for graft tunnel placement.

We prefer the muscle-splitting approach for its ease of exposure of the medial capsule, low risk of muscle denervation, and potentially lower postoperative morbidity. In addition, if the preoperative examination indicates ulnar neuropathy, anterior subcutaneous ulnar nerve transposition can be achieved easily through this approach. However, if the surgeon prefers a submuscular transposition of the nerve, the flexor–pronator muscle mass turndown as described by Jobe et al. is the best approach for combining these procedures.[12] The surgeon must take care to preserve the motor branches to the flexor carpi ulnaris muscle.

Graft fixation is achieved through bony tunnels in the ulna and in the medial epicondyle. For fixation in the ulna, we continue to use the technique that Jobe et al. originally described; it entails placing convergent drill holes at the anterior and posterior margins of the sublime tubercle of the ulna separated by a 1-cm bone bridge (Fig. 7.13).[12] The hard cortical surface of the tubercle provides an excellent bone bridge for graft fixation. The surgeon connects the holes under the bridge using a small, curved curette, taking care to preserve the bone bridge.

For graft fixation in the medial epicondyle, Jobe and associates described fashioning divergent drill holes from a single entry hole on the anterior portion of the distal epicondyle (Fig. 7.13).[12] Using this technique, the surgeon advances the graft into one tunnel, around the epicondyle, and back through the second tunnel in a figure-of-eight fashion. The graft is tensioned and secured to itself.

We have developed an alternative technique of countersinking the proximal ends of the graft into one unicortical drill hole at the anterior portion of the distal epicondyle (or the origin of the anterior bundle) and tensioning the graft over bone-bridge sutures on the prox-

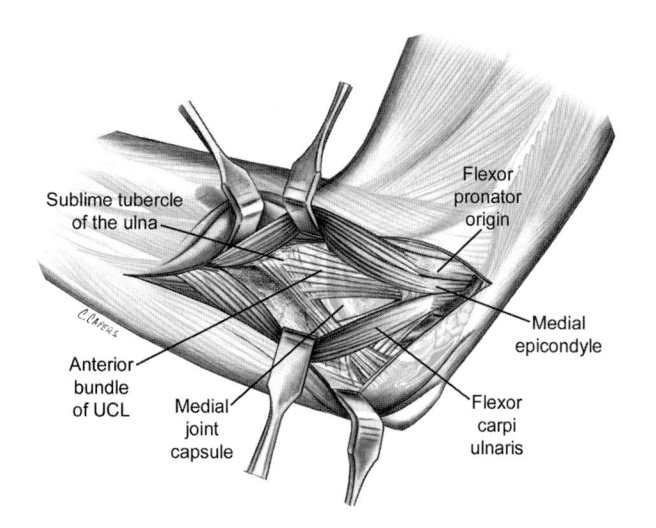

FIGURE 7.12. The muscle-splitting approach to the ulnar collateral ligament demonstrating the insertion of the anterior bundle on the sublime tubercle of the ulna. UCL, ulnar collateral ligament.

Phase VI: Weeks 10 to 13

The patient continues aggressive upper-body strengthening and begins plyometric training. He or she continues endurance training. Restoration of normal flexibility is emphasized.

Further Rehabilitation

After completion of this initial rehabilitation interval, throwing is initiated under the surgeon's supervision and is advanced between weeks 14 and 20. The patient begins light tossing (i.e., from 30 to 40 ft without a windup) for 10 to 15 minutes during each of two or three sessions weekly.

The distance is increased to 60 ft at 5 months after surgery, and an easy windup is added at 6 months. Flexibility exercises are continued, and a total upper-body exercise program using normal training principles is started. The patient applies ice to the elbow after each training or throwing session to reduce inflammation. At 7 or 8 months after surgery, pitchers can return to the mound. The duration of the throwing sessions increases to 25 min, and effort progresses from 50% to 70% velocity by the eighth or ninth month. During the tenth and eleventh months, rehabilitation focuses on body mechanics and technique. The patient participates in longer throwing sessions and begins game simulation. Competitive throwing is permitted at 12 months if upper-body range of motion and strength are normal and if the arm is pain free. Elite-level pitchers might need 18 months to fully regain preoperative rhythm and accuracy.

RESULTS

Of the various sport participants who have had UCL reconstruction, baseball pitchers are the most difficult to return to their previous level of function. However, most athletes who participate in sports involving overhead-throwing motions and who have UCL reconstruction are able to return to their previous level of function. Jobe and associates reported that 68% of overhead athletes, most of whom were baseball players, in their series returned to their previous level of participation after UCL reconstruction.[12] Fifty percent of the repair group returned to their previous level. The time to recovery differed between the two groups; the repair group averaged 9 months, and the reconstruction group averaged 12 months. Athletes who had previous elbow operations had a lower chance of returning to their previous level of participation than athletes who had not had previous elbow operations.

COMPLICATIONS

The most common postoperative complications following UCL reconstruction include trauma to the medial antebrachial cutaneous nerve and trauma to the ulnar nerve. In one series, researchers noted that ulnar nerve irritation occurred in 21% of patients who had a reconstruction.[11] Seven patients who had ulnar nerve transpositions with the primary reconstruction needed another procedure to treat ulnar nerve problems.

When using the muscle-splitting approach, we do not routinely transpose or release the ulnar nerve and have found that most of our patients do not require ulnar nerve procedures. When the ulnar nerve is addressed, gentle handling and preservation of its vascular supply are essential. Meticulous hemostasis can prevent postoperative hematoma formation.

We routinely address intra-articular injuries, such as loose bodies or osteophytes, with preliminary arthroscopy to avoid the need for a posterior arthrotomy near the ulnar nerve. Careful subcutaneous dissection during the approach with preservation of branches of the medial antebrachial cutaneous nerve can prevent inadvertent transection and development of paresthesias or painful neuromas. Mild postoperative flexion deformities do not appear to preclude an excellent functional result.[10]

CONCLUSION

Reconstruction of the ulnar collateral ligament has proved to be a successful method of restoring the valgus stability to the elbow of the overhead-throwing athlete with ligament incompetence or rupture. Although many athletes can rehabilitate and return to sports without reconstruction of an incompetent UCL, overhead-throwing athletes, such as baseball players, often require stabilization to return to their previous level of play. A thorough preoperative history and physical examination are essential in the management of the athletes, and imaging studies such as MRI are extremely helpful in defining the articular and periarticular anatomy. Associated injuries, such as articular cartilage damage or ulnar nerve injury, must be identified preoperatively and addressed appropriately for a successful result.

Surgical technique and graft selection vary depending on the surgeon's experience and the patient's associated disorders and anatomy. A careful elbow examination under anesthesia and arthroscopy combined with the reconstruction procedure allow for improved joint and ligament evaluation and should be left to an experienced elbow surgeon.

The patient–athlete should be made aware of the prolonged recovery period after ligament reconstruction. To return to the previous level of throwing, he or she must remain committed to a graduated rehabilitation program of 12 to 18 months. This recovery process should be supervised by the surgeon and involve close collaboration among the athlete, coaches, trainers, and physical therapists.

REFERENCES

1. Hotchkiss RN, Weiland AJ. Valgus stability of the elbow. *J Orthop Res* 1987;5:372–377.
2. Morrey BF. Applied anatomy and biomechanics of the elbow joint. *Instructional Course Lect* 1986;35:59–68.
3. Morrey BF, An K-N. Articular and ligamentous contributions to the stability of the elbow joint. *Am J Sports Med* 1983;11:314–319.
4. Morrey BF, An K-N. Functional anatomy of the ligaments of the elbow. *Clin Orthop* 1985;201:84–90.
5. Regan WD, Korinek SL, Morrey BF, et al. Biomechanical study of ligaments around the elbow joint. *Clin Orthop* 1991;271:170–179.
6. Sojbjerg JO, Ovesen J, Nielsen S. Experimental elbow instability after transection of the medial collateral ligament. *Clin Orthop* 1987;218:186–190.
7. Tullos HS, Schwab G, Bennett JB, et al. Factors influencing elbow instability. *Instructional Course Lect* 1981;31:185–199.
8. Morrey BF, Tanaka S, An K-N. Valgus stability of the elbow: A definition of primary and secondary constraints. *Clin Orthop* 1991;265:187–195.
9. Protzman RR. Dislocation of the elbow joint. *J Bone Joint Surg* 1978;60A:539–541.
10. Andrews JR, Whiteside JA. Common elbow problems in the athlete. *J Orthop Sports Phys Ther* 1993;17:289–295.
11. Conway JE, Jobe FW, Glousman RE, et al. Medial instability of the elbow in throwing athletes. Treatment by repair or reconstruction of the ulnar collateral ligament. *J Bone Joint Surg* 1992;74A:67–83.
12. Jobe FW, Stark H, Lombardo SJ. Reconstruction of the ulnar collateral ligament in athletes. *J Bone Joint Surg* 1986;68A:1158–1163.
13. Norwood LA, Shook JA, Andrews JR. Acute medial elbow ruptures. *Am J Sports Med* 1981;9:16–19.
14. Timmerman LA, Andrews JR. Undersurface tears of the ulnar collateral ligament in baseball players: A newly recognized lesion. *Am J Sports Med* 1994;22:33–36.
15. Wilson FD, Andrews JR, Blackburn TA, et al. Valgus extension overload in the pitching elbow. *Am J Sports Med* 1983;11:83–88.
16. Timmerman LA, Andrews JR. Histology and arthroscopic anatomy of the ulnar collateral ligament of the elbow. *Am J Sports Med* 1994;22:667–673.
17. O'Driscoll SW, Jaloszynski R, Morrey BF, et al. Origin of the medial ulnar collateral ligament. *J Hand Surg* 1992;17A:164–168.
18. London JT. Kinematics of the elbow. *J Bone Joint Surg* 1981;63A:529–535.
19. Morrey BF, Chao EYS. Passive motion of the elbow joint. *J Bone Joint Surg* 1976;58A:501–508.
20. Schwab GH, Bennett JB, Woods GW, et al. Biomechanics of elbow instability: The role of the medial collateral ligament. *Clin Orthop* 1980;146:42–52.
21. Tullos HS, King JW. Throwing mechanism in sports. *Orthop Clin North Am* 1973;4:7709–7720.
22. Barnes DA, Tullos HS. An analysis of 100 symptomatic baseball players. *Am J Sports Med* 1978;6:62–66.
23. King JW, Brelsford HJ, Tullos HS. Analysis of the pitching arm of the professional baseball pitcher. *Clin Orthop* 1969;67:116–123.
24. Feltner M, Dapena J. Dynamics of the shoulder and elbow joints of the throwing arm during a baseball pitch. *J Sport Biomech* 1986;2:235–259.
25. Werner SL, Fleisig GS, Dillman CS, et al. Biomechanics of the elbow during baseball pitching. *J Orthop Sports Phys Ther* 1993;17:274–278.
26. Glousman RE, Barron J, Jobe FW, et al. An electromyographic analysis of the elbow in normal and injured pitchers with medial collateral ligament insufficiency. *Am J Sports Med* 1992;20:311–317.
27. Veltri DM, O'Brien SJ, Field LD, et al. The milking maneuver—A new test to evaluate the MCL of the elbow in the throwing athlete. *J Shoulder Elbow Surg* 1995;4:S10, 22.
28. Albright JA, Jokl P, Shaw R, et al. Clinical study of baseball pitchers: Correlation of injury with method of delivery. *Am J Sports Med* 1978;6:15–21.
29. Timmerman LA, Schwartz ML, Andrews JR. Preoperative evaluation of the ulnar collateral ligament by magnetic resonance imaging and computed tomography arthrography. *Am J Sports Med* 1994;22:26–31.
30. Mirowitz SA, London SL. Ulnar collateral ligament injury in baseball pitchers: MR imaging evaluation. *Radiology* 1992;185:573–576.
31. Hamilton CD, Glousman RE, Job FW, et al. Dynamic stability of the flexor pronator group and the extensor group in pitchers with valgus instability. *J Shoulder Elbow Surg* 1995;5:347–354.
32. Smith GR, Altchek DW, Pagnani MJ, et al. A muscle-splitting approach to the ulnar collateral ligament of the elbow. Neuroanatomy and operative technique. *Am J Sports Med* 1996;24:575–580.

CHAPTER 8

Lateral Collateral Ligament Reconstruction

Mark S. Cohen

INTRODUCTION

Posterolateral rotatory instability is a recently described condition resulting from insufficiency of the lateral ligamentous and muscular support of the elbow.[1,2] Lateral joint laxity allows the proximal forearm (i.e., ulna and radius) to subluxate away from the humeral trochlea when loaded in supination. Unlike medial collateral instability that manifests as medial elbow pain with laxity to valgus stress, posterolateral instability is rarer and is not associated with a specific activity, such as overhead throwing. It often presents with subtle findings on history and examination, and thus the diagnosis requires a high index of suspicion. In this chapter, we review the pertinent anatomy, pathophysiology, and surgical treatment of posterolateral rotatory instability of the elbow.

FUNCTIONAL ANATOMY

Lateral elbow instability is most commonly a posttraumatic condition. In most instances, the injury involves a combination of axial compressive, external rotatory, and valgus forces applied to the elbow.[3,4] Researchers also have proposed varus extension as a mechanism of injury.[1] It also may have an iatrogenic origin, because this instability has been reported following overly aggressive debridement of the lateral soft tissues for recalcitrant lateral epicondylitis, or tennis elbow.[1,5]

This instability pattern involves rotatory subluxation of the elbow without dislocation. The proximal radioulnar relationship remains undisturbed. The proximal radius and ulna subluxate as a unit, resulting in lateral gaping at the ulnohumeral joint and posterior translation of the radial head in relation to the capitellum. This result occurs primarily when the elbow is loaded in supination, which places stress on the lateral soft tissues opposing the posterolateral subluxation of the proximal forearm. The instability is greatest at approximately 40° of elbow flexion and reduces with forearm pronation and elbow flexion.

Both ligamentous and musculotendinous restraints are responsible for stabilizing the relationship between the proximal forearm and humerus. Researchers recently have elucidated the anatomy and functional contribution of these structures.[6] The radial collateral ligament originates along the base of the lateral epicondylar teardrop. It extends distally and blends with the annular ligament to form a broad, common insertion onto the proximal ulna along the supinator crest.[6,7] The proximal margin of this conjoined ligamentous insertion is at the most proximal aspect of the radial head. The insertion spans distally approximately 2 cm in either a single or bilobed fashion (Fig. 8.1).[6] The fibers of the supinator cross obliquely from distal to proximal over this ligamentous complex. The extensor muscles of the lateral portion of the elbow cover this deep tissue layer (Fig. 8.2).

The lateral collateral and annular ligament complex represents the primary restraint to posterolateral elbow instability. This structure maintains the ulnohumeral and radiocapitellar joints in a reduced position when the elbow is loaded in supination. Principal secondary restraints of the lateral elbow consist of the extensor muscles with their fascial bands and intermuscular septa.[6] By virtue of their course alone, the extensor muscles serve to independently support the forearm unit from laterally rotating away from the humerus. In supination, they provide a static and dynamic vector supporting the lateral

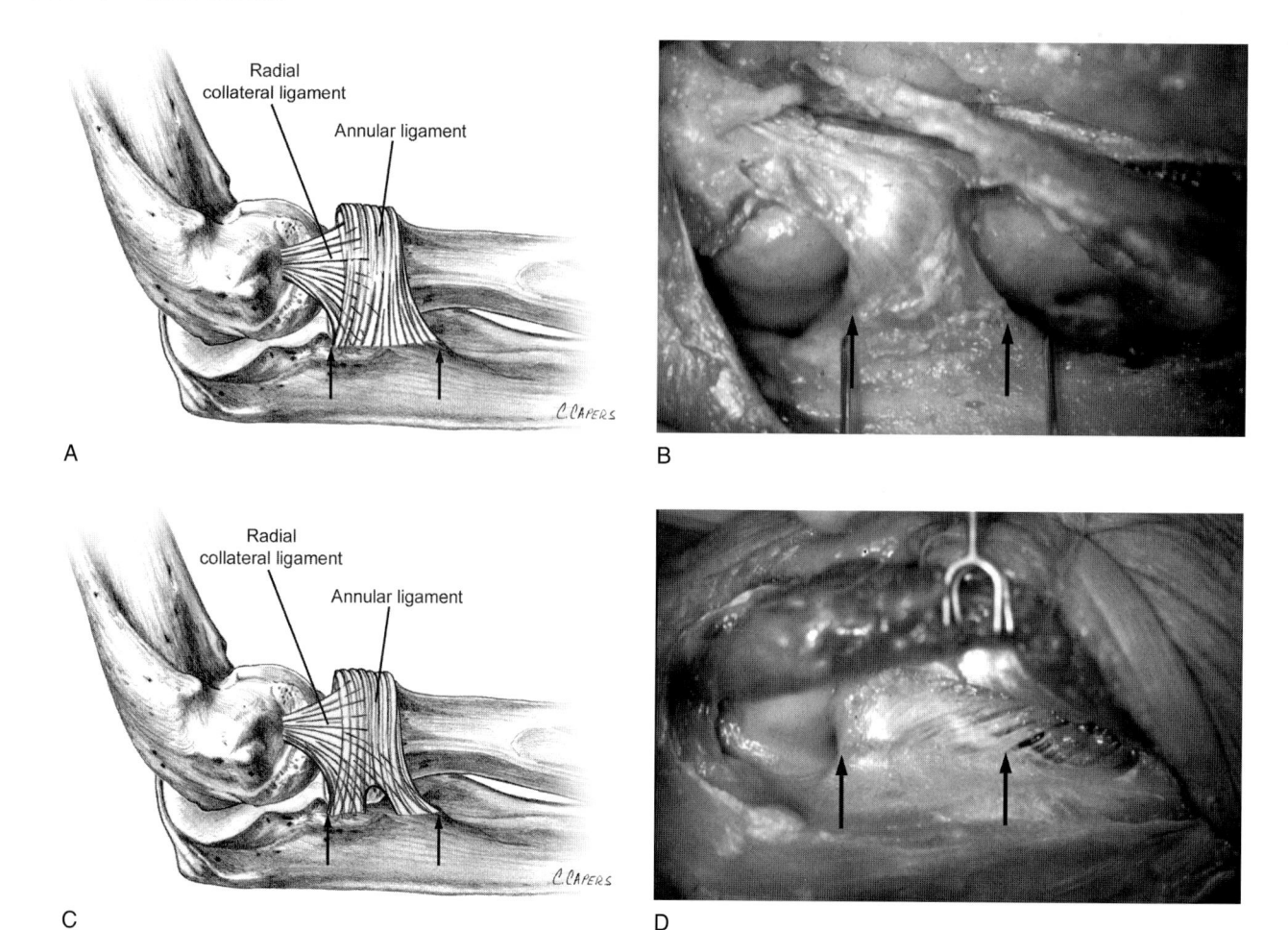

FIGURE 8.1. (A) Drawing and (B) cadaveric specimen depicting the anatomy of the lateral collateral and annular ligament complexes. (C) Drawing and (D) cadaveric specimen depicting a bilobed ulnar insertion. In both cadaveric specimens, the overlying extensor muscles and supinator fibers have been removed. Note how the collateral ligament blends with the annular ligament to form a conjoined insertion (arrows) on the proximal ulna.

portion of the joint. An additional stout intermuscular septum between the extensor digitorum communis and extensor digiti quinti muscular compartments (which defines the axis of rotation of the elbow) tightens in forearm supination, providing further lateral support.[6]

The extensor carpi ulnaris is the most proximal of the extensor muscles and thus has the best mechanical advantage in supporting the proximal forearm. This muscle has a consistent fascial band on its undersurface that originates at the inferior epicondyle and inserts onto the ulna approximately 5 cm distal to the radial head (Fig. 8.3).[6,8–10] The extensor carpi ulnaris fascial band becomes taut in supination and, with the extensor tendon origins and septa, it can provide significant lateral elbow support.[6]

Clinically, posterolateral elbow rotatory instability requires insufficiency of both the ligamentous and musculotendinous origins about the lateral elbow. Both clinical and experimental studies show that the most common mechanism of injury involves proximal attenuation or avulsion of these structures from the lateral epicondyle during a traumatic injury.[6,11–14]

DIAGNOSIS

Patients who have lateral elbow instability present with a variable history and symptoms. Previous trauma can involve a documented dislocation of the elbow or an injury without dislocation. Patients report a sensation of their elbow intermittently "giving way" or "going out." Common mechanical symptoms include popping, catching, or snapping of the elbow. The symptoms typically manifest during loading of the joint in a slightly flexed position with the forearm in supination, such as when picking up a heavy briefcase. In patients whose elbows are more unstable, these episodes can occur with very minor loading, such as when turning over in bed during sleep.

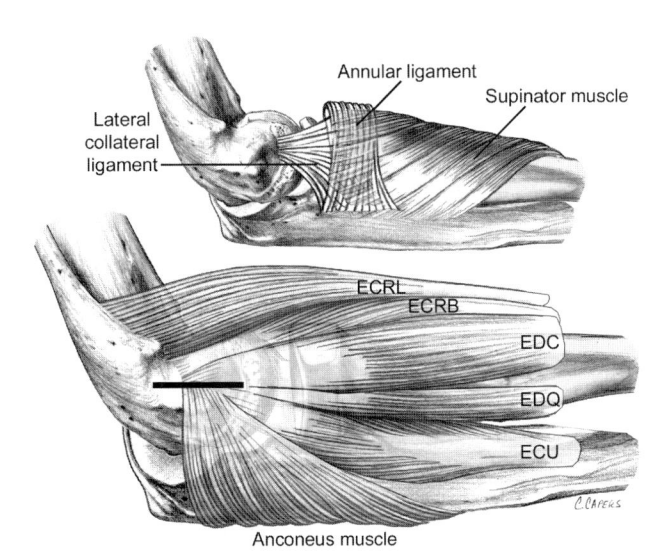

FIGURE 8.2. The deep (above) and superficial (below) layers supporting the lateral elbow. The deep layer consists of the lateral collateral and annular ligament complex with the tightly opposed overlying tendinous fibers of the supinator muscle. The superficial layer comprises the extensor tendons and their intermuscular fascia and septa. Note that the axis of the elbow is defined by the intermuscular septum between the extensor digitorum communis (EDC) and the extensor digiti quinti (EDQ). The extensor carpi ulnaris (ECU), with its broad fascial band, has the best mechanical advantage of the extensors in resisting posterolateral rotatory instability of the elbow. ECRL, extensor carpi radialis longus; ECRB, extensor carpi radialis brevis.

The physical examination is characteristically benign with respect to range of motion (although a slight loss of extension can be observed) and motor and sensory evaluations. Grip strength is typically normal as well. If the patient's initial injury occurred long before this examination, he or she might only have minimal discomfort when the examiner palpates the bony or soft tissue structures of the lateral portion of the elbow. The elbow is clinically stable to varus and valgus stress. Plain radiographs (anteroposterior and lateral views) are usually negative, but the examiner might observe a small lateral avulsion fragment off the lateral epicondyle (Fig. 8.4).

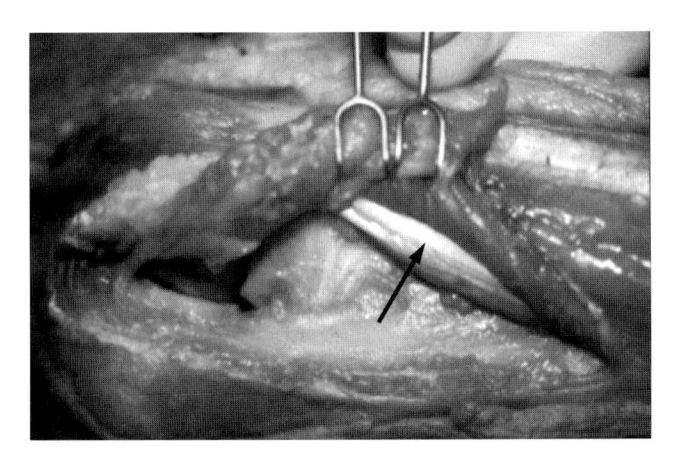

FIGURE 8.3. Cadaveric specimen depicting the broad fascial band on the undersurface of the extensor carpi ulnaris (ECU) (arrow). This band originates on the inferior aspect of the humeral epicondyle and runs along the undersurface of the ECU at its inferior margin to insert onto the ulna. With the extensor muscles and intermuscular septa, it provides a secondary restraint to posterolateral elbow instability.

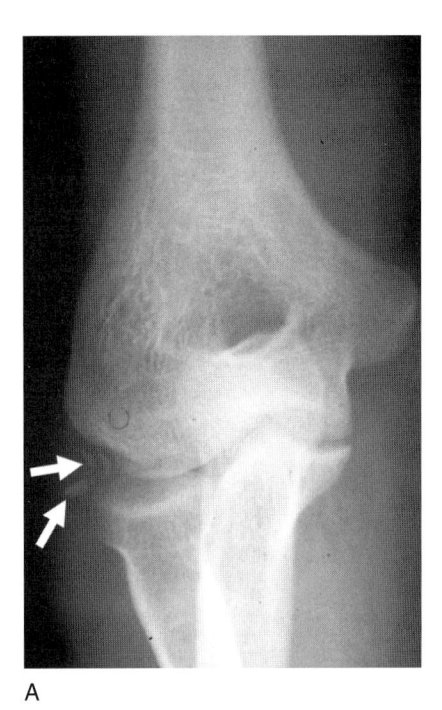

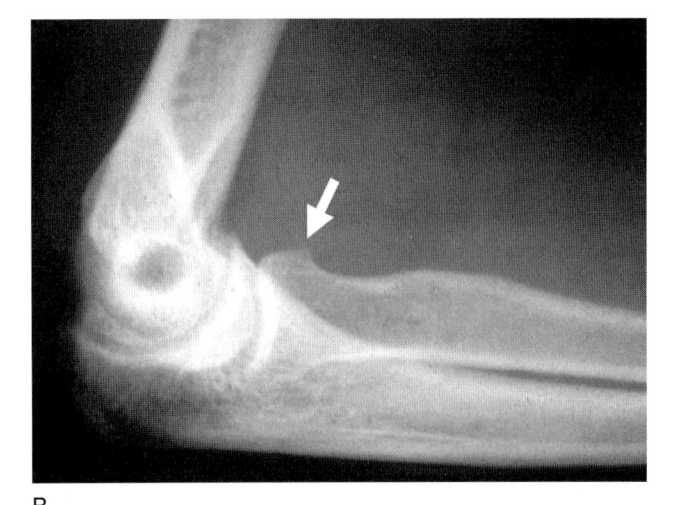

FIGURE 8.4. (A) Anteroposterior and (B) lateral radiographs of a patient with posttraumatic rotatory instability of the elbow. Note the small avulsion fragments (arrows) seen adjacent to the radial head from proximal failure of the collateral and extensor tendon origins at the lateral epicondyle. The lateral radiograph reveals a concentrically reduced joint. Small lateral avulsion fractures are occasionally associated with this condition.

Often, several physicians may have examined the patient, but may not have made a specific diagnosis.

Although clinically demonstrating frank posterolateral instability is difficult, the appropriate provocative maneuver often can reproduce subtle subluxation of the lateral portion of the elbow. One such maneuver is the posterolateral rotatory instability test.[2] The examiner conducts this test with the patient's arm in adduction, forearm in supination, and elbow in approximately 40° to 45° of flexion. The examiner stabilizes the humerus with one hand, placing his or her fingers along the lateral ulnohumeral joint line. The examiner's contralateral arm applies a slight axial and valgus force while loading the patient's proximal forearm in supination. Gaping at the ulnohumeral articulation as the ulna and radial head subluxate from the humerus demonstrates instability (Fig. 8.5). This maneuver results in a posterolateral prominence as the radial head subluxates with the ulna away from the capitellum. The elbow subluxates during this maneuver but does not dislocate. Pronating and slightly flexing the joint reduce the ulnohumeral articulation. A palpable "clunk" occasionally accompanies reduction.

A positive posterolateral rotatory instability test is difficult to elicit in patients who are not anesthetized, especially in individuals who have well-developed musculature. Patients who have lateral rotatory instability characteristically resist this provocative maneuver. Guarding, in effect, constitutes a positive apprehension test. The clinician can conduct the examination most easily when the patient is anesthetized because the muscles are relaxed. Lateral stress radiographs aid in the diagnosis. A true lateral elbow film can be taken with the forearm maximally supinated or during the posterolateral rotatory instability test (Fig. 8.5B). This film might reveal a widened ulnohumeral articulation with an inferiorly subluxated radial head that is now posterior to the midline of the capitellum. Although not typically used to make the diagnosis, magnetic resonance imaging commonly reveals a disruption of the lateral collateral and tendinous origins at the humeral epicondyle. The clinician sometimes can observe subluxation of the lateral joint as well (Fig. 8.6).

SURGICAL REPAIR

The most common abnormality leading to posterolateral instability of the elbow is disruption of the collateral ligament and musculotendinous extensor origins at the humeral epicondyle. In children, a simple reefing of the lateral soft tissues might successfully treat the instability. However, in adults, reconstruction of the collateral ligament with a free autogenous tendon graft typically is necessary to stabilize the lateral portion of the elbow.[14] The palmaris longus tendon is most commonly harvested for this purpose.

The surgeon may perform the procedure while the patient is under regional anesthesia with a long-acting axillary block. To confirm the diagnosis of posterolateral rotatory instability of the elbow, he or she conducts an examination under anesthesia. Next, an extended Kocher incision is made that begins along the supracondylar humeral ridge and passes distally over the radiocapitellar joint toward the ulna.[15] The interval between the anconeus and the extensor carpi ulnaris is defined. The anconeus is reflected posteriorly with the triceps along the supracondylar humeral ridge (Fig. 8.7). The extensor carpi ulnaris is retracted anteriorly, revealing the deep

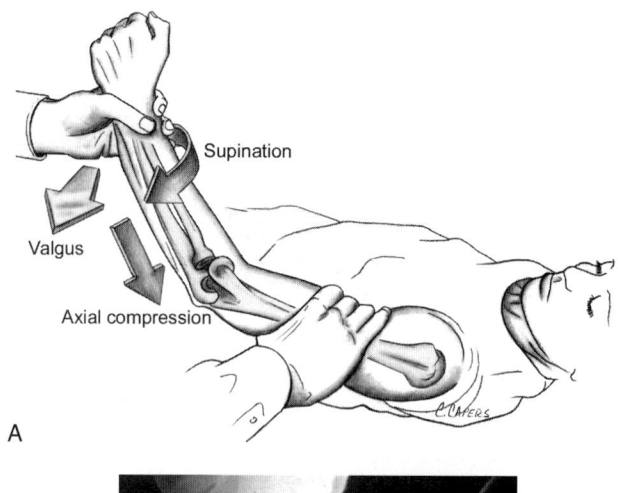

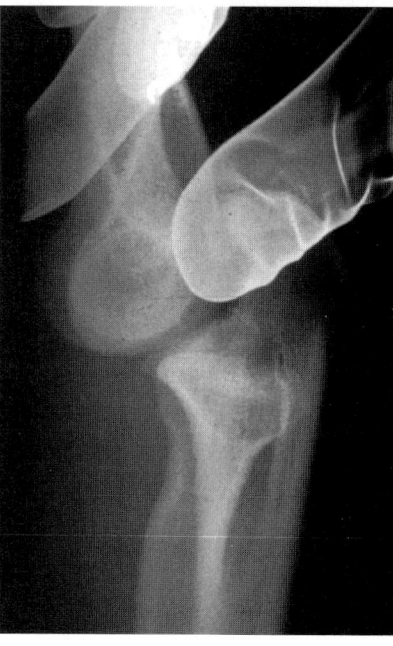

FIGURE 8.5. (A) The posterolateral rotatory instability test. In patients who have posterolateral instability, the examiner can elicit guarding or frank joint subluxation with this maneuver. (B) Lateral stress radiograph depicting this provocative maneuver in a patient who has posterolateral elbow instability. This radiograph shows gaping at the ulnohumeral articulation and posterior translation of the radial head now projecting posterior to the center of the capitellum.

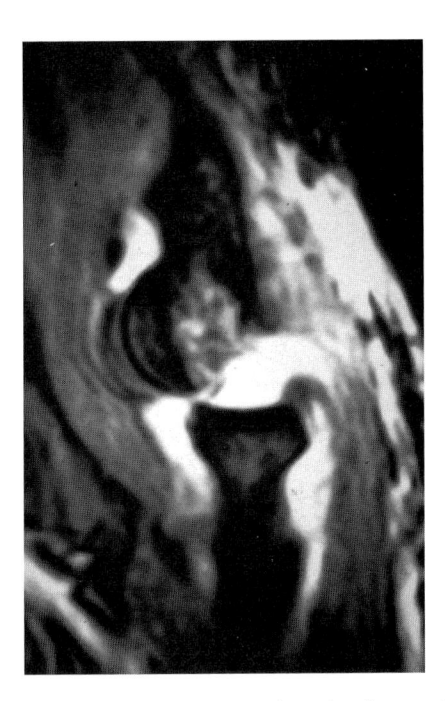

FIGURE 8.6. Magnetic resonance imaging in a patient who has documented posterolateral instability of the elbow. Note the posterior subluxation of the radiocapitellar joint. This scan also depicts altered signal intensity and decreased definition of the origin of the collateral ligament and common extensor tendon origins at the lateral humeral epicondyle.

collateral and annular ligament layer with the overlying fibers of the supinator.

The ulnohumeral and inferior radiocapitellar articulations can be inspected by incising the posterior joint capsule in the soft spot, which is in the triangular area formed by the palpable epicondyle, radial head, and ulna. This capsular tissue is very thin and of little functional importance.[6] The cartilage surfaces can be inspected, and any synovitis within the joint can be excised. Care must be taken to incise the capsule only up to the most proximal margin of the radial head. This margin marks the proximal extent of the fibers of the radial collateral and annular ligamentous complex (see Fig. 8.1).

The dissection of the extensor carpi ulnaris is carried back to the humeral epicondyle, and the entire common extensor tendon and ligamentous origin can be reflected anteriorly off the epicondyle. This origin is best released from posterior and inferior to anterior and superior. The release allows full exposure of the capitellum and epicondyle. The origin later is advanced and repaired back to the humerus. A burr can be used to roughen up the area of origin down to bleeding subchondral bone to aid in healing. Distally, the proximal ulna must be exposed adequately to identify the supinator crest just posterior to the radial head. Maximum supination of the forearm clearly demonstrates subluxation of the ulnohumeral and radiocapitellar joints due to insufficient lateral joint support.

Next, the surgeon drills holes for placement of the free tendon graft (Fig. 8.7B). The center of rotation, or isometric origin, of the lateral ligamentous complex of the elbow is at the base of the epicondylar teardrop where the epicondyle flattens onto the lateral aspect of the capitellum. This point is at the center of the trochlea and capitellum and is at the intersection of a line connecting the anterior cortex of the humerus with the center of the radial head when reduced.[16,17] An entry hole is placed with its distal margin at the isometric point and drilled out posteriorly and superiorly using sequential drill bits. A second posterior hole is positioned inferior to the first and connected to the isometric entry hole. The surgeon uses curettes to create tunnels that are approximately 4 mm in diameter. The free tendon graft then can be threaded through the isometric point posteriorly, through the second hole, and back into the isometric point, allowing for a two-ply graft at this point (Fig. 8.7C). A suture placed through the end of the graft and a ligature passer aid in threading the graft.

When fashioning the ulnar tunnels, the surgeon must understand the normal insertion of the lateral collateral and annular ligament complex. The ligament inserts along the supinator crest of the proximal ulna only several millimeters posterior to the proximal radioulnar joint. Using sequential drill bits, the surgeon makes an entry hole several millimeters distal to the proximal margin of the radial head. An exit hole is created along the supinator crest approximately 1.5 cm distal to the first hole. The osseous bridge should be at least 1 cm long to provide stability. Curettes are used to create a tunnel between these drill holes. If the surgeon has not had experience defining the proximal isometric point on the humerus, a free suture can be used for this purpose once the ulnar tunnel has been drilled[1] (Fig. 8.7B).

The free tendon graft is then threaded through the ulnar tunnel. Usually, the length of the graft is adequate to pass each free end through the tunnel (i.e., one end passed distal to proximal and one end passed proximal to distal), allowing a four-ply tendon graft. Care must be taken to clean these tunnels adequately to allow a crossed passage of the graft (Fig. 8.7E). Alternatively, if the length is insufficient, the graft can be passed once distally, yielding a three-ply graft.

We reattach the original collateral ligament and extensor tendon origin before final securing of the graft. The forearm is flexed to approximately 45° and fully pronated, reducing the posterolateral joint subluxation. With the aid of suture anchors (i.e., one placed slightly distal and one placed just anterior to the isometric point) or drill holes through bone, the ligament and tendon origin is advanced and repaired back to the humerus (Fig. 8.7E). Next, the tendon graft is sutured to itself when pulled taut. The graft strands can be sutured to one another and to the underlying capsule and adjacent collateral ligament complex to reinforce the reconstruction

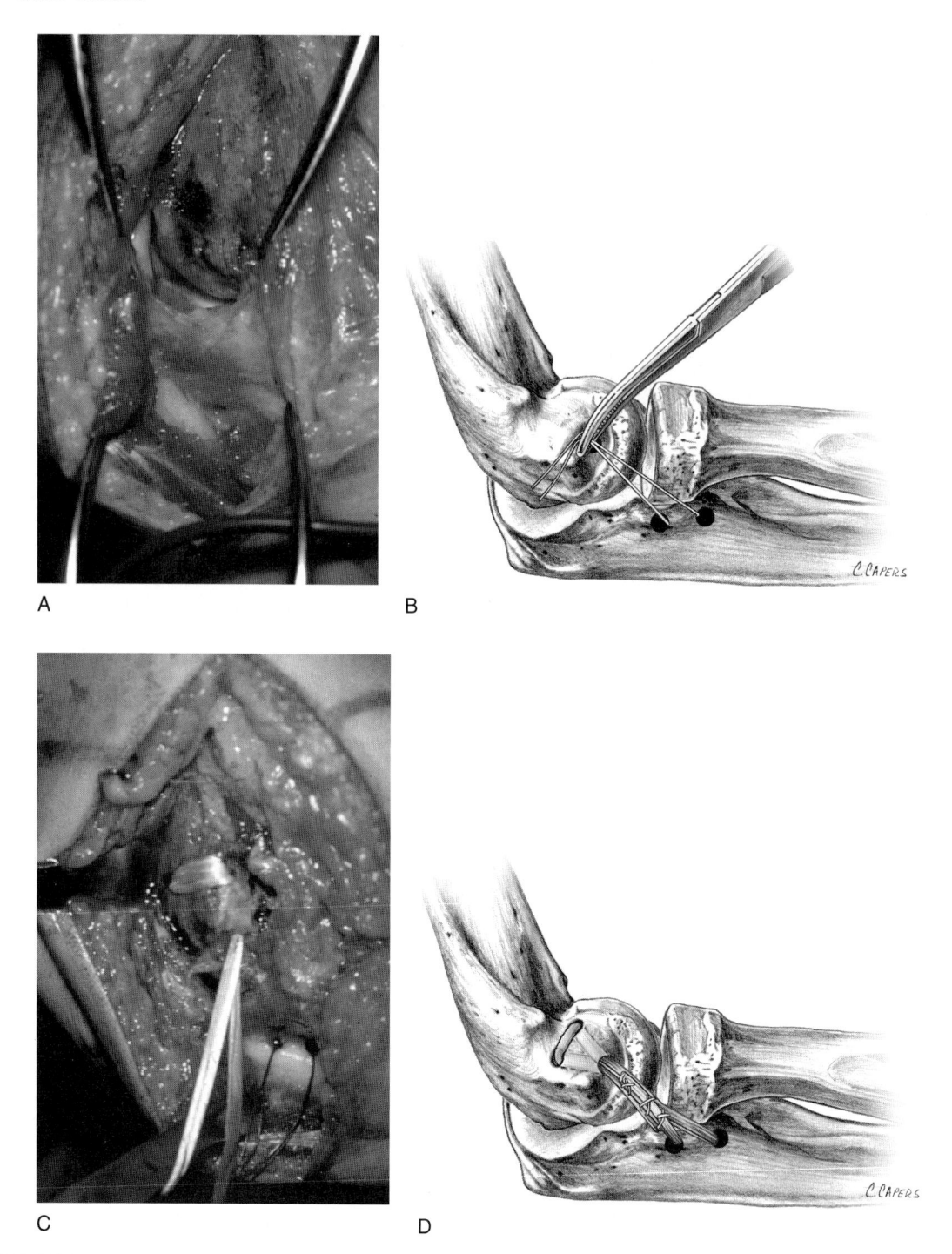

FIGURE 8.7. (A) Intraoperative photograph during reconstruction for posterolateral instability of the elbow. The anconeus and triceps have been reflected posteriorly. The posterior joint capsule has been opened, allowing inspection of the ulnohumeral joint and the posterior aspect of the radiocapitellar articulation. The capsule can be released distally to the proximal margin of the radial head, which marks the most proximal aspect of the lateral collateral and annular ligament complex. (B) Tunnel placement and course of the free tendon graft. The ulnar tunnel is placed just posterior to the radiocapitellar joint along the supinator crest of the ulna. (C) Intraoperative photograph of the free tendon graft that has been passed through the isometric point, out posteriorly, and back through the isometric point, yielding a two-ply graft at this point. Note the suture that has been placed through the ulnar tunnel to aid in graft passage. (D) Final graft and tunnel placement. (*Continues*)

(Fig. 8.7F). The elbow can be taken through a range of motion once the graft is secured. The surgeon now can appreciate the function of the graft, which acts as a reinforcement to the radial collateral and annular ligament complex. It holds up the proximal ulna to the humeral trochlea, and it provides a restraint to the radial head because it prevents the radial head from subluxating laterally from the capitellum in supination. The anconeus and

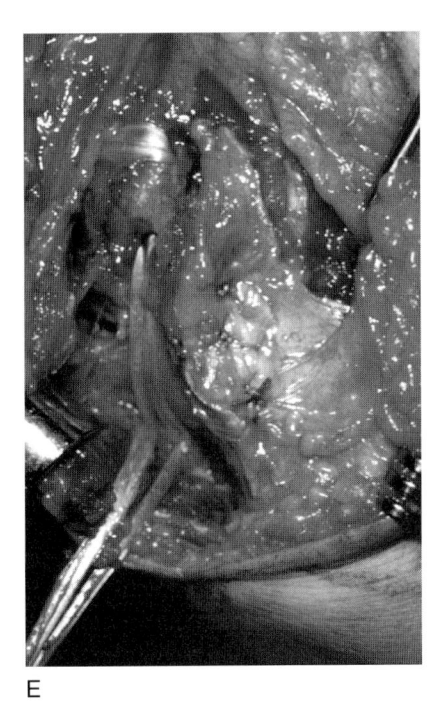

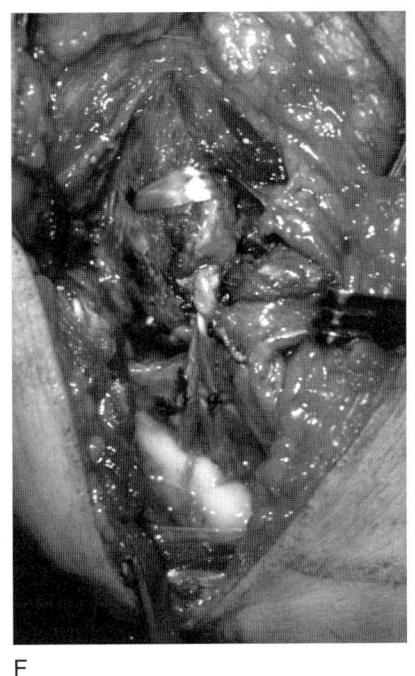

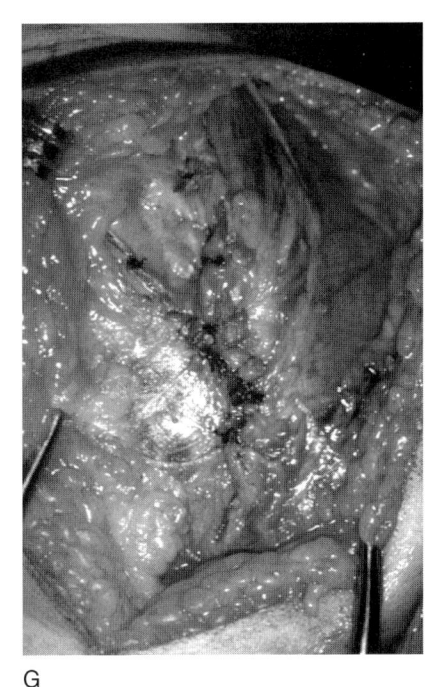

FIGURE 8.7. (*Continued*) (E) The graft has now been passed through the ulnar tunnel (one arm from proximal to distal and one from distal to proximal), which now results in a four-ply graft for reconstruction. The common extensor and collateral ligament origins have been advanced and repaired back to the humerus with the aid of bone suture anchors once the joint has been reduced in pronation. Note the running, locking sutures used to reinforce this repair. (F) The tendon graft has now been secured to itself and to the adjacent lateral ligamentous tissues for reinforcement. (G) The triceps and anconeus fasciae are brought anteriorly and repaired to the brachialis and extensor fasciae, completing the reconstruction. The elbow should now be stable throughout a full range of motion without evidence of instability when gently stressed.

extensor fasciae are repaired securely, and the skin is closed in layers (Fig. 8.7G).

A compressive dressing applied with plaster splints maintains the elbow in at least 90° of flexion and neutral or slight pronation. We immobilize the elbow in this position with a cast or splint for 2 or 3 weeks. At the end of this time, a progressive range-of-motion program is initiated with interval splinting for protection and support. Active supination is allowed with the elbow flexed past 90°, which locks the lateral joint, and no passive extension or supination is permitted initially. Gradual extension is allowed in pronation, limiting the last 30° of extension for approximately 4 to 6 weeks after surgery. The patient is weaned from the splint at 2 to 3 months after surgery. Strengthening or loading of the elbow is not permitted until approximately 4 to 6 months following reconstruction.

RESULTS

In 1992, Nestor et al. reported the results of eleven patients who had reconstruction of the lateral elbow for recurrent posterolateral rotatory instability.[1] In the five patients who had reconstruction with a palmaris longus tendon graft (the currently preferred method), three had an excellent result. The authors believed that a previous operation to the lateral elbow was a possible negative prognostic factor to a good or excellent result.

Using the aforementioned technique, we have performed this reconstruction in six patients who had isolated posterolateral elbow instability. Symptoms of instability resolved in all patients. Elbow motion returned by approximately 3 to 4 months after surgery. All patients regained full elbow flexion and forearm rotation, but lost 5° to 15° of terminal elbow extension. This loss of extension was not a functional problem.

CONCLUSION

Insufficiency of the lateral elbow stabilizers leads to rotatory subluxation of the ulna and forearm unit away from the trochlea when loaded in supination. This instability pattern is rare and easily can be missed if the examiner does not consider this diagnosis when a patient presents with a characteristic history and physical findings. The diagnosis primarily is made clinically with the aid of a provocative test for posterolateral rotatory instability of the elbow. Reconstruction requires an understanding of the normal anatomic relationships about the lateral portion of the elbow and can lead to successful stabilization of the joint with maintenance of a functional arc of motion.

REFERENCES

1. Nestor BJ, O'Driscoll SW, Morrey BF. Ligamentous reconstruction for posterolateral rotatory instability of the elbow. *J Bone Joint Surg* 1992;74A:1235–1241.
2. O'Driscoll SW, Bell DF, Morrey BF. Posterolateral rotatory instability of the elbow. *J Bone Joint Surg* 1991;73A:440–446.
3. O'Driscoll SW, Morrey BF, Korinek S, et al. Elbow subluxation and dislocation: A spectrum of instability. *Clin Orthop* 1992;280:186–197.
4. Sojbjerg JO, Helmig P, Kjaersgaard–Andersen P. Dislocation of the elbow: An experimental study of the ligamentous injuries. *Orthopedics* 1989;12:461–463.
5. Morrey BF. Reoperation for failed surgical treatment of refractory lateral epicondylitis. *J Shoulder Elbow Surg* 1992;1:47–55.
6. Cohen MS, Hastings H II. Rotatory instability of the elbow: The anatomy and role of the lateral stabilizers. *J Bone Joint Surg* 1997;79A:225–233.
7. Martin BF. The annular ligament of the superior radio-ulnar joint. *J Anat* 1958;92:473–482.
8. Grant JCB. *Anatomy*, 6th ed. Baltimore: Williams & Wilkins; 1972.
9. Langman J, Woerdeman MW. *Atlas of medical anatomy*. Philadelphia: WB Saunders; 1978.
10. Rohen JW, Yokochi C. *Color atlas of anatomy: A photographic study of the human body*. New York: Igaku-Shoin; 1983.
11. Cohen MS, Hastings H II. Acute elbow dislocation: Evaluation and management. *J Am Acad Orthop Surg* 1998;6:15–23.
12. Josefsson PO, Gentz CF, Johnell O, et al. Surgical versus nonsurgical treatment of ligamentous injuries following dislocation of the elbow. *J Bone Joint Surg* 1987;69A:605–608.
13. Josefsson PO, Johnell O, Wendeberg B. Ligamentous injuries in dislocations of the elbow joint. *Clin Orthop* 1987;221:221–225.
14. Morrey BF, O'Driscoll SW. Lateral collateral ligament injury. In: Morrey BF, ed. *The elbow and its disorders*, 2nd ed. Philadelphia: WB Saunders; 1993:573–580.
15. Crenshaw AH. Surgical approaches. In: Crenshaw AH, ed. *Campbell's operative orthopaedics*, 7th ed. St. Louis, MO: CV Mosby; 1987:92–93.
16. An KN, Morrey BF. Biomechanics of the elbow. In: Morrey BF, ed. *The elbow and its disorders*, 2nd ed. Philadelphia: WB Saunders; 1993:53–73.
17. Morrey BF. Applied anatomy and biomechanics of the elbow joint. *Instructional Course Lect* 1986;35:59–68.

CHAPTER 9

Biceps Tendon and Triceps Tendon Ruptures

Bruce M. Leslie and Helen Ranger

INTRODUCTION

The most common tendon ruptures about the elbow are of the biceps and triceps tendons. The biceps tendon rupture is the more frequent of the two, but neither is particularly common.

Biceps tendon ruptures are always associated with weakness of supination and are frequently associated with ecchymosis. Weakness of elbow flexion and proximal migration of the muscle belly sometimes occur in these patients. The biceps tendon may or may not be present in the antecubital fossa. Radiographs are usually normal. Partial and complete tears should be treated operatively. Anatomic repair improves supination strength and restores the normal muscle contour of the upper arm.

Triceps tendon ruptures are always associated with weakness of elbow extension and are frequently associated with ecchymosis and swelling. A palpable defect can sometimes be palpated proximal to the olecranon. Radiographs frequently show calcific or bony fragments. Partial tears can be treated nonoperatively. Anatomic repair of complete tears restores extension strength.

BICEPS TENDON RUPTURES

The biceps brachii muscle has two attachments on the arm: a proximal tendinous attachment on the glenoid and coracoid and a distal tendinous attachment on the radial tuberosity. Both attachments are subject to acute or chronic stress. Disruption of the muscle–tendon–bone interface results in a rupture. Ninety to ninety-seven percent of biceps tendon ruptures occur at the proximal attachment.[1] Ruptures at the distal biceps tendon attachment are considered uncommon. Johnson in 1897 and Acquaviva in 1898 were the first to describe distal biceps tendon ruptures.[2,3] This injury most often occurs in men who are in their fifth or sixth decade of life; however, it can occur in patients at any age after the early twenties.[4–6] The muscles in these patients tend to be well developed, but the patients do not need to have the build of a weight lifter to be at risk for rupture. Ruptures can occur in any persons who have reasonably developed muscles in their arms.

The mechanism of injury is an eccentric loading of the biceps muscle that can occur as a result of actions, such as suddenly lifting a heavy load, catching a heavy load, carrying an unbalanced object, or reaching up to prevent a fall. Ruptures also occur following relatively routine activities, such as throwing a football, carrying a large sheet of plywood, or going for a slap shot while playing hockey. The association of biceps tendon ruptures with relatively routine activities suggests that the problem may be due to chronic attritional tears that eventually weaken the distal biceps tendon. Degeneration of the tendon identified at the time of surgery and shreds of tendinous material still attached to the radial tuberosity support this supposition.[5,7,8]

Clinical Anatomy

The biceps brachii muscle originates on the scapula at the glenoid rim and coracoid process. It is the most superficial muscle belly, lying in the anterior portion of the middle third of the humerus. This muscle joins the distal tendon in the lower third of the arm. The tendon passes distally into the antecubital fossa. The antecubital fossa is defined by the brachioradialis radially and the pronator teres ulnarly. A sheath surrounds the biceps tendon as it passes through the antecubital fossa toward its insertion on the radial tuberosity. The lateral antebrachial cutaneous nerve lies superficially in the subcutaneous tissue of the antecubital fossa. The nerve parallels the brachioradialis. An incision along the anterior edge of the brachioradialis can injure the nerve. While still superficial, the tendon is contiguous with the lacertus fibrosis that becomes confluent medially with the fascia overlying the flexor–pronator mass. The brachial artery lies just beneath the lacertus fibrosis at the level of the elbow flexion crease. The tendon travels just lateral (radial) to the median nerve within the antecubital fossa and passes beneath the recurrent radial artery before it attaches to the radial tuberosity. Full forearm supination allows visualization of the tendinous insertion on the radial tuberosity.

Physical Examination

Patients who have an acute distal biceps tendon rupture often describe the sensation at the time of injury as tearing, ripping, popping, or electric. The sensation is usually sudden and dramatic. The pain is not excruciating, and it often subsides after several days. Chronic pain in the region of the distal biceps tendon suggests an incomplete or partial tear. Range of motion is normal following an acute distal biceps tendon rupture. Significant swelling and ecchymosis about the medial and anterior elbow regions are common (Fig. 9.1). Ecchymosis is due to the bleeding associated with the rupture from the radial tuberosity. Ecchymosis typically does not appear until 1 or 2 days after injury and begins to resolve within 1 or 2 weeks. It can vary from a small patch that forms in the region of the flexor–pronator origin to an area that extends from the distal third of the medial forearm to the middle portion of the medial upper arm.

Because the biceps muscle is the strongest supinator in the upper extremity, weak supination after tendon rupture is always present. Rupture of the distal biceps tendon makes resisting attempts at passive forearm pronation while the elbow is flexed difficult for even the most muscularly well-developed patient. Weak elbow flexion is not always present. Any of the other muscles that cross the anterior aspect of the elbow can contribute to elbow flexion; therefore, patients who have complete ruptures of the distal biceps tendon may appear to have normal strength when resisted elbow flexion is tested. However, a computerized muscle evaluation, such as Cybex® testing (Cybex II & Human Software, Ronkonkoma, New York), usually demonstrates marked differences in strength between the injured arm and the uninjured arm. The difference is more marked when testing supination than when testing elbow flexion.

Usually, but not always, the biceps brachii muscle belly migrates proximally with a complete distal biceps tendon rupture (Fig. 9.2). When the muscle migrates proximally, a palpable defect exists in the antecubital fossa. In patients who have muscularly well-developed arms, the defect may be difficult to appreciate; however, when the elbow is supported and the arm is relaxed, the difference between the injured and uninjured arm is apparent. The injured arm no longer has the gentle convex curve associated with an intact biceps tendon. The retracted muscle gives a more rounded appearance to the mid-third portion of the arm, creating the so-called Popeye arm.

The absence of proximal migration does not rule out the diagnosis of a distal biceps tendon rupture. A tendon may be detached completely from the radial tuberosity, but adherent to either the tendon sheath or the lacertus fibrosis. A tendon also may be ruptured almost completely, but still have enough fibers attached to the radial tuberosity to prevent proximal migration. In either case, careful examination reveals thickening about the biceps tendon in the antecubital fossa or softening of the distal portion

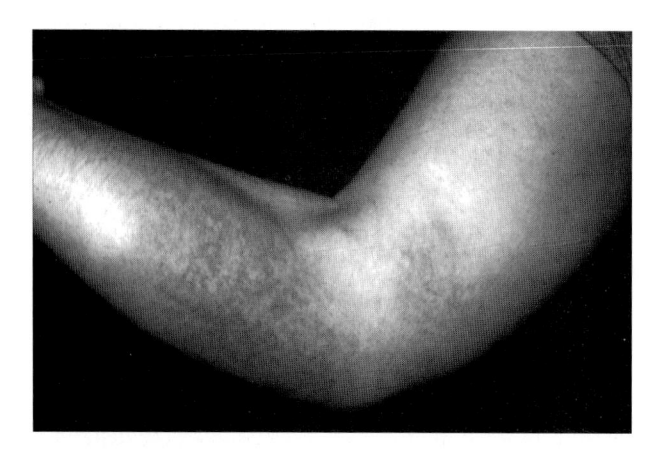

FIGURE 9.1. Ecchymosis along the medial aspect of the elbow.

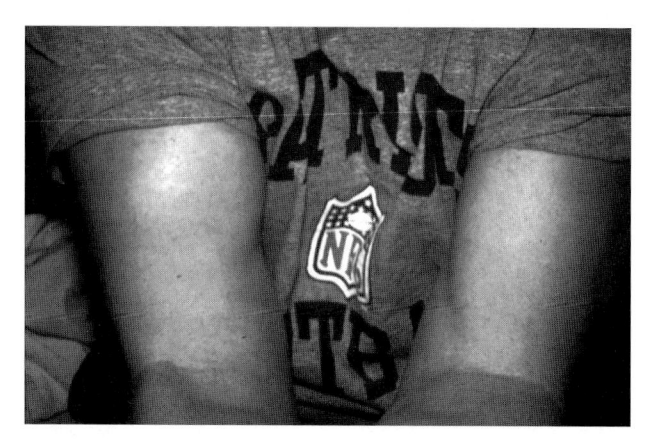

FIGURE 9.2. The right arm shows proximal migration of the biceps brachii muscle belly. Note the loss of fullness in the antecubital fossa due to retraction of the biceps tendon and the compensatory contracture of the brachioradialis with resisted elbow flexion.

of the biceps muscle. The thickening may be subtle, but comparing one arm with the other reveals the loss of the normal sharp edge to the medial and lateral aspects of the biceps tendon. The thickening is due to the bleeding and swelling along the tendon sheath. The softening is detected while palpating the distal portion of the biceps muscle while the patient resists elbow flexion. The softening also can be subtle, but comparison with the uninvolved arm assists the examiner in making the diagnosis.

Radiographs

Radiographs usually are not helpful in making the diagnosis of a distal biceps tendon rupture. Despite the presence of histologic calcifying tendinopathy,[8] which suggests a chronic degenerative process, calcification usually is not seen on radiographs. Some authors have identified mineralization or irregularity adjacent to the radial tuberosity on lateral oblique radiographs when a ruptured tendon is present.[5,7] Calcification is not a common finding.

Magnetic resonance imaging (MRI) scans are more helpful than plain radiographs in diagnosing distal biceps tendon ruptures, because the swelling and bleeding associated with a tendon rupture are usually apparent.[9] MRI scans are not necessary to confirm the diagnosis if the patient has an appropriate history, medial ecchymosis, and weak supination. MRI scans can help the examiner to diagnose a partial distal biceps tendon rupture, but incomplete tears are not easily interpreted, because the tendon can be attached to the tuberosity by a few intact tendinous fibers or by a pseudotendon of mature scar tissue.

Treatment

Nonoperative Treatment

In the past, nonoperative management of distal biceps tendon ruptures was popular.[2,4,6,7,10–12] Authors of numerous case reports suggested that early motion and strengthening exercises could restore normal strength. Authors of subsequent studies in which they used dynamometers demonstrated the deficits of nonoperative treatment.[4,6] They found that patients who were treated nonoperatively for their distal biceps tendon ruptures had weaker supination and flexion than patients who had the ruptured tendon reattached to the bicipital tuberosity.

If supination strength is not important, nonoperative treatment can be considered. A surprising degree of elbow flexion strength can be restored by strengthening the other muscles that cross the anterior aspect of the elbow. If the distal biceps tendon becomes tethered distally, it too may add to the variable elbow flexion strength that develops.

Although the treatment for each patient must be considered individually, nonoperative treatment generally yields unsatisfactory results. Using Cybex testing of nonoperatively treated patients, Baker and Bierwagen demonstrated objective deficits of biceps weakness, with endurance affected more than strength.[4] Patients in a study by Morrey et al. noted that, while they did not find their weakness debilitating, they did reach fatigue more easily with repeated, forceful supination activity.[6] Muscularly well-developed patients, particularly those involved in body-building competition, may occasionally prefer to be treated nonoperatively to avoid scarring.

Indications for Operative Treatment

The main indication for operative repair is restoration of supination strength. Without an anatomic repair, the arm's twisting motions, such as when using a screwdriver, will be weak. Patients who can effectively meet the demands of daily living without significant disability or restriction do not require surgery.

Another indication for surgery is improvement of the cosmetic appearance of the arm. A completely ruptured distal biceps tendon can cause proximal migration of the muscle belly, giving an unacceptable appearance to the arm. Anatomic restoration restores the normal contour to the arm. In a patient who desires surgery for cosmesis, the incision should not cross the antecubital fossa. Incisions that do so usually widen and are less cosmetic than those that avoid the anterior elbow flexion crease.

Delayed diagnosis can be a relative contraindication to repair.[6] Anatomic reattachment to the bicipital tuberosity is harder with contracture or scarring of the biceps muscle.[7] For such situations, some authors have advocated attachment of the tendon to the brachialis or use of a tendon graft.[5–7,13] In our own series, we have found that most delayed repairs can be reattached anatomically, even in patients whose injuries had occurred more than 6 months earlier.[14] In some cases, the tendon could only be secured with the elbow flexed 45° to 60°, but full extension was ultimately restored.

Operative Techniques

Repairs of distal biceps tendon ruptures fall into one of two groups: anatomic and nonanatomic. The earlier operations tended to be nonanatomic repairs. This type of repair was favored because of concerns about injury to the vital structures in the region of the antecubital fossa. At that time, surgeons avoided the deeper dissections associated with anatomic repair and secured the ruptured distal biceps tendon to either the lacertus fibrosis or the brachialis.[5,15] Authors of the earlier literature suggested that they could obtain a good result by attaching the ruptured tendon to the brachialis muscle. Their conclusions, however, were not based on objective measurements.

Most modern surgeons recommend anatomic reattachment. The differences in modern techniques center around the number of incisions, the site of tendon reattachment, the type of fixation device, and the use of grafts.

Initially, the tendon was reattached through an anterior incision,[16,17] but the number of reported neurovascular complications dampened the enthusiasm for this approach.[5,15] In 1961, Boyd and Anderson reported a method of reattaching the distal end of the ruptured biceps tendon using two approaches.[16,18] They used an anterior incision to retrieve the ruptured tendon and a posterior incision to reattach the tendon to the tuberosity. The tendon was passed posteriorly between the radius and ulna and was retrieved through a posterior incision. Silk sutures were passed through the tendon and out the avulsed end. The forearm was pronated to expose the radial tuberosity. A "trap door" was made in the radial tuberosity by elevating the cortex and drilling holes opposite the cortical hinge. The tendon was advanced into the trap door and the sutures tied outside the cortical drill holes. The Boyd–Anderson approach avoided the dangers of deep dissection in the antecubital fossa, but required dissection of the muscles off the lateral aspect of the olecranon. Modifications of this approach avoid the ulna by approaching the tuberosity through a posterior muscle-splitting incision and by using a high-speed burr to make the trough.[6]

The development of suture anchors has rekindled interest in the anterior approach. Le Huec et al.[9] and Lintner and Fischer[19] used a single anterior incision and reattached the tendon end with suture anchors placed into the radial tuberosity. The authors of both studies reported excellent results with no nerve injuries.

In some patients, the distal end of the ruptured distal biceps tendon cannot be brought down easily to the tuberosity. Although such instances are rare, they usually occur in patients who present many months after the complete rupture. In such situations, the distal end of the ruptured biceps tendon may be either extended or augmented with fascia lata or palmaris longus tendon graft.[7] If augmentation is not an option, the tendon can be attached to the brachialis muscle.[5]

Authors' Preferred Technique

The senior author (BML) prefers to use a modified two-incision technique to reattach the ruptured distal biceps tendon to the radial tuberosity. Most of the dissection is done through an anterior incision. A small posterolateral incision is used to tie the knot. The surgeon positions the patient supine on the operating table and extends the patient's upper extremity on a hand table. A pneumatic tourniquet is placed close to the axilla; a sterile tourniquet generally is not needed. A 6- to 8-cm oblique incision is made along the anterior edge of the flexor–pronator muscle mass and distal to the elbow flexion crease (Fig. 9.3). Placing the incision medially reduces the possibility of injury to the lateral antebrachial cutaneous

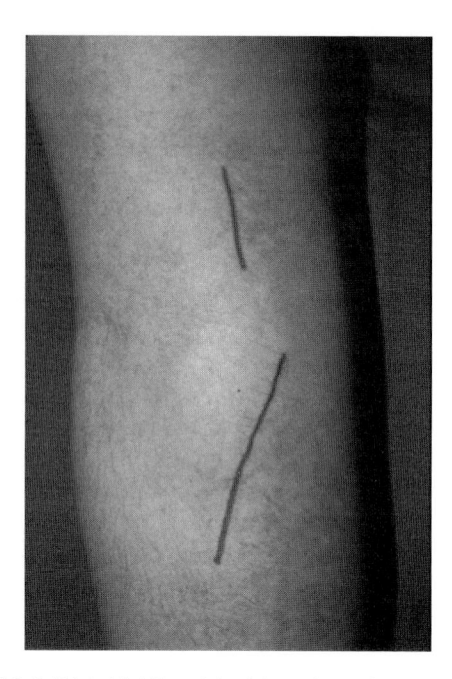

FIGURE 9.3. Distal (oblique) incision along the anterior edge of the flexor–pronator mass and the supplemental proximal incision used for tendon retrieval.

nerve. Dissection is carried down through the subcutaneous tissue to the deep forearm fascia. If the tendon rupture is partial, the tendon may appear intact and course deep toward the radial tuberosity. If the tendon rupture is complete, the tendon may have migrated proximally. If the tendon has migrated proximally, division of the lacertus fibrosis facilitates tendon exposure. At times, a swollen, fluid-filled tendon sheath obscures the tendon. Incising the sheath usually releases serosanguineous fluid. If the tendon still is not visible, milking and flexing the arm may advance the tendon into view. Sometimes the tendon can be brought down by inserting a finger proximally and medially in the incision. If the surgeon can palpate the tendon, he or she may be able to expose the end of the tendon with deep retractors and grasp it with a Kocher clamp (Fig. 9.4). Alternatively, the surgeon can make a small incision proximal and medial to the elbow flexion crease to retrieve the tendon (see Fig. 9.3). The tendon then can be passed safely into the distal incision. The use of two separate incisions, rather than a standard S-shaped incision that crosses the anterior elbow, usually provides a more cosmetically pleasing result.

After passing the tendon into the distal incision, a Kocher clamp is placed transversely at the distal end of the ruptured tendon. Traction is applied for a few minutes to overcome muscle contracture and tendinous adhesions. Blunt digital dissection usually is adequate to release the peritendinous adhesions. Two Keith needles are threaded on a no. 5 nonabsorbable suture. The suture is

9: Biceps Tendon and Triceps Tendon Ruptures / 113

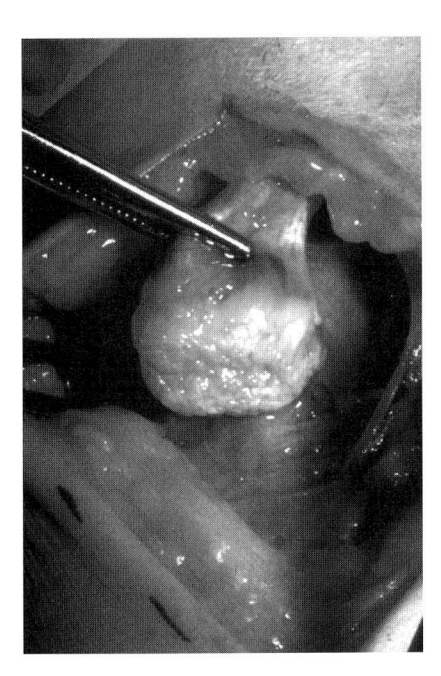

FIGURE 9.4. The distal end of the ruptured biceps tendon. Note the thickened, swollen, nodular appearance suggestive of chronic inflammation.

passed transversely near the musculotendinous junction. A Bunnell suture is placed with which to grasp the tendon. The needles should be passed simultaneously so that the suture material is not cut (Fig. 9.5). Small cuts on the medial and lateral aspects of the distal end of the ruptured tendon allow the surgeon to pass the Keith needles out of the freshly debrided tendon while still grasping the tendon with the Kocher clamp. After passing the needles and suture through the distal stump, the surgeon can safely divide the residual tendon, which is being held firmly in the Kocher clamp (Fig. 9.6). Unless the Keith needles are swagged onto the suture, small clamps should be kept on the ends of the suture to prevent the needles from sliding off. The Keith needles and suture ends then are wrapped in towels and set aside to prevent accidental puncture of the protective drapes or injury to the operating room personnel.

The next step is exposure of the radial tuberosity. If the tendon sheath is still visible, a Kelly clamp can be passed down the sheath to the tuberosity. Slow, careful dissection about the clamp exposes the radial tuberosity. Frequently, however, the tendon sheath is not visible. In this case, the tuberosity can be exposed safely by dissecting lateral to the midline and close to the extensor muscle mass. Generally, two or three veins and a branch of the recurrent radial artery must be ligated. Once the vessels are ligated, a blunt-tipped cobra retractor can be placed around the radial neck. The cobra retractor is crucial to the exposure of the radial tuberosity because it protects the medial neurovascular structures (Fig. 9.7). If the tissue is dissected lateral to the midline, the median nerve usually cannot be seen. Inadvertent dissection medial to the midline exposes the median nerve. The forearm is supinated, and the radial tuberosity is visualized. Shreds of tendon often still are attached to the tuberosity. If the patient has a partial tear, serosanguineous fluid is released as the tuberosity is approached. Careful inspection of the

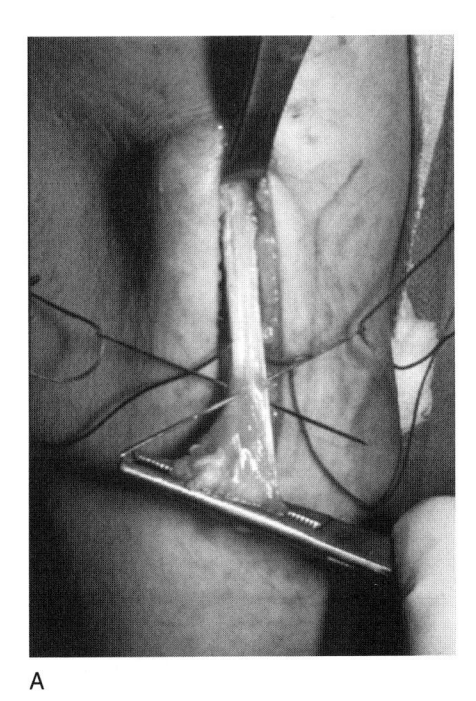

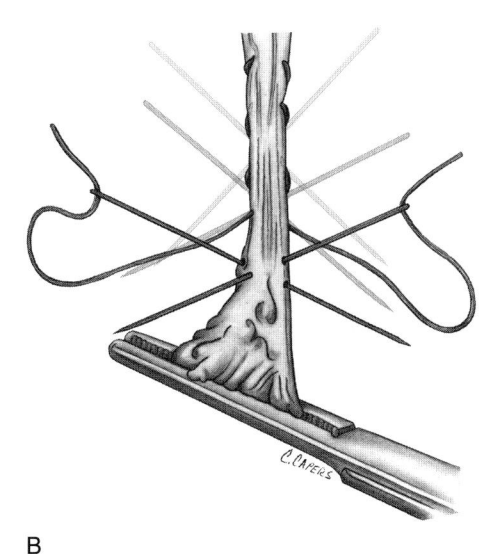

A B

FIGURE 9.5. (A) Keith needles are passed simultaneously for placement of the Bunnell suture through the distal end of the biceps tendon. (B) At least three separate passes can be made.

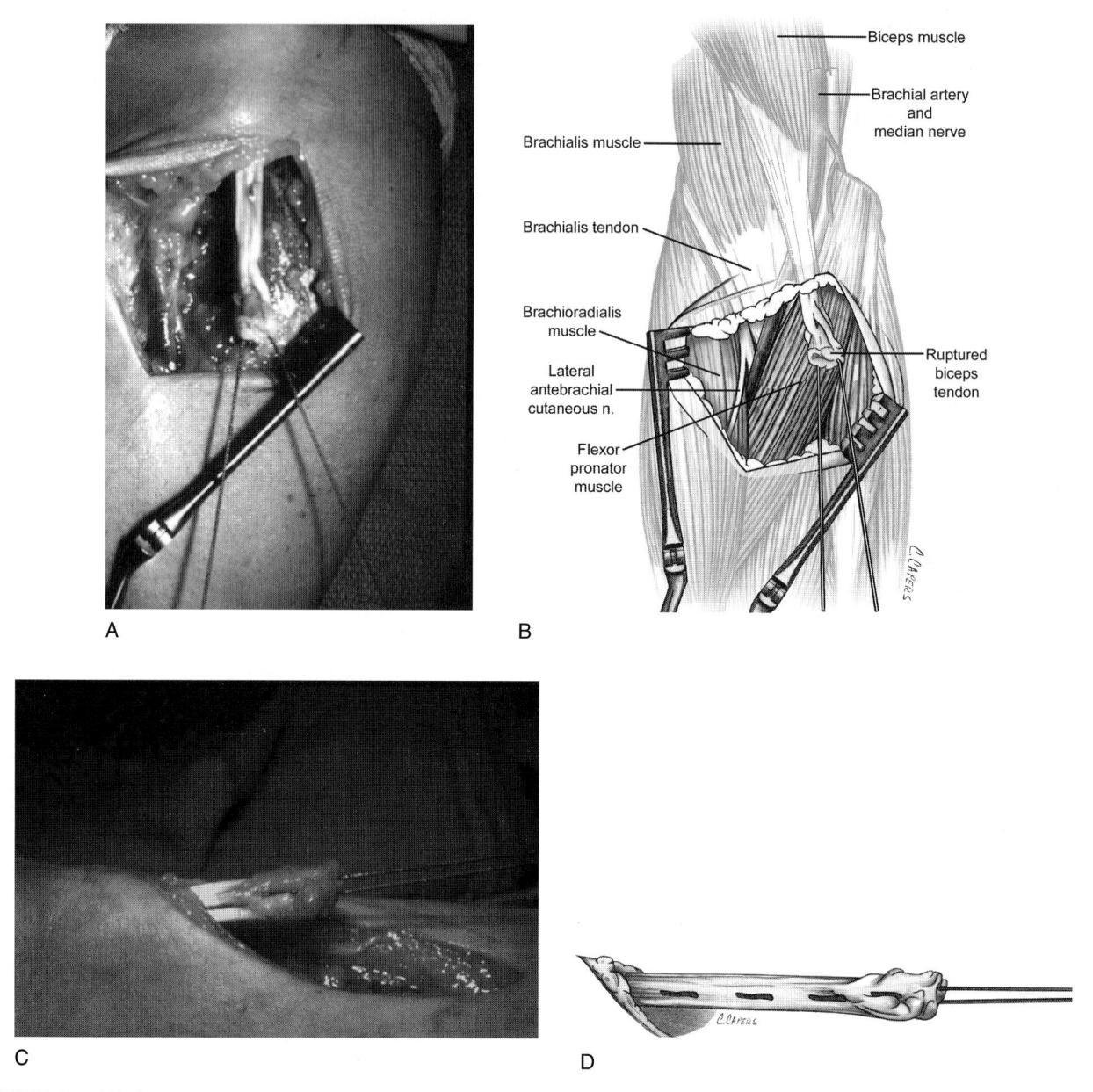

FIGURE 9.6. (A) Suture exiting from the freshly debrided end of distal biceps tendon. (B) Ruptured biceps tendon is brought out through the distal incision. (C) and (D) Lateral views of the tendon with the Bunnell sutures woven through it.

distal attachment can demonstrate nearly complete detachment of the tendon from the tuberosity. If a portion of the tendon is still attached, it generally is attached at the proximal end of the tuberosity. In nearly complete ruptures, the small remaining fibers are divided to facilitate repair.

Using a rongeur, the surgeon removes bursal and tendinous tissue from the radial tuberosity. Next, he or she makes a trough in the radial tuberosity either with a power burr or with drill holes. Because burrs usually have small shanks, I prefer to use drill bits. An awl is used to make two or three holes in a straight line over the tuberosity. The distance between the awl holes should be approximately $\frac{1}{4}$ in., which is usually the diameter of the largest drill bit that can be inserted comfortably into the tuberos-

ity. Any bridging bone between the holes can be removed with a rongeur, creating a trough that comfortably contains the end of the distal biceps tendon. The surgeon secures the biceps tendon in the trough by making two holes in the posterior cortex.

The drill holes in the posterior cortex of the radial neck are made with 0.062 smooth Kirschner wires (K-wires). The K-wires are directed posteriorly and aiming toward the posterior edge of the extensor muscle mass. This edge is one or two fingerbreadths anterior to the posterior edge of the subcutaneous proximal ulna. While maintaining a finger over the posterior edge of the extensor muscle mass and holding the patient's arm in full supination, the surgeon makes a hole in the posterior cortex with a 0.062 smooth K-wire. Directing the wire toward the postero-

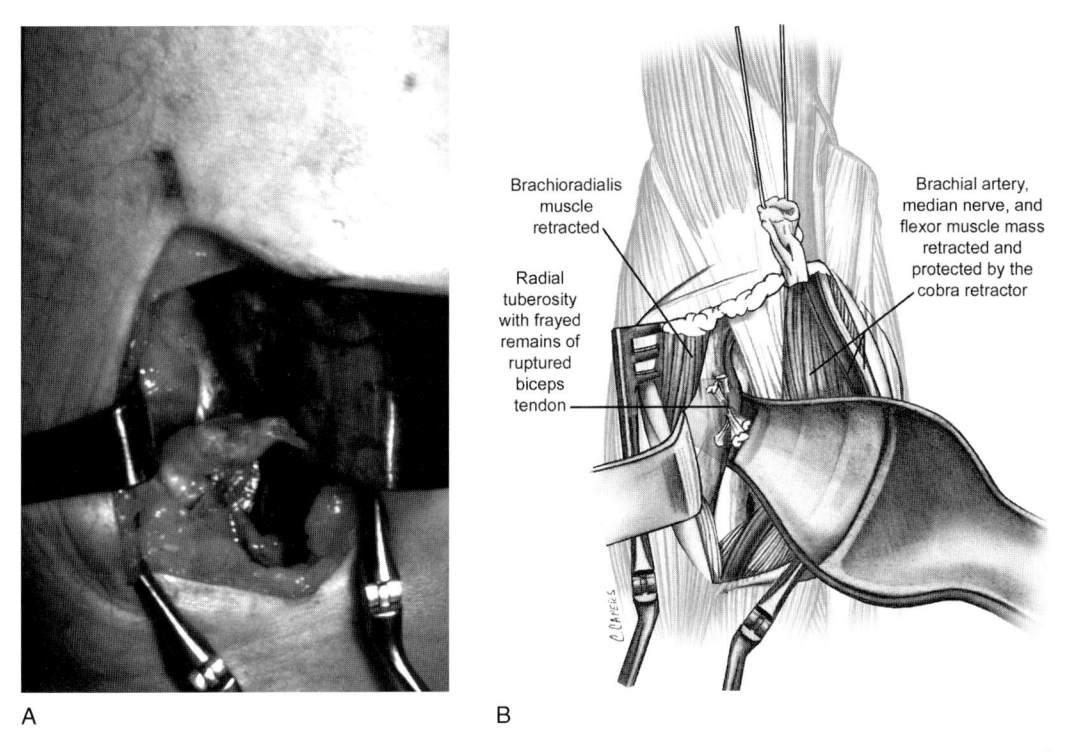

FIGURE 9.7. (A) Placing the cobra retractor around the medial aspect of the proximal radius protects the medial neurovascular structures and exposes the radial tuberosity. (B) The biceps tendon is retracted. Note that the frayed shreds of biceps tendon are still attached to the tuberosity.

lateral edge of the proximal ulna helps to avoid injury to the more anterior posterior interosseous nerve. The K-wire is left in place as a directional guide. A similar wire is placed more distal following the general direction of the first wire, but converging posteriorly (Fig. 9.8). The holes generally are placed proximally and distally in the posterior cortex to provide an adequate bony bridge. The K-wires are removed, and a Keith needle is passed

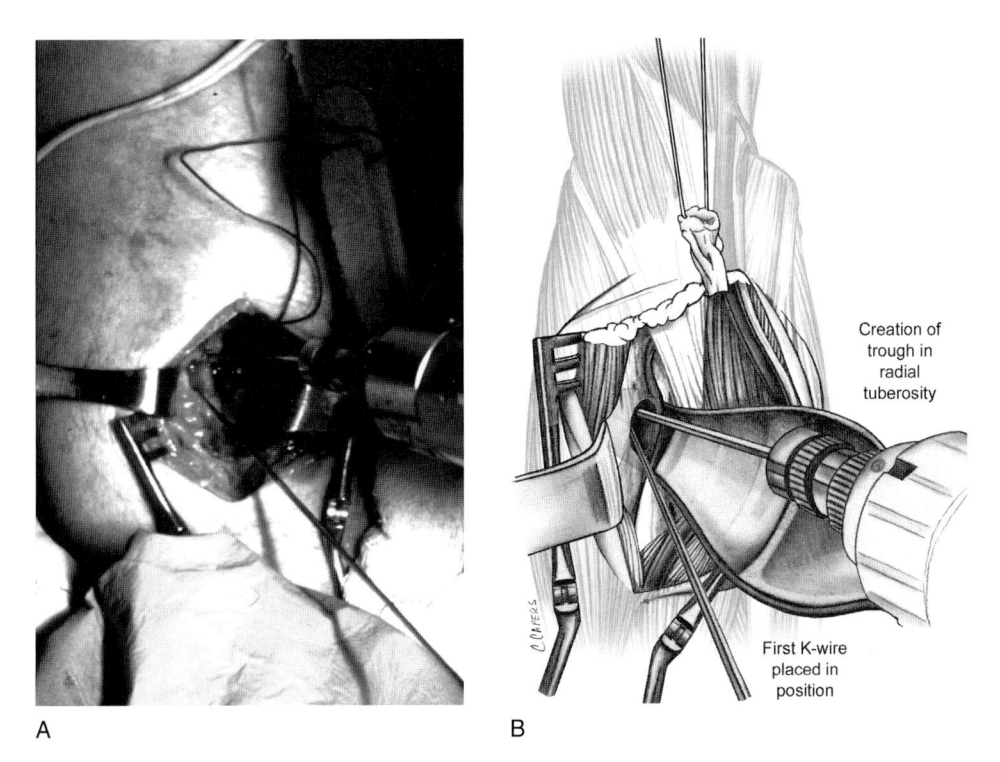

FIGURE 9.8. (A) The trough has been created in the tuberosity, and the first 0.062 K-wire is in place. (B) Note the distance between the K-wires and the convergence posteriorly.

through each drill hole and pushed posteriorly through the soft tissues (Fig. 9.9).

The sutures are retrieved by flexing the patient's elbow and making a small incision over the protruding Keith needles. The incision only needs to be large enough to allow the surgeon to retrieve the sutures and tie a knot. The needles are removed and traction is applied to the sutures, bringing the tendon end into the bony trough (Fig. 9.10). While the patient's elbow is flexed and supinated, the sutures are tied. No attempt is made to dissect down to the posterior cortex of the radius. The sutures are tied directly over the posterior muscle mass. Most of the time, the end of the tendon lies within the intramedullary cavity of the radius; however, sometimes it rests at the entrance to the trough. Either position is acceptable and has not been shown to affect the clinical outcome.

After tying the sutures, the surgeon should measure the passive elbow range of motion. Full pronation and supination and full flexion should be expected. However, flexion contractures of 20° to 30° are relatively common. With delayed repairs, the flexion contracture may be more than 45°. The degree of contracture should be noted because it affects postoperative mobilization.

The anterior and posterior wounds are closed. A long-arm splint is applied with the patient's forearm in supination and elbow flexed slightly more than the recorded flexion contracture.

Table 9.1 outlines the postoperative regimen.[20-23] At 7 to 10 days after surgery, the sutures are removed and a long-arm cast is applied with the patient's arm in a posture similar to that of the postoperative splint. The cast is removed at 3 to 4 weeks after surgery, and the elbow

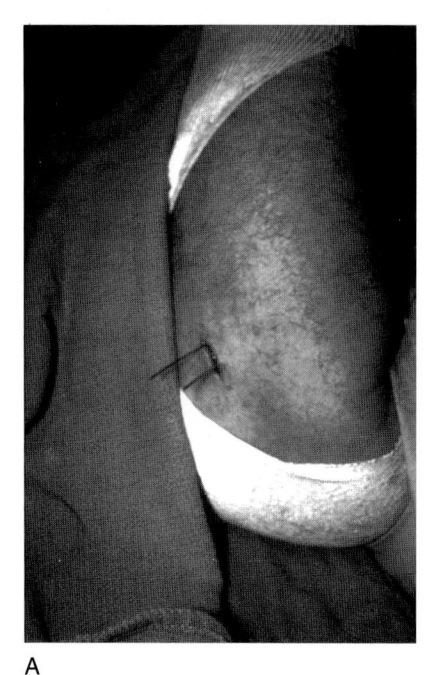

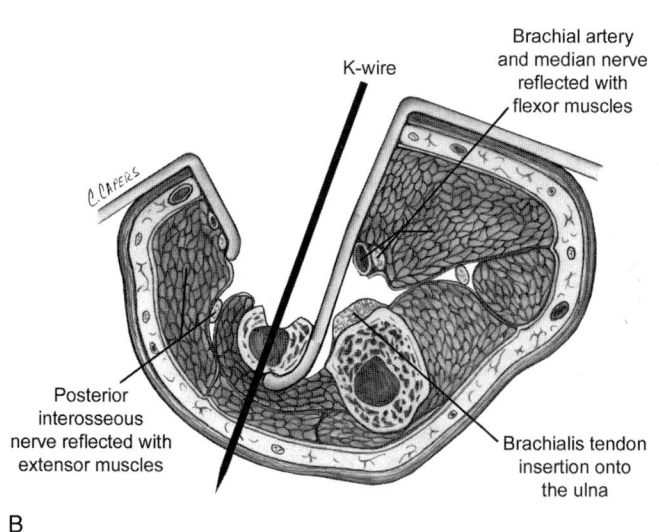

FIGURE 9.9. (A) Passage of the Keith needles through the skin posteriorly. (B) Cross-sectional anatomy in the region of the tuberosity shows the course of the K-wires in relation to the surrounding vital structures. Note proximity of the posterior interosseous nerve. (C) Drawing demonstrates the close association between the distal biceps tendon and nearby vital structures.

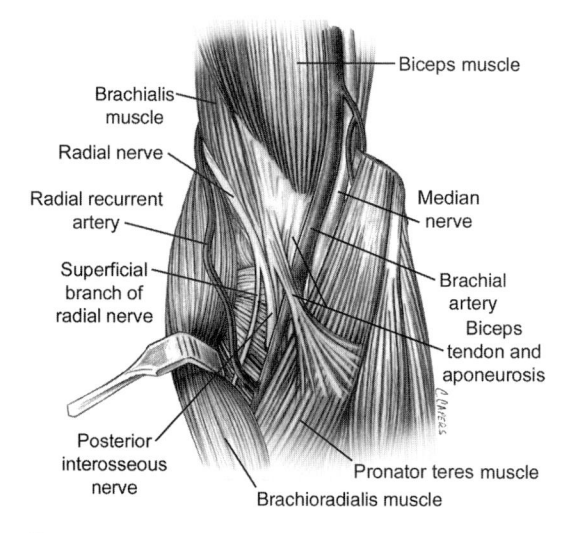

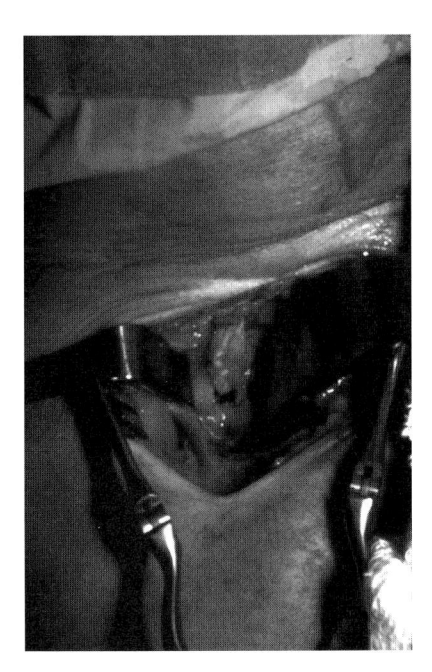

FIGURE 9.10. The tendon end is drawn into the bony trough with distal traction on the posterior sutures.

is gently put through a range of motion. At this point, patients usually demonstrate a slight loss of supination and continue to demonstrate a loss of elbow extension. The arm then is placed in a hinged brace with an extension stop at the degree of terminal elbow extension noted at the 3- to 4-week visit. The extension stop is decreased gradually until full extension is reached. The patient begins isotonic and isokinetic strengthening exercises 8 weeks after surgery. Return to all activities is allowed at 12 to 16 weeks after surgery.

Results

Anatomic repair of the ruptured distal biceps tendon to the radial tuberosity is the treatment of choice. In the absence of complications, the results are universally good, with normal range of motion and restoration of strength.[24,25] In repair of acute ruptures, flexion and supination strength generally return completely.[4,6,14] However, some studies have shown that repaired nondominant arms have persistent isokinetic deficits of 15% to 50%.[20–22] Attachment of the ruptured tendon to the brachialis muscle results in nearly normal return of flexion strength, but can leave as much as a 50% loss of supination strength.[6]

The senior author (BML) reviewed his last 25 patients (25 injuries) who had a distal biceps tendon rupture repaired by the described technique. Four of the tears were partial. All the patients were men with an average age of 45 years (range, 32 to 61 years). The dominant arm was injured in seven patients (six right and one left arm) and the nondominant arm in eighteen patients (four right and fourteen left arms). The incidence of injury in the nondominant arm was statistically significant ($p = 0.003$).

TABLE 9.1. *Clinical guidelines for rehabilitation of distal biceps tendon repairs*

Phase I: Protection and promotion of healing (0 to 3 weeks)	Cast immobilization: elbow in 90° of flexion, forearm in supination, wrist in neutral Activity modification: Lifting limited to 5 lb Maintain uninvolved joint mobility
Phase II: Restoration of motion (3 to 8–12 weeks)	Cast removed Hinged elbow brace applied, 30° extension block to full extension; decrease extension block by 10° per week Brace is worn at all times except for exercising A/PROM of wrist, forearm, and elbow Soft-tissue stretch to tolerance Aerobic conditioning using lower extremities Activity modification continues; return-to-work restriction to 5-lb lifting limit Control swelling and inflammation
Phase III: Restoration of strength and endurance (8 to 16 weeks)	Hinged elbow brace discontinued Functional activities progressed to tolerance Isotonic strengthening; initial biceps curl 5 lb Isokinetic strengthening for supination and elbow flexion Upper extremity aerobic conditioning; UBE, rowing
Phase IV: Return to function (4 to 6–9 months)	Endurance and neuromuscular retraining: controlled to uncontrolled environment Work hardening Return to work Isokinetic testing

Source: Harris and Dyrek,[20] O'Sullivan and Schmitz,[21] Seiler et al.,[22] Wilk et al.[23]

The time from injury to repair averaged 41.3 days (range, 2 to 330 days). The results of postoperative isokinetic testing varied with arm dominance. Patients whose dominant arm was repaired had normal work production, but had a 6.5% deficit in supination strength and a 12% deficit in flexion strength. Patients whose nondominant arm was repaired had normal work production with their arm in flexion, but a 19% deficit when it was in supination. Patients had no deficit in supination strength of their repaired nondominant arm, but had a 15% deficit in flexion strength. Average pain, subjective weakness, and work or activity limitation were 1.4, 1.2, and 1.2, respectively (1.0, none present; 5.0, extreme pain). The average patient satisfaction was 4.5 on a 5-point scale (5, extremely satisfied). No statistically significant correlation existed with patient age or delay in diagnosis.

Complications

Fortunately, complications from distal biceps tendon repair are uncommon. Postoperative infections and tendon reruptures are rare. Irritation of the lateral antebrachial cutaneous nerve can be avoided by making a more medial skin incision. Injuries to the radial nerve typically are transient, but can be devastating.[5,15] The author has seen a patient who had a high median nerve palsy that occurred when the biceps tendon was placed inadvertently medial to the median nerve. The nerve recovered when the surgical repair was redone with the tendon placed lateral to the median nerve. Sporadic cases of proximal radioulnar synostosis continue to be reported and seem to be more common with the two-incision technique.[6,26–28] Limiting soft-tissue dissection and not exposing the ulna appear to reduce the risk of this complication. Heterotopic calcification continues to be a problem, but probably represents the intrinsically chronic nature of the injury, rather than specific soft-tissue damage.

In my experience with repair of more than 40 distal biceps tendon ruptures, the modified two-incision technique that I use has caused no injuries to the posterior interosseous nerve. Postoperative irritation of the medial antebrachial cutaneous nerve has been transient. One patient presented with decreased sensation in the distribution of the medial antebrachial cutaneous nerve as a result of inflammation associated with the tendon rupture. Two patients demonstrated radiographic heterotopic calcification in the region of the musculotendinous junction. In one of the two patients, the calcification interfered with supination, but the patient was still able to return to his job as a laborer.

TRICEPS TENDON RUPTURES

Triceps tendon ruptures are extremely rare.[29] Anzel et al. reviewed 1014 tendon injuries treated at the Mayo Clinic.[30] Eighty-five percent of the injuries involved the upper extremity, but only eight (less than 0.8%) involved the triceps, and four of the eight were lacerations. Given the small number of reported cases, the male-to-female ratio is difficult to gauge, but estimates range from 2:1[31] to 2:3.[13] The injury has been reported in patients ranging in age from 13 to 72 years, but the average age is 33 years.[13,31–37] Viegas reported two adolescents who presented with an avulsion fracture from a maturing olecranon,[31] and Clayton and Thirupathi reported the injury in a 72-year-old patient.[34]

Various disorders have been associated with triceps tendon rupture. Chronic renal failure and hyperparathyroidism have been associated with tendon ruptures.[35,36,38] Clayton and Thirupathi attributed the rupture in their patient to chronic olecranon bursitis.[34] Other authors believe that a combination of trauma and osteogenesis imperfecta can contribute to a triceps tendon rupture.[39] We found one case report of a rupture associated with ulnar neuritis, but the patient was a competitive powerlifter who previously had undergone an ulnar neurolysis and had a history of taking anabolic steroids.[40]

The mechanism of injury is either an eccentric loading of the triceps tendon or a direct blow to the posterior aspect of the arm. Fractures of the ipsilateral radial neck and head and of the distal radius have been reported with triceps tendon ruptures.[41] Rupture most frequently occurs at the tendo-osseous junction; however, it can occur anywhere along the length of the musculotendinous unit.[42]

Clinical Anatomy

The triceps tendon represents the confluence of the long, lateral, and medial triceps muscles in the distal third of the posterior aspect of the arm. The long head originates from the infraglenoid tubercle of the scapula. The lateral head arises from the posterior aspect of the humeral shaft. The medial head originates inferior to the lateral border of the humerus. Superior to the medial head is an oblique shallow groove that passes from superomedial to inferolateral. This groove is known as the spiral groove and contains the radial nerve. Two aponeurotic layers enclose the tendon that attaches broadly upon the posterosuperior surface of the olecranon. A lateral band passes from the triceps tendon to the anconeus and blends with the dorsal forearm fascia. The radial nerve lies deep to the triceps muscle. In the distal third of the arm, the nerve passes laterally and anteriorly to pierce the lateral intermuscular septum and enter the anterior compartment of the arm.

Physical Examination

Patients who have a triceps tendon rupture initially experience sudden acute pain along the course of the rup-

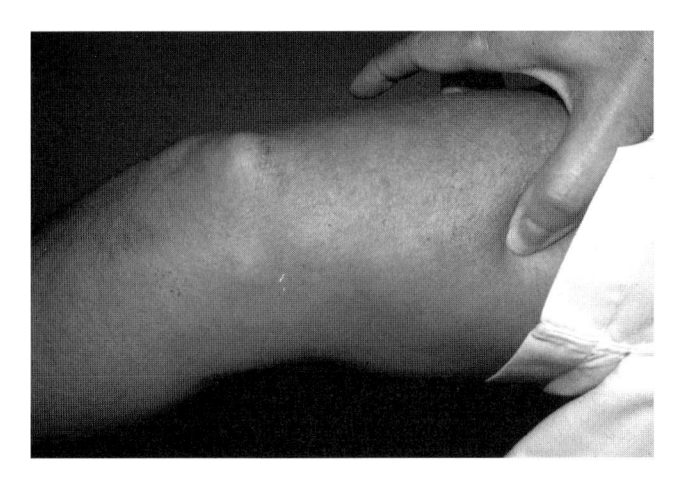

FIGURE 9.11. The modified Thompson test is performed with the elbow flexed to 90° and the arm abducted to eliminate the effect of gravity on elbow extension. The examiner squeezes the triceps muscle belly and observes the elbow for extension motion. If none is present, a complete tear probably has occurred.

tured tendon. Ecchymosis may be present. If an avulsion fracture is also present, the proximal olecranon may be tender. With a complete rupture, elbow extension is either weak or absent. A palpable defect may be felt in the tendon, but is not always present.[40] With a partial rupture, elbow motion and extension against resistance may be maintained.[38] Viegas writes that the "modified" Thompson test is helpful in making the diagnosis of a complete tear[31] (Fig. 9.11).

In the case of a distal triceps tendon rupture, unlike that of a distal biceps tendon rupture, radiographs of the elbow should be obtained because they frequently demonstrate calcific or bony fragments.[33,34,36–38] Radiographs also enable the examiner to determine the presence or absence of a fracture. A nondisplaced avulsion fracture may indicate a partial tear.[38]

Treatment

Nonoperative Treatment

A partial rupture of the triceps tendon can be treated nonoperatively. The patient can obtain normal range of motion and strength through participation in a rehabilitation program. The patient should begin this program as soon as the acute pain has subsided.[38] No consensus has been reached regarding the best way to position the elbow during the period of immobilization. Several authors have commented on the way the ruptured ends are approximated when the elbow is extended.[32,42] This approximation has usually been confirmed in patients treated operatively. Most authors, however, prefer to place the elbow in slight flexion to facilitate recovery.[36,38,42]

Indications for Operative Treatment

Complete tears are debilitating and should be repaired surgically. Initially, the examiner can miss the diagnosis of a complete rupture because the patient's elbow is swollen and the patient cannot fully extend it. Nonoperative treatment of a complete tear results in incomplete extension and weakness.[32,37,43] Therefore, the examiner must be careful to make the correct diagnosis.

Operative Techniques

All described surgical repairs of ruptured triceps tendons involve anatomic reapproximation of the tendon to its attachment on the proximal ulna. The triceps tendon usually retracts no more than 3 to 5 cm. The tendon does not need to be grasped with a clamp, but the distal edge should be trimmed back a few millimeters to provide fresh tissue. Securing the tendon in drill holes placed in the proximal ulna facilitates the repair.[37] This repair can be augmented or protected by closing the periosteum over the tendon[32,38] or oversewing a proximally based flap of forearm fascia[33] or a distally based, partial-thickness flap of triceps.[34] If an avulsion fracture of sufficient size is present, it can be fixed with a screw and washer,[31] but the fragment should be at least three times the diameter of the screw. Sherman et al. and Levy used surgical tape to secure the tendon to the olecranon.[43,44] Others have augmented the repair with either fascia lata or palmaris longus passed through drill holes in the olecranon.

Authors' Preferred Technique

The repair of the ruptured triceps tendon may be accomplished with the patient either positioned supine or prone. The senior author prefers to position the patient supine with a large bolster rolling the patient forward (Fig. 9.12). Rolling the patient forward allows the arm to be placed on the abdomen or chest, but still allows comfortable ex-

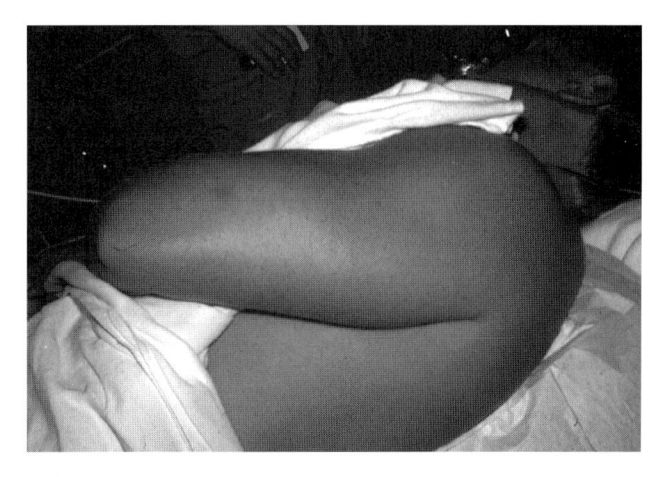

FIGURE 9.12. Patient positioning for triceps tendon repair. The patient is rolled into the lateral decubitus position.

posure of the distal aspect of the upper arm. Unlike the approach for repairing a ruptured biceps tendon, which requires a deeper dissection, the approach for repairing a ruptured triceps tendon is relatively superficial. Consequently, a tourniquet is not always necessary. If bleeding becomes a problem, a sterile tourniquet can be applied during surgery.

The surgeon makes a straight longitudinal incision over the posterior aspect of the elbow and the palpable tendon defect (Fig. 9.13). If skin integrity is a concern, the surgeon can make a curvilinear incision to avoid the bony prominence of the proximal portion of the olecranon. The ruptured end of the tendon usually can be identified after the subcutaneous dissection is complete (Fig. 9.14). In partial tears the central portion of the tendon is disrupted. A no. 5 nonabsorbable suture is secured in the end of the tendon with either a Krakauer or Bunnell stitch (Fig. 9.15). In acute ruptures, the tendon usually can be brought down to the olecranon. The surgeon ties a knot in the nonabsorbable suture to secure it to drill holes made in the ulna (Fig. 9.16). The knot should be placed on the radial side of the ulnar ridge. Placing the knot directly posterior can cause postoperative irritation, and placing the knot ulnad can irritate the ulnar nerve. The surgeon should move the patient's elbow through a range of motion. Full extension should be obtained easily. The elbow should flex to 90°; some springiness is acceptable.

If the surgeon cannot bring the tendon down to the olecranon without sacrificing passive flexion, he or she must consider lengthening the tendon or using intercalated tissue. Elevating the triceps muscle off the posterior humerus sometimes can yield length. Care must be taken with this maneuver, because the radial nerve is vulnerable to injury in the spiral groove at the junction of the middle and distal thirds of the humerus. In chronic ruptures, mobilizing the proximal end still may be difficult.

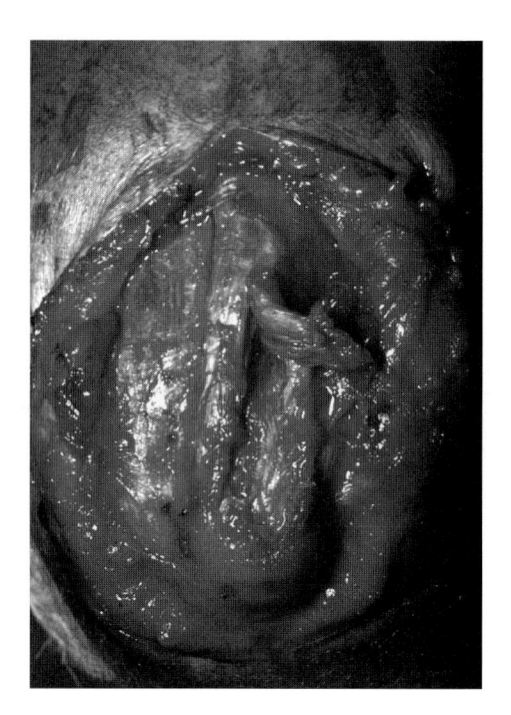

FIGURE 9.14. Triceps tendon tear. The central portion of the tendon is detached, but the medial and lateral portions of the tendon are still attached to the olecranon.

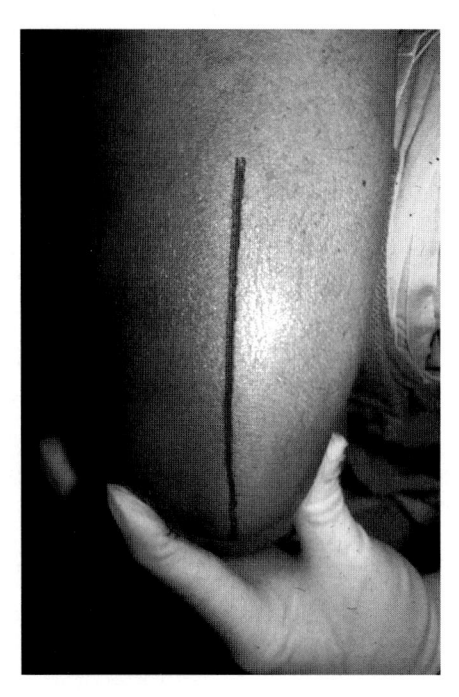

FIGURE 9.13. Posterior incision over the distal aspect of the upper arm.

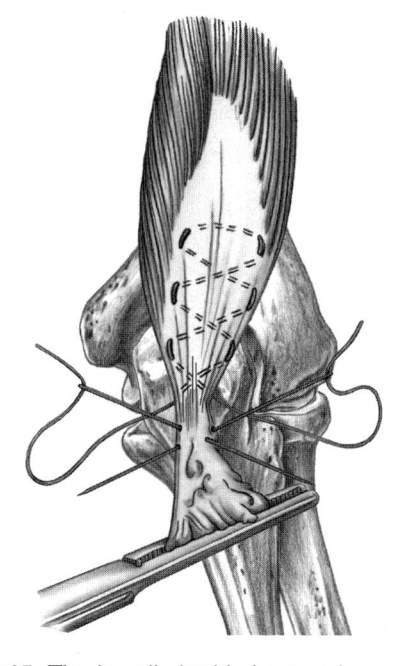

FIGURE 9.15. The heavily braided suture is secured to the triceps tendon rupture.

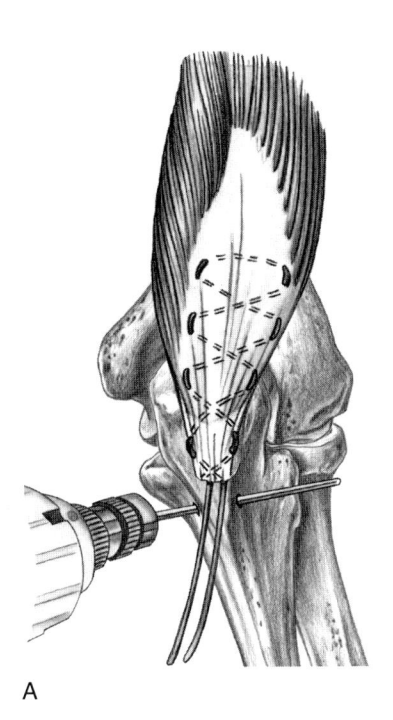

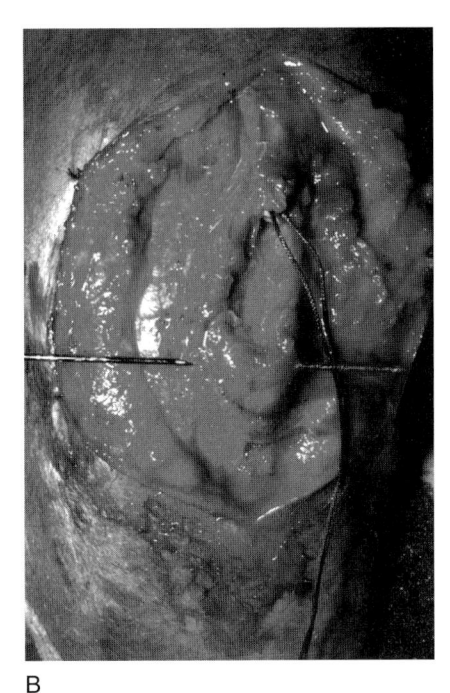

FIGURE 9.16. (A) A smooth Steinmann pin is passed transversely through the proximal olecranon. (B) One limb of the suture will be passed through the hole made by the pin, and the suture will be tied on the radial side of the olecranon.

Creating a distally based, partial-thickness flap, as Clayton and Thirupathi described, provides 2 to 4 cm of length.[34] Additional length can be gained by modifying the Vulpius Achilles tendon lengthening technique. A V-shaped incision can be made proximal to the musculotendinous junction in the superficial triceps fascia. Sometimes, two incisions may be necessary. However, the use of V-shaped incisions generally weakens the triceps. In one patient I treated, the repair was augmented with a slip of the palmaris longus to bridge the gap between the olecranon and the triceps.

After surgery, the patient's arm is placed into a posterior splint with the elbow flexed from 45° to 90°. The patient begins elbow motion 3 weeks after surgery and begins strengthening exercises 6 to 8 weeks after surgery. The patient can return to full activities 12 weeks after surgery.

Results

The results of triceps tendon rupture repair generally are good.[37,38,43,44] The surgeon can expect the patient to regain almost full range of motion, possibly with the loss of a few degrees of elbow extension. The problems with nerve injury, decreased rotation, and heterotopic bone that are seen with biceps tendon repairs do not seem to plague triceps tendon repairs.

Although not measured with isokinetic testing, extension strength seems to return to normal. Complications are few and generally are treatable, leading to a good end result.

CONCLUSION

Distal biceps tendon rupture can lead to significant functional deficits. Anatomic repair of the tendon to the radial tuberosity reliably restores strength and endurance; however, the results may be better in injured dominant arms. Surgical treatment for partial tears also is effective at relieving pain and restoring strength. Complications are uncommon and can be avoided by paying careful attention to elbow anatomy and by limiting soft-tissue dissection.

Triceps tendon ruptures are rare injuries, but they are diagnosed easily by history and physical examination. Partial ruptures should be treated nonoperatively with an aggressive physical therapy program. Complete ruptures should be treated with surgical repair of the tendon to its attachment on the proximal ulna. Appropriately treated patients can expect good functional results with a low incidence of complications.

REFERENCES

1. Bourne MH, Morrey BF. Partial rupture of the distal biceps tendon. *Clin Orthop* 1981;271:143–148.
2. Johnson AB. Avulsion of biceps tendon from the radius. *NY Med J* 1897;66:261.
3. Acquaviva. Rupture du tendon inferieur du biceps brachial droit a son insertion sur la tuberosite bicipitale: Tenosuture succes operatoire. *Marseilles Med* 1898;35:570.
4. Baker BE, Bierwagen D. Rupture of the distal tendon of the biceps brachii. Operative versus non-operative treatment. *J Bone Joint Surg* 1985;67A:414–417.

5. Dobbie RP. Avulsion of the lower biceps brachii tendon: Analysis of 51 previously unreported cases. *Am J Surg* 1941;51:662–683.
6. Morrey BF, Askew LJ, An KN, Dobyns JH. Rupture of the distal tendon of the biceps brachii. A biomechanical study. *J Bone Joint Surg* 1985;67A:418–421.
7. Hovelius L, Josefsson G. Rupture of the distal biceps tendon. Report of five cases. *Acta Orthop Scand* 1977;8:280–282.
8. Kannus P, Jozsa L. Histopathological changes preceding spontaneous rupture of a tendon. A controlled study of 891 patients. *J Bone Joint Surg* 1991;73A:1507–1525.
9. Le Huec JC, Moinard M, Liquois F, et al. Distal rupture of the tendon of biceps brachii. Evaluation by MRI and the results of repair. *J Bone Joint Surg Br* 1996;78:767–770.
10. Bauman GI. Rupture of the biceps tendon. *J Bone Joint Surg* 1934;16:966–967.
11. Lee HG. Traumatic avulsion of tendon of insertion of biceps brachii. *Am J Surg* 1951;82:290–292.
12. Rogers SP. Avulsion of tendon of attachment of biceps brachii. A case report. *J Bone Joint Surg* 1939;21:197.
13. Morrey BF. Tendon injuries about the elbow. In: Morrey BF, ed. *The elbow and its disorders*, 2nd ed. Philadelphia: WB Saunders; 1993: 492–504.
14. Leslie BM. Experience with distal biceps tendon ruptures. *ASSH Correspondence Newsletter* 1997:38.
15. Meherin JM, Kilgore ES. The treatment of ruptures of distal biceps brachii tendon. *Am J Surg* 1960;99:636–640.
16. Anderson LD. Affections of muscles, tendons, and tendon sheaths. In: Crenshaw AH, ed. *Campbell's operative orthopaedics*, 5th ed. St. Louis, MO: CV Mosby; 1971:1459–1503.
17. Fischer WR, Shepanec LA. Avulsion of the insertion of the biceps brachii. Report of a case. *J Bone Joint Surg* 1956;38A:158–159.
18. Boyd HB, Anderson LD. A method for reinsertion of the distal biceps brachii tendon. *J Bone Joint Surg* 1961;43A:1041–1043.
19. Lintner S, Fischer T. Repair of the distal biceps tendon using suture anchors and an anterior approach. *Clin Orthop* 1996; 322:116–119.
20. Harris BA, Dyrek DA. A model of orthopaedic dysfunction for clinical decision making in physical therapy practice. *Phys Ther* 1989;69:548–553.
21. O'Sullivan S, Schmitz T. Physical rehabilitation: Assessment and treatment. Philadelphia: FA Davis; 1988:143–156.
22. Seiler JG III, Parker LM, Chamberland PD, et al. The distal biceps tendon. Two potential mechanisms involved in its rupture: arterial supply and mechanical impingement. *J Shoulder Elbow Surg* 1995;4:149–156.
23. Wilk K, Arrigo C, Andrews JR. Rehabilitation of the elbow in the throwing athlete. *J Orthop Sports Phys Ther* 1993;17: 305–317.
24. Agins HJ, Chess JL, Hoekstra DV, Teitge RA. Rupture of the distal insertion of the biceps brachii tendon. *Clin Orthop* 1988; 234:34–38.
25. D'Alessandro DF, Shields CL Jr, Tibone JE, Chandler RW. Repair of distal biceps tendon ruptures in athletes. *Am J Sports Med* 1993;21:114–119.
26. Leighton MM, Bush-Joseph CA, Bach BR Jr. Distal biceps brachii repair. Results in dominant and nondominant extremities. *Clin Orthop* 1995;317:114–121.
27. Davison BL, Engber WD, Tigert LJ. Long term evaluation of repaired distal biceps brachii tendon ruptures. *Clin Orthop* 1996;333:186–191.
28. Failla JM, Amadio PC, Morrey BF, Beckenbaugh BD. Proximal radioulnar synostosis after repair of distal biceps brachii rupture by the two-incision technique. Report of four cases. *Clin Orthop*. 1990;253:133–136.
29. Waugh RL, Hathcock TA, Elliot JL. Ruptures of muscles and tendons. *Surgery* 1949;25:370–392.
30. Anzel SH, Covey KW, Weiner AD, et al. Disruption of muscles and tendons: An analysis of 1,014 cases. *Surgery* 1959; 45:406–414.
31. Viegas SF. Avulsion of the triceps tendon. *Orthop Rev* 1990; 19:533–536.
32. Anderson KJ, LeCocq JF. Rupture of the triceps tendon. *J Bone Joint Surg* 1957;39A:444–446.
33. Bennett BS. Triceps tendon rupture. Case report and a method of repair. *J Bone Joint Surg* 1962;44A:741–744.
34. Clayton ML, Thirupathi RG. Rupture of the triceps tendon with olecranon bursitis. A case report with a new method of repair. *Clin Orthop* 1984;184:183–185.
35. Murphy KJ, McPhee I. Tears of major tendons in chronic acidosis with elastosis. *J Bone Joint Surg*. 1965;47A:1253–1258.
36. Preston FS, Adicoff A. Hyperparathyroidism with avulsion of three major tendons. Report of a case. *N Engl J Med* 1962; 266:968.
37. Tarsney FF. Rupture and avulsion of the triceps. *Clin Orthop* 1972;83:177–183.
38. Farrar EL III, Lippert FG III. Avulsion of the triceps tendon. *Clin Orthop* 1981;161:242–246.
39. Match RM, Corrylos EV. Bilateral avulsion fracture of the triceps tendon insertion from skiing with osteogenesis imperfecta tarda. A case report. *Am J Sports Med* 1983;11:99–102.
40. Herrick RT, Herrick S. Ruptured triceps in a powerlifter presenting as cubital tunnel syndrome. A case report. *Am J Sports Med* 1987;15:514–516.
41. Holleb PD, Bach BR Jr. Triceps brachii injuries. *Sports Med* 1990;10:273–276.
42. Penhallow DP. Report of a case of ruptured triceps due to direct violence. *NY Med J* 1910;91:76.
43. Sherman OH, Snyder SJ, Fox JM. Triceps tendon avulsion in a professional body builder. A case report. *Am J Sports Med* 1984;12:328–329.
44. Levy M. Repair of triceps tendon avulsions or ruptures. *J Bone Joint Surg* 1987;69:115.

CHAPTER 10

Valgus Extension Overload Syndrome

James R. Andrews and Eric P. Launer

INTRODUCTION

Valgus extension overload syndrome is one entity within a spectrum of elbow injuries seen most commonly in competitive baseball pitchers and to a lesser extent in other throwing athletes, such as football quarterbacks and javelin throwers. The term **valgus extension overload** (VEO) is commonly associated with medial compartment distraction, lateral compartment compression, and posterior compartment impingement. This spectrum of elbow injuries has been well documented.[1-14] One of the most common ways that VEO presents is with pain secondary to impingement in the posteromedial olecranon and medial aspect of the trochlea. The impingement produces degenerative changes in the posterior compartment of the elbow as a result of forces placed on the elbow during repetitive throwing or during participation in sports requiring similar motions. The abnormalities produced in the posterior compartment of the elbow are the subject of this chapter.

History, physical examination, and radiographic studies are used to make the diagnosis of VEO. The treatment of this disorder requires an in-depth understanding of throwing biomechanics, elbow anatomy, arthroscopic techniques, and rehabilitation and conditioning protocols. The surgeon who treats this lesion can expect good results with arthroscopic techniques combined with an aggressive and progressive rehabilitation program.

HISTORY

Degenerative changes in the elbow of throwing athletes have interested researchers for the past 60 years. Waris[13] credited Heiss and Baetzner with recognizing radiographic changes in the elbows of throwing athletes as early as the 1930s, and in 1946 he correlated the clinical findings with the radiographic features of elbow abnormalities in overhead throwing athletes in his study on javelin throwers. Bennett[5] is credited with first describing specific injuries in the pitcher's elbow in 1941. In addition, he anecdotally reported the successful removal of loose bodies and the return of the athletes to competition. In 1959, he described spurs in the posterior compartment that he believed were part of the spectrum of lesions he had noted 18 years earlier.[6] King et al.[10] pointed out that about 50% of baseball pitchers have flexion contractures and 30% have cubitus valgus deformity. They coined the term **medial elbow stress syndrome**. Their description of the olecranon osteophyte and medial olecranon fossa hypertrophy leading to impingement is similar to VEO as it is recognized today. Slocum[11] recognized the repetitive stresses that were placed on the elbow during pitching and the associated clinical and radiographic changes that result from these stresses. He categorized these changes into three types of abnormalities: medial tension overload, lateral compression, and extensor mechanism overload. In 1983, Wilson et al. published their first article on the open treatment of VEO in which they described confirmed success with surgical treatment and return of athletes to their premorbid level of competition.[14]

RELEVANT ANATOMY AND PATHOPHYSIOLOGY

The anatomy that ultimately is affected in VEO is the medial aspect of the posterior compartment. The posterior compartment includes the overlying capsule, posterior aspect of the trochlea and the olecranon fossa, the proximal two-thirds of the olecranon process, and the posterior aspect of the radiocapitellar joint. The ulnar nerve runs subcutaneously through the cubital tunnel just medial to the olecranon process and also may be involved clinically. Symptoms of ulnar nerve irritation may be present. The soft-tissue structures on the medial aspect of the elbow (i.e., the ulnar collateral ligament and the flexor–pronator mass) also play a role in the pathophysiology of this entity. The physician's ability to diagnose and treat this lesion depends on his or her understanding of the relevant anatomy, biomechanics, and pathophysiology in the elbow of a throwing athlete.[15]

The biomechanics of throwing has been well described, and baseball pitching is recognized as one of the most demanding activities on the elbow in sports.[16,17] The acceleration phase of throwing has been implicated in VEO (see Chapter 2). With repetitive valgus stress incurred during the acceleration phase over time, the ulnar collateral ligament (UCL), the humeroulnar articulation, and the flexor–pronator mass can weaken. As a result, when the elbow is brought into extension, the olecranon is wedged against the medial aspect of the trochlear groove and olecranon fossa. Because of this contact, impingement, chondromalacia, osteophyte production, and loose-body formation can occur (Fig. 10.1). Similar lesions can be seen, although less commonly, in the elbows of other athletes, such as tennis and volleyball players who place similar stresses on their elbows.

PHYSICAL EXAMINATION AND DIAGNOSIS

Because the injuries occurring in throwing athletes are complex and subtle, the treating physician needs to take a detailed history and complete a thorough physical examination of the injured athlete. Finding concomitant shoulder and elbow pain in the thrower is common. The patient may have only slight discomfort with throwing, but may have a subjective and documented decrease in velocity, distance, or control. Commonly, pitchers who have VEO report early release, high pitches, and pain during ball release.

Inspection of the elbow may reveal increased valgus alignment and usually reveals a flexion contracture ranging from 5° to 20°. Palpation of the posteromedial aspect of the elbow in full extension reveals tenderness on the olecranon tip and in the olecranon fossa. This tenderness is best appreciated with the elbow in 45° of flexion. Tenderness in the posterior region that is more proximal or distal to the olecranon tip is present in triceps tendinitis or in an olecranon stress fracture,[18] respectively. Palpable loose bodies in the posterior compartment may be an additional finding. The examiner should palpate the ulnar nerve along its course, checking for subluxation and positive signs of nerve compression. A valgus stress test at 20° and 30° of elbow flexion should be performed on both elbows and should be compared for subtle differences in UCL integrity. The VEO test, or valgus extension snap maneuver,[19] reveals the most consistent finding. To perform this provocative test, the examiner places moderate valgus stress on the seated athlete's elbow and simultaneously palpates the posteromedial tip of the olecranon. Next, he or she moves the elbow from 30° of flexion to full extension (Fig. 10.2). This maneuver acts to simulate the impingement that occurs during the throwing motion and to reproduce the symptoms of posterior elbow pain.

Standard radiographs should include anteroposterior, lateral, and oblique views, as well as the axial view. The lateral view may demonstrate an osteophyte at the tip of the olecranon, and the axial view[14] may reveal characteristic osteophytes at the posteromedial aspect of the olecranon (Fig. 10.3). To obtain the axial view (see Chapter 3) the elbow should be flexed to 110°, and the beam

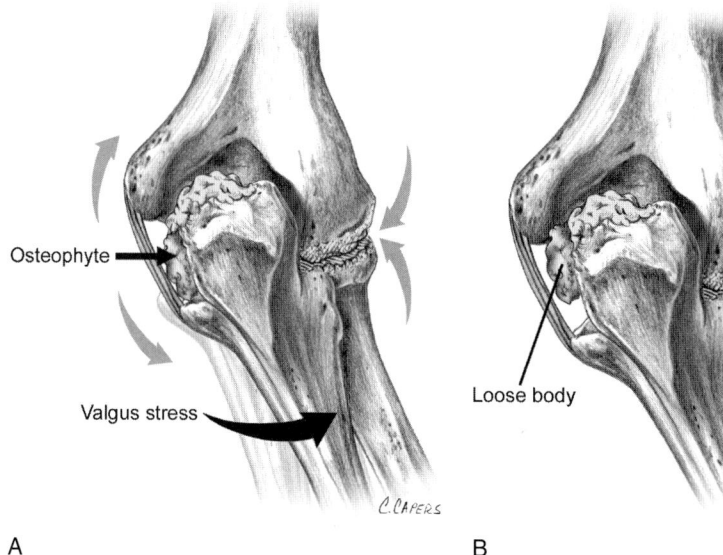

FIGURE 10.1. (A) Posterior aspect of the elbow with valgus stress during acceleration. (B) Osteophyte breaks off to form a loose body. (Adapted from Andrews JR and Craven WM.[2])

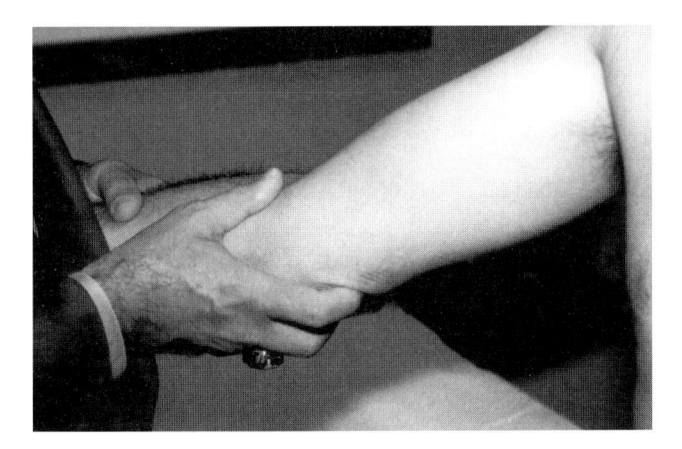

FIGURE 10.2. Technique for performing the VEO test.

should be directed 45° to the long axis of the ulna. The lesions may not be appreciated on radiographs in about 35% of these patients,[3] and they are confirmed visually only at the time of surgery. Radiographic stress views of the elbow also are used frequently to assess the integrity of the UCL. Contrast-enhanced magnetic resonance imaging[20] may be helpful when the diagnosis is unclear. It is highly specific for injuries of the ulnar collateral ligament and also can reveal cartilaginous loose bodies or articular surface defects that cannot be visualized on standard radiographs.

NONOPERATIVE TREATMENT

Before recommending surgery, the physician should treat the patient nonoperatively for 3 to 6 months. During this time, the patient begins treatment with an initial period of rest (lasting from 1 to 3 weeks), progresses through the rehabilitation phase, and progresses back into throwing. The nonoperative treatment is similar to the postoperative protocol that is used for elbow arthroscopy in the throwing athlete.[21] Specific goals for the patient to achieve include full, nonpainful range of motion; absence of pain and tenderness on physical examination; and the ability to demonstrate satisfactory muscle strength, power, and endurance. The initial period of rest should be allowed so that synovitis and inflammation can resolve. After this period, the patient begins wrist and elbow flexor and extensor muscle stretching and strengthening exercises. This program is progressed to plyometrics. Finally, the patient begins an interval-throwing program. Nonsteroidal anti-inflammatory drugs may be used. In addition to the stretching and strengthening exercises, therapeutic modalities, such as moist heat, ultrasound, massage, and phonophoresis, may be used. Ice should be applied to the elbow after throwing in practice or games for the athlete who is not restricted from these activities.

OPERATIVE TREATMENT

Indications and Contraindications

For a throwing athlete, the indications for operative intervention are clinical evidence of a posterior compartment lesion with posteromedial pain during throwing, posteromedial tenderness on examination, a positive VEO test, and radiographic evidence of impingement. Patients who have these findings and who do not improve with nonoperative management are deemed good candidates for arthroscopic surgery unless it is contraindicated.

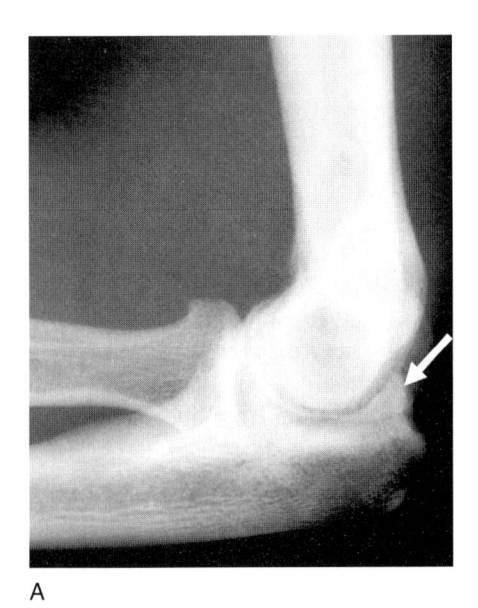

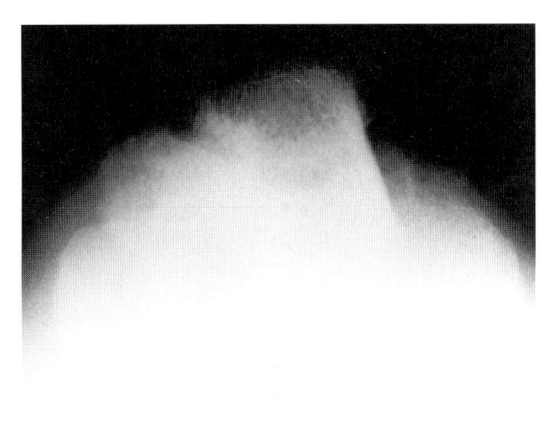

FIGURE 10.3. (A) Radiographic appearance of an osteophyte (arrow) at the tip of the olecranon as seen on a 90° lateral radiograph. (B) Axial radiograph that shows an osteophyte on the medial aspect of the olecranon and trochlea.

Relative contraindications to arthroscopic treatment include severe bony or fibrous ankylosis or previous surgery that has distorted the native anatomy, such as a previous ulnar nerve transposition. In these situations, open resection may be required.

Operative Techniques

Elbow arthroscopy has made open resection of olecranon osteophytes primarily a point of historic interest. However, occasions still exist when an open procedure may and should be performed. The determining factor in this decision should be whether a contraindication to elbow arthroscopy is present. If a contraindication is present, the posterior compartment may be accessed through an open posteromedial or open posterolateral approach. The decision as to which approach is used should be based on the nature or existence of concomitant elbow abnormalities.

The posteromedial approach to the elbow is used when concomitant UCL reconstruction, ulnar nerve transposition, or exploration of a previously transposed ulnar nerve is to be accomplished in conjunction with removal of posteromedial osteophytes. The surgeon places the patient supine. The shoulder is abducted 90° and externally rotated on a hand table. The medial antebrachial cutaneous nerve always should be identified and preserved. The ulnar nerve always is protected and mobilized, and vessel loops are placed both proximally and distally. If UCL reconstruction is necessary, posterior compartment lesions should be addressed before reconstruction. Usually, exploration of the ligament is done, and then attention is turned to the posterior compartment. A small capsular incision just proximal to the posterior band of the UCL is made, and the posteromedial olecranon and medial aspect of the trochlea and olecranon fossa are identified and inspected. If an osteophyte is present, a $\frac{1}{4}$-in. osteotome is used to resect the proximal 1 cm of the olecranon and the medial osteophyte. The debridement should be completed with a rongeur to smooth the resected edges. The medial aspect of the distal humerus should be inspected, and any chondromalacia should be smoothed out. Before closure, the joint should be irrigated thoroughly.

Before the advent of elbow arthroscopy, the open posterolateral elbow approach was used to treat VEO. It still may be employed if concomitant radiocapitellar chondromalacia must be addressed and arthroscopy is contraindicated. Additionally, in the absence of abnormality in the medial aspect of the elbow, a posterolateral approach avoids mobilization of the ulnar nerve. To begin this approach, the surgeon makes a straight incision that is centered over the lateral supracondylar ridge of the humerus. This incision is extended 4 to 5 cm distally. Dissection through the edge of the triceps tendon and the anconeus is done sharply, and these fibers are elevated from the supracondylar ridge. Retraction of the triceps exposes the posterior compartment. Additional dissection of overlying synovial tissue may be required to fully expose the proximal tip of the olecranon. Flexion and extension of the elbow further aid in visualization. After the exposure is adequate and the lesion is identified, the $\frac{1}{4}$-in. osteotome is used to resect the osteophytes in the same fashion as described for the posteromedial approach (Fig. 10.4). This approach requires additional caution because the ulnar nerve lies within close proximity to the osteotome or the biting end of the rongeur when the medial osteophyte is debrided from this angle. As with the posteromedial approach, the surgeon smoothes the resected edges with a rongeur and irrigates the joint. Closure is done in a typical fashion.

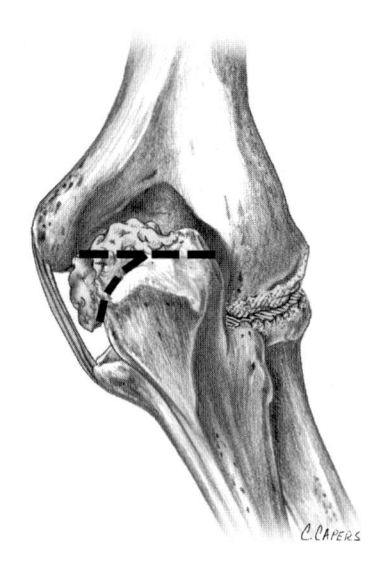

FIGURE 10.4. Broken lines indicate posteromedial olecranon lesion and area that is removed surgically. (Adapted from Wilson FD, Andrews JR, and Blackburn TA, et al.[14])

Authors' Preferred Technique

Arthroscopic treatment of VEO has evolved as arthroscopic techniques and understanding of arthroscopic anatomy of the elbow have evolved.[22-27] The primary advantages are the small incisions; direct visualization and access to the medial aspect of the olecranon fossa; and thorough evaluation of the entire elbow joint for additional abnormalities, such as aberrant loose bodies, and for evaluation of the UCL and medial compartment under stress. The procedure can be done with the patient placed either in the supine or prone position. The setup for surgery and the arthroscopic evaluation are described in Chapter 14.

The surgeon always should accomplish a general arthroscopic examination of the elbow even when he or she believes that the abnormality is localized to a specific compartment. This examination ensures that no coexistent abnormality is missed. For example, the surgeon needs to examine the UCL using the arthroscopic stress view in patients who have VEO and to document the presence or absence of laxity. The sequence of evaluation should be orderly and done in the same fashion each time.

After evaluating the elbow joint, the surgeon begins arthroscopic treatment of VEO. He or she initially uses the 3.5-mm, full-radius resector to debride the soft tissue and synovitis of the posterior compartment. This debridement facilitates visualization of the bony margins and osteophytes. The surgeon uses a $\frac{1}{4}$-inch, straight osteotome to remove posterior and posteromedial osteophytes (Fig. 10.5). Next, he or she smoothes the resected edges with a high-speed burr. The full-radius resector is reintroduced through the straight posterior portal, and any areas of chondromalacia (i.e., "kissing lesions") (Fig. 10.6) of the trochlea are debrided to a smooth surface. The elbow is put through its full range of motion to ensure that no further impingement or loose fragments of articular cartilage exist. An intraoperative lateral radiograph should be obtained at this point to visualize the resection (Fig. 10.7). The posterior compartment is irrigated copiously, and a medium hemovac drain is placed. The wounds are closed with sterile adhesive strips or butterfly-type bandages, and a soft, bulky dressing is applied.

A postoperative exercise protocol is outlined in Table 10.1. The exercises are very similar to those used in nonoperative management; however, Table 10.1 reflects the

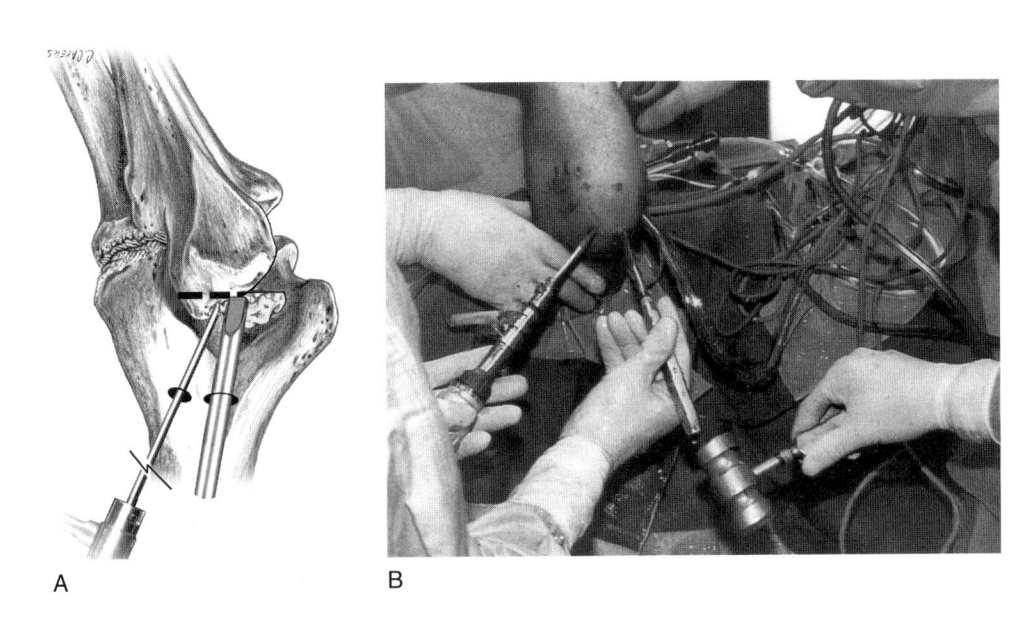

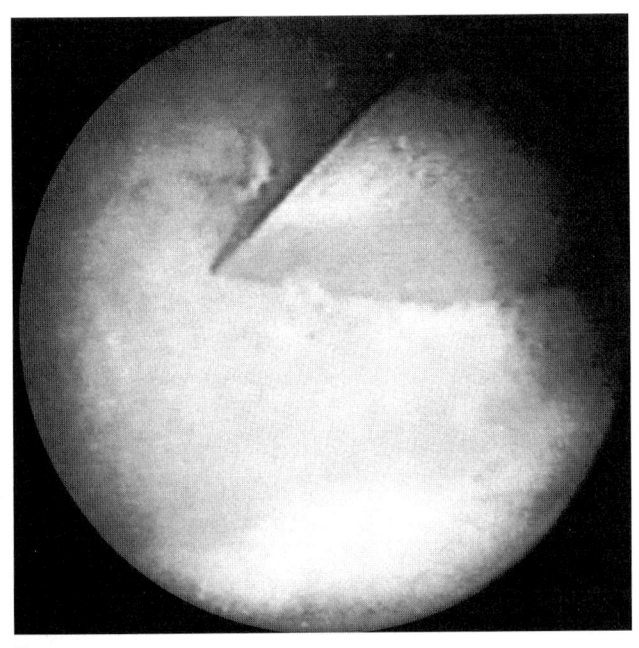

FIGURE 10.5. (A) and (B) Osteophyte removal in a patient with valgus extension overload. (Adapted from Andrews JR and McKenzie PJ.[23]) (C) Arthroscopic view from the posterolateral portal. The spur has been debrided, and an osteotome is in place to remove more of the spur. The osteotome is placed through the straight posterior portal. (Used with permission from Timmerman LA.[27])

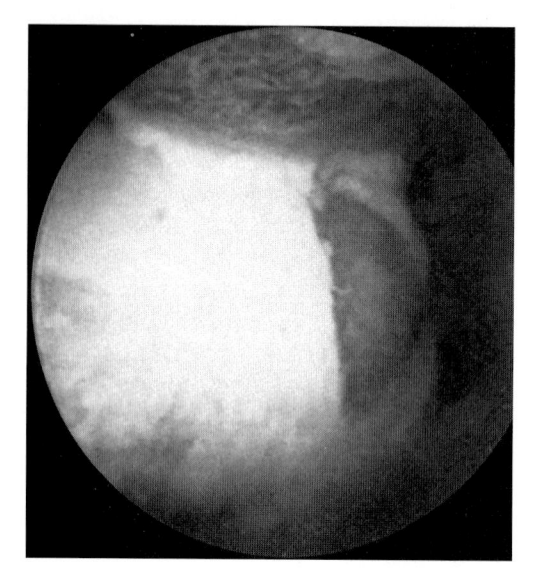

FIGURE 10.6. Once the spur is removed, the area of corresponding chondromalacia of the trochlea, or the "kissing lesion," is seen. (Used with permission from Timmerman LA.[27])

timing of progression to account for the initial period of recovery from surgery. The athlete should be prepared to embark on an aggressive rehabilitation program with the goal of beginning an interval throwing program 6 to 8 weeks after surgery.

RESULTS AND EXPECTATIONS

Athletes who have isolated posterior compartment lesions usually return to their premorbid level of competition. At our clinic, we have found that 71% of athletes

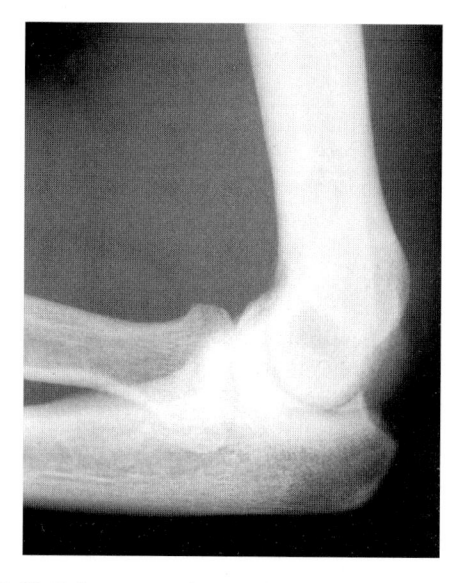

FIGURE 10.7. Intraoperative lateral radiograph of the elbow after arthroscopic excision of the osteophyte.

TABLE 10.1. *Postoperative rehabilitative protocol for elbow arthroscopy.*

I. Initial phase (week 1)
  Goal: Full wrist and elbow ROM, decrease swelling, decrease pain, retardation of muscle atrophy
  A. Day of surgery
    1. Begin gently moving elbow in bulky dressing
  B. Postoperative days 1 and 2
    1. Remove bulky dressing; replace with elastic bandages
    2. Immediate postoperative hand, wrist, and elbow exercises
      a. Putty/grip strengthening
      b. Wrist flexor stretching
      c. Wrist extensor stretching
      d. Wrist curls
      e. Reverse wrist curls
      f. Neutral wrist curls
      g. Pronation/supination
      h. A/AAROM elbow extension/flexion
  C. Postoperative days 3 through 7
    1. PROM elbow extension/flexion (motion to tolerance)
    2. Begin PRE exercises with 1-lb weight
      a. Wrist curls
      b. Reverse wrist curls
      c. Neutral wrist curls
      d. Pronation/supination
      e. Broomstick roll-up
II. Intermediate phase (weeks 2 through 4)
  Goal: Improve muscular strength and endurance; normalize joint arthrokinematics
  A. Week 2 ROM exercises (overpressure into extension)
    1. Addition to biceps curl and triceps extension
    2. Continue to progress PRE weight and repetitions as tolerable
  B. Week 3
    1. Initiate biceps and triceps eccentric exercise program
    2. Initiate rotator cuff exercise program
      a. External rotators
      b. Internal rotators
      c. Deltoid
      d. Supraspinatus
      e. Scapulothoracic strengthening
III. Advanced phase (weeks 4 through 8)
  Goal: Preparation of athlete for return to functional activities
  Criteria to progress to advanced phase:
    1. Full nonpainful ROM
    2. No pain or tenderness
    3. Isokinetic test that fulfills criteria to throw
    4. Satisfactory clinical exam
  A. 3 through 6 weeks
    1. Continue maintenance program, emphasizing muscular strength, endurance, and flexibility
    2. Initiate interval-throwing program phase I

Used with permission from Wilk KE, Azar FM, and Andrews JR.[21]

ROM, range of motion; AAROM, active-assistive range of motion; PROM, passive range of motion; PRE, passive resistance exercise.

returned to participation at the same or higher level of competition for an average of 3.3 years. Patients should be counseled that this procedure is palliative, and recurrence of osteophytes or increased symptoms of instability may occur. Recently, questions have been raised regarding the possible stabilizing effect of the posteromedial osteophyte. Underlying incompetence of the UCL may be partially responsible for the development of the posteromedial osteophyte, and resection of the osteophyte may lead to increased stress on the ligament. Some patients may require subsequent reconstruction of the UCL. A recent follow-up study[3] showed that the rate of revision elbow surgery was about 30% in professional baseball pitchers. Fifteen percent of these patients needed repeat osteophyte excision, and 15% needed UCL reconstruction. Patients who have revision elbow surgery have about a 50% chance of returning to their previous level of competition.

COMPLICATIONS

The complications related to surgery to treat VEO are similar to any open or arthroscopic procedure on the elbow: damage to neurovascular structures either by direct injury or by the compressive phenomenon of fluid extravasation, damage to articular surfaces from instrumentation, infection, breakage of instruments, or tourniquet-related problems. The other complication is formation of early heterotopic bone or scar tissue in the posterior compartment in a small percentage (less than 10%) of patients. This complication often occurs when the recovery period is accelerated and early throwing is pushed. Damage to neurovascular structures is the most common complication of elbow arthroscopy.[28] Thus, the surgeon must have a thorough knowledge of the technique and of elbow anatomy as seen during arthroscopic surgery.

SUMMARY

VEO is a well-recognized entity in the spectrum of elbow injuries in competitive baseball pitchers. Other athletes involved in throwing or in sports requiring similar motions may be predisposed as well. History, physical examination, and radiographs help the surgeon to make the diagnosis. Before treating VEO through arthroscopic surgery, the surgeon should diligently evaluate the patient for coexistent shoulder or other elbow abnormalities. A supervised physical therapy program and arthroscopic surgical decompression are the mainstays of treatment. In the absence of other shoulder or elbow abnormalities, the athlete's likelihood of return to his or her premorbid level of competition is high.

REFERENCES

1. Andrews JR. Bony injuries about the elbow in the throwing athlete. *Instructional Course Lect* 1985;34:323–331.
2. Andrews JR, Craven WM. Lesions of the posterior compartment of the elbow. *Clin Sports Med* 1991;10:637–652.
3. Andrews JR, Timmerman LA. Outcome of elbow surgery in professional baseball players. *Am J Sports Med* 1995;23:407–413.
4. Barnes DA, Tullos HS. An analysis of 100 symptomatic baseball players. *Am J Sports Med* 1978;6:62–67.
5. Bennett GE. Shoulder and elbow lesions of the professional baseball pitcher. *JAMA* 1941;117:510–514.
6. Bennett GE. Elbow and shoulder lesions of baseball players. *Am J Surg* 1959;98:484–492.
7. DeHaven KE, Evarts CM. Throwing injuries of the elbow in athletes. *Orthop Clin North Am* 1973;4:801–808.
8. Indelicato PA, Jobe FW, Kerlan RK, et al. Correctable elbow lesions in professional baseball players: A review of 25 cases. *Am J Sports Med* 1979;7:72–75.
9. Jobe FW, Nuber G. Throwing injuries of the elbow. *Clin Sports Med* 1986;5:621–636.
10. King JW, Brelsford HS, Tullos HJ. Analysis of the pitching arm of the professional baseball pitcher. *Clin Orthop* 1969;67:116–123.
11. Slocum DB. Classification of elbow injuries from baseball pitching. *Tex Med* 1968;64:48–53.
12. Tullos HS, King JW. Throwing mechanism in sports. *Orthop Clin North Am* 1973;4:709–720.
13. Waris W. Elbow injuries of javelin throwers. *Acta Chir Scand* 1946;93:563–575.
14. Wilson FD, Andrews JR, Blackburn TA, et al. Valgus extension overload in the pitching elbow. *Am J Sports Med* 1983;11:83–88.
15. Guerra JJ, Timmerman LA. Clinical anatomy, histology, and pathomechanics of the elbow in sports. *Oper Tech Sports Med* 1996;4:69–76.
16. Fleisig GS, Andrews JR, Dillman CJ, et al. Kinetics of baseball pitching with implications about injury mechanisms. *Am J Sports Med* 1995;23:233–239.
17. Fleisig GS, Escamilla RF. Biomechanics of the elbow in the throwing athlete. *Oper Tech Sports Med* 1996;4:62–68.
18. Nuber GW, Diment MT. Olecranon stress fractures in throwers. A report of two cases and a review of the literature. *Clin Orthop* 1992;278:58–61.
19. Andrews JR, Whiteside JA, Buettner CM. Clinical evaluation of the elbow in throwers. *Oper Tech Sports Med* 1996;4:77–83.
20. Timmerman LA, Schwartz ML, Andrews JR. Preoperative evaluation of the ulnar collateral ligament by magnetic resonance imaging and computed tomography arthrography. Evaluation in 25 baseball players with surgical confirmation. *Am J Sports Med* 1994;22:26–31.
21. Wilk KE, Azar FM, Andrews JR. Conservative and operative rehabilitation of the elbow in sports. *Sports Med Arthr Rev* 1995;3:237–258.
22. Andrews JR, Carson WG. Arthroscopy of the elbow. *Arthroscopy* 1985;1:97–107.
23. Andrews JR, McKenzie PJ. Surgical techniques "supine" with arthroscopic surgical treatment of elbow pathology. In: McGinty JB, Caspari RB, Jackson RW, Poehling GG, eds. *Operative arthroscopy*, 2nd ed. Philadelphia: Lippincott-Raven; 1996:877–885.

24. Andrews JR, St Pierre RK, Carson WG Jr. Arthroscopy of the elbow. *Clin Sports Med* 1986;5:653–662.
25. Soffer SR. Diagnostic arthroscopy of the elbow. In: Andrews JR, Timmerman LA, eds. *Diagnostic and operative arthroscopy*. Philadelphia: WB Saunders; 1997:169–181.
26. Soffer SR, Andrews JR. Arthroscopic surgical procedures of the elbow: Common cases. In: Andrews JR, Soffer SR, eds. *Elbow arthroscopy*. St. Louis, MO: CV Mosby; 1994:59–86.
27. Timmerman LA. Operative arthroscopy of the elbow. In: Andrews JR, Timmerman LA, eds. *Diagnostic and operative arthroscopy*. Philadelphia: WB Saunders; 1997:182–189.
28. Carson WG Jr, Meyers JF. Diagnostic arthroscopy of the elbow: Supine position surgical technique, arthroscopic and portal anatomy. In: McGinty JB, Caspari RB, Jackson RW, Poehling GG, eds. *Operative arthroscopy*, 2nd ed. Philadelphia: Lippincott-Raven; 1996:851–868.

CHAPTER 11

Cubital Tunnel Syndrome

Glenn C. Terry and Todd E. Zeigler

INTRODUCTION

Compressive neuropathies are caused by forces that increase tissue pressure in the involved area of a peripheral nerve. Any increase in pressure about a nerve may cause venous congestion and result in circulatory compromise. Researchers believe that this ischemic change is the primary lesion of entrapment neuropathies.[1–3] Ischemia results in edema, which causes further compression. Ischemia and compression also affect the axoplasmic flow, which is vital to nerve function. The chronically ischemic axon then develops an altered ionic environment, loss of cell membrane integrity, and impairment of conduction along the nerve fiber. Many authors believe that, through this mechanism, external compression affects the function of a nerve.[1–4]

When a peripheral nerve is subject to abnormal compression, the patient may experience a variety of effects. Patients typically report pain at the affected area and often distally along the course of the nerve, as well. Paresthesias are also common and usually are noted distally in the area of distribution of an affected sensory nerve. Patients also may report weakness in the muscles that a compressed motor nerve serves. When a significant deficit is chronic, the innervated muscles eventually become atrophic.

Compression of the ulnar nerve is the most common entrapment neuropathy about the elbow. Commonly referred to as cubital tunnel syndrome, this condition is the second most frequently occurring compressive neuropathy in the upper extremity; only carpal tunnel syndrome occurs more often. In addition to being caused by forces of compression, irritation of the ulnar nerve at the elbow also may result from conditions that repeatedly stretch or apply friction to the nerve.

In 1816, Earle initially described surgical treatment for ulnar nerve neuropathy at the elbow.[5] His radical treatment consisted of excising a segment of the nerve. Other procedures, such as excision of a segment of the nerve and then repairing the nerve, deepening the epicondylar groove in an attempt to improve the bed of the nerve followed.

The first effective procedure to treat ulnar nerve compression at the elbow was described by Curtis in 1898.[6,7] He performed transposition of the nerve. Buzzard recommended decompression without transposition in 1922, and in 1928, Platt popularized intramuscular transposition, a procedure that Adson had proposed in 1918.[6,7] Learmonth introduced submuscular transposition in 1932, and King and Morgan described medial epicondylectomy in 1950.[6,7] Currently, several different, widely used procedures are available for the surgical treatment of cubital tunnel syndrome.[7]

In this chapter, we discuss the causes and treatment of cubital tunnel syndrome. We emphasize the importance of the differential diagnosis and of tailoring treatment to each patient's specific circumstances.

CLINICAL ANATOMY AND ETIOLOGY

Compression of the ulnar nerve at the elbow occurs from approximately 10 cm proximal to the joint to 5 cm distal to it.[4] The most common sites of compression occur where the nerve passes behind the medial epicondyle in the epicondylar groove and where it passes between the heads of the flexor carpi ulnaris muscle (Fig. 11.1). In 1958, Feindel and Stratford named this latter passage the "cubital tunnel."[8] Although it technically refers to a specific anatomic location, the term **cubital tunnel syndrome** is used to describe a compressive neuropathy of the ulnar nerve anywhere in the region of the elbow joint. Several other specific anatomic areas exist where ulnar nerve compression can occur about the elbow.

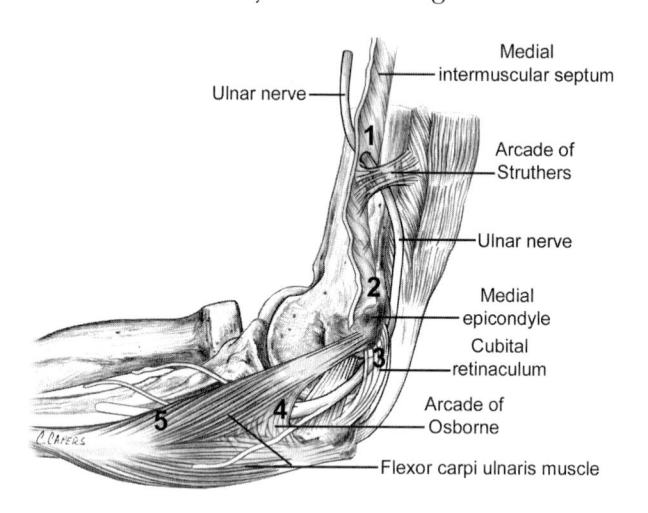

FIGURE 11.1. Potential sites of ulnar nerve compression: (1) intermuscular septum, (2) medial epicondyle, (3) epicondylar groove, (4) cubital tunnel, and (5) exit from flexor carpi ulnaris muscle.

More proximally in the arm, the nerve passes into the posterior muscular compartment through the medial intermuscular septum. Here, the arcade of Struthers may impinge on it. This arcade is a musculofascial band formed by the medial intermuscular septum, medial triceps, and deep investing fascia of the arm.[9] This structure should not be confused with the ligament of Struthers, which can be a cause of median nerve compression on the lateral side of the arm. In an anatomic study, the arcade of Struthers was present in 70% of cadaveric specimens.[10] Even in the absence of the arcade of Struthers, the nerve may be stretched across the medial intermuscular septum. This situation is most often encountered as a complication of anterior transposition of the nerve, which is performed to treat cubital tunnel syndrome. The medial head of the triceps also can impinge on the nerve in this region if the muscle is hypertrophied, such as occurs in body builders.

Another cause of ulnar neuropathy is valgus deformity of the elbow, usually due to a previous distal humeral fracture. Growth abnormality at the lateral condylar physis or a malunited supracondylar fracture can predispose to this problem. This condition is commonly called **tardy ulnar palsy**.[11] In this situation, the nerve is stretched along the distal end of the humerus because of the valgus deformity at the elbow.

The nerve becomes superficial at the elbow as it passes in the epicondylar groove behind the medial epicondyle. The floor of this groove is formed by the medial epicondyle, the olecranon, and the medial collateral ligament of the elbow. The nerve is covered and held in the groove by a fibroaponeurotic band. Due to the superficial location of the nerve in this region, simple direct external pressure on the medial aspect of the elbow can cause transient symptoms in the ulnar nerve distribution. Patients who lean on their elbows regularly may be prone to symptoms. Splints, casts, or braces applied for unrelated problems may cause nerve irritation. The nerve is also most susceptible to compression by mass lesions, such as osteoarthritic spurs protruding from the elbow joint in this area. Other mass lesions that can affect the ulnar nerve include ganglion cysts, lipomas, osteochondromas, and rheumatoid synovium.[4]

Hypermobility or subluxation of the nerve can also cause ulnar nerve irritation. Nerve hypermobility may be congenital or due to previous trauma. In these conditions, the nerve may migrate repeatedly from a position posterior to the medial epicondyle to one medial or anterior to it due to laxity of Osborne's ligament, which is described later. This subluxation is usually a transient event that occurs in positions of elbow flexion with activity. The nerve is compressed as it is stretched over the epicondyle during repeated episodes. Subsequent nerve fibrosis and a decrease in nerve elasticity can develop.[12]

After the ulnar nerve leaves the epicondylar groove, it passes between the humeral and ulnar heads of the flexor carpi ulnaris, the anatomic area of the cubital tunnel. The fibroaponeurotic covering of the epicondylar groove continues distally. At this point, it is called the ligament of Osborne. With flexion of the elbow, the ligament of Osborne becomes taut and decreases the space available to the nerve in the tunnel (Fig. 11.2). The ulnar collateral ligament of the elbow also bulges outward with elbow flexion, further decreasing the space available to the nerve. The tunnel changes from an oval to a flattened ellipse[5] with flexion, and pressures within the tunnel may increase by seven times.[13]

The throwing athlete is vulnerable to compression of the ulnar nerve at the elbow. Pressures in the cubital tunnel can increase six times over the resting pressure when the arm is placed in the cocking position of throwing, with the elbow flexed and the wrist extended.[14] Any attenuation of the ulnar collateral ligament allows subtle

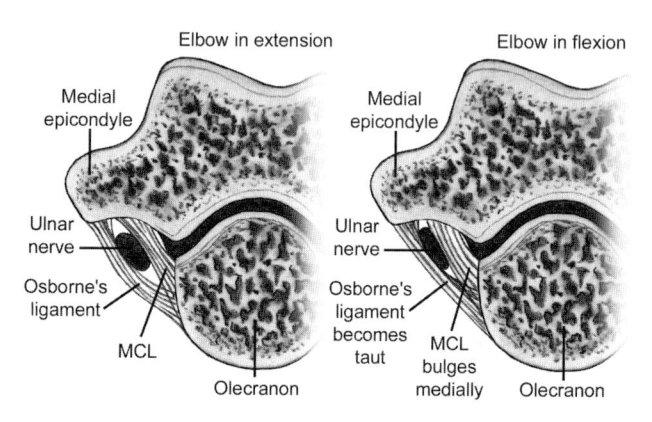

FIGURE 11.2. Bird's-eye view of the elbow and the cubital tunnel with the elbow in extension and flexion (MCL, medical collateral ligament).

opening of the medial elbow with stress, further stretching the already compressed ulnar nerve.[15] Any resultant thickening of the ulnar collateral ligament or degenerative spurring of the medial elbow also contributes to compression.

Prolonged positioning of the arm with the elbow in flexion may cause ulnar nerve symptoms by the same mechanism. Positional problems can occur iatrogenically from flexed positioning of the elbow during unrelated surgical procedures or from upper-extremity immobilization in flexion after an unrelated injury. Patients may have subclinical neuropathy that then becomes symptomatic due to these factors.[16]

The muscle fascia of the humeral and ulnar heads of the flexor carpi ulnaris represent another potential site of compression. The nerve remains intramuscular for approximately 5 cm and, when it leaves the flexor carpi ulnaris, it again may be compressed by the muscle fascia. This anatomic structure is referred to as the deep flexor pronator aponeurosis.[17]

Any scarring along the course of the nerve from previous surgery or injury can be problematic. The ulnar nerve normally moves as much as 10 mm proximal to and 6 mm distal to the medial epicondyle with elbow motion.[18] The medial head of the triceps also can displace the proximal nerve up to 7 mm medially.[19] For these normal, necessary motions to be possible, the nerve must remain free to alter its shape and position. Any tethering of the nerve by adhesions can cause traction, and scar bands may also have a direct compressive effect.

DIFFERENTIAL DIAGNOSIS

Any lesion proximal to the elbow that affects the nerve fibers that go on to compose the ulnar nerve can cause symptoms that can be confused with cubital tunnel syndrome. A lesion can occur in the spinal cord, cervical roots (C8, T1), or brachial plexus (medial cord). Examples of such diseases include cervical disc protrusion, brachial plexopathy, spinal cord mass-effect lesions, syringomyelia, and thoracic outlet syndrome. Distally, the nerve may be compressed in Guyon's canal, causing ulnar nerve symptoms only in the hand. This entity is commonly referred to as ulnar tunnel syndrome. It is not uncommon for the nerve to be affected at multiple levels. Compression at one level may make the nerve more susceptible to further compression distally.

Any systemic disease that affects peripheral nerves also must be considered. Diabetes mellitus, alcoholism, hypothyroidism, malignancies, and vitamin deficiencies can all cause peripheral neuropathies. Remember that patients who have such conditions probably are more susceptible to nerve compression and also may have a concomitant compressive neuropathy.

History, physical examination, and diagnostic testing should be used to identify and rule out these other processes. This evaluation also helps to accurately identify the anatomic area of the nerve entrapment, which is an important fact when considering any surgical treatment.

PHYSICAL EXAMINATION

The classic presentation of cubital tunnel syndrome is pain at the medial elbow and along the proximal medial portion of the forearm.[4,20] Pain most commonly radiates distally but also may radiate proximally. Sensory problems often occur in the ulnar one and one-half digits and in the dorsoulnar portion of the hand. Patients who have sensory problems may report difficulty or fatigue performing motor tasks with the hand. Patients should be questioned about their participation in any activities that are known to cause ulnar nerve neuritis. Prolonged or repeated direct pressure on the medial elbow may elicit symptoms. Prolonged elbow flexion also can cause ulnar nerve transient compression. Any previous elbow injury or surgery must be noted, and previous treatment should be identified. Questions must be directed toward uncovering other local and systemic conditions that mimic external nerve compression in the cubital tunnel.

The physical examination must extend from the cervical spine to the hand. A general examination should be performed to identify findings that suggest a systemic disease that may be a contributing factor.

If ulnar nerve compression is significant, the ulnar-innervated intrinsic muscles in the hand may be weak. This weakness is noted by testing the first dorsal interosseous muscle against resistance and by simultaneously palpating its substance. The findings should be compared with findings for the uninvolved side. With long-standing compression, atrophy of the ulnar-innervated intrinsic muscles of the hand is commonly noted. Atrophy and weakness of the ulnar-innervated forearm muscles are less often seen and are less useful clinically. Weakness of the flexor digitorum profundus to the little finger is the most readily detectable extrinsic muscle deficit. Severe, long-standing compression may result in clawing of the ring and little fingers and hyperextension of the metacarpophalangeal joint of the thumb.

If present, altered sensation in the ulnar nerve distribution is noted in the ulnar one and one-half digits and the dorsoulnar portion of the hand. The dorsal sensory branch of the ulnar nerve supplies sensation to the dorsoulnar aspect of the hand. This branch typically leaves the main nerve 5 to 6 cm proximal to the ulnar styloid before the main nerve enters Guyon's canal at the wrist. If sensation in the dorsoulnar aspect of the hand is intact, the clinician must consider ulnar tunnel syndrome as the diagnosis. Sensation can be measured grossly or by more specific means. Vibratory sensation and light touch assessment using graded monofilaments may be the most sensitive sensory tests.[4] Findings should again be compared with the opposite, unaffected side.

The clinician should measure the elbow carrying angle and range of motion. He or she should palpate the ulnar nerve along its course around the elbow, noting any masses, swellings, or tender areas. The nerve should be palpated at the epicondylar groove with active and passive range of motion and also with resisted flexion and extension. Any subluxation of the nerve anteriorly that is different from the uninvolved side may be significant.

A provocative test to aid in diagnosis of ulnar nerve compression at the cubital tunnel is the elbow flexion test. The elbow is held in full flexion with the forearm supinated and the wrist extended for 1 to 3 min to see if symptoms are reproduced. This test is somewhat analogous to Phalen's test of the median nerve at the wrist and is also more sensitive than specific.[21]

Direct percussion of the nerve just posterior to the medial epicondyle also may reproduce symptoms and indicate neuritis in this area. The clinician should perform a thorough examination of the neck, upper extremity, and other extremities as indicated by the initial evaluation. Physical examination can be very helpful in ruling in or out the other entities described in the differential diagnosis.

Diagnostic Studies

Electrical studies are often helpful in localizing the lesion. These tests include measures of the motor and sensory nerve conduction velocities and include electromyographic examination. Any segment of the nerve that is compressed may show delayed conduction. In addition, the distribution of muscles with altered electromyographic potentials may be helpful in localizing the lesion. It is possible for patients to have significant symptoms with equivocal findings on electrical tests. Some patients only have symptoms with a certain position of the elbow or during certain activities involving flexion of the elbow or direct pressure on the nerve. If these patients are tested with the elbow in a nonprovocative position, the nerve may not be affected at this time, and findings may be normal. In patients, such as throwing athletes, testing of the nerve in the provocative position may be impossible. For this reason, the results of electrodiagnostic testing must be combined with a history and physical examination before a diagnosis is made or surgical treatment is considered. In addition, note that the ulnar nerve can be compressed at more than one site[22]; the surgeon should always consider this possibility before planning treatment. Electrical testing may be helpful in the differential diagnosis by identifying conditions such as brachial neuritis, thoracic outlet syndrome, and cervical radiculopathy.

Plain radiographs of the elbow should be obtained to aid in evaluation. A posteroanterior axial view of the distal humerus and cubital tunnel profiling the epicondylar groove may show bony prominences that could be implicated in compression. See Figure 3.22.

Other diagnostic studies may be needed based on the findings of the initial evaluation. These studies may include more involved imaging studies of the elbow, such as magnetic resonance imaging, to evaluate a suspected mass lesion. If indicated, laboratory testing for systemic disease should be obtained.

NONOPERATIVE TREATMENT

To treat a patient who has external compressive syndrome of the ulnar nerve,[23] the clinician should remove the cause of the external compression. Any external splints, casts, or braces pressing on the medial elbow should be removed. The patient should avoid any activities requiring prolonged flexion or leaning on the elbows; this activity modification may be sufficient to resolve symptoms. The patient's work environment should be investigated and altered, if necessary.

Sleeping with the elbow in flexion or repeated flexion activities can also be a causative factor. Both of these situations may be addressed by splinting the elbow in limited flexion (30° to 40°) continuously for several weeks to allow the neuritis to resolve. The wrist may be immobilized to limit contraction of the flexor carpi ulnaris. Care must be taken not to put any direct pressure on the medial elbow with the splint; therefore, anterior splinting may be best. Nonsteroidal anti-inflammatory medications often are used as an adjunct.

OPERATIVE TREATMENT

Indications and Contraindications

If symptoms do not resolve with nonoperative measures, operative treatment may be considered. The clinician should not accomplish surgical decompression unless he or she has fully evaluated the patient to rule out other causes for the symptoms. He or she should attempt to localize the lesion to the elbow region with physical examination and electrodiagnostic measures as described earlier; however, the decision to operate should not be based solely on the results of electrodiagnostic studies.

If a lesion at the elbow causes refractory pain or sensory symptoms, surgical decompression of the nerve can be considered. If the patient has muscle weakness, he or she should be followed closely for any change in condition. Persistent mild weakness or worsening weakness is an indication for surgery. In a patient who has severe persistent sensory deficits, marked weakness, or perceptible muscle atrophy, surgery is clearly indicated. In a long-standing neuropathy, nonoperative treatment is less likely to be effective, and surgery may be recommended for pain relief. In this chronic setting, the patient should be counseled that surgical decompression has a variable effect, especially on weakness and atrophy. Even so, surgery still may be indicated for pain relief and for attempted recovery of some sensory and motor function.

Operative Techniques

The most commonly performed operative treatments for cubital tunnel syndrome involve releasing the nerve from its fascial sheath and transposing it anterior to the medial epicondyle. A limited decompression at the epicondylar groove and cubital tunnel without transposition may be performed, but this procedure does not address all potential areas of nerve compression in the elbow region. If the nerve is released from its sheath without a planned transposition, it may subluxate anteriorly, causing recurrent symptoms and a failed procedure. For these reasons, a surgical procedure involving both decompression and transposition usually is recommended. By transposing the nerve, the surgeon removes it from any abnormality present in its native location. The nerve also is effectively lengthened so that it no longer is placed under tension with elbow flexion.

Decompression in Situ

Decompression in situ without transposition is recommended in a few specific situations. Limited release can be considered for patients who have local or systemic diseases that make them poor candidates for operations involving extensive soft-tissue dissection. Probably the best candidate for the limited procedure is a patient, such as a violinist, who has symptoms due to prolonged and repetitive contraction of the flexor carpi ulnaris muscle.[6] In the limited procedure, the sheath over the nerve should only be released distal to a line drawn from the medial epicondyle to the olecranon.[9] More proximal release can predispose the nerve to subluxation. The finding of an indentation in the nerve at the edge of the fascia overlying the heads of the flexor carpi ulnaris may indicate a good prognosis for recovery after limited release in this area.

This procedure may be performed with the patient under general, regional, or local anesthesia. The incision is made halfway between the medial epicondyle and the olecranon tip overlying the ulnar nerve and is carried distally about 5 cm along the course of the nerve. The surgeon isolates the nerve proximally and divides the fascia over it as he or she traces the nerve distally between the two heads of the flexor carpi ulnaris muscle.[9]

Postoperatively, the patient's elbow is placed in a soft dressing, and elbow range of motion is begun after the initial postoperative swelling subsides.

Full Exposure and Release of the Ulnar Nerve

Full exposure and release of the ulnar nerve are typically performed with the patient under regional or general anesthesia and the patient's arm under tourniquet control. The incision for exposure of the ulnar nerve at the elbow begins 8 to 10 cm proximal to the medial epicondyle directly over the intermuscular septum. The incision should extend distally along the course of the nerve, passing just behind the medial epicondyle. Leaving the scar directly over the prominence of the medial epicondyle is undesirable. The incision should not be too far posterior, because anterior transposition procedures require exposure in front of the medial epicondyle. Distally, the incision should extend 5 to 7 cm distal to the medial epicondyle along the area that is the medial border of the forearm when the forearm is supinated. Care should be taken during the creation of the full-thickness skin and subcutaneous flaps, because branches of the medial antebrachial cutaneous nerve cross this region. These branches cross in the region spanning from 6 cm proximal to the medial epicondyle to 6 cm distal to it.[24]

The surgeon should mobilize the flaps with most of the dissection done anteriorly to expose the deep fascia in anticipation of anterior transposition. The ulnar nerve is identified proximal to the cubital tunnel by penetrating the deep fascia of the arm just posterior to the intermuscular septum. The nerve then is followed along its course into the flexor carpi ulnaris. This may be done safely within the approximately 15 cm of the described region without compromising the vascular supply.

At the distal edge of the intermuscular septum, a plexus of vessels typically lies adjacent to the nerve. These vessels should be mobilized carefully from the nerve and should be cauterized carefully, if necessary, to prevent postoperative bleeding. The nerve should be freed carefully from any scar. Any constricting bands of epineurium should be released. The surgeon should carefully inspect the walls of the cubital tunnel for any mass lesions or other abnormalities. The first branches off the nerve are small articular branches to the elbow joint. These branches often must be sacrificed to allow transposition of the nerve. Often, the branches in this area are actually the first motor branches to the flexor carpi ulnaris.[25] In this case, these branches should be dissected distally and preserved if possible.

With any of the anterior transposition techniques, placing the nerve in front of the medial epicondyle subjects it to impingement by the medial intermuscular septum of the arm (Fig. 11.3). The distal portion of the septum should be resected to prevent this problem. Distally, the nerve should be followed through the flexor carpi ulnaris to the deep flexor pronator aponeurosis. Any fascia impinging on the nerve after it is placed in its new location must be divided or resected.

After the nerve is fully exposed along its course at the

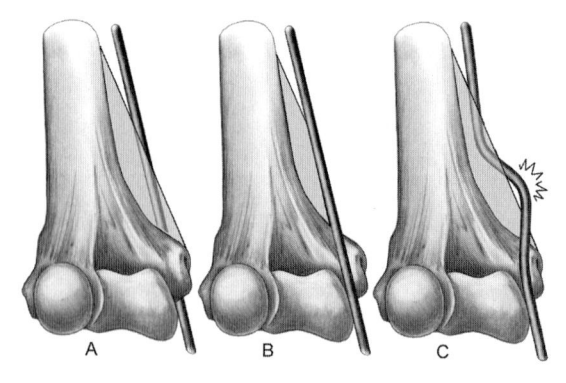

FIGURE 11.3. (A) The ulnar nerve typically lies posterior to the intermuscular septum. (B) After ulnar nerve transposition, it lies in front of the medial epicondyle. (C) The intermuscular septum should be excised distally to prevent compression.

elbow and released from its bed, several options are available for repositioning the nerve to prevent recurrent problems. These options include subcutaneous transposition, intramuscular transposition, and submuscular transposition.

Subcutaneous Transposition

Subcutaneous transposition is the most common surgical procedure performed for treatment of ulnar neuropathy at the elbow. This simple procedure is the method of choice for nerve transposition done in conjunction with elbow trauma surgery or total elbow replacement. Very thin individuals may not be good candidates for this procedure because the nerve may still be subjected to external forces in its new location.

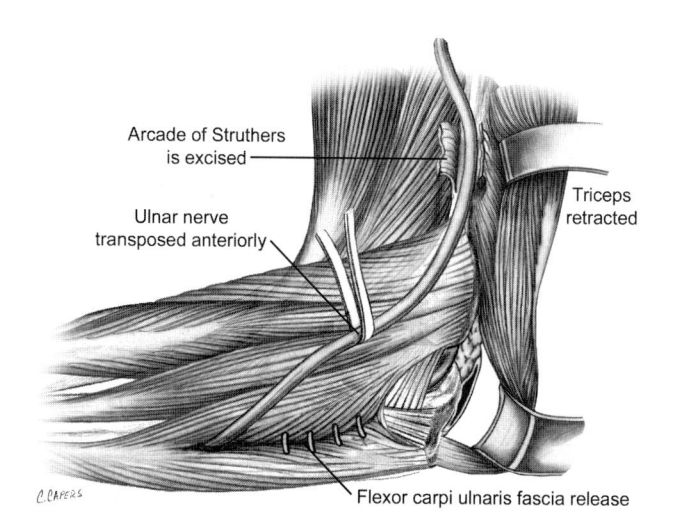

FIGURE 11.4. After subcutaneous transposition, the nerve must lie in a smooth course on the flexor–pronator mass with adequate release of the medial intermuscular septum, the arcade of Struthers, and the fascia of the flexor carpi ulnaris.

The nerve is exposed as described earlier. The anterior full-thickness flap is raised off the muscle fascia so that the nerve can be positioned anterior to the medial epicondyle. The surgeon places the nerve so that it follows a smooth course across the elbow. Care is taken to ensure that the nerve is not bent sharply or kinked. If the distal intermuscular septum is not resected as described earlier, it may become a new site of nerve compression. The fascia of the flexor carpi ulnaris also must be released sufficiently so that it does not impinge on the nerve in this new position (Fig. 11.4).

Some authors recommend methods to ensure that the nerve remains in its new location and does not slip back posteriorly onto the apex of, or behind, the medial epicondyle. The creation of a fasciodermal sling is the preferred procedure.[26] In this procedure, a 1.5-cm rectangular flap of fascia from the flexor–pronator muscle is raised and sutured to the overlying subcutaneous tissue. This is done so that the flap prevents migration of the nerve medially. Care must be taken to not make a constricting band on the nerve when performing this adjunctive procedure.

Postoperatively, the elbow may be immobilized in 45° of flexion for 2 weeks to allow soft-tissue healing. After 2 weeks, range of motion is encouraged to prevent elbow stiffness.

Intramuscular Transposition

The intramuscular transposition involves placing the nerve into a groove in the flexor–pronator muscle mass. This placement provides more protection against external forces than the subcutaneous position provides and requires less dissection than submuscular transposition requires. Some authors warn that excessive scarring occurs with use of this procedure.[27–29] However, in one animal study, researchers found no more scar formation with intramuscular transposition than with submuscular transposition.[30] Clinical studies have demonstrated acceptable results with this procedure.[31]

With this method, the procedure is performed just as for the subcutaneous transposition. Next, a groove is cut 0.5 to 1.0 cm deep into the muscle along the path where the nerve lies. Any fibrous septae within the muscle substance must be divided so that they do not impinge on the nerve. The muscle fascia over the nerve is closed. After surgery, the upper extremity is immobilized with the forearm pronated and the elbow in 90° of flexion for 3 weeks. Range-of-motion exercises begin after this period.

Submuscular Transposition

Submuscular transposition is the method most often recommended for serious athletes because it best protects the nerve from external and traction forces. The nerve is placed under the entire origin of the flexor–pronator mass.

This technique should not be used for trauma, arthroplasty, or in the presence of other conditions, such as severe arthritis, that deform the joint or joint capsule.

After exposing the nerve, the surgeon releases the flexor–pronator muscle mass from its origin on the medial epicondyle. Several techniques have been described for this. Most often, the muscle is sharply released directly from the bone or is released except for a 1-cm cuff of soft tissue that is left to facilitate reattachment.[29] Some authors advocate a step-cut Z-plasty of the muscle to lengthen it.[32,33] This technique is designed to decrease the pressure of the reattached muscle on the nerve. With any of these techniques, care must be taken not to damage the underlying medial collateral ligament.

Next, the nerve is placed along the brachialis muscle, anterior to the elbow capsule and medial to the medial epicondyle. A small portion of the flexor carpi ulnaris may be released from the ulna to allow the nerve to pass into the muscle in a straight path.

When the surgeon removes the muscle directly from the bone, he or she reattaches it with braided suture passed through drill holes in the epicondyle. Otherwise, the surgeon repairs it to the soft-tissue cuff that is left on the epicondyle. Another method involves detaching the entire medial epicondyle with its attached flexor–pronator muscle.[34] The risk of this technique is complications related to the reattachment of the epicondyle. With any of the techniques, the surgeon must be sure that, when it is reattached, the muscle does not compress the nerve.

Postoperatively, the upper extremity is immobilized with the elbow in 45° of flexion, the forearm in slight pronation, and the wrist in neutral flexion–extension. After 3 weeks, the patient begins active motion. To allow healing of the detached muscle, he or she should wait 6 weeks after surgery to begin gradual resistive exercises. The patient should not attempt athletic activities involving the arm or heavy lifting until at least 3 months after surgery. In throwing athletes, full recovery may take 6 to 9 months.

Medial Epicondylectomy

A variation of the decompression in situ procedure is the medial epicondylectomy. This procedure is designed to eliminate some of the problems associated with other procedures. The epicondyle is removed so that the nerve cannot subluxate (as it can after limited release of the nerve or after subcutaneous transposition). After the epicondyle is removed, the surgeon allows the nerve to lie in whatever position appears best. This technique also helps to avoid scarring, which is a concern with intramuscular and submuscular transpositions.

The surgeon exposes the nerve in the epicondylar groove and the cubital tunnel. Significant proximal and distal dissection usually are not performed, because the nerve is not translocated from its bed. The soft tissues are dissected subperiosteally off the epicondyle. The flexor–pronator muscles are dissected anteriorly, and the periosteum is elevated posteriorly. With the nerve protected, the epicondyle is removed, and the cut surface is smoothed (Fig. 11.5). The soft-tissue cuffs are closed over the cut bone surface. If sufficient bone has been removed, the nerve should move freely forward with elbow flexion. Further release of the soft tissues must be done proximally or distally if compression of the nerve is noted in either of these locations. The skin and subcutaneous tissue are closed over the nerve. Care must be taken not to remove so much of the bone that the medial collateral ligament is disrupted. Disruption of this ligament may result in elbow instability and even dislocation.[35]

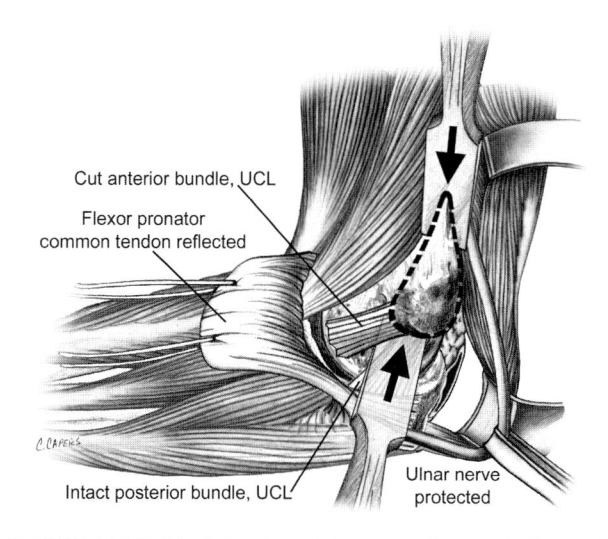

FIGURE 11.5. Medial epicondylectomy. Arrows indicate the proper plane of the osteotomy to remove the epicondyle (UCL, ulnar collateral ligament).

Neurolysis

After release and exposure, the nerve may be enlarged with thickened epineurium noted at the site of the compression. Careful localized external neurolysis often is recommended in this situation to relieve compression on the fascicles.[6] Internal neurolysis is not recommended because of the risk of injury to the rich interfascicular plexus of the nerve at the elbow.[9]

RESULTS

All the surgical techniques that we have described have been reported to yield acceptable results.[4,6,7] Often, the decision to employ one technique instead of another is based on the personal preference of the operating surgeon.

Dellon reviewed the literature up to 1988 to examine

the reported results of nonoperative and operative treatment of ulnar nerve compressive neuropathy at the elbow.[36] In the literature, he found 1435 patients who could be grouped into three stages of ulnar nerve compression. Patients whose neuropathy was classified as mild had transient paresthesias and subjective weakness only. The moderately affected group had measurable weakness. The severely affected group had persistent paresthesias and muscle atrophy.

In the group with mild compressive neuropathy, 50% of the patients were treated successfully with nonoperative means. Any of the operative techniques yielded excellent results in 90% of patients. In patients who had moderate compression, nonoperative treatment and simple decompression were not effective. Medial epicondylectomy gave 50% excellent results and had the highest recurrence rate; anterior submuscular transposition gave 80% excellent results and had the lowest recurrence rate. For severe cases, the literature lacked a large series of patients on which to report. The authors did note that the anterior intermuscular technique had the highest recurrence rate in this group. Among patients who had recurrent ulnar nerve compression, anterior submuscular transposition with internal neurolysis provided the greatest percentage of excellent results.

COMPLICATIONS

Few authors have reported major complications of procedures performed for treatment of ulnar nerve compressive neuropathy at the elbow. The most obvious mistake is when a procedure is performed to address compression of the ulnar nerve at the elbow when the true abnormality lies elsewhere. As discussed earlier, proper diagnostic evaluation must be done for all patients to be sure that the patient's symptoms are caused by abnormalities involving the nerve in the region of the elbow. Patients obviously do not benefit from surgery of the ulnar nerve at the elbow when the actual disorder is cervical radiculopathy or compression at Guyon's canal.

Patients who have compromised skin or vascular problems in the affected extremity may be at risk for wound complications. During surgery, the ulnar nerve must be treated carefully to avoid iatrogenic injury. Dissection of the nerve from its bed and of any associated scar tissue should only be performed under excellent visualization, with proper equipment, and without placing any significant traction on the nerve. The nerve should be protected carefully throughout the remainder of the surgical procedure. Meticulous soft-tissue dissection and hemostasis should be employed. Any postoperative immobilizing devices must be fitted carefully to avoid external compression of the nerve, especially if it has been placed in a superficial location.

Injury to the sensory branches of the medial antebrachial cutaneous nerve during superficial dissection can cause painful neuroma formation. These nerve branches should always be identified and protected. With medial epicondylectomy, the ulnar collateral ligament of the elbow must not be compromised, because elbow instability can result. If the surgeon dissects the flexor–pronator mass off its attachment for submuscular transposition, he or she must use proper postoperative protection to prevent failure of the muscular repair.

Recurrence of symptoms is the major postoperative problem. The most common cause of recurrence is reported to be insufficient decompression at the original surgery.[37] Most episodes of recurrence can be avoided by meticulous attention to surgical technique. All the potential sites of compression, from the arcade of Struthers proximally to the flexor carpi ulnaris aponeurosis distally, must be addressed to perform a complete decompression. If the nerve is moved from its bed, it must be inspected carefully in its new location to ensure that new sites of compression have not been created. The most common sites for this problem to occur are the medial intermuscular septum and the fascial edge of the flexor carpi ulnaris muscle.

If a limited decompression in situ is performed, the nerve may be prone to subluxate anteriorly because its overlying aponeurosis has been divided. If subluxation is problematic, repeat surgery with full transposition of the nerve to an anterior position may be necessary.

SUMMARY

Compressive neuropathy of the ulnar nerve at the elbow is a common problem, and many acute cases resolve with nonoperative treatment. Before considering operative treatment for chronic cases, the surgeon must consider differential diagnoses and must localize the lesion to the elbow. The type of procedure chosen depends on many factors. There is a paucity of good comparative studies in the literature to aid the surgeon in selection of the most effective procedure. The surgical treatment must be tailored to each case after determining the cause of the neuropathy and after examining patient factors, such as occupation, activity level, and coexisting systemic conditions. Often, the type of surgery performed is the one with which the surgeon has the most experience and is most comfortable. Recurrent problems most often are due to failure to relieve the true source of compression at the original procedure. Repeat exploration to address all potential areas of compression, with subsequent submuscular transposition, is effective in most of these difficult cases.

REFERENCES

1. Lundborg G. Ischemic nerve injury. Experimental studies on intraneural microvascular pathophysiology and nerve function

in a limb subjected to temporary circulatory arrest. *Scan J Plast Reconstr Surg Suppl* 1970;6:3–113.
2. Eversmann WW Jr, Ritsick JA. Intraoperative changes in motor nerve conduction latency in carpal tunnel syndrome. *J Hand Surg* 1978;3:77–81.
3. Sunderland S. The nerve lesion in the carpal tunnel syndrome. *J Neurol Neurosurg Psychiatry* 1976;39:615–626.
4. Posner MA. Compressive ulnar neuropathies at the elbow: I. Etiology and diagnosis. *J Am Acad Orthop Surg* 1998;6:282–288.
5. Adelaar RS, Foster WC, McDowell C. The treatment of the cubital tunnel syndrome. *J Hand Surg* 1984;9A:90–95.
6. Posner MA. Compressive ulnar neuropathies at the elbow: II. Treatment. *J Am Acad Orthop Surg* 1998;6:289–297.
7. Posner MA. Compressive ulnar neuropathies of the ulnar nerve at the elbow and wrist. *Instr Course Lect* 2000;49:305–317.
8. Feindel W, Stratford J. The role of the cubital tunnel in tardy ulnar palsy. *Can J Surg* 1958;1:287–300.
9. Eversmann WW Jr. Entrapment and compression neuropathies. In: Green DP, ed. *Operative hand surgery*, 3rd ed. New York: Churchill Livingstone; 1993:1356–1365.
10. Spinner M, Kaplan EB. The relationship of the ulnar nerve to the medial intermuscular septum in the arm and its clinical significance. *Hand* 1976;8:239–242.
11. Hunt JR. Tardy or late paralysis of the ulnar nerve. A form of chronic progressive neuritis developing many years after fracture dislocation of the elbow joint. *JAMA* 1916;66:11–15.
12. Lazaro L III. Ulnar nerve instability: Ulnar nerve injury due to elbow flexion. *South Med J* 1977;70:36–40.
13. Werner C-O, Ohlin P, Elmqvist D. Pressures recorded in ulnar neuropathy. *Acta Orthop Scand* 1985;56:404–406.
14. Pechan J, Julis I. The pressure measurement in the ulnar nerve. A contribution to the pathophysiology of the cubital tunnel syndrome. *J Biomech* 1975;8:75–79.
15. Jobe FW, Fanton GS. Nerve injuries. In: Morrey BF, ed. *The elbow and its disorders*. Philadelphia: WB Saunders, 1985: 497.
16. Alvine FG, Schurrer ME. Postoperative ulnar-nerve palsy. Are there predisposing factors? *J Bone Joint Surg* 1987;69A:255–259.
17. Amadio PC, Beckenbaugh RD. Entrapment of the ulnar nerve by the deep flexor–pronator aponeurosis. *J Hand Surg* 1986; 11:83–87.
18. Wilgis EF, Murphy R. The significance of longitudinal excursion in peripheral nerves. *Hand Clin* 1986;2:761–766.
19. Butters KP, Singer KM. Nerve lesions of the arm and elbow. In: DeLee JC, Drez D Jr, eds. *Orthopaedic sports medicine: Principles and practice*. Philadelphia: WB Saunders; 1994:802.
20. James GH. Nerve lesions about the elbow [abstract]. *J Bone Joint Surg* 1956;38B:589.
21. Rayan GM, Jensen C, Duke J. Elbow flexion test in the normal population. *J Hand Surg* 1992;17A:86–89.
22. Upton AR, McComas AJ. The double crush in nerve entrapment syndromes. *Lancet* 1973;2:359–362.
23. Wadsworth TG. The external compression syndrome of the ulnar nerve at the cubital tunnel. *Clin Orthop* 1977;124:189–204.
24. Dellon AL, Mackinnon SE. Injury to the medial antebrachial cutaneous nerve during cubital tunnel surgery. *J Hand Surg* 1985;10B:33–36.
25. Watchmaker GP, Lee G, Mackinnon SE. Intraneural topography of the ulnar nerve in the cubital tunnel facilitates anterior transposition. *J Hand Surg* 1994;19A:915–922.
26. Eaton RG, Crowe JF, Parkes III JC. Anterior transposition of the ulnar nerve using a non-compressing fasciodermal sling. *J Bone Joint Surg* 1980;62A:820–825.
27. Broudy AS, Leffert RD, Smith RJ. Technical problems with ulnar nerve transposition at the elbow: Findings and results of reoperation. *J Hand Surg* 1978;3:85–89.
28. Gabel GT, Amadio PC. Reoperation for failed decompression of the ulnar nerve in the region of the elbow. *J Bone Joint Surg* 1990;72A:213–219.
29. Leffert RD. Anterior submuscular transposition of the ulnar nerves by the Learmonth technique. *J Hand Surg* 1982;7A: 147–155.
30. Dellon AL, Mackinnon SE, Hudson AR, et al. Effect of submuscular versus intramuscular placement of ulnar nerve. Experimental model in the primate. *J Hand Surg* 1986;11B:117–119.
31. Kleinman WB, Bishop AT. Anterior intramuscular transposition of the ulnar nerve. *J Hand Surg* 1989;14A:972–979.
32. Dellon AL. Operative technique for submuscular transposition of the ulnar nerve. *Contemp Orthop* 1988;16:17–24.
33. Pasque CB, Rayan GM. Anterior submuscular transposition of the ulnar nerve for cubital tunnel syndrome. *J Hand Surg* 1995; 20B:447–453.
34. Mass DP, Silverberg B. Cubital tunnel syndrome: Anterior transposition with epicondylar osteotomy. *Orthopedics* 1986; 9:711–715.
35. Cole RJ, Jemison DM, Hayes CW. Anterior elbow dislocation following medial epicondylectomy: A case report. *J Hand Surg* 1994;19A:614–616.
36. Dellon AL. Review of treatment results for ulnar nerve entrapment at the elbow. *J Hand Surg* 1989;14A:688–700.
37. Rogers MR, Bergfield TG, Aulicino PL. The failed ulnar nerve transposition. Etiology and treatment. *Clin Orthop* 1991;269: 193–200.

CHAPTER 12

Pronator Syndrome

N. George Kasparyan and Andrew J. Weiland

INTRODUCTION

Median nerve compressive neuropathy in the proximal forearm occurs in predictable locations that are associated with specific anatomic structures. Pronator syndrome was first described in the literature in 1951. Seyffarth[1] presented a series of 17 patients who were treated nonoperatively. In his initial work, he described the site of compression as being between the two heads of the pronator teres muscle or by the flexor digitorum superficialis arch. Since then, numerous authors have confirmed and further clarified the causes of median nerve entrapment near the elbow. In this chapter, we discuss these causes, the diagnostic criteria and studies, nonoperative treatment, our operative technique, and the results and complications of treatment.

HISTORY

The classic presentation of pronator syndrome is aching, dull pain in the volar aspect of the proximal forearm. In some patients, the pain radiates distally toward the wrist. A focus of pain also may occur at the distal aspect of the humerus with proximal radiation. The pain may be associated with a specific provocative event or may appear with gradual onset without a history of trauma. The patient often reports worsening symptoms with repetitive use of the forearm, specifically in pronation. Pain at night appears to be uncommon. A painful, tender mass may be noticed in the proximal volar forearm. Patients often report diminished sensibility or paresthesia in the radial three and one-half digits. In long-standing cases, the individual may demonstrate weakened grasp or loss of fine dexterity with small objects.[2–4]

The incidence of pronator syndrome in the general population is much lower than the incidence of carpal tunnel syndrome. Women appear to be approximately four times more likely than men to develop it, and the preponderance of cases occur in the fifth decade. Most patients experience symptoms from 9 to 24 months before a physician makes a diagnosis.[2]

CLINICAL ANATOMY

The median nerve is formed from contributions of both the lateral and medial cords of the brachial plexus. As the two cords merge to form the median nerve, they partially envelope the distal aspect of the axillary artery. As the median nerve progresses distally, it is juxtaposed to the medial aspect of the brachial artery at the level of the antecubital fossa, lying on the anterior surface of the brachialis muscle. At the level of the antecubital fossa, the median nerve passes posterior to the bicipital aponeurosis and usually underneath the origin of the flexor pronator muscle mass. Just distal to the elbow joint, the median nerve passes between the two heads of the pronator teres. Here, it crosses over to the lateral side of the ulnar artery. The median nerve is separated from the ulnar artery by the deep head of the pronator teres. From this position, the nerve moves more dorsally and runs between the flexor digitorum superficialis and flexor digitorum profundus muscle bellies. The nerve continues distally down the forearm on the undersurface of the deep fascia of the flexor digitorum superficialis. The median nerve eventually emerges in the distal third of the forearm along the radial aspect of the superficialis muscle, finally passing beneath the flexor retinaculum and transverse carpal ligament at the wrist.[2–7]

The median nerve rarely has major branches proximal to the elbow. The most common initial branching of the median nerve occurs in a variable pattern of three to four separate innervations, usually at or just distal to the elbow flexion crease. These branches enter the pronator teres, flexor carpi radialis, palmaris longus, and flexor digitorum superficialis. A number of very small articular branches of the median nerve innervate the ulnohumeral and proximal radioulnar joint. These articular branches rarely are seen during routine dissection of the nerve.[2–7]

The most important branch of the median nerve, the anterior interosseous nerve, decussates at the level of the two heads of the pronator teres. The anterior interosseous nerve emerges posteriorly from the median nerve at the same level as the motor branches of the flexor–pronator mass. The anterior interosseous artery, which is a branch of the ulnar artery, accompanies the anterior interosseous nerve along the interosseous membrane between the radius and ulna. The anterior interosseous nerve supplies innervation to the flexor pollicis longus, pronator quadratus, and flexor digitorum profundus to the index finger; in some individuals, it provides variable innervation to the flexor digitorum profundus to the long finger. The anterior interosseous nerve also may supply small articular branches to the ulnohumeral and proximal radioulnar joints.[2–7]

The location of the median nerve in relation to the two heads of the pronator teres varies. The median nerve actually lies between the two heads of the pronator teres in approximately 80% of dissections. In some people, the nerve lies dorsal to both heads of the pronator and lies posterior to a superficial head, with no deep head present. The nerve, at times, may pierce the substance of one or both heads of the pronator.[2–7]

Pronator syndrome can be associated with four specific anatomic sites of compression of the median nerve in the proximal forearm. The first, and most proximal, region of compression is the distal third of the humerus beneath the supracondyloid process and the ligament arising from it (Fig. 12.1). This ligament, known as the ligament of Struthers, becomes confluent with the superficial head of the pronator teres muscle. The second site of proximal median nerve compression is the lacertus fibrosus, which is a thin fibrous band covering the median nerve at the elbow joint (Fig. 12.2). In certain instances, the median nerve is uncovered from its muscular bed and is exposed directly to the lacertus fibrosus. This exposure results in impingement, particularly in excessive pronation. Moving distally, the third location of compression is the pronator teres muscle itself. Direct compression by the pronator teres can be due to hypertrophy of the muscle or to compression by the aponeurotic fascia of the superficial or deep head of the muscle against the nerve. The fourth, and most distal, site of median nerve compression about the elbow is at the arch of the flexor digitorum superficialis (Fig. 12.1). The median nerve passes deep to the flexor digitorum superficialis and continues distally between the flexor digitorum superficialis and flexor digitorum profundus.[2–7]

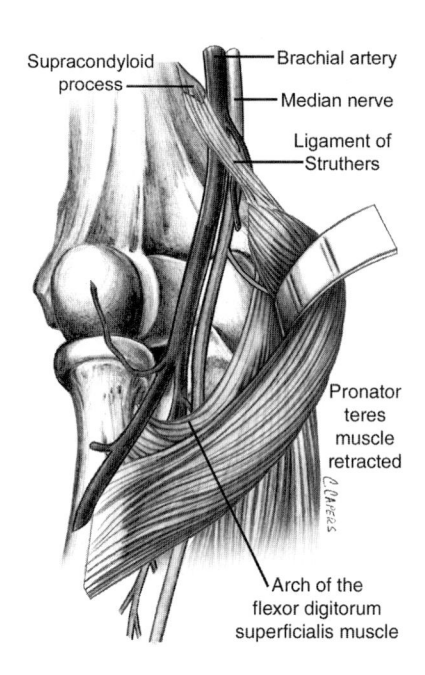

FIGURE 12.1. The ligament of Struthers can act as a conjoined origin for the pronator teres, thereby compressing the median nerve.

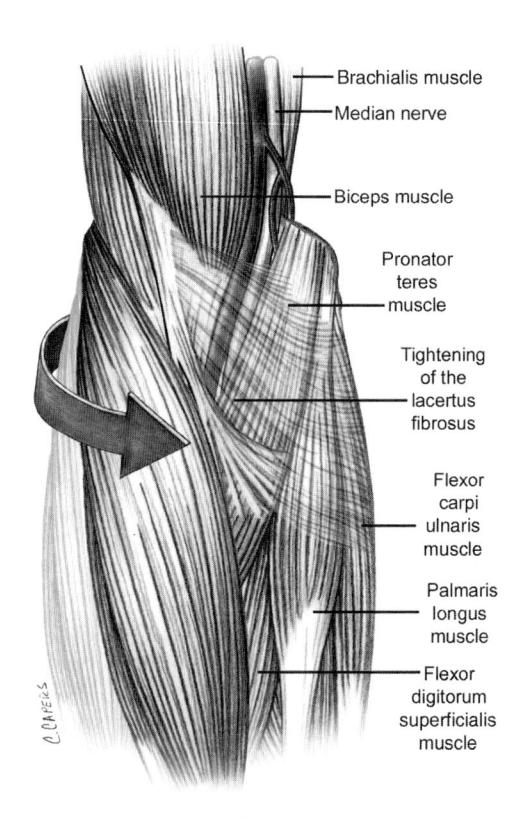

FIGURE 12.2. Pronation of the forearm may cause tightening of the lacertus fibrosus. This tightening can compress the median nerve if the nerve does not lie fully protected beneath the flexor–pronator muscle mass.

PHYSICAL EXAMINATION

Clinical examination of the patient who has pronator syndrome rarely demonstrates atrophy of thenar or forearm musculature. Often, patients report tenderness to palpation over the pronator muscle group. Hartz et al.[8] reported a 95% incidence of this physical finding in their series. Direct and constant pressure over the proximal aspect of the pronator teres may reproduce pain, and the muscle itself may be significantly firmer than the muscle on the unaffected side. After 4 to 5 months of symptoms, patients may begin to experience a positive Tinel sign at the proximal or distal edge of the muscle.[2-7]

The distal aspect of the humerus on the medial side should be palpated for the presence of a supracondyloid process (Fig. 12.1). In the presence of a supracondyloid process, the ligament of Struthers may be more likely to cause compression. However, because of its location, the ligament of Struthers may be the offending compressive structure in the absence of the supracondyloid process.

Some authors have reported tenderness in the thenar region, but this symptom has not been a consistent finding.[2-7] In our experience, a Phalen test is often negative. However, even with proximal compression of the median nerve, 50% of patients showed a positive Phalen test at the wrist distally in one study.[8]

Reports of sensory deficits in patients who have pronator syndrome vary widely in the literature. Morris and Peters[9] reported a diminished sensibility in 88% of patients in their study. Werner et al.[10] found that all patients in their series had normal two-point discrimination. The disparity in the literature may be due to specific provocative maneuvers causing the sensory deficit.[2-7]

Authors also have shown variable motor nerve deficits in both intrinsic and extrinsic muscles.[9] A meticulous physical examination of both the affected and unaffected sides exposes subtle differences in strength. In their series, Morris and Peters[9] showed consistent findings of weakness in the flexor pollicis longus and abductor pollicis brevis muscles. Contrary to these findings, Johnson and Spinner[11] found no evidence of motor dysfunction in a series of 71 patients.

The following provocative testing can be extremely useful in eliciting a diagnosis.

1. If pain becomes exaggerated by flexion of the elbow between 120° and 130°, the likely site of compression is at the ligament of Struthers approximately 4 cm proximal to the elbow joint.

2. According to Stern and Fassler,[2] the lacertus fibrosus exhibits its greatest compressive force on the median nerve when the elbow is flexed in a supinated position. Eversmann stated that compression of the median nerve by the lacertus fibrosus only becomes significant when the median nerve is superficial to the flexor muscle mass and the flexor muscle origin or when the nerve lies just lateral to the edge of the flexor muscle mass (Fig. 12.2).[3,4]

3. To test the pronator muscle mass itself as the cause of compression, the elbow should be fixed flat in extension on a table (Fig. 12.3). The patient pronates against resistance with the arm in neutral rotation and the wrist flexed (to relax the flexor digitorum superficialis).

4. Resisted flexion of the flexor digitorum superficialis of the middle finger that elicits pain may indicate compression of the median nerve at the superficialis arch.[2-7]

Diagnostic Criteria

From a study with a series of 103 patients, Johnson and Spinner[11] found that a positive diagnosis of pronator syndrome can be made if most of the following criteria are established in the patient.

1. Tenderness and firmness to palpation of the pronator teres muscle

2. A positive Tinel sign over the proximal or distal border of the pronator

3. Increased paresthesia of the radial three and one-half digits with compression of the pronator

4. Variable weakness of the forearm and hand muscles that the median nerve innervates

5. Reproduction of paresthesias with one or more of the provocative tests described earlier

6. Conduction defect or abnormal electromyogram localizing the lesion to the pronator area

7. Muscle spasms and cramping in the forearm with repetitive pinching-type exercises

8. Absence of symptoms at night

9. Reproduction of symptoms after a blood pressure cuff is inflated above the diastolic pressure.

DIAGNOSTIC STUDIES

Electromyography and nerve conduction velocities are infrequently diagnostic for a proximal median nerve compressive neuropathy. Johnson and Spinner[11] did not report conduction deficits in their series. However, Hartz et al.[8] demonstrated that 23% of the patients in their series of 40 forearms showed evidence of delayed sensory and motor conduction changes. Only two of these patients had clear electrodiagnostic evidence of pronator syndrome. In a thorough review of the literature, Stern and Fassler[2] stated that slowing of motor or sensory conduction from the wrist to the elbow is neither specific nor sensitive for proximal compressive neuropathy of the median nerve.

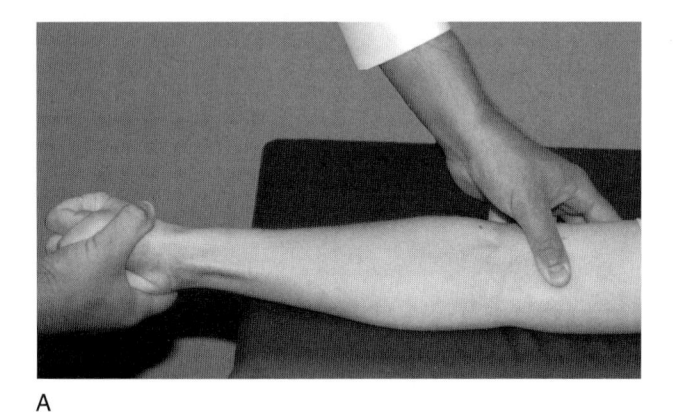

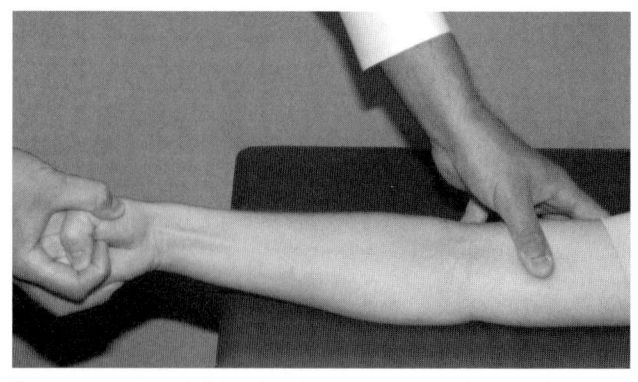

FIGURE 12.3. Testing of the pronator teres. (A) With the elbow extended, the patient actively pronates against resistance. (B) Active pronation of the forearm with active flexion of the wrist tests for pronator teres compression only and isolates the flexor digitorum superficialis. (C) Resisted flexion of the flexor digitorum superficialis tests for compression beneath the superficialis arch.

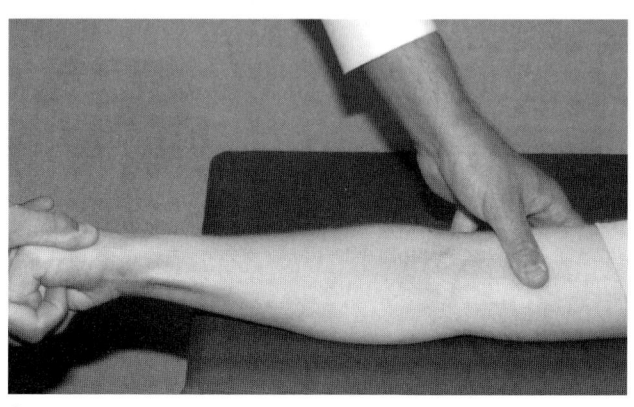

Gessini et al.[12] demonstrated that needle electromyography is the most useful portion of the overall electrodiagnostic test. Stern and Fassler[2] stated that precise localization of the site of proximal entrapment is very difficult and usually is not possible. A diagnosis of proximal compressive neuropathy is much more likely if denervation potentials are localized to both extrinsic and intrinsic muscles. However, even with the densest neuropathy, the branches to the pronator teres muscle usually are spared. When denervation of the pronator teres is noted, it usually indicates compression at the pronator or superficialis arch.[2–7]

Generally, the greatest value of using electrodiagnostic studies in suspected pronator syndrome is the ability to rule out other maladies with comparable clinical presentations. These studies also can enable the examiner to seek out other sites of compression of the median nerve more proximal or distal to the elbow. To most accurately localize the compressive lesion, the study must include needle electromyography of the hand and forearm musculature and motor and sensory conduction studies across the pronator.[2–7]

Nerve conduction velocity determinations of the median nerve in the antecubital region are affected by a number of variables, including age of the patient, obesity of the extremity, physical condition of the arm, and level of edema. These factors can render the nerve conduction velocity either difficult to interpret or, at times, useless. Therefore, electromyography of the pronator teres, flexor carpi radialis, and flexor digitorum sublimis is more reliable. Even these tests may need to be repeated one or two times at 4- to 6-week intervals to confirm the diagnosis.[2–7]

Even in the most technically capable hands, serial electromyography and nerve conduction velocity may be normal in the face of a clearly positive physical examination for median nerve compression at the elbow. This situation is similar to the classic scenario that occurs in the evaluation for radial tunnel syndrome (proximal compressive neuropathy of the posterior interosseous nerve). Because of this situation, surgical exploration is the final option for confirming the diagnosis and simultaneously alleviating the problem.[2–7,13,14]

NONOPERATIVE TREATMENT

After the diagnosis has been made, nonoperative treatment usually is indicated. Splinting the elbow in a custom-molded orthoplast splint and prescribing a course of nonsteroidal anti-inflammatory drugs can be useful. Johnson and Spinner[11] noted that nonoperative measures helped completely to alleviate symptoms in 50% of patients. In a small group of patients, Morris and Peters[9] found that steroid injection in the region of the pronator teres was beneficial in 72% of patients.

The difficulty in nonoperative treatment lies in the patient population that does not improve. The literature does not specify the length of time that nonoperative measures should be employed before moving forward with surgical decompression. Delaying operative intervention is reasonable in patients who have a recent onset of symptoms, but is unreasonable in patients presenting with long-standing symptoms or a delay in diagnosis.[2–7]

OPERATIVE TREATMENT

Indications

Although authors disagree on when to initiate surgery, firm indications for operative intervention include (1) a clinical diagnosis supported by a strong history of symptoms and physical examination of compressive neuropathy at the elbow, (2) clear evidence of proximal median nerve compression confirmed by electrodiagnostic studies, (3) failure of nonoperative measures after a reasonable course of time (usually 6 to 12 weeks), and (4) symptoms that are severely disabling to the patient and thus warrant a surgical procedure.[2–7]

Authors' Preferred Technique

The approach begins with a skin incision approximately 5 to 6 cm proximal to the elbow flexion crease. The incision should be centered slightly anteromedially directly over the neurovascular bundle proximal to the elbow. As the approach progresses distally, a zigzag incision at 60° angles should be made over the antecubital region. The incision courses distally on the anterior surface of the forearm between the flexor and extensor muscle groups.[2–7]

If a supracondyloid process is evident on plain radiographic films, inspection for the ligament of Struthers originating from this bony prominence should begin at this level and move distally. When the supracondyloid process is present, the ligament of Struthers lies over the median nerve, brachial artery, and brachial vein (Fig. 12.1). The median nerve is usually medial to the vascular structures at this level. The ligament of Struthers courses distally and blends into the humeral head of the pronator teres fascia, which originates at the most superior aspect of the medial epicondyle. In our experience, release of the ligament of Struthers and resection of the supracondyloid process, when present, yield the best results.[2–7,15–17]

Once the proximal compressive structures are released, the nerve can be followed distally to the second region of possible compression, the lacertus fibrosus. We have found that the lacertus fibrosus varies considerably in thickness in each individual. We release the fibers of the lacertus over the nerve and, if the lacertus is markedly thickened, recommend a segmental resection of a small portion of the lacertus fibers directly over the course of the nerve. The lacertus fibrosus usually causes a compressive neuropathy of the median nerve when the nerve lies along the lateral edge of the pronator muscle group and is not covered fully by the flexor muscle mass. When this anatomic variation occurs, the reason that the lacertus impinges directly on the median nerve is clearly evident.[2–7]

The nerve is followed distally to the third compressive region in the proximal forearm. During the course distally, all muscular branches arise medially, and even the large anterior interosseous branch arises medially or posteromedially.[18–20] The dissection is best carried out on the lateral aspect of the nerve's path. All branches arising medially should be identified and explored to their muscular innervation. The median nerve enters the forearm through the two heads of the pronator teres. In our experience, the most common cause of compression at this level is hypertrophy of the pronator teres. If significant hypertrophy is noted, a partial release of the superficial head of the pronator teres from its origin is indicated. However, thickened fascial slips at the edge of the underlying aponeurotic head or overlying superficial head of the pronator teres may be the cause of compression at this site. The surgeon needs to explore for and release these fascial slips. Next, the superficial head is elevated distally from its conjoined tendon to the deep head, is separated along the course of its fibers, and is retracted in an ulnar direction.[2–7,21–23]

After elevating the superficial head of the pronator, the surgeon exposes the fourth site of possible compression, the flexor digitorum superficialis arch (Fig. 12.4). The deep portion of the flexor digitorum superficialis arises from the medial epicondyle. It has a common conjoined site of origin with the medial collateral ligament of the elbow. The superficial origin of the flexor digitorum superficialis arises from the radial tuberosity. This superficial head origin of the flexor digitorum superficialis forms a fibrous aponeurotic arch under which the median nerve passes. This superficial flexor digitorum superficialis arch is the last site of possible compression of the median nerve in pronator syndrome and the last site that requires surgical release.[2–7]

In their review on this subject, Stern and Fassler[2] pointed out that a more limited decompression of the median nerve than what earlier authors described is inadequate. Any one or more of the four compression regions in this syndrome may be the actual cause of the patient's symptoms. Accurately assessing which specific structure is playing the greatest role in compression is nearly im-

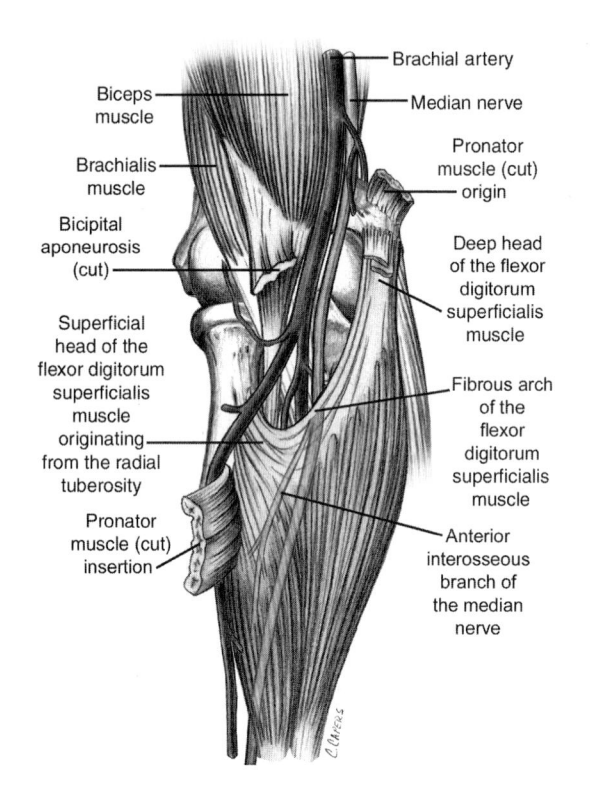

FIGURE 12.4. The arch of the flexor digitorum superficialis can act as a constrictive band. Its radial origin can be elevated to expose the anterior interosseous branch of the median nerve, which runs deep to it.

possible; therefore, leaving any one site unattended is not advisable.[2–7]

POSTOPERATIVE TREATMENT

Recommendations for postoperative treatment vary slightly in the literature. Eversmann recommended applying a soft bulky dressing for 3 to 5 days and then initiating gradual, full range of motion even if the pronator has been elevated.[3,4] Stern and Fassler[2] recommended 1 week of immobilization in a posterior splint followed by gradual flexion and extension. According to Stern and Fassler,[2] pronation and supination can be started simultaneously if the pronator teres has not been detached and repaired. If the pronator teres has been released, they recommend delaying these motions for 2 weeks.

We recommend applying a posterior splint for 1 week and delaying pronation and supination exercises for 2 weeks if the pronator teres has been released from its origin and repaired. If we have not released and repaired the pronator teres, we do not apply a splint, and we initiate full range-of-motion exercises at 3 to 5 days. The patient advances to strengthening activities at 2 weeks. In our experience, using a running subcuticular closure of non-reactive 4.0 Monocryl or Maxon suture for skin minimizes postoperative scar formation.

RESULTS

According to the literature, the results after surgical decompression demonstrate a 90% good to excellent outcome.[2–4,8,11] Almost all patients who underwent decompression for paresthesia in the median nerve distribution had a normalization of sensory deficits. Other symptoms, including pain and rare motor dysfunction, often resolve at a later time than sensory deficits. As with many compressive neuropathies, certain authors found that postoperative clinical improvement was closely related to the presence of a clearly identifiable constrictive lesion.[2–7] Hartz et al.[8] found that patients without an obvious compressive lesion on surgical exploration were less likely to demonstrate a good to excellent outcome.

COMPLICATIONS

Few authors have reported on complications related to surgical decompression of pronator syndrome. The reoperation rate for failed surgical decompression is relatively low. Hartz et al.[8] revised 6 of 39 patients, and Johnson and Spinner[11] reported four failed releases in 51 patients. Stern and Fassler[2] pointed out that inaccurate diagnosis, incomplete decompression of the nerve, and subsequent development of other compressive neuropathies are the most common causes of failure and reoperation after the primary procedure.

SUMMARY

Pronator syndrome is the most common median nerve entrapment neuropathy proximal to the carpal canal. Obtaining a detailed history and performing a meticulous physical examination usually enable the physician to diagnose pronator syndrome. Although electrodiagnostic studies are helpful when they are positive, they are often normal, even in patients who subsequently present with a clear site of compression at surgery. However, due to equivocal findings on electrophysiologic testing, most clinicians first treat their patients nonoperatively. Certainly, a nonoperative approach is a prudent initial step in the management of pronator syndrome, particularly if the symptoms have been present for less than 2 to 3 months.

Although electrodiagnostic studies are often negative, we still recommend their use. We recommend surgical exploration from 3 to 6 months after initiating nonoperative measures. Deciding when to initiate surgery must be tailored according to the severity of the patient's symptoms and personal responsibilities.

Patients who have pronator syndrome often demonstrate evidence of a "double crush" of the median nerve at a proximal or distal site. These patients should have all sites of median nerve compression released at the time of pronator syndrome decompression. The surgeon must consider this diagnosis as he or she examines the patient. Pronator syndrome may be present in a patient who has sensory deficits in the median nerve distribution, but maintains a negative Phalen test and a negative Tinel sign. This presentation, combined with pain and firmness in the proximal volar aspect of the forearm, should alert the clinician to consider pronator syndrome in the differential diagnosis.

REFERENCES

1. Seyffarth H. Primary mycoses in the m. pronator teres as cause of the lesion of the n. medianus. *Acta Psychiatr Scand Suppl* 1951;74:251–254.
2. Stern PJ, Fassler PR. Pronator syndrome. In: Gelberman R, ed. *Operative nerve repair and reconstruction.* Philadelphia: Lippincott; 1991:995–1002.
3. Eversmann WW. Proximal median nerve compression. *Hand Clin* 1992;8:307–315.
4. Eversmann WW Jr. Entrapment and compression neuropathies. In: Green DP, Hotchkiss RN, eds. *Operative hand surgery,* 3rd ed. New York: Churchill-Livingstone; 1993:1342–1344.
5. Beaton LE, Anson BJ. The relation of the median nerve to the pronator teres muscle. *Anat Rec* 1939;75:23–26.
6. Dellon AL. Musculotendinous variations about the medial humeral epicondyle. *J Hand Surg* 1986;11B:175–181.
7. Dellon AL, Mackinnon SE. Musculoaponeurotic variations along the course of the median nerve in the proximal forearm. *J Hand Surg* 1987;12B:359–363.
8. Hartz CR, Linscheid RL, Gramse RR, et al. The pronator teres syndrome: Compressive neuropathy of the median nerve. *J Bone Joint Surg* 1981;63A:885–890.
9. Morris HH, Peters BH. Pronator syndrome: Clinical and electrophysiological features in seven cases. *J Neurol Neurosurg Psychiatry* 1976;39:461–464.
10. Werner CO, Rosen I, Thorngren KG. Clinical and neurophysiological characteristics of the pronator syndrome. *Clin Orthop* 1985;197:231–236.
11. Johnson RK, Spinner M. Median nerve compression in the forearm: The pronator tunnel syndrome. In: Szabo RM, ed. Nerve compression syndromes: Diagnosis and treatment. Thorofare, NJ: Slack; 1989:137–151.
12. Gessini L, Jandolo B, Pietrangeli A. The pronator teres syndrome. Clinical and electrophysiological features in six surgically verified cases. *J Neurosurg Sci* 1987;31:1–5.
13. Buchthal F, Rosenfalck A, Trojaborg W. Electrophysiological findings in the entrapment of the median nerve at the wrist and elbow. *J Neurol Neurosurg Psychiatry* 1974;37:340–360.
14. Cho DS, MacLean IC. Pronator syndrome: Establishment of electrophysiological parameters. *Arch Phys Med Rehab* 1981;62:531–535.
15. Barnard LB, McCoy SM. The supracondyloid process of the humerus. *J Bone Joint Surg* 1946;28:845–850.
16. Bell GE Jr, Goldner JL. Compression neuropathy of the median nerve. *South Med J* 1956;49:966–972.
17. Kessel L, Rang M. Supracondylar spur of the humerus. *J Bone Joint Surg* 1966;48B:765–769.
18. Farber JS, Bryan RS. The anterior interosseous nerve syndrome. *J Bone Joint Surg* 1968;50A:521–523.
19. Fearn CB d'A, Goodfellow JW. Anterior interosseous nerve palsy. *J Bone Joint Surg* 1965;47B:91–93.
20. Spinner M, Spencer PS. Nerve compression lesions of the upper extremity. A clinical and experimental review. *Clin Orthop* 1974;104:46–67.
21. Wiggins CE. Pronator syndrome. *South Med J.* 1982;75:240–241.
22. Esposito GM. Peripheral entrapment neuropathies of upper extremity. *NY State J Med* 1972;72:717–724.
23. Kopell HP, Thompson WA. Pronator syndrome: A confirmed case and its diagnosis. *N Engl J Med* 1958;259:713–715.

CHAPTER 13

Radial Nerve Compression about the Elbow

David C. Rehak

INTRODUCTION

Compression of the radial nerve in the elbow region most commonly occurs after the nerve divides into the superficial sensory branch and the deep posterior interosseous motor branch distal to the radiocapitellar joint. Compression of the superficial sensory branch is uncommon around the elbow except when a space-occupying lesion is present. Compression of the radial nerve in the elbow region usually involves its deep motor branch: the posterior interosseous nerve (PIN). Two clinical syndromes result from compression of the PIN at this level. **Posterior interosseous nerve compression syndrome** is a partial or complete motor paralysis of any or all muscles that the PIN innervates. Pain is an unusual symptom, but may occur temporarily in the early stages. **Radial tunnel syndrome** consists of pain at the site of the PIN in this region. The patient has no muscle weakness. Neither syndrome causes sensory disturbances. When nerve compression results from a space-occupying lesion (e.g., a mass or cyst) or from proliferative synovitis as seen in rheumatoid arthritis, compression should be considered as a secondary problem to the underlying primary diagnosis. The key to diagnosing PIN compression syndrome and, in particular, radial tunnel syndrome is having a high index of suspicion. The key to surgically treating these syndromes is having a thorough understanding of the clinical anatomy.

The purpose of this chapter is to describe radial nerve compression about the elbow, focusing on clinical presentation, physical examination, and operative treatment.

CLINICAL ANATOMY

In the elbow region, the radial nerve passes from the dorsal–posterior compartment of the arm, pierces the lateral intermuscular septum, and enters the volar–anterior compartment 10 to 12 cm proximal to the lateral humeral epicondyle.[1] It follows the same path as the radial collateral artery.[2] As it courses distally and anteriorly, the nerve lies between the brachialis medially and the brachioradialis laterally. The radial nerve organizes, but does not bifurcate, into its two terminal branches before piercing the lateral intermuscular septum.[3] Proximal to this point, the nerve innervates the triceps, anconeus, brachialis, brachioradialis, and extensor carpi radialis longus. In the radiocapitellar joint region, it bifurcates into the PIN (motor) and the superficial sensory nerve. In this region, the motor branch to the extensor carpi radialis brevis also becomes an individual branch; however, the exact level at which it exits is variable, and it can originate from the radial nerve itself, the PIN, or the sensory branch.[4] The superficial sensory branch of the radial nerve courses deep to the brachioradialis muscle after the bifurcation. At this level, the PIN enters the radial tunnel.

The radial tunnel comprises five structures that can potentially cause compression, resulting in either PIN compression syndrome or radial tunnel syndrome (Fig. 13.1). Proximally, the first site of compression is a *fibrous band of tissue* anterior to the radiocapitellar joint.[5,6] The PIN passes beneath this fascial tissue, which when tensed or thickened can compress the nerve. Distal to this level, branches from the radial recurrent artery

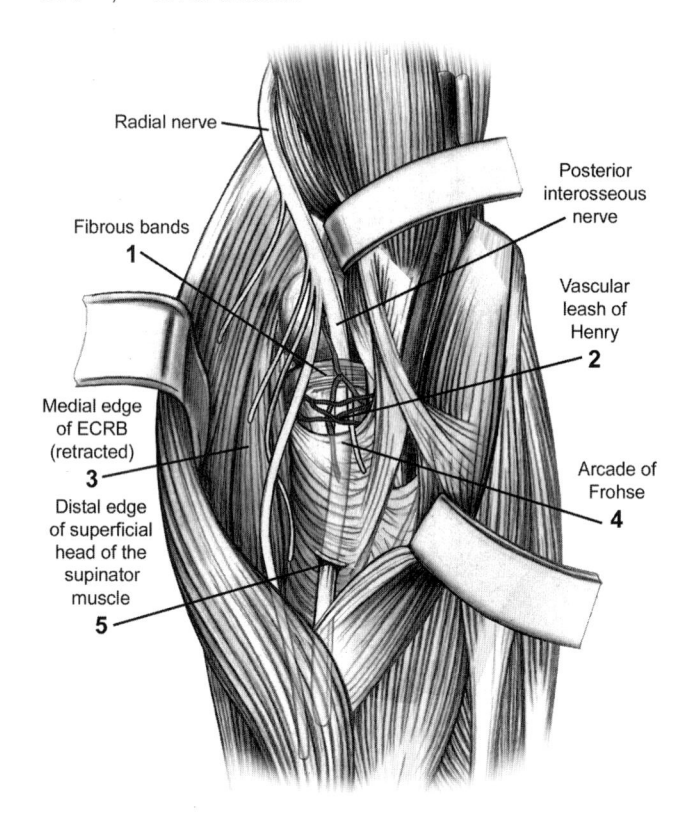

FIGURE 13.1. Potential sites of posterior interosseous nerve compression within the radial tunnel. ECRB, extensor carpi radialis brevis.

CLINICAL PRESENTATION

PIN Compression Syndrome

PIN compression syndrome can be preceded by trauma to the proximal forearm. However, the onset is typically insidious, and symptoms may go unnoticed for a period of time. The key clinical feature is weakness (ranging from partial to complete paralysis) of muscles that the PIN innervates. PIN compression syndrome may be complete (involving all the muscles that the PIN innervates) or incomplete (involving only a portion of these muscles).[1] Pain can be present early, but it usually subsides and is not considered to be part of this syndrome, thus distinguishing it from radial tunnel syndrome. Usually, patients have no sensory abnormalities unless a space-occupying lesion is present.

PIN compression syndrome can involve any of the muscles that this nerve innervates and can present with the following motor deficits, ranging from weakness to total paralysis: (1) weakness or radial deviation of wrist extension (extensor carpi radialis brevis and ulnaris muscles); note that wrist extension is never completely absent because the radial nerve innervates the extensor carpi radialis longus before the PIN enters the radial tunnel;[1] (2) weakness or absent extension of the index, middle, ring, and little finger metacarpophalangeal joints (extensor digitorum communis muscle); and (3) weakness or absent extension of the thumb metacarpal joint (abductor pollicis longus muscle) and an inability to bring the thumb up into the plane of the palm (extensor pollicis longus muscle). Loss of supination is usually not appreciated because the biceps brachii is the primary supinator. Active extension of the proximal and distal interphalangeal joints remains possible because of the ulnar innervation to the intrinsic muscles. When partial paralysis involves only the ring and little fingers, the differential diagnosis becomes more complex, and PIN palsy must be distinguished from tendon rupture, particularly in patients who have rheumatoid arthritis.[4]

Radial Tunnel Syndrome

Radial tunnel syndrome causes pain at the radial tunnel. Patients present with a deep aching pain on the anterolateral aspect of the proximal forearm. The pain is usually distal to and must be differentiated from lateral epicondylar pain (tennis elbow). If present, weakness is secondary to pain.[4] The patient has no motor losses, thus distinguishing radial tunnel syndrome from PIN compression syndrome. There are no sensory losses. Radial tunnel syndrome can be exacerbated by motion, which increases the tension on the extensor carpi radialis brevis or supinator muscles, or both.[8,10] Consequently, passive

and their accompanying veins pass anterior to the nerve. These vessels, known as the *leash of Henry*,[7] can compress the nerve. During exercise, these vessels may become distended, exacerbating the neural compression.[3] In the radial tunnel, the PIN passes beneath the deep fibrous edge of the *extensor carpi radialis brevis*. The thin, rigid medial edge of this muscle can compress the nerve.[6] This compression may be more significant during forearm pronation and wrist flexion.[8] The nerve then passes between the superficial and deep heads of the supinator muscle, encountering its last two potential sites of compression. Proximally, the nerve enters the supinator by passing beneath a fibrous arch known as the *arcade of Frohse*.[6,8,9] This fibrous edge may be tendinous, firm, or abnormally thickened. Distally, the PIN passes through the supinator muscle and encounters fibrous bands, including the *distal edge of the supinator muscle*. This area is the distalmost extent of the radial tunnel. After exiting from the supinator muscle belly, the PIN does not encounter other common sites of compression.

forearm pronation and wrist flexion or active forearm supination and wrist dorsiflexion, particularly against resistance, can reproduce the pain. This pain may be exacerbated when the elbow is in extension because both of these muscles also cross this joint.

PHYSICAL EXAMINATION

PIN Compression Syndrome

The examiner inspects the upper extremity for atrophy of the muscles that the PIN innervates (Fig. 13.2) and for swelling or the presence of a mass. Palpation over the radial tunnel may reveal tenderness or a mass. The lateral epicondylar region should always be palpated in an attempt to distinguish lateral epicondylar tenderness from tenderness associated with the PIN, which runs more distally and anteriorly. Motor evaluation should include each muscle that the radial nerve innervates in the wrist and fingers. The strength of the triceps muscle should be evaluated to assess the radial nerve motor function proximal to the elbow, distinguishing a high radial nerve lesion from a low PIN problem. Active extension of the wrist should be evaluated to determine if any weakness or radial deviation is present. Active extension of the finger and thumb metacarpophalangeal joints should also be tested with and without resistance. Excellent tests of PIN function include maneuvers such as actively making a claw hand (metacarpophalangeal joint hyperextension combined with interphalangeal joint flexion), hyperextending the metacarpophalangeal joints with the palm and hand flat on a table, and bringing the thumb up into and above the plane of the palm. Incomplete PIN compression syndrome involving a limited number of muscles, such as the common extensors to the ring and little fingers or the extensor pollicis longus, must be distinguished from tendon rupture by assessing for the tenodesis effect of these tendons.[11] When the wrist is passively flexed, the metacarpophalangeal joints of the fingers and thumb should extend, indicating continuity of the tendons. Lack of extension of one or more digits suggests the possibility of a tendon rupture.

Radial Tunnel Syndrome

Examination for radial tunnel syndrome includes the examination described for PIN compression syndrome. Palpation along the course of the nerve in the region of the radial tunnel is a key component of this examination. Maneuvers that increase the tension in the extensor carpi radialis brevis or supinator muscles can place pressure on the PIN, thus reproducing the patient's pain. Palpation of any nerve can elicit tenderness, and the involved and uninvolved sides should always be compared. The middle finger resistance test also can be helpful.[6] To perform this test, the examiner instructs the patient to extend his or her elbow and metacarpophalangeal joints and to actively resist dorsal pressure, which the examiner applies, to the proximal phalanx of the middle finger. This maneuver increases tension along the extensor carpi radialis brevis, which inserts into the base of the third metacarpal, and may reproduce the patient's pain. Resisted forearm supination or passive pronation with the elbow extended may also reproduce pain by increasing tension in the supinator muscle directly over the PIN. Again, lateral epicondylitis should be ruled out.

Diagnostic Studies

Plain radiographs should be taken to evaluate the elbow for acute injuries, including fractures, radial head dislocation, and presence of internal fixation. Chronic conditions, such as radial head dislocation and arthritis of the elbow (particularly in the patient who has rheumatoid arthritis), may be present. Use of electrodiagnostic studies can help confirm the diagnosis of PIN compression. Increased fibrillation potentials, insertional activity, and positive waves can be seen approximately 3 weeks after denervation. This study is usually normal when radial tunnel syndrome is present.[12] A normal electrodiagnostic study should never be used to exclude the diagnosis of radial tunnel syndrome in the presence of a classic his-

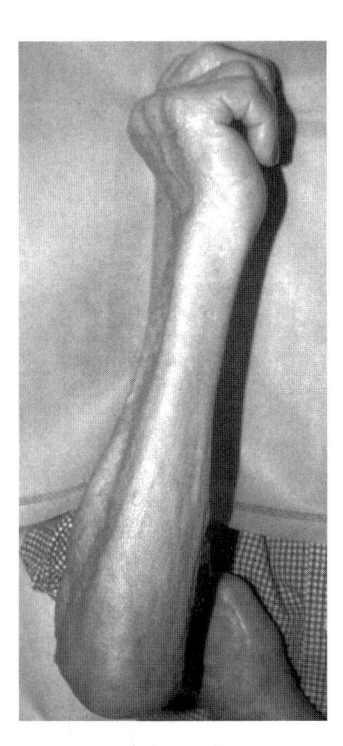

FIGURE 13.2. Severe atrophy of all extensor muscles innervated by the posterior interosseous nerve.

tory and physical examination. Use of magnetic resonance imaging or computed tomography can help to reveal the presence of a mass.

NONOPERATIVE TREATMENT

PIN Compression Syndrome

Nonoperative treatment of PIN compression syndrome is usually indicated in the initial 8 to 12 weeks, beginning from the date on which the symptoms first occurred. However, the presence of a mass or penetrating trauma is an indication for operative exploration and decompression.[13] Nonoperative treatment is designed to eliminate tension in the extensor carpi radialis brevis and supinator muscles and to eliminate repetitive trauma to the nerve. A stretching program for these muscles should also be started. The elbow should be immobilized in flexion; the forearm, in neutral to supination; and the wrist, in extension.[1] Repetitious use of the forearm and wrist should be avoided. Patients treated nonoperatively should be followed at 4-week intervals with physical examinations and electrodiagnostic studies. If improvement occurs, nonoperative treatment can be continued. If the syndrome progresses clinically or electrodiagnostically during the initial 8 to 12 weeks of symptoms, surgical exploration and decompression of the nerve should be performed. Unnecessary delay of surgical treatment can lead to permanent muscle weakness.

Radial Tunnel Syndrome

In radial tunnel syndrome, the patient has no muscle weakness or corresponding electrodiagnostic changes. Consequently, nonoperative treatment is usually indicated initially unless a space-occupying lesion or other underlying cause of the nerve compression can be determined. The nonoperative treatment for radial tunnel syndrome is similar to that for PIN palsy; however, no maximum time period has been established. If lateral epicondylitis exists concurrently, it should also be treated. If the patient's symptoms and physical findings are persistent and consistent with the diagnosis of radial tunnel syndrome, surgical decompression should be considered.

OPERATIVE TREATMENT

The surgical exploration and decompression of the PIN is the same for PIN compression syndrome and radial tunnel syndrome. Determining the exact anatomic structure responsible for compression within the radial tunnel is extremely difficult. If the surgeon can determine the presence of a space-occupying lesion or other underlying cause of focal nerve compression, he or she should address it, thus decompressing the nerve.[11,13,14] If, however, PIN compression syndrome or radial tunnel syndrome exists, the entire radial tunnel must be explored, releasing each of the potential sites of compression.[10,12] All five potential sites of PIN compression should be explored and decompressed, including the fibrous tissue anterior to the radiocapitellar joint, vascular leash of Henry, leading edge of the extensor carpi radialis brevis, arcade of Frohse, and the entire supinator muscle belly. Several techniques, each with its advantages and disadvantages, are available for exposing and decompressing the PIN.[4,15–17] Some authors recommend combined approaches, maximizing the advantages and minimizing the disadvantages. All procedures are accomplished using tourniquet control. Bipolar electrocautery and loupe magnification are also recommended.

Anterior Approach to the Radial Nerve

The most proximal potential site of PIN compression is at the level of the radiocapitellar joint and is related to the fibrous bands of tissue found at this level. Consequently, the exposure and decompression do not necessarily require dissection proximal to the elbow. However, with the anterior approach, the radial nerve often is identified most easily between the brachioradialis and the bra-

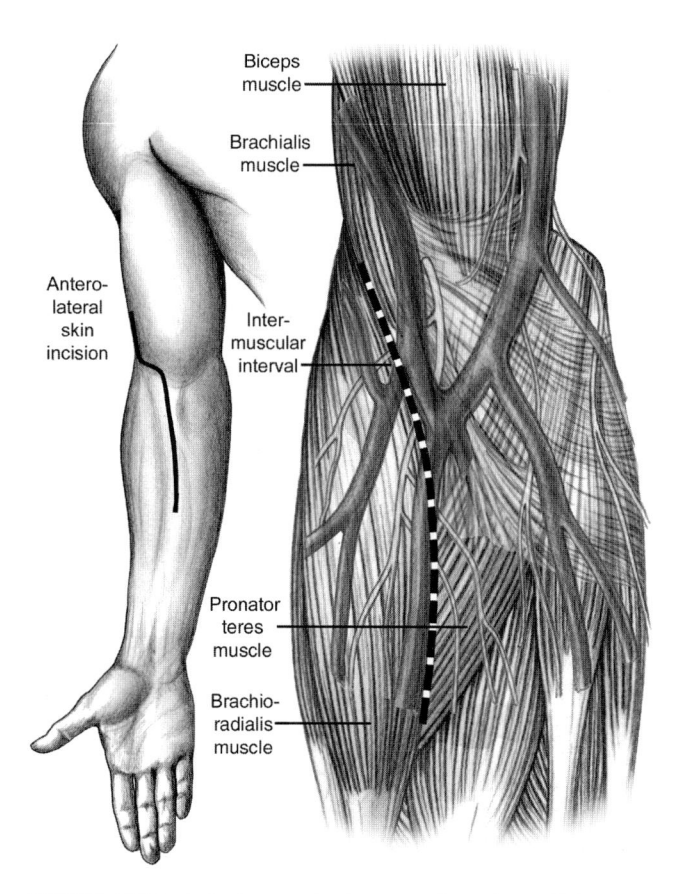

FIGURE 13.3. Anterior surgical approach to the radial nerve.

chialis muscle bellies at the elbow or just proximal to it. Consequently, the surgeon may choose to extend the incision more proximally to identify the nerve and then to continue distally. The surgeon can determine at which level to begin his or her approach.

The incision begins 2 cm proximal to the elbow flexion crease between the brachioradialis laterally and the brachialis and biceps muscle bellies medially (Fig. 13.3). This longitudinal portion of the incision proceeds distally to the region of the elbow flexion crease. At this point, the incision is curved medially so that it will not cross the elbow flexion crease at 90°. Next, the incision is curved distally and continues between the brachioradialis laterally and the flexor pronator muscles medially. If the incision is extended more than 2 cm proximal to the elbow flexion crease, the lateral antebrachial cutaneous nerve of the forearm should be identified and protected.

Full-thickness subcutaneous flaps should be mobilized from the muscle fascia. The cephalic vein or its tributaries often are encountered and may need to be ligated for exposure. The medial border of the brachioradialis muscle belly should be identified, and its fascia should be incised. Retract the brachioradialis laterally and the brachialis medially to identify the radial nerve deep between the muscle bellies (Fig. 13.4). This plane should be developed distally. In this region, the superficial sensory branch should depart from the radial nerve and should follow the deep surface of the brachioradialis muscle belly. Unless clinical signs of sensory loss are present, the superficial branch does not need to be dissected further except to identify, retract, and protect it. Often, the motor branch to the extensor carpi radialis brevis also exits the nerve at this level. The brachioradialis muscle belly and the sensory nerve should be carefully retracted laterally. The PIN should be identified.

At the level of the radiocapitellar joint, the fibrous bands of tissue should be dissected carefully. As the exploration proceeds distally, the plane of dissection lies between the brachioradialis laterally and the pronator teres medially. The next potential site of compression is the vascular leash of Henry (Fig. 13.5). Bipolar electrocautery should be used to carefully remove each of these vessels from the anterior surface of the nerve. Postoperative bleeding from these vessels can result in hematoma

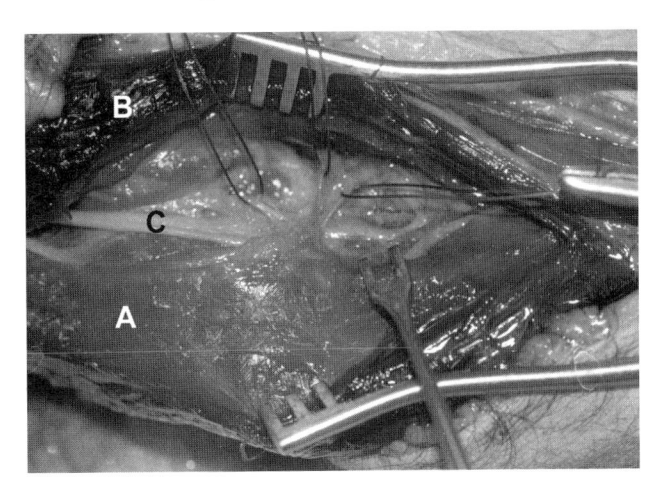

FIGURE 13.5. Lateral retraction of the brachioradialis muscle (A) and medial retraction of the pronator teres muscle (B) expose the posterior interosseous nerve (C) and allow identification of the vascular leash of Henry (marked with suture tags).

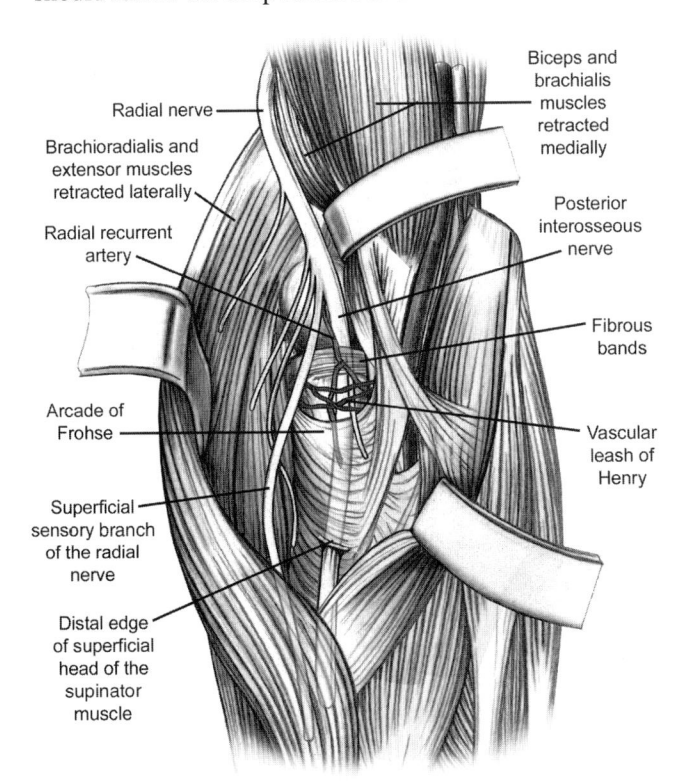

FIGURE 13.4. Surgical exposure of the radial nerve. Deep dissection exposes the radial nerve where it bifurcates into the PIN and the superficial sensory branch of the radial nerve.

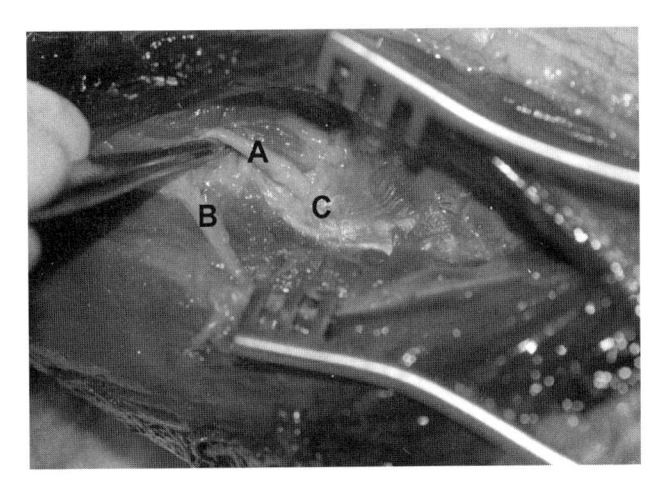

FIGURE 13.6. Incision exposes the posterior interosseous nerve (A), the superficial sensory branch of the radial nerve (B), and the arcade of Frohse (C).

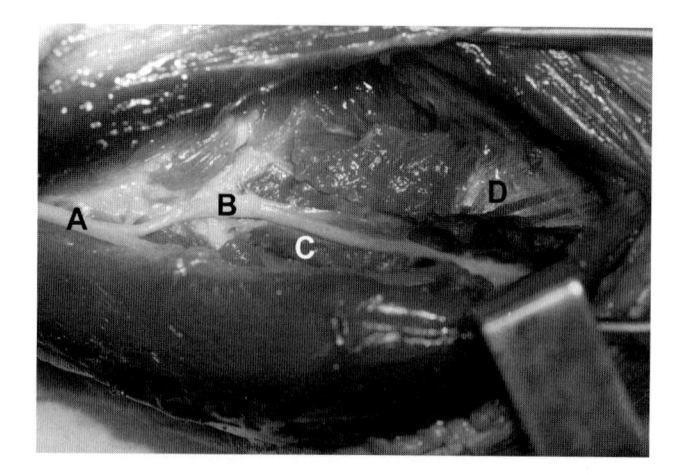

FIGURE 13.7. Completely decompressed radial nerve: radial nerve proper (A), posterior interosseous nerve (B), proximal portion of the supinator muscle (C), distal (released) supinator muscle (D).

formation and additional nerve compression. Proceeding distally, the next potential site of compression is the edge of the extensor carpi radialis brevis muscle. The surgeon should excise the fascia where it encounters the nerve. Placing the patient's elbow in extension and passively flexing the wrist sometimes help the surgeon appreciate this site of compression. At this point, the nerve passes through the arcade of Frohse and the supinator muscle belly (Fig. 13.6). The arcade of Frohse should be released completely into the muscle belly (Fig. 13.7). The surgeon can facilitate this release, particularly in the middle and distal portions of the supinator muscle, by pronating the patient's forearm. To visualize the distal edge of the supinator, he or she must elevate and retract the mobile wad.[7,17] The anterior approach is extensile and allows exposure of all five potential sites of compression and can be extended proximally. However, this approach may leave an undesirable scar,[6] and access to the distal edge of the supinator muscle is difficult.

Posterior Approach to the Posterior Interosseous Nerve

The surgeon begins the posterior approach to the PIN by making a straight incision in the proximal two-thirds of the forearm along a line that extends from a point just anterior to the lateral epicondyle down toward Lister's tubercle[16,17] (Fig. 13.8). The internervous plane between the extensor carpi radialis brevis muscle (radial nerve) and the extensor digitorum communis muscle (PIN) is identified easily in the distal portion of the wound (Fig. 13.9). The abductor pollicis longus and extensor pollicis brevis muscle bellies also pass between this interval. Incise the deep fascia and continue the dissection proximally. The extensor carpi radialis brevis and longus and the brachioradialis are retracted anteriorly, and the extensor digitorum communis is retracted posteriorly (Fig. 13.10). When retracting the extensor digitorum, do not place unnecessary traction on the PIN. The supinator muscle can be identified in the proximal third of the forearm. The PIN should be identified, emerging between the superficial and deep heads of the supinator muscle 1 cm proximal to the distal edge of the muscle. The superficial head of the supinator is completely incised longitudinally. At this point, the arcade of Frohse and fibrous edge of the extensor carpi radialis brevis should be released. The vessels composing the vascular leash of Henry can be ligated, and the fibrous bands of tissue at the level of the radiocapitellar joint can be released. The proximal extent of the radial tunnel is difficult to access by the posterior approach and often involves detaching the extensor digitorum communis muscle from the lateral epicondyle.

Brachioradialis Splitting Approach

The incision begins at the level of the elbow and extends 6 cm distally directly over the brachioradialis muscle belly. The brachioradialis muscle can be bluntly separated because of its more proximal innervation. The superficial radial nerve is identified on its deep surface. The brachioradialis split is lengthened proximally and distally, exposing the radial tunnel to the mid-supinator level. At this point, the exposure is similar to the anterior approach. This approach is advantageous because it offers the most direct access to the nerve in the radial tunnel region where the nerve is most commonly compressed. Therefore, a dissection over a shorter interval is required. The disadvantages of this approach include the splitting of the brachioradialis muscle, the potential for postoperative pain and hemorrhage, and the inability to adequately access the distal edge of the supinator.

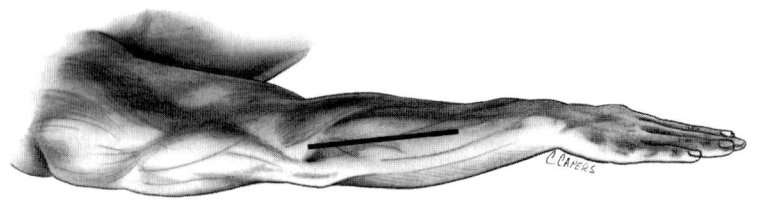

FIGURE 13.8. Posterior surgical approach to the posterior interosseous nerve.

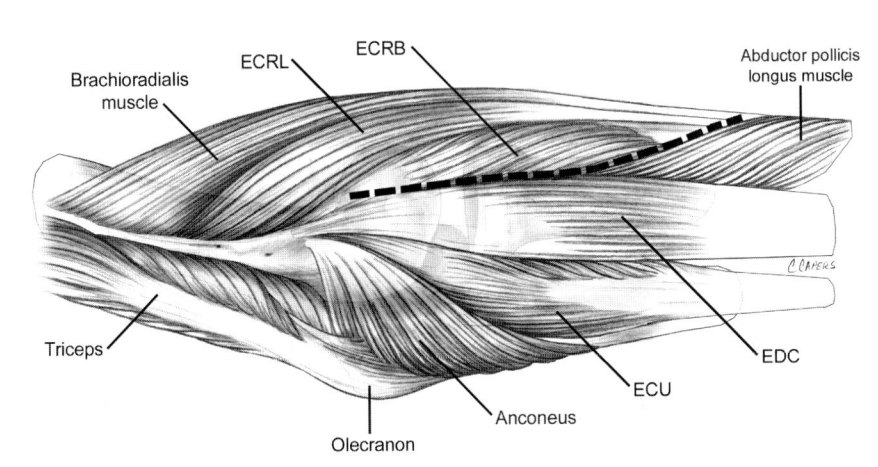

FIGURE 13.9. Incision at the internervous plane. ECRL, extensor carpi radialis longus; ECRB, extensor carpi radialis brevis; ECU, extensor carpi ulnaris; EDC, extensor digitorum communis.

Brachioradialis–Extensor Carpi Radialis Longus Interval

Hall et al. initially described the brachioradialis–extensor carpi radialis longus interval approach.[18] The incision should be marked preoperatively with the patient awake. The patient is asked to actively flex the elbow against forearm resistance to assist the surgeon in identifying the interval. A curvilinear incision is marked centered on this interval between the brachioradialis anteromedially and the extensor carpi radialis longus muscle posterolaterally. Identifying and marking the interval preoperatively greatly aids the surgeon in placement of the incision and intraoperative identification of the interval.

The incision begins proximal to the radial head and lateral to the biceps tendon and extends 6 cm distally. The fascia overlying the mobile wad is incised. The interval between the brachioradialis and the extensor carpi radialis longus is identified and bluntly separated, exposing the superficial and deep branches of the radial nerve. Care must be taken to identify and protect the branches to the extensor carpi radialis brevis muscle. The brachioradialis muscle is retracted anteriorly and medially, and the extensor carpi radialis longus muscle is retracted laterally and posteriorly. From this point forward, the procedure is the same as with the anterior approach. This approach uses a bloodless plane between the brachioradialis and the extensor carpi radialis longus muscles. It provides the same exposure as the brachioradialis splitting approach and increases the ability to expose the distal portion of the supinator muscle.

Some authors prefer combining the posterior approach for complete exposure of the PIN throughout the entire length of the supinator muscle with one of the other approaches for complete exposure of the remaining proximal portion of the PIN.[4,5]

POSTOPERATIVE MANAGEMENT

The surgeon applies a bulky, compressive, postoperative dressing and sling immobilization. Instruct the patient to elevate, ice, and rest the elbow for 24 to 48 hours. After this time, he or she can remove the sling several times a day and can begin gentle, active range-of-motion exercises. The patient begins formal physical therapy within the first week after surgery. The goals of this therapy, in order, include decreasing pain and swelling, reestablish-

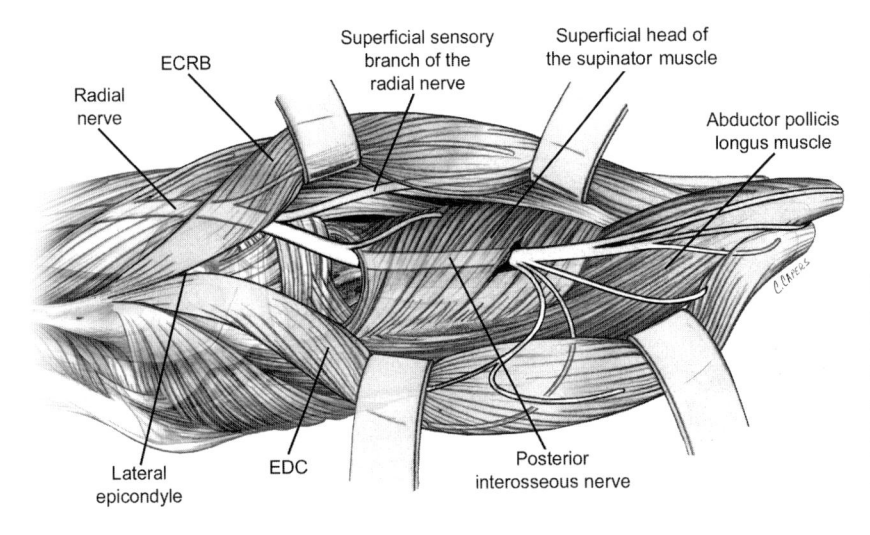

FIGURE 13.10. Retraction of the extensor carpi radialis brevis (ECRB) and the brachioradialis muscles anteriorly and the extensor digitorum communis (EDC) muscle posteriorly reveals the posterior interosseous nerve in the distal portion of the wound.

ing range of motion, and regaining strength. Use of the extremity is significantly restricted until pain and swelling have resolved and range of motion has been restored, which occurs after approximately 4 to 6 weeks. Significant lifting and repetitive motion are avoided for approximately 12 weeks.

COMPLICATIONS

Complications following surgical decompression of the PIN are uncommon, but they can occur. One complication is a direct injury to the nerve due to traction that results in temporary alteration in the superficial sensory distribution or paralysis, or both.[8,10] Postoperative bleeding and hematoma formation with potential nerve compression can also occur. Additional complications include reflex sympathetic dystrophy, unsightly scar formation, and epicondylitis.

RESULTS

Results of surgical decompression of the radial nerve vary, with good to excellent results ranging from approximately 50% to more than 90%.[7] Lawrence et al. found better results in women and in patients who had positive nerve conduction tests.[10] They reported 70% good or excellent results overall. Most of their patients who had poor or fair results had signs of additional abnormalities unrelated to the nerve. Lister et al.[6] reported that, after surgery, most of their patients had almost immediate relief of symptoms. In reviewing the literature and their own surgical cases, Lister et al. reported an "overall significant improvement" in 91.7% of cases. Moss and Switzer[19] reported good or excellent results in 14 of 15 patients, and Roles and Maudsley[8] reported 92% good or excellent results. Ritts et al.[20] reported that 70% of their patients were improved, but only 51% were able to obtain previous activity levels. Eighty percent of their patients who experienced significant relief of pain after diagnostic anesthetic injection had good surgical results. The remaining 20% had poor surgical results. Their workers' compensation patients had poorer results than their nonworkers' compensation patients.

CONCLUSION

In reviewing the literature, as well as in my own experience, I have found that straightforward cases of radial tunnel syndrome and PIN syndrome without secondary gain issues, previous surgeries, and unrelated concurrent diagnoses can be treated successfully with surgical decompression.

REFERENCES

1. Eaton CJ, Lister GD. Radial nerve compression. *Hand Clin* 1992;8:345–357.
2. Snell RS. *Clinical anatomy for medical students*, 2nd ed. Boston: Little, Brown; 1981.
3. Lister GD. Radial tunnel syndrome. In: Gelberman RH, ed. *Operative nerve repair and reconstruction*, Volume 2. Philadelphia: Lippincott; 1991:1023–1037.
4. Szabo RM. Entrapment and compression neuropathies. In: Green DP, Hotchkiss RN, Pederson WC, eds. *Green's operative hand surgery*, Volume 2, 4th ed. New York: Churchill Livingstone; 1999:1431–1447.
5. Steichen JB, Christensen AW. Posterior interosseous nerve compression syndrome. In: Gelberman RH, ed. *Operative nerve repair and reconstruction*, Volume 2. Philadelphia: Lippincott; 1991:1005–1022.
6. Lister GD, Belsole RB, Kleinert HE. The radial tunnel syndrome. *J Hand Surg* 1979;4:52–59.
7. Henry AK. *Extensile exposure*, 2nd ed. London: E & S Livingstone; 1966:99–115.
8. Roles NC, Maudsley RH. Radial tunnel syndrome. Resistant tennis elbow as a nerve entrapment. *J Bone Joint Surg* 1972;54B:499–508.
9. Spinner M. The arcade of Frohse and its relationship to posterior interosseous nerve paralysis. *J Bone Joint Surg* 1968;50B:809–812.
10. Lawrence T, Mobbs P, Fortems Y, et al. Radial tunnel syndrome. A retrospective review of 30 decompressions of the radial nerve. *J Hand Surg* 1995;20B:454–459.
11. Millender LH, Nalebuff EA, Holdsworth DE. Posterior interosseous-nerve syndrome secondary to rheumatoid synovitis. *J Bone Joint Surg* 1973;55A:753–757.
12. Verhaar J, Spaans F. Radial tunnel syndrome. An investigation of compression neuropathy as a possible cause. *J Bone Joint Surg* 1991;73A:539–544.
13. Ritts GD, Wood MB, Linscheid RL. Posterior interosseous palsy caused by ganglions of the proximal radial ulnar joint. *J Hand Surg* 1988;13A:725–728.
14. Marmor L, Lawrence JF, Dubois EL. Posterior interosseous nerve palsy due to rheumatoid arthritis. *J Bone Joint Surg* 1967;49A:381–383.
15. Spinner M, Linscheid RL. Nerve entrapment syndromes. In: Morrey BF, ed. *The elbow and its disorders*, 2nd ed. Philadelphia: WB Saunders; 1993:815–831.
16. Spinner M. *Injuries to the major branches of peripheral nerves of the forearm*, 2nd ed. Philadelphia: WB Saunders; 1978:80–157.
17. Hoppenfeld S, de Boer P. *Surgical exposures in orthopaedics: The anatomic approach*. Philadelphia: Lippincott; 1984.
18. Hall HC, MacKinnon SE, Gilbert RW. An approach to the posterior interosseous nerve. *Plastic Reconst Surg* 1984;74:435–437.
19. Moss SH, Switzer HE. Radial tunnel syndrome: A spectrum of clinical presentations. *J Hand Surg*? 1983;8:414–420.
20. Ritts GD, Wood MB, Linscheid RL. Radial tunnel syndrome. A ten-year surgical experience. *Clin Orthop* 1987;219:201–205.

CHAPTER 14

Arthroscopy of the Elbow
Setup and Portal Anatomy

Arlon H. Jahnke Jr. and Nicholas Yokan

INTRODUCTION

Arthroscopy of the elbow was first described by Burman[1] in the 1930s. However, only in recent years has it been used with increased frequency. The lack of popularity for the procedure can be attributed to its technical demands, limited clinical indications, and relative risk of injury to neurovascular structures. Recently, there have been improvements in equipment, advances in operative techniques, and a better overall understanding of the surgical anatomy about the elbow. These factors have led to a renewed interest in arthroscopy of the elbow, and the procedure is used more commonly for both diagnosis and treatment of disorders that affect the elbow joint. Still, the procedure remains technically demanding. A precise knowledge of portal anatomy and the proximity to neurovascular structures is imperative to minimize complications. In this chapter, we discuss the typical equipment used in elbow arthroscopy, describe the operating room setup including patient positioning, and describe different surgical portals used in diagnostic and operative elbow arthroscopy.

OPERATING ROOM SETUP

The operating room should be arranged to allow the surgeon ready access to the extremity without interference from anesthetic or operative equipment. The patient is placed on the operating room table in the supine, prone, or lateral decubitus position. The anesthetist and his or her equipment are located at the patient's head (Fig. 14.1). The operative extremity is flexed to 90° and placed over a bolster. The surgeon and assistant stand lateral to the flexed elbow. The arthroscopic equipment, monitor, and tower are located on the other side of the patient's body, allowing the surgeon to directly visualize the monitor and equipment. The scrub assistant and the operative instruments should be located behind the operating surgeon or at the foot of the operating table. This setup within the operating room theater allows the surgeon ready access to the extremity and comfort while viewing the video monitor. In addition, anesthetic equipment and operating room personnel cause no interference.

Equipment

Elbow arthroscopy can be performed with the standard arthroscopic equipment commonly used for arthroscopy of the knee or shoulder. Although many surgeons use a 2.7-mm arthroscope, we prefer to use 4.0-mm 30° and 70° arthroscopes. Because of the relatively small volume of the elbow joint, the arthroscope often must be positioned at or near the capsular entrance of the portal. The cannula for the arthroscope should not have a large bevel located at the tip of the instrument. Using an instrument with a large bevel causes unnecessary extravasation of fluid from the arthroscope into soft tissues surrounding the elbow. Cannula systems with incorporated rubber dams also prevent unnecessary fluid leakage. We prefer to use only blunt-tipped trocars. We also frequently use Wissinger rods and switching sticks to assist in maintaining portal position.

Elbow arthroscopy can be accomplished with gravity irrigation, but we prefer to use a pulsed irrigation system with a pump. Most irrigation pump systems offer pressure and flow regulation, but the surgeon must be aware

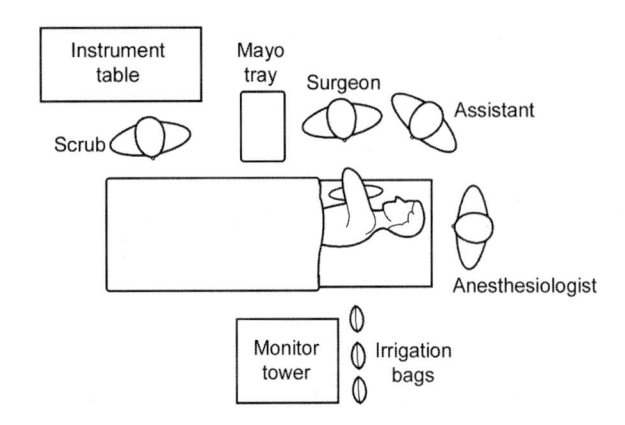

FIGURE 14.1. Operating room setup.

of the possibility of fluid extravasation. Close monitoring of soft-tissue distention is always important when performing elbow arthroscopy.

A standard arthroscopic shaving apparatus is used with a variety of blades measuring 3.5 to 4.5 mm. If necessary, other standard arthroscopic instruments (e.g., probes, graspers, biters) can be used.

Patient Positioning

Initially, elbow arthroscopy was done with the patient in the supine position and with the patient's operative arm in overhead traction. This position can lead to technical difficulties and can be frustrating for the operating surgeon. The overhead suspension of the patient's arm allows the surgeon access to the medial and lateral aspects of the elbow; however, the arm is unstable and swings like a pendulum. Furthermore, access to the posterior compartments is restricted and awkward for the surgeon. Finally, with the patient in the supine position, the anterior neurovascular structures are brought closer to the operative portals by gravity, thus potentially increasing the risk of injury to these structures.

The prone position, which Poehling et al.[2] introduced in 1989, offers advantages for both the patient and the surgeon. In this position, the operative arm rests over a padded bolster. This position of the upper extremity improves the mobility of the arthroscope within the joint, facilitates manipulation of the joint, provides a more complete intra-articular examination of the elbow joint, and eliminates the need for an overhead suspension device to support the extremity. Furthermore, this position facilitates access to the posterior compartments. The arm is stable, and the elbow is maintained in a flexed position. Gravity and the fluid within the joint distend the anterior cubital fossa, thereby displacing the neurovascular structures further from the surgical portals.

We prefer to place the patient in the lateral decubitus position (Fig. 14.2). This position offers all the advantages of the prone position, and it allows for a more convenient position for the anesthetist to manage the patient's airway. When using the prone or lateral decubitus position, use a well-padded bolster to support the operative arm. A standard leg holder commonly used for knee arthroscopy can be used; however, this holder tends to be bulky and can interfere with the arthroscope and instruments. We prefer the use of a simple padded post or bolster placed in the horizontal position (Fig. 14.3).

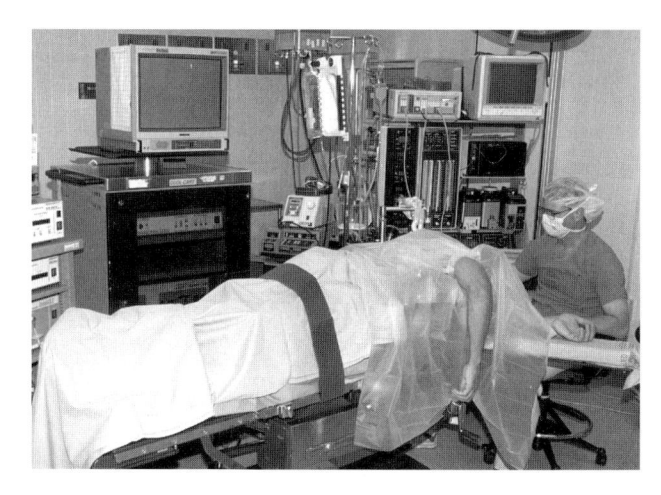

FIGURE 14.2. Operating room setup with the patient in the lateral decubitus position. The affected extremity is placed over a bolster to allow free access to the elbow and upper extremity.

PORTALS AND SURGICAL ANATOMY

Elbow arthroscopy requires a complete understanding of the regional anatomy. The surgeon needs to have a thor-

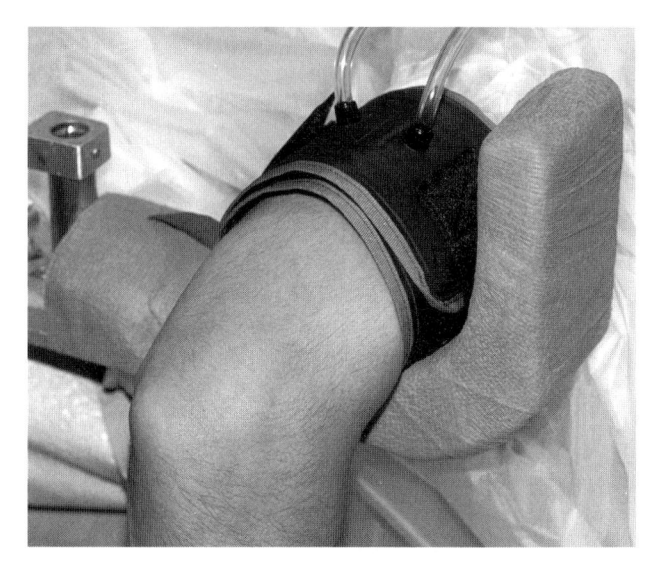

FIGURE 14.3. The upper extremity is placed over a padded leg holder or bolster. This placement allows access to the entire elbow and upper extremity.

ough knowledge of both the superficial neurovascular anatomy and the intra-articular anatomy in order to minimize injury to these structures. The surgeon draws superficial landmarks on the skin, including the olecranon, the medial and lateral humeral epicondyles, the radial head, medial intermuscular septum, and coursing neurovascular structures. The proposed portal sites also are marked on the skin.

After routine preparation and draping are completed, a sterile tourniquet is applied to the patient's upper arm. The hand and forearm are wrapped with an elastic bandage to prevent forearm swelling. This wrapping is continued almost to where the portals will be established. This combination of forearm wrapping and tourniquet application limits the intraoperative fluid swelling to the region of the elbow and, at the end of the procedure, it permits rapid diffusion of any accumulated fluid from the elbow region to the other parts of the limb. Next, the extremity is exsanguinated, and the tourniquet is inflated. The elbow is distended with 15 to 25 mL of sterile normal saline instilled through the *soft spot*, which is located in the center of a triangle created by lines connecting points on the olecranon, lateral humeral epicondyle, and radial head. Distention of the elbow displaces the vital neurovascular structures anteriorly, creating a greater distance between the surgical portals and these structures.[3]

Authors have described many different portals for performing arthroscopy of the elbow.[2,4–11] Advantages and disadvantages for each of the portals have been described. We prefer to use five basic portals: a medial portal, a lateral portal, a midlateral (or direct lateral) portal, and two posterior portals. We describe each of these portals in detail, outlining the techniques of creating the portal, the advantages and disadvantages of the portal, the pertinent anatomy and structures that are at risk when using the portal, and the intra-articular structures that are visualized with the portal.

Medial Portal

In arthroscopic surgery of the elbow, the first portal can be placed on either the medial[2,4–6,12,13] or lateral[7–9] side of the joint. We begin by accessing the medial side of the joint. The basic medial portals that can be used are the proximal medial and the anteromedial portals. The proximal medial portal is located 2 cm proximal to the medial humeral epicondyle.[2] The anteromedial portal is created at a point 2 cm anterior and 2 cm distal to the medial humeral epicondyle.[7] We prefer to use the proximal medial portal.

We start the proximal medial portal by incising only the skin about 2 cm proximal to the medial humeral epicondyle and just anterior to the medial intermuscular septum (Fig. 14.4). Hemostats are used to bluntly dissect soft tissues to the anterior aspect of the distal humerus. A blunt

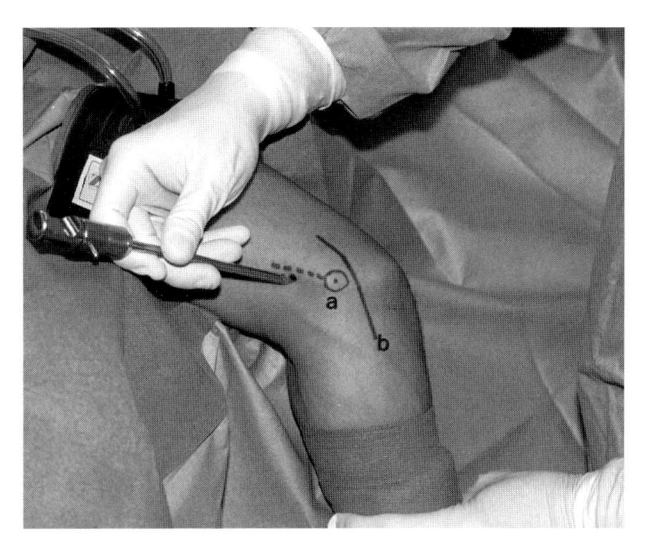

FIGURE 14.4. The proximal medial portal is started approximately 2 cm proximal and just anterior to the intermuscular septum. Preoperative evaluation should rule out the presence of a subluxating ulnar nerve. The trocar should be directed toward the radial head. (a) Medial epicondyle. (b) Ulnar nerve.

trocar with the arthroscopic cannula is directed toward the center of the joint. Care is taken to guide the trocar, ensuring it is anterior to the intermuscular septum. The trocar is guided along the anterior aspect of the humerus until the joint capsule is pierced. Next, the trocar is removed, and backflow of fluid confirms placement of the cannula into the joint.

The risks of medial portal placement include potential injury to the median nerve, brachial artery, ulnar nerve, and medial antebrachial nerve. In their study, Lynch et al.[3] used an anteromedial portal that was 2 cm anterior and 2 cm distal to the medial humeral epicondyle. These authors noted that with the joint empty the median nerve and brachial artery are 4 and 9 mm, respectively, from the portal site; with the joint maximally distended, they are 14 and 17 mm, respectively, from the portal site.

Using a more proximal medial portal, Lindenfeld[5] found the median nerve an average distance of 22 mm from the portal site. He explained that the distances he found differed from those that Lynch et al.[3] found because of the more proximal placement of the portal and the direction with which the trocar is guided with this more proximal portal. A more proximal portal allows the surgeon to guide the trocar in a direction more parallel to the course of the median nerve (Fig. 14.5). With the joint distended, the trocar is closest to the median nerve at the skin puncture. The distance from the trocar to the median nerve is greatest when the tip of the trocar is at the ulnar–humeral articulation.

The medial antebrachial cutaneous nerve is close to the medial portal sites. Lynch et al.[3] found that this nerve is as close as 1 mm to the portal site. Injury to this nerve

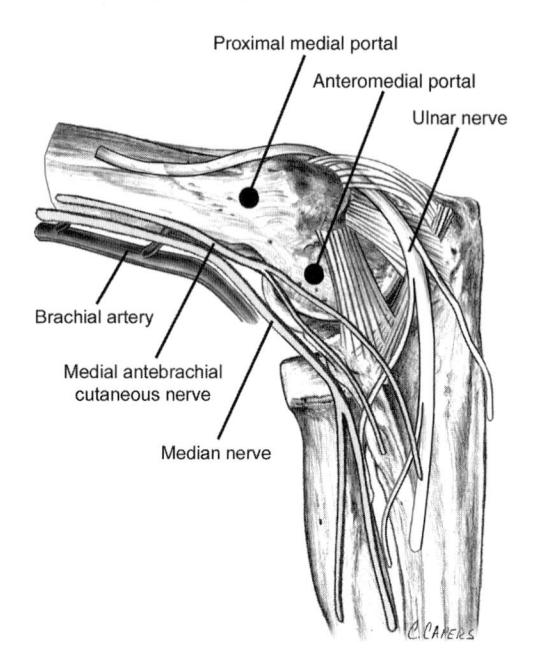

FIGURE 14.5. Anatomy of the medial side of the elbow with portal placements noted.

can be minimized by making the incision through skin only and by bluntly dissecting the soft tissues with a hemostat.

The ulnar nerve is relatively safe and lies an average distance of 25 mm from the proximal medial portal. However, the ulnar nerve may be at risk for injury in two situations. The first situation involves the patient who has an ulnar nerve that subluxes anteriorly from the cubital tunnel. In this patient, subluxation usually occurs at about 120° of elbow flexion. The surgeon should examine the elbow before surgery to ensure that the patient does not have this variant. In a patient who has a subluxating ulnar nerve, the portal can be made safely by limiting the elbow flexion to 90° and by manually positioning the ulnar nerve posterior to the medial epicondyle in the cubital tunnel.

The other situation in which the ulnar nerve is at risk is in the patient who has had an anterior transposition of the ulnar nerve. The use of either of the medial portals in this patient is relatively contraindicated.

The capitellum and radial head are best seen from the medial portal. Pronating and supinating the forearm facilitate the examination of the radial head. The lateral aspect of the trochlea and the coronoid process can be seen with careful retraction of the arthroscope and direction of the light source toward the ulna. A variety of abnormalities involving the lateral aspect of the elbow includes loose bodies, radial head fractures, and osteochondral injuries to the capitellum.

Lateral Portal

Andrews and Carson[7] described placing an anterolateral portal 3 cm distal and 1 cm anterior to the lateral humeral epicondyle. Several authors have recognized the proximity of the radial nerve to this portal and have recommended placing the lateral portal more proximal.[5,6,10] O'Driscoll and Morrey[9,11] and Baker and Brooks[4] have recommended placing the portal exactly in the sulcus that is felt anteriorly between the radial head and capitellum. This portal is approximately 1 cm anterior and 1 cm distal to the lateral humeral epicondyle. Recently, Stothers et al.[6] recommended placing a lateral portal proximal to the lateral humeral epicondyle. This portal lies from 1 to 2 cm proximal to the lateral epicondyle and lies directly on the anterior surface of the humerus. Using an inside-out technique, we prefer to create a lateral portal that is just proximal and anterior to the radial head. This results in a position approximately 1 cm anterior and 1 cm proximal to the lateral epicondyle.

After making the proximal medial portal, the surgeon identifies and inspects the radial head and capitellum. He or she identifies the capsule that is located just proximal and anterior to the radial head. Under direct vision, the arthroscope is advanced toward this point on the capsule. Next, the arthroscope is removed, keeping the arthroscopic sheath in place and tented against the lateral elbow capsule. A Wissinger rod is advanced through the arthroscopic sheath, gently piercing the lateral capsule. The rod is easily seen tenting the skin over the anterolateral aspect of the elbow joint. The skin is incised, allowing the rod to exit through the skin (Fig. 14.6). An arthroscopic cannula with a rubber dam is introduced over the rod into the lateral aspect of the joint. Diagnostic and operative procedures are completed with the arthroscope in the proximal medial portal. The arthroscope is placed into the lateral portal using switching sticks.

The neurovascular structure most at risk for injury during elbow arthroscopy is the radial nerve, which lies over the radial head directly adjacent to the elbow joint capsule. The classic anterolateral portal, which is located 3 cm distal and 1 cm anterior to the lateral humeral epicondyle, places the radial nerve at significant risk. Lynch et al.[3] noted a mean distance between the portal and the radial nerve of 4 mm without joint distention and 11 mm with joint distention. Stothers et al.[6] and Lindenfeld[5] have recognized the nerve to be closer, citing a mean distance of 4.9 and 3 mm, respectively, from this portal with the elbow flexed and the joint distended. The recommended distance of 3 cm distal from the lateral epicondyle results in an entry point that is distal to the radiocapitellar joint in most patients and even distal to the joint in smaller patients. The posterior interosseous nerve, which is relatively fixed as it passes through the arcade of Frohse just distal to the joint, is at risk for injury because it is poorly

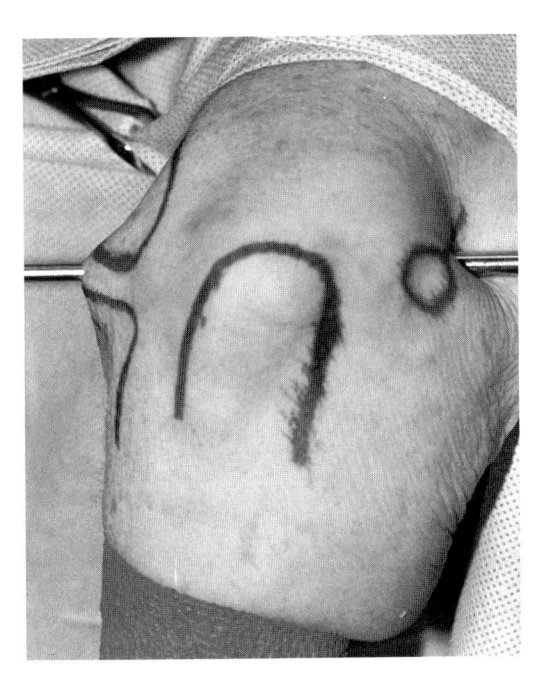

FIGURE 14.6. Creating the lateral portal using an inside-out technique. A Wissinger rod introduced into the cannula penetrates the capsule and tents the skin anterolaterally. The rod is brought out through the skin, and a second cannula is placed over the Wissinger rod and brought into the joint.

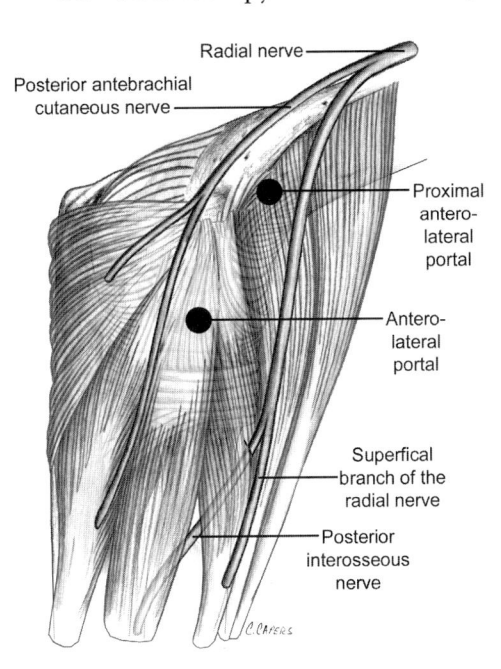

FIGURE 14.7. Anatomy of the lateral aspect of the elbow with portal placements noted.

protected. Furthermore, this portal is close to the distal capsular attachment, and the radial nerve is not protected from elbow flexion and joint distention at this point.

Stothers et al.[6] also recognized that more proximal placement of the portal increases the protective distance between the nerve and the portal by a factor of 2. We also have noted this relationship during cadaveric dissections, recognizing relative safety in portal placement if the surgeon stays proximal to the radial head (Fig. 14.7).

The structures best seen from the anterolateral portal include the coronoid process; the trochlear region of the distal humerus; and the anterior, superior, and medial capsules of the elbow joint. A portion of the radial head and capitellum can be seen by gently pulling the arthroscope back and directing the light source toward the distal humerus. The portal is used primarily as a working portal, because most problems requiring elbow arthroscopy affect the lateral aspect of the joint.

Midlateral, or Direct Lateral, Portal

The midlateral, or direct lateral, portal has been described by several authors[7,9,11] and is located within the triangle formed by the olecranon, lateral humeral epicondyle, and radial head (Fig. 14.8). It is commonly used for distending the joint with fluid before starting elbow arthroscopy.

O'Driscoll and Morrey[11] recommend that this portal be the initial portal made in diagnostic arthroscopy. In our experience, as well as that of others,[6] leakage of fluid into surrounding soft tissue can be troublesome with this por-

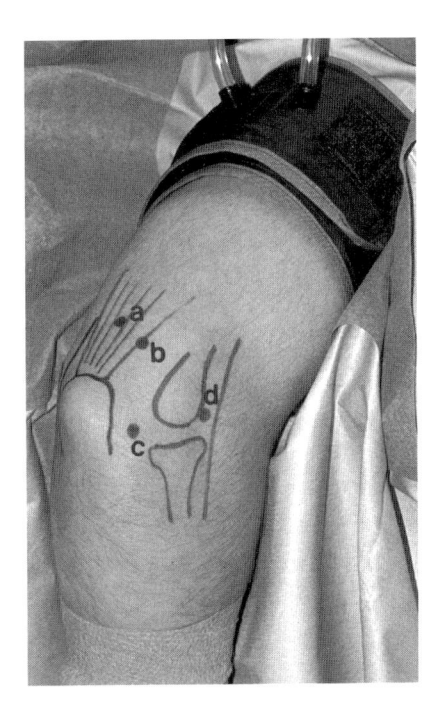

FIGURE 14.8. Arthroscopic portals along the lateral and posterolateral aspects of the elbow joint are marked on the skin: (a) direct posterior, (b) posterolateral, (c) midlateral, and (d) anterolateral portals. The portals are shown in relation to the radial nerve, lateral humeral epicondyle, and the radial head.

tal, and we prefer to use this portal, if needed, toward the end of the procedure. This portal provides relatively little room within the capsule, and care must be taken to keep the arthroscope within the joint. If this portal is needed, the surgeon may find the smaller, 2.7-mm arthroscope useful.

The midlateral portal is relatively safe because no vital neurovascular structures are in its proximity. The portal pierces the anconeus muscle and joint capsule over the lateral aspect of the elbow. Intra-articular structures visualized through this portal include the posterolateral aspect of the radial head and capitellum, ulnohumeral joint, olecranon, and posterior joint capsule. We reserve the use of the midlateral portal for patients who may have an abnormality involving the posterior aspect of the capitellum.

Posterior Portals

Access to the posterior aspect of the elbow joint is relatively safe compared with access to the anterior aspect of the joint. Access to the posterior aspect of the joint may be obtained through the direct posterior and posterolateral portals. We prefer to use these two posterior portals for routine elbow arthroscopy. Most disorders involving the posterior aspect of the joint can be approached and treated using them.

The direct posterior portal is created approximately 2 cm proximal to the tip of the olecranon, just medial to the midline. The elbow is placed in 30° to 45° of flexion to relax the triceps, and the trocar is advanced gently into the olecranon fossa. This portal is safe, with the ulnar nerve approximately 20 mm medial to the portal. It is used most commonly as a working portal with the arthroscope in the posterolateral portal; however, the arthroscope can be placed in this portal, and the posterolateral portal can be used for the working instruments. Through the posterior portal, the surgeon can visualize the structures of the posterior aspect of the joint: olecranon tip, olecranon fossa, and posterior aspect of the capsule.

The posterolateral portal is created approximately 2 to 3 cm from the olecranon tip, along the lateral border of the triceps tendon. Again, the elbow is placed in 30° to 45° of flexion to relax the posterior structures. The trocar is directed toward the olecranon fossa and is passed lateral to or through the lateral aspect of the triceps muscle to reach the capsule. This portal also is relatively safe, with the nearest neurovascular structure 15 to 20 mm from the portal site.

SUMMARY

Arthroscopy of the elbow remains a technically demanding procedure. The potential for injury to major neurovascular structures is greater with this procedure than with arthroscopic procedures of the knee, shoulder, and ankle. An understanding of regional anatomy and the proximity of major neurovascular structures to the anterior portals is essential. Injury to these structures can be minimized by incising the skin only, using blunt dissection and blunt trocars, distending the joint, and placing the anterior portals in a more proximal position. Arthroscopy of the elbow offers major advantages in the treatment of many disorders of the elbow, particularly in the athlete. The technique can be performed safely using the portals outlined and principles discussed.

REFERENCES

1. Burman MS. Arthroscopy or the direct visualization of joints: An experimental cadaver study. *J Bone Joint Surg* 1931;13: 669–695.
2. Poehling GG, Whipple TL, Sisco L, et al. Elbow arthroscopy: A new technique. *Arthroscopy* 1989;5:222–224.
3. Lynch GJ, Meyers JF, Whipple TL, et al. Neurovascular anatomy and elbow arthroscopy: Inherent risks. *Arthroscopy* 1986; 2:191–197.
4. Baker CL, Brooks AA. Arthroscopy of the elbow. *Clin Sports Med* 1996;15:261–281.
5. Lindenfeld TN. Medial approach in elbow arthroscopy. *Am J Sports Med* 1990;18:413–417.
6. Stothers K, Day B, Regan WR. Arthroscopy of the elbow: Anatomy, portal sites, and a description of the proximal lateral portal. *Arthroscopy* 1995;11:449–457.
7. Andrews JR, Carson WG. Arthroscopy of the elbow. *Arthroscopy* 1985;1:97–107.
8. Andrews JR, Baumgarten TE. Arthroscopic anatomy of the elbow. *Orthop Clin North Am* 1995;26:671–677.
9. O'Driscoll SW, Morrey BF. Arthroscopy of the elbow. Diagnostic and therapeutic benefits and hazards. *J Bone Joint Surg* 1992;74A:84–94.
10. Field LD, Altchek DW, Warren RF, et al. Arthroscopic anatomy of the lateral elbow: A comparison of three portals. *Arthroscopy* 1994;10:602–607.
11. O'Driscoll SW, Morrey BF. Arthroscopy of the elbow. In: Morrey BF, ed. *The elbow*. New York: Raven Press; 1994: 21–34.
12. Verhaar J, van Mameren H, Brandsma A. Risks of neurovascular injury in elbow arthroscopy: Starting anteromedially or anterolaterally? *Arthroscopy* 1991;7:287–290.
13. Day B. Elbow arthroscopy in the athlete. *Clin Sports Med* 1996;15:785–797.

CHAPTER 15

Diagnostic Arthroscopy of the Elbow

Matthew L. Ramsey and R. John Naranja

INTRODUCTION

Arthroscopic surgery of the elbow has emerged as an important tool in the diagnosis and treatment of various elbow disorders. The value of elbow arthroscopy as a diagnostic tool lies in its ability to allow the surgeon to directly visualize normal and abnormal intra-articular structures. However, diagnostic arthroscopy is not a substitute for a careful history, physical examination, and radiographic evaluation.

Arthroscopy of the elbow has proved safe, effective, and reproducible when it is used for the proper indications. Diagnostic elbow arthroscopy is a technically demanding procedure. More than with any other joint, an understanding of the neurovascular anatomy and attention to detail are critical to avoiding complications.

INDICATIONS

The value of elbow arthroscopy as a diagnostic tool lies in its ability to document the presence or, at times, absence of intra-articular abnormalities. Diagnostic arthroscopy provides useful information about the presence or absence of loose bodies; allows direct assessment of the quality of the articular cartilage, joint capsule, and synovium; and allows the surgeon to visualize joint instability while he or she applies varus, valgus, and rotational stresses.

The ideal indications for diagnostic arthroscopy of the elbow are a history of pain or mechanical symptoms and a physical examination and radiographic studies that demonstrate intra-articular abnormalities. Injuries in patients who have a history of pain with no physical findings or radiographic studies suggesting intra-articular abnormalities are infrequently diagnosed through arthroscopy.[1] Occasionally, diagnostic arthroscopy helps the surgeon to document the absence of intra-articular abnormalities as the cause of a pain in this group of patients.

Other indications for diagnostic arthroscopy are a suspected loose body; locking, clicking, or catching of the elbow; chronic or undiagnosed elbow pain; and the need to obtain tissue for biopsy.

CONTRAINDICATIONS

Elbow arthroscopy has relatively few absolute contraindications. The surgeon should avoid arthroscopy when severe capsular contracture or frank ankylosis prevents the protection of the neurovascular structures through adequate joint distention. Any process that distorts the normal anatomy of the elbow is a relative contraindication to elbow arthroscopy. Congenital anomalies, posttraumatic deformity, or surgical alteration of normal anatomy (e.g., ulnar nerve transposition) can alter anatomic relationships to such a degree that the risk of neurovascular injury is unacceptably high.

SURGICAL TECHNIQUE

Arthroscopy of the elbow joint as a diagnostic and therapeutic modality is well established. Although the joint is easily accessible for examination, the risk of neurovascular injury is greater in the elbow than in any other joint; therefore, the surgeon must pay attention to details throughout the surgical procedure.

As with arthroscopy in any other joint, a systematic approach to visualization of the intra-articular structures creates a routine that becomes familiar and easily reproducible. This routine results in minimal time of diagnostic arthroscopy and maximal diagnostic and therapeutic benefit. A thorough arthroscopic examination of the elbow requires evaluation of all compartments of the joint.

Patient Position

Alternatives for positioning include placing the patient in the supine, prone, or lateral decubitus position. As Andrews and Carson described, the supine position offers easy access to the airway for anesthesia and allows excellent access to the anterior aspect of the elbow joint.[2] The joint is oriented anatomically, making arthroscopy less confusing for the novice arthroscopic surgeon. Disadvantages of this position include the requirement for an overhead traction device, awkward positioning for access to the posterior aspect of the elbow, and a somewhat unstable working base, because the arm is suspended in the air.

Popularized by Poehling et al., the prone position affords easy access to the anterior and posterior compartments of the elbow and allows the surgeon to work from a stable base.[3] Because no accessory traction devices are required, the elbow is easily taken through a full range of motion without restrictions. The disadvantage of this technique is the anesthetic difficulties associated with placing the patient face down.

We prefer to place the patient in the lateral decubitus position. This position appears to alleviate the disadvantages and to maintain the advantages of both the supine and prone positions.[1] The affected arm hangs free over a padded support, permitting free flexion and extension of the elbow joint (Fig. 15.1).

Portal Anatomy

A detailed discussion of portal anatomy was presented in Chapter 14; therefore, we only briefly discuss it here. The principles of establishing arthroscopic portals are the same for the elbow as for other joints, with the exception that, in the elbow, closer attention to the relationship of local neurovascular structures must be maintained from the outset. To avoid injuring the patient's neurovascular structures, the surgeon must have an appreciation of the topographical anatomy of the elbow and the relationship of the neurovascular structures to these external landmarks. The position of the olecranon, medial and lateral epicondyles, radial head, and radial and ulnar nerves are outlined on the skin with a sterile marker before joint distention.

Regardless of the portal used, the risk of injury to the neurovascular structures exists at all levels of portal placement, from the skin incision to joint penetration. A variety of anterior and posterior portals has been described.[1-6] Portal placement has evolved to decrease the risks of cutaneous and deep neurovascular injury and to provide adequate intra-articular visualization of the elbow joint.

Authors' Preferred Technique

The patient receives a general anesthetic and is placed in the lateral decubitus position with the involved extremity up. A tourniquet is placed high on the arm. The arm is supported and stabilized on a padded bolster, with the shoulder abducted to 90° and the elbow flexed to 90°.

The operative extremity is prepped and draped free to allow the surgeon to manipulate it intraoperatively. The forearm is wrapped with an elastic bandage from the fingers to just below the portal sites to minimize fluid extravasation into the forearm. The topographical anatomy of the elbow and the portal sites are marked on the skin before joint distention. The limb is exsanguinated with an Esmarch bandage, and the tourniquet is inflated to 250 mm Hg.

An 18-gauge spinal needle is inserted into the elbow joint through the lateral "soft spot," and the elbow is distended with 15 to 20 mL of sterile fluid. The soft spot is located at the center of the triangle defined by the radial head, the lateral epicondyle, and the olecranon process. Overdistention of the joint with more than 15 to 20 mL of fluid risks capsular rupture and the resultant fluid extravasation during arthroscopy.[7] Free backflow of fluid is confirmed after joint distention.

The proximal medial portal is established first for initial arthroscopic examination. A no. 11 scalpel blade is used to nick only the skin. Plunging the knife through tissue places the cutaneous nerves at risk for injury. A blunt, straight hemostat completes dissection to the joint capsule. A 4.5-mm arthroscopic cannula with the blunt trocar is advanced toward the center of the joint until the surgeon feels a pop, which signifies entrance of the cannula into the joint. The cannula must not contain side fenestrations that would allow extracapsular fluid extravasation into the soft tissues (Fig. 15.2).

A 4.0-mm, 30° arthroscope is used for routine diag-

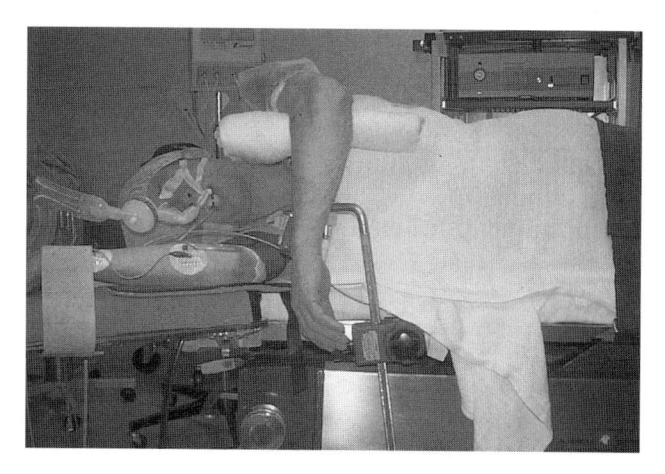

FIGURE 15.1. The patient is positioned in the lateral decubitus position for arthroscopy. A tourniquet is placed high on the arm. The arm hangs free over a padded bolster with the elbow flexed to 90°.

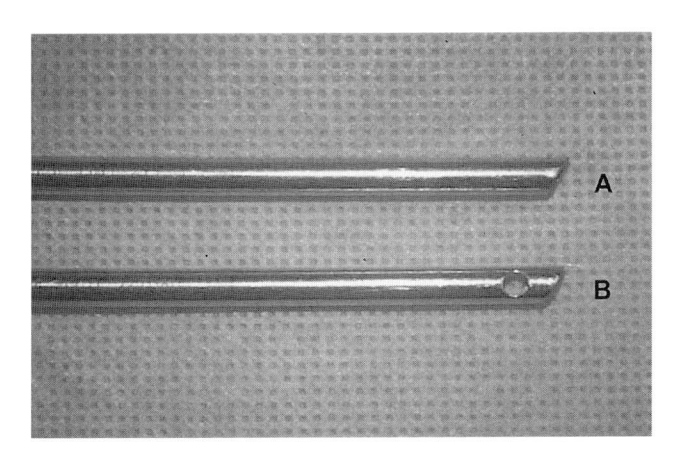

FIGURE 15.2. (A) The arthroscopic cannula should have no side fenestrations. (B) Side fenestrations allow extracapsular fluid extravasation.

nostic elbow arthroscopy. Occasionally, a 2.7-mm, 30° or a 4.0-mm, 70° arthroscope is useful, but we have not found it necessary for routine diagnostic arthroscopy. Inflow is established through the arthroscope by an arthroscopic pump set at 50 mm Hg. Higher pump pressures risk capsular rupture, with the attendant fluid extravasation into the soft tissues and difficult maintenance of capsular distention. Failure to maintain capsular distention during arthroscopy places the neurovascular structures about the elbow at risk for injury.

When viewing the joint from the proximal medial portal, the initial intra-articular landmark is the radial head and the radiocapitellar articulation (Fig. 15.3). The structures that need to be examined in the anterolateral portion of the joint include the concave articular surface of the radial head; the articular margin of the radial head; the radial fossa; the superior aspect of the capitellum; the anterolateral joint capsule and synovium; and, if possible, the annular ligament. To view the articular margin of the radial head, the surgeon takes the patient's forearm from pronation to supination (Fig. 15.4). Approximately three-fourths of the articular margin of the radial head can be examined in this manner. Because the lateral ligaments of the elbow are more lax than the medial ligaments, especially with the forearm in pronation, the radiocapitellar joint can be distracted slightly with a varus force to visualize the concave articular surface of the radial head.

The anterior and superior portions of the capitellum are easily visualized from the proximal medial portal. With elbow extension, more of the anterior surface of the capitellum can be visualized. However, continued elbow extension limits anterior compartment visualization because the anterior capsule tightens and closes down on the arthroscope. The radial fossa is easily viewed above the capitellum and is inspected for impinging osteophytes.

Visualization of the entire lateral collateral ligament complex is not possible. Occasionally, the annular ligament is seen distal to the articular margin of the radial head. However, the lateral collateral ligament and the lateral ulnar collateral ligament cannot be visualized from the anterior portal. The surgeon withdraws the arthroscope while visualizing the ulnohumeral articulation and proximal radioulnar joint.

After completing the initial diagnostic evaluation of the anterolateral compartment, the surgeon establishes an anterolateral portal under direct visualization from within the joint. We prefer proximal placement of the anterolateral portal. It provides excellent visualization of the anterior compartment. In addition, the radial nerve can be

FIGURE 15.3. The radiocapitellar joint is the initial landmark in the lateral aspect of the anterior compartment. The capitellum is visualized with elbow flexion and extension. A portion of the concave articular surface of the radial head usually can be seen.

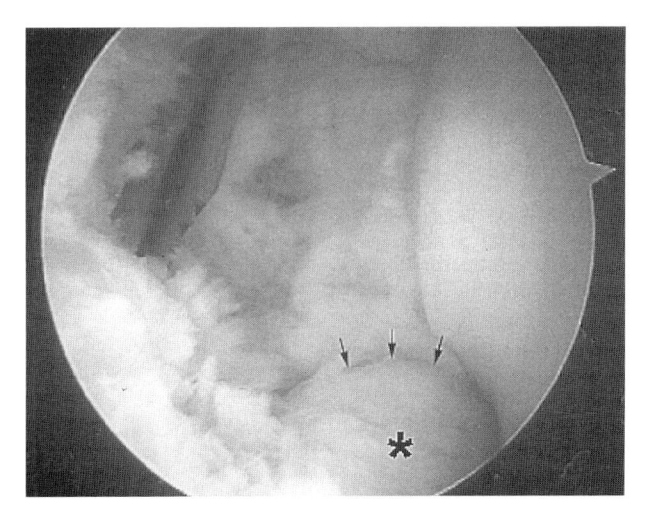

FIGURE 15.4. The proximal radioulnar joint is visualized as the arthroscope is withdrawn (arrows). The surgeon can view the marginal circumference of the radial head by taking the arm from pronation to supination (*).

maintained at a greater distance with this portal than with other anterolateral portals.[5] With the elbow held in 90° of flexion and capsular distention maintained, an 18-gauge spinal needle is inserted toward the center of the joint from this portal. The surgeon switches the arthroscope to the proximal anterolateral portal and examines the medial aspect of the anterior compartment.

The ulnohumeral articulation is the initial landmark in the medial aspect of the anterior compartment (Fig. 15.5). The structures in the medial aspect of the anterior compartment of the joint that are evaluated include the coronoid process, coronoid fossa, trochlea, and medial capsule. The coronoid process is inspected for any osteophytes projecting from the superior margin. The surgeon flexes and extends the patient's elbow to evaluate the ulnohumeral articulation and the trochlear articular surface. The coronoid fossa proximal to the trochlea is evaluated for osteophytes and loose bodies. The medial capsule, including the medial collateral ligament, is visualized. Only the anteriormost aspect of the anterior bundle of the medial collateral ligament is seen arthroscopically.[8,9] The arthroscope is withdrawn, allowing visualization of the trochleocapitellar groove and the anterior capsule. This step completes diagnostic arthroscopy of the anterior compartment. The cannula in the proximal medial portal is left in place as an inflow cannula.

A posterolateral portal is established for initial arthroscopic examination of the posterior compartment. Because soft tissue in the posterior compartment of the elbow often obscures visualization, the surgeon needs a second working posterior portal. A straight posterior portal allows easy access to the posterior compartment for soft-tissue debridement. With improved visualization, the

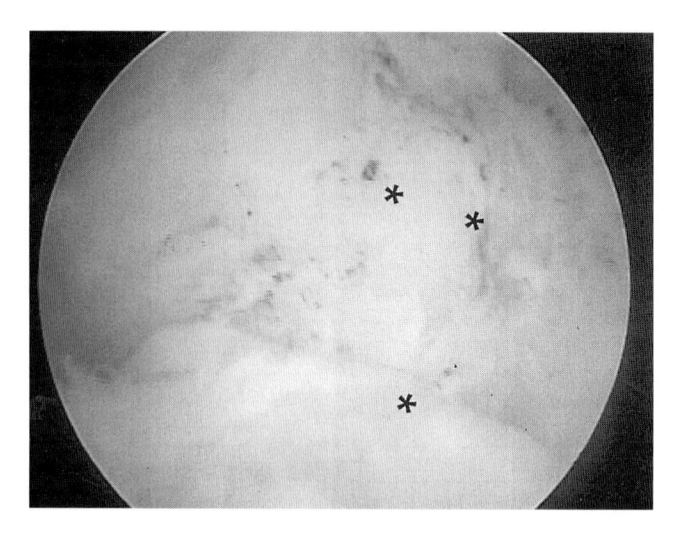

FIGURE 15.6. The articulation between the olecranon process (*) and the trochlea is visualized in the posterior compartment. The articular surface of the posterior aspect of the trochlea is best visualized in flexion. With the elbow in extension, the articulation between the olecranon and the olecranon fossa (**) is assessed.

surgeon can accomplish a systematic examination of the posterior compartment. With the arthroscope in the posterolateral portal, he or she examines the posterior aspect of the trochlea, olecranon fossa, and tip of the olecranon (Fig. 15.6). A thorough examination of the posterior compartment is mandatory because this compartment is a common site for loose bodies, which can be easily missed.

The olecranon process is examined for impinging osteophytes. The medial aspect of the olecranon process is a common site for osteophyte formation in valgus extension overload, with a mated "kissing lesion" on the posteromedial aspect of the trochlea. The articulation between the olecranon process and olecranon fossa is examined in extension to evaluate any bony or soft tissue impingement that limits extension.

The surgeon advances the arthroscope into the lateral gutter to examine the lateral aspect of the ulnohumeral articulation and the inferior aspect of the capitellum. Visualization of these structures is sometimes difficult from a proximal posterolateral portal. The direct lateral, or soft-spot, portal is better suited for visualization of these structures.

The posteromedial aspect of the posterior compartment is examined next. The arthroscope is switched to the straight posterior portal and advanced toward the medial gutter. The posterior bundle of the medial collateral ligament can be seen from this location and is visualized best with the elbow in 70° to 90° of flexion.[8] Remember, only a thin capsular layer and synovium lie between the arthroscope and the ulnar nerve; therefore, the surgeon must take care when arthroscopically examining this region.[10]

The surgeon completes diagnostic arthroscopy through

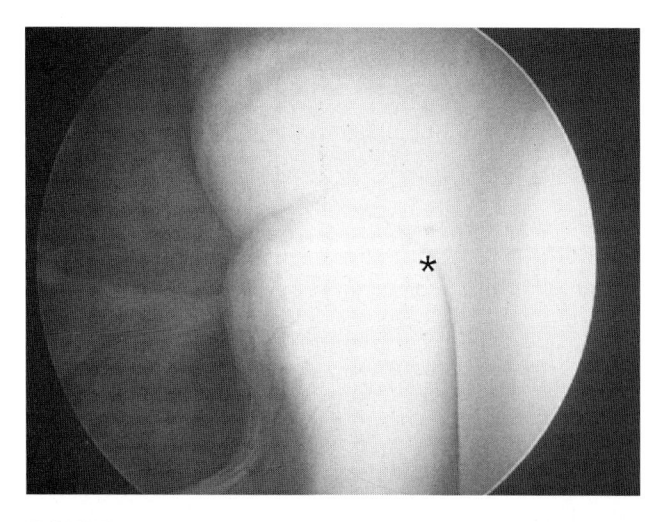

FIGURE 15.5. The initial landmark in the medial aspect of the anterior compartment is the ulnohumeral articulation. The coronoid process (*) should be inspected for osteophytes, and the articulation between the coronoid fossa and trochlea should be examined. Extension of the elbow allows visualization of a portion of the trochlear articular surface.

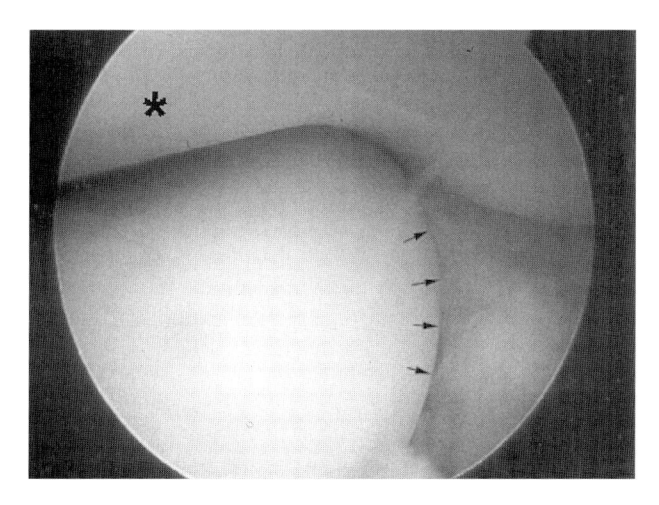

FIGURE 15.7. The inferior portion of the capitellum (*) and inferior aspect of the proximal radioulnar joint (arrows) are best visualized from the direct lateral (soft spot) portal.

the direct lateral portal. Through this portal, he or she can visualize the undersurface of the margin of the radial head, the inferior aspect of the capitellum, and the inferior portion of the proximal radioulnar joint (Fig. 15.7). This region is also a common location for loose bodies. The direct lateral portal allows the surgeon to evaluate suspected posterolateral rotatory instability. If present, this instability can be seen when the surgeon supinates the partially flexed elbow, causing opening of the ulnohumeral articulation with posterior subluxation of the radial head (Fig. 15.8).

With the diagnostic arthroscopy complete, the instruments are removed from the elbow. Thorough irrigation of the joint flushes out any debris. The portals are closed with interrupted nylon suture. This closure is particularly important for the direct lateral portal. Little tissue is present between the joint and the skin, and persistent portal drainage and formation of a synovial fistula have been reported.[1,11]

The elastic bandage is removed from the arm, allowing any fluid in the tissues about the elbow to diffuse into the remainder of the forearm and hand. With the elbow flexed to 90°, the extremity is immobilized in a bulky dressing to absorb any portal drainage. After 1 to 2 days, the dressing is removed, and range-of-motion exercises are begun.

RESULTS

Although arthroscopy is an established procedure for the treatment of intra-articular abnormalities of the elbow, the diagnostic benefit of elbow arthroscopy has received little attention in the literature. O'Driscoll and Morrey evaluated the diagnostic and therapeutic benefits of elbow arthroscopy in their series of 71 consecutive elbow arthroscopies (70 patients).[1] Patients realized a diagnostic benefit from arthroscopy when an incorrect preoperative diagnosis was changed to a correct diagnosis, a diagnosis was established when no preoperative diagnosis existed, or the diagnosis was expanded or confirmed when the preoperative diagnosis was incomplete or uncertain. Of the 71 arthroscopies, 56 (80%) were performed in some part for diagnosis: 30% for diagnosis alone and 50% for diagnosis and treatment. Thirty-six patients (64%; 36 arthroscopies) derived a diagnostic benefit from their arthroscopic procedure. Interestingly, when the authors reviewed the results of arthroscopy based on the indications for surgery, they found that only 29% of patients who had pain and had normal physical examination and radiographic studies benefited from arthroscopy of the elbow. Excluding these patients from the evaluation improved the diagnostic and therapeutic benefit from 64% to 78%.[1]

COMPLICATIONS

The risk of neurovascular injury during elbow arthroscopy is an ever-present concern because of the proximity of superficial and deep neurovascular structures to standard arthroscopic portals.[2,5,6,12–17] Although attention is focused on the neurovascular complications of elbow arthroscopy because of the devastating nature of these injuries, other complications do occur and must be appreciated so that they can be avoided. Most complications from elbow arthroscopy are easily avoided by paying careful attention to the technical details of the surgery and by understanding the local neurovascular anatomy.

The overall complication rate following elbow arthroscopy in two large series was approximately 7%.[1,11] O'Driscoll and Morrey[1] reported eight complications in 71 arthroscopies (11%), and Savoie[11] reported 15 com-

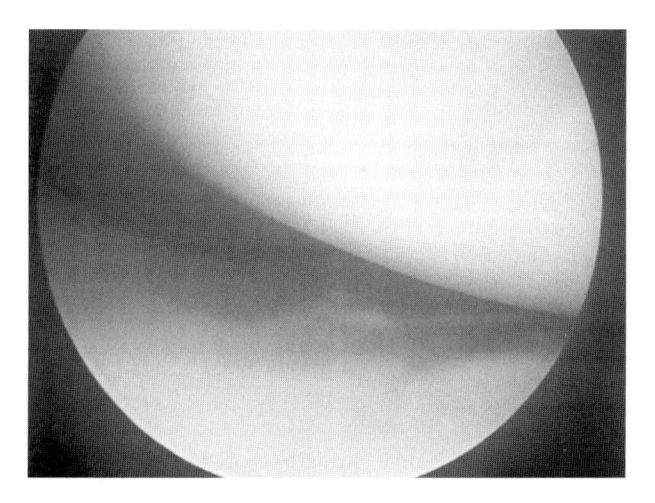

FIGURE 15.8. In a patient who has posterolateral rotatory instability, the ulna rotates away from the distal humerus when the forearm is in forced supination. This rotation is visualized well from the direct lateral portal.

plications in 247 elbow arthroscopies (6%). Most complications of elbow arthroscopy involve neurovascular injury. For this reason, complications typically are classified as neurologic and nonneurologic.

Neurologic Complications

None of the nerves surrounding the elbow is immune from injury during arthroscopic surgery. A number of transient nerve injuries have been reported in the literature.[1,2,11,13,18–21] Most of these injuries are related to technique and have resulted in technique modifications in an attempt to minimize their occurrence.

Extravasation of local anesthetics has been implicated as the cause of transient nerve palsy of the median[2,13] and radial nerves.[1] Transient nerve palsies caused by local anesthetic extravasation are easily avoided by eliminating the use of local anesthetics in elbow arthroscopy. Lynch et al.[13] reported a transient, low radial nerve palsy that they attributed to overdistention of the elbow joint. Other authors have reported that aggressive intra-articular manipulation with the arthroscope and arthroscopic instruments causes a transient posterior interosseous nerve injury.[20] Other nerve injuries for which no cause was mentioned include transient radial sensory nerve injury[18,21] and transient ulnar sensory nerve injury.[11]

Permanent neurologic injuries have devastating implications and can occur as an outside-in injury when establishing arthroscopic portals and instrumenting the elbow or as an inside-out injury when performing surgical arthroscopy.[10,15]

Nerve injuries can occur in routine arthroscopic procedures of the elbow[22] as well as in advanced arthroscopic procedures.[23,24] As more complicated surgery of the elbow is performed arthroscopically, the risk of nerve injury increases, because the normal anatomic relationships that are required for safe elbow arthroscopy are often distorted.

Inside-out nerve injuries can occur when arthroscopic surgery is performed in the vicinity of a nerve. Casscells reported injury to the ulnar nerve when he used a motorized arthroscopic shaver in the medial gutter.[10] Because of the proximity of the ulnar nerve to the medial joint capsule, aggressive debridement of the anteromedial and posteromedial gutter puts the ulnar nerve at risk for injury. Miller et al.[15] reported transection of the median nerve when they performed an arthroscopic synovectomy. Procedures performed along the capsular margin of the elbow joint and away from bone can injure nerves if the joint capsule is violated.[15] Elbow joint insufflation with the elbow in flexion increases the distance between the distal humerus and the radial and median nerves, but does not increase the distance between the capsule and nerves.[15] The surgeon must pay careful attention to the integrity of the joint capsule when performing any arthroscopic procedure against the joint capsule.

Nonneurologic Complications

The nonneurologic complications of elbow arthroscopy are similar to the complications reported in other arthroscopic procedures. These complications include intra-articular breakage of arthroscopic instruments,[19] superficial wound infection,[23] hematoma formation,[11] reflex sympathetic dystrophy,[11] loss of motion (arthrofibrosis),[1,11,24] and persistent drainage from the portal sites.[1,11]

CONCLUSION

Arthroscopy of the elbow has evolved rapidly over the last decade into a powerful diagnostic and therapeutic tool. The value of elbow arthroscopy as a diagnostic tool lies in the surgeon's ability to directly evaluate intra-articular structures that he or she can only indirectly evaluate with physical examination and radiographic studies. The diagnostic benefit of elbow arthroscopy is greatest in a patient who has a history of elbow pain or mechanical symptoms and has physical findings and radiographic studies documenting elbow abnormalities. However, by enabling the surgeon to document the absence of intra-articular abnormalities, diagnostic elbow arthroscopy benefits patients who have chronic pain and no physical findings or radiographic studies revealing intra-articular abnormalities.

The proximity of vital neurovascular structures demands attention to the details of arthroscopy from the outset. Establishing a reproducible routine for performing a diagnostic arthroscopy minimizes the risk of complications and maximizes the benefit to the patient.

REFERENCES

1. O'Driscoll SW, Morrey BF. Arthroscopy of the elbow. Diagnostic and therapeutic benefits and hazards. *J Bone Joint Surg* 1992;74A:84–94.
2. Andrews JR, Carson WG. Arthroscopy of the elbow. *Arthroscopy* 1985;1:97–107.
3. Poehling GG, Whipple TL, Sisco L, et al. Elbow arthroscopy: A new technique. *Arthroscopy* 1989;5:222–224.
4. Boe S. Arthroscopy of the elbow. Diagnosis and extraction of loose bodies. *Acta Orthop Scand* 1986;57:52–53.
5. Field LD, Altchek DW, Warren RF, et al. Arthroscopic anatomy of the lateral elbow: A comparison of three portals. *Arthroscopy* 1994;10:602–607.
6. Lindenfeld TN. Medial approach in elbow arthroscopy. *Am J Sports Med* 1990;18:413–417.
7. O'Driscoll SW, Morrey BF, An KN. Intraarticular pressure and capacity of the elbow. *Arthroscopy* 1990;6:10–103.
8. Field LD, Callaway GH, O'Brien SJ, et al. Arthroscopic as-

sessment of the medial collateral ligament complex of the elbow. *Am J Sports Med* 1995;23:396–400.
9. Timmerman LA, Andrews JR. Histology and arthroscopic anatomy of the ulnar collateral ligament of the elbow. *Am J of Sports Med* 1994;22:667–673.
10. Casscells SW. Editor's comment. Neurovascular anatomy and elbow arthroscopy: Inherent risks. *Arthroscopy* 1986;2:190.
11. Savoie FH III. Complications. In: Savoie FH III, Field LD, eds. *Arthroscopy of the elbow*. New York: Churchill Livingstone; 1996:151–156.
12. Adolfsson L. Arthroscopy of the elbow joint: A cadaveric study of portal placement. *J Shoulder Elbow Surg* 1994;3:53–61.
13. Lynch GJ, Meyers JF, Whipple TL, et al. Neurovascular anatomy and elbow arthroscopy: Inherent risks. *Arthroscopy* 1986;2:190–197.
14. Marshall PD, Fairclough JA, Johnson SR, et al. Avoiding nerve damage during elbow arthroscopy. *J Bone Joint Surg* 1993;75B:129–131.
15. Miller CD, Jobe CM, Wright MH. Neuroanatomy in elbow arthroscopy. *J Shoulder Elbow Surg* 1995;4:168–174.
16. Stothers K, Day B, Regan WR. Arthroscopy of the elbow: Anatomy, portal sites, and a description of the proximal lateral portal. *Arthroscopy* 1995;11:449–457.
17. Verhaar J, van Mameren H, Brandsma A. Risks of neurovascular injury in elbow arthroscopy: Starting anteromedially or anterolaterally? *Arthroscopy* 1991;7:287–290.
18. Guhl JF. Arthroscopy and arthroscopic surgery of the elbow. *Orthopedics* 1985;8:1290–1296.
19. Kim SJ, Kim HK, Lee JW. Arthroscopy for limitation of motion of the elbow. *Arthroscopy* 1995;11:680–683.
20. Papilion JD, Neff RS, Shall LM. Compression neuropathy of the radial nerve as a complication of elbow arthroscopy. A case report and review of the literature. *Arthroscopy* 1988;4:284–286.
21. Rupp S, Tempelhof S. Arthroscopic surgery of the elbow. Therapeutic benefits and hazards. *Clin Orthop* 1995;313:140–145.
22. Thomas MA, Fast A, Shapiro D. Radial nerve damage as a complication of elbow arthroscopy. *Clin Orthop* 1987;215:130–131.
23. Redden JF, Stanley D. Arthroscopic fenestration of the olecranon fossa in the treatment of osteoarthritis of the elbow. *Arthroscopy* 1993;9:14–16.
24. Jones GS, Savoie FH III. Arthroscopic capsular release of flexion contractures (arthrofibrosis) of the elbow. *Arthroscopy* 1993;9:277–283.

CHAPTER 16

Arthroscopic Removal of Loose Bodies in the Elbow

Mark S. Schickendantz

INTRODUCTION

The use of the arthroscope for the diagnosis and treatment of intra-articular abnormalities of the elbow has become accepted widely. Over the past decade, improvements in arthroscopic equipment and operative techniques have allowed the orthopaedic surgeon a greater comfort level and more confidence in using the arthroscope in the elbow. Historically, one of the most common indications for elbow arthroscopy has been for the diagnosis and removal of intra-articular loose bodies.[1–6] In this chapter, I outline my surgical techniques for the arthroscopic removal of loose bodies from the elbow.

HISTORY

In addition to pain, loose bodies of the elbow typically cause mechanical symptoms of catching and locking of the joint.[4] Although less common, swelling and stiffness also may be present.[4]

While one single traumatic injury can lead to the creation of a loose body of the elbow, a more typical history is one of repetitive overuse, such as in the overhead-throwing athlete who develops valgus extension overload syndrome.[7] In this disease, repetitive valgus and extension stress of the elbow leads to the development of osteophyte formation of the posterior medial olecranon. A corresponding "kissing" lesion typically develops in the underlying olecranon fossa where the posterior medial spur chronically impinges on it. Loose bodies can form from fragmentation of the posterior medial olecranon osteophyte or from chondral or osteochondral defects generated in the trochlear groove by the repetitive rubbing of the osteophyte in this area. Usually, a large amount of synovitis is present in this region as well. It has been demonstrated that inflamed synovium may fragment into smaller pieces and may become soft-tissue loose bodies within the joint.[8]

Loose bodies in the adolescent athlete's elbow are most often the result of osteochondritis dissecans of the capitellum (Fig. 16.1).[9–13] This entity, often called Panner's disease or Little Leaguer's elbow, is caused by repetitive valgus stress of the elbow, resulting in compressive forces across the radiocapitellar joint and a presumed disruption of blood supply to the capitellum.[14] While some authors debate the existence of a separate idiopathic variety of osteochondritis dissecans of the capitellum, these problems most likely represent different stages of progression of a single disease process.[12,14] As in the knee, progression of the disease from early osteochondrosis to an actual osteochondritic lesion of the joint surface with resultant fragmentation and loose-body formation probably depends on the age of the patient at the onset of the disease and any overlying trauma that may occur to the joint.

Primary or posttraumatic osteoarthrosis also may lead to loose-body formation in the adult's elbow either in the form of loose fragments of articular cartilage or fragmentation of marginal osteophytes.[5]

IMAGING

Authors have demonstrated that plain radiographic evaluation of the elbow for the diagnosis of loose bodies is less than ideal.[15–17] Particularly, loose bodies in the posterior compartment of the elbow often are missed with standard anteroposterior (AP) and lateral radiographs. In

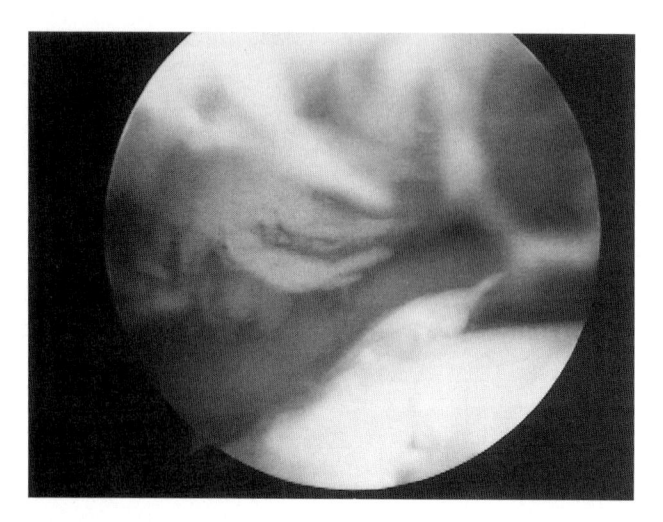

FIGURE 16.1. Arthroscopic appearance, as viewed from the anterolateral portal, of osteochondritis dissecans. Fragmentation of articular cartilage from the capitellum is seen in the bottom half of the field of view. Above, synovitis is prevalent.

a review of 70 patients who underwent arthroscopy of the elbow, O'Driscoll and Morrey reported that 7 of 23 patients who had loose bodies at the time of surgery failed to demonstrate loose bodies on preoperative AP and lateral radiographs.[15] All these loose bodies were found in the posterior compartment of the elbow.

Computed tomography and magnetic resonance imaging may be more useful than plain radiography for determining the presence and location of loose bodies (Fig. 16.2).[17,18] In our experience, the addition of contrast agents, such as gadolinium, enhances the sensitivity of these tests even further.

PHYSICAL EXAMINATION

Physical findings in the adult who has loose bodies of the elbow almost always include mechanical catching or locking of the elbow with active or passive range of motion. Posterior lesions typically block full extension, and attempts at full extension are often painful. Loose bodies in the radiocapitellar articulation may produce limitations in pronation and supination, as well as associated pain, with these maneuvers.

Athletes who have valgus extension overload syndrome usually lack full extension of the elbow, which also causes pain. Valgus stress with the elbow flexed to approximately 30° can reproduce the symptoms that the athlete experiences while throwing, posterior medial pain and catching.[7]

In the adolescent athlete who has radiocapitellar osteochondrosis, valgus stress on the flexed elbow places a compressive load across the radiocapitellar joint and may re-create symptoms of pain and catching. Often the athlete has tenderness directly over the joint and may have pain with pronation and supination of the forearm.

NONOPERATIVE TREATMENT

Patients who present with mechanical symptoms of catching and locking in the elbow joint in all likelihood need arthroscopic evaluation and treatment. If a diagnosis of loose bodies has been made, no nonoperative treatment is available to treat this problem. Continued catching and locking of the joint can damage the articular surfaces. Persistent inability to extend the elbow fully can lead to permanent flexion contracture. Failure to recognize and treat Panner's disease may result in cortical flattening and deformity of the capitellum, with permanent restrictions in elbow motion and resultant functional limitations.[12]

OPERATIVE TREATMENT

Indications

Virtually any patient who presents with mechanical symptoms of catching and locking as a result of loose bodies in the elbow is a candidate for elbow arthroscopy.

Contraindications for proceeding with arthroscopic removal of loose bodies from the elbow include active elbow sepsis, active systemic sepsis, and medical conditions that preclude the safe and successful completion of this procedure.

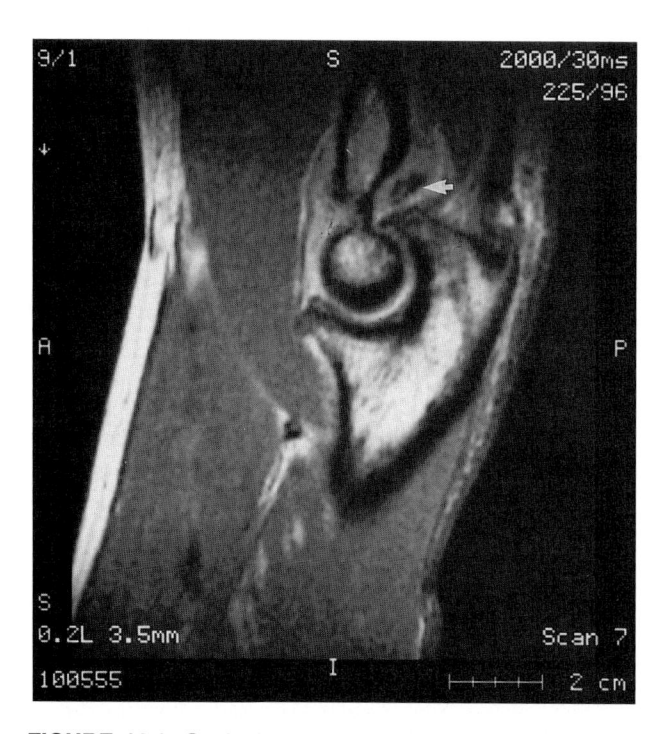

FIGURE 16.2. Sagittal magnetic resonance image through the mid-portion of the ulnohumeral joint demonstrating a large loose body in the posterior compartment (white arrow).

Techniques

Several different patient positions currently are used for arthroscopy of the elbow.[5,6,9] Although each of these positions has certain advantages and disadvantages, I have found that the supine position with the arm held in traction is very useful.

The patient is placed supine on the operating table. Although intravenous block anesthesia can be used, the double-tourniquet technique often leaves the more distal tourniquet in the way and therefore may not be convenient for many surgical cases. An alternative is to use a sterile tourniquet distally. For most procedures, however, a general anesthetic is used. A well-padded tourniquet is placed on the upper arm of the affected side. The arm is suspended with 10 lb of traction in 90° of abduction (Fig. 16.3). Initially, the elbow is flexed to 90° to provide maximum clearance of the anterior neurovascular structures away from the joint. The elbow is prepared and draped free in a sterile fashion.

The surgeon inspects the anterior compartment in a systematic fashion, beginning laterally and working medially. With the arthroscope in the anterolateral portal, the surgeon cannot visualize the entire radiocapitellar joint. However, approximately half of this articulation can be visualized by pointing the lens down toward the joint surface. Rotation of the forearm easily confirms visualization of the radial head. Lesions of the radiocapitellar joint can be visualized partially from this vantage point.

The anterolateral viewing portal gives the best view of the ulnohumeral articulation. The surgeon easily can visualize the coronoid process as it articulates with the trochlea. Pushing the arthroscope farther medially and looking down along the medial gutter may reveal a hiding place for small loose bodies. Authors have shown that the medial collateral ligament is visible from this vantage point as well.[19,20] While viewing medially, the surgeon applies valgus stress to the elbow, which is now flexed to approximately 60°. Significant increase in the space between the ulna and the humerus medially may indicate insufficiency of the medial collateral ligament.[19,21]

Small loose bodies may be found in the synovium that is attached to the anterior capsule both proximally and distally within the joint (Fig. 16.4). A probe introduced through the medial cannula should be used to palpate the synovium for a more thorough examination.

If small (i.e., 3 mm or less) loose bodies are found and are truly nonadherent, they can be flushed out the medial cannula. Larger or partially adherent loose bodies are removed with grasping forceps (Fig. 16.5). Very large fragments often are best removed in a piecemeal fashion. A shaver or burr may be used to reduce the size of the loose body. Large pieces may need to be removed without the cannula in place. The portal also may have to be enlarged. Ideally, however, once portals are established, they should be maintained. If the surgeon needs to remove a

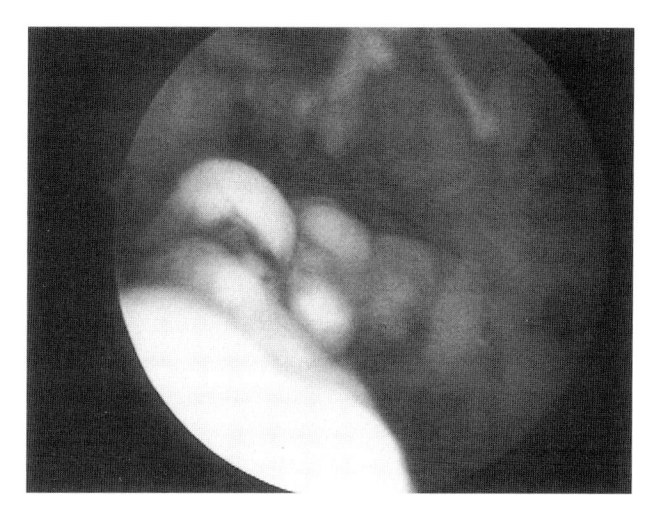

FIGURE 16.4. Small osteochondral loose bodies adherent to synovium in the anteromedial aspect of the elbow as viewed from the anterolateral portal.

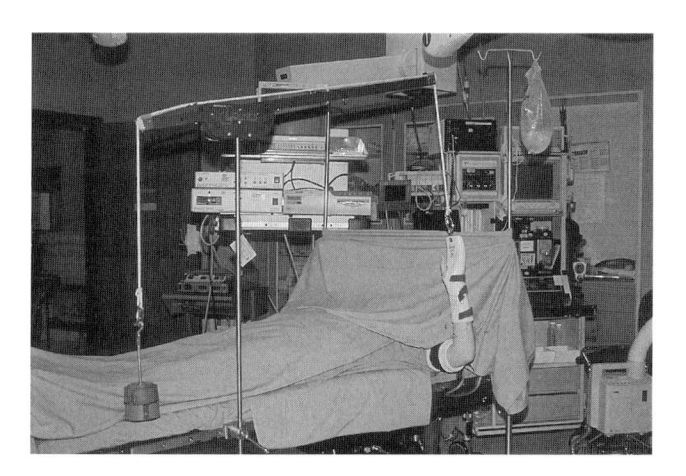

FIGURE 16.3. Operating room setup and patient positioning. The patient's arm is suspended with 10 lb of traction in 90° of flexion.

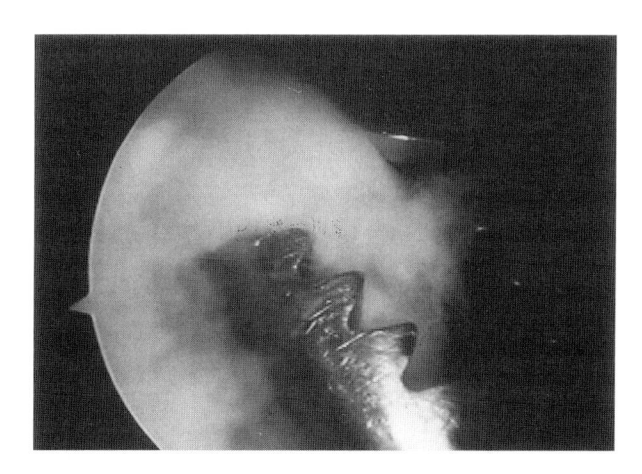

FIGURE 16.5. Removal of large loose body using a grasping forceps.

large loose fragment without the cannula in place, he or she removes the cannula, carefully enlarges the skin incision to the appropriate size, uses a hemostat to enlarge the deeper aspects of the portal and capsule, and grasps and removes the loose body. The cannula is reinserted to maintain patency of the portal site.

The radiocapitellar joint can be more thoroughly visualized with the arthroscope in the anteromedial portal. Visualization is facilitated by the use of switching sticks or Wissinger rods. The rods are placed through the corresponding cannulas. The arthroscope is introduced anteromedially, and outflow is established anterolaterally. Loose bodies found in this region are removed in a similar manner. If the surgeon finds significant articular surface damage to the capitellum (as is found in osteochondritis dissecans), he or she can address it from this perspective as well.

Next, a straight or direct lateral portal is created in the soft spot. The arthroscope is removed from its sheath in the anteromedial portal, and a Wissinger rod is placed through the arthroscope cannula, which subsequently is replaced by a small outflow cannula. If desired, the surgeon can maintain patency of the anterolateral portal with a blunt Steinmann pin.

A spinal needle is used to help localize the direct lateral portal and the soft spot. Outflow of fluid through the spinal needle confirms intra-articular placement. The site is injected with a local anesthetic, and a no. 11 blade is used to create a small stab incision in the skin. The surgeon carries out blunt dissection through the joint capsule and introduces the arthroscope. Visualization of the remainder of the radiocapitellar joint is possible from this portal. The radioulnar and lateral ulnohumeral articulations also can be easily seen. Small loose bodies sometimes can be found in this region and often can be flushed out through one of the posterior portals, which are described next.

With the arthroscope in the direct lateral portal, the lens is turned to view the posterior capsule, and the elbow is extended to about 30° of flexion. A spinal needle is introduced in the posterolateral corner of the elbow immediately lateral to the triceps tendon and approximately 2 to 3 cm proximal to the tip of the olecranon. The portal track is infiltrated as the spinal needle is withdrawn. The surgeon makes a small stab incision and introduces a 4.5-mm cannula with a blunt trocar. This posterolateral portal can be used as a working portal if visualization is adequate with the arthroscope in the direct lateral portal. However, a better view of the posterior compartment can be achieved with the arthroscope placed into the posterolateral portal with subsequent creation of the straight posterior portal. This straight posterior portal is approximately 1 to 2 cm more medially and 1 to 2 cm more distally located than the posterolateral portal. To avoid injury to the ulnar nerve, the surgeon must not place the straight posterior portal medial to the posterior midline.

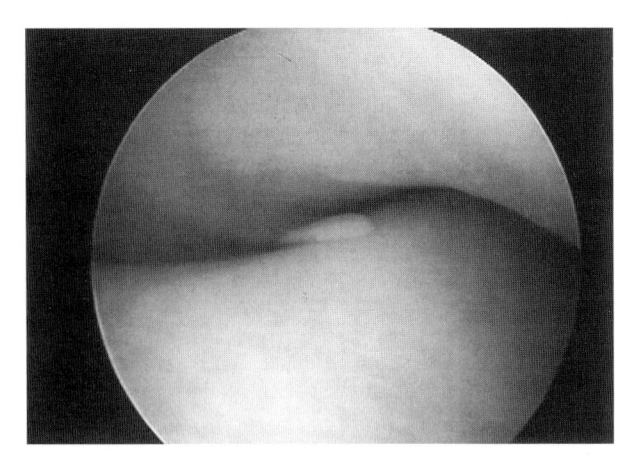

FIGURE 16.6. Small loose body in the ulnohumeral joint as viewed through the posterolateral portal.

To create the straight posterior portal, the surgeon uses the same technique described for the posterolateral portal.

With the arthroscope in the posterolateral portal, the straight posterior portal provides an excellent working portal for the posterior compartment. Most loose bodies in the elbow are found in this area, particularly proximal in the olecranon fossa. They may be caught up in and partially adherent to the synovium. A 3.5-mm full-radius resector or incisor blade on the shaver may be used to carry out synovectomy in this region. Small loose bodies can be flushed out (Fig. 16.6). Larger bodies may need to be grasped with grasping forceps and, depending on their size, may need to be removed either through the cannula or directly through the skin (Fig. 16.7). A technique that is useful in the posterior compartment, but not safe to use anteriorly, involves placing a spinal needle into a large loose body in order to hold it in place; the surgeon reduces the loose body in size with a shaver or burr so that he or she can remove it without having to expand the portal sites significantly. Care must be taken to avoid the ulnar nerve by staying lateral to the midline.

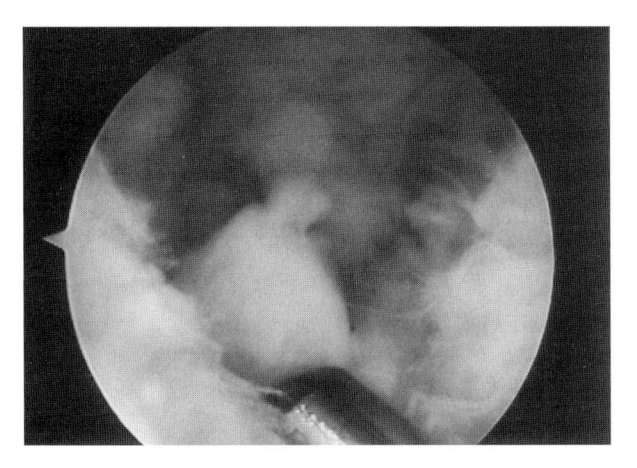

FIGURE 16.7. Large loose body in the posterior compartment as viewed from the posterolateral portal.

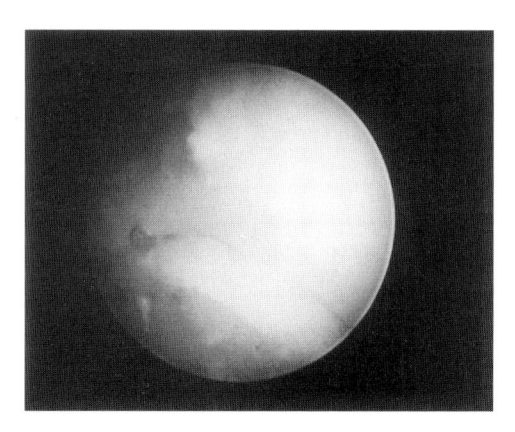

FIGURE 16.8. Posteromedial osteophyte in the elbow of a throwing athlete as viewed from the posterolateral portal.

In cases of a valgus impingement overload, the posteromedial osteophyte that develops may be removed with a burr or even with a small osteotome placed through the straight posterior portal (Fig. 16.8). The surgeon must remove all particulate debris.

Once the surgeon is satisfied that all abnormalities have been addressed appropriately, he or she flushes the elbow until it is clear of all particulate debris and removes the arthroscope and instruments from the elbow. Portals are closed with subcuticular 3-0 plain suture and adhesive strips. A bulky sterile bandage and Cryocuff (Aircast, Inc., Summit, New Jersey) are applied. The tourniquet is removed, and the arm is let down out of traction and placed into a sling.

Postoperatively, the patient uses a sling for comfort as needed. Early active range of motion is encouraged. A structured physical therapy program is prescribed to control pain and swelling initially and to restore range of motion. Strengthening and functional exercises are added gradually. Depending on the primary abnormality, return to vocation or sports is variable. Athletes who have valgus extension overload are not allowed to throw for at least 6 weeks after surgery. At that time, a progressive interval throwing program is begun.

RESULTS

Arthroscopic removal of loose bodies from the elbow is generally a very safe and effective procedure.[2–4,11,15,16] Most patients report a significant decrease in mechanical symptoms and pain and improvement in function. The highest rates of success are reported in patients who have isolated loose bodies of the elbow. O'Driscoll and Morrey reported improvement in all 20 of their patients who had arthroscopic surgery for removal of isolated loose bodies of the elbow.[15,16] Additionally, three of three patients who had osteochondritis dissecans and loose bodies also showed significant improvement. Alternatively, patients who had posttraumatic arthritis, degenerative joint disease, and other abnormalities were not improved significantly. Postoperative improvement in range of motion is particularly unpredictable.[4]

Complications related to the arthroscopic removal of loose bodies from the elbow are the same as those seen with diagnostic arthroscopy of the elbow. The only exception might be the result of careless extension of a portal site in an effort to extract a very large loose body.

SUMMARY

Arthroscopic removal of loose bodies from the elbow is a relatively safe and efficacious procedure. Knowledge of elbow anatomy and attention to proper surgical techniques are critical to avoiding potential neurovascular complications. Patients who have isolated loose bodies of the elbow can be expected to benefit the most from this procedure. Expectations should be tempered in cases of posttraumatic arthritis, degenerative arthritis, and other associated abnormalities.

REFERENCES

1. McGinty JB. Arthroscopic removal of loose bodies. *Orthop Clin North Am* 1982;13:313–328.
2. Boe S. Arthroscopy of the elbow: Diagnosis and extraction of loose bodies. *Acta Orthop Scand* 1986:57:52–53.
3. O'Driscoll SW. Elbow arthroscopy for loose bodies. *Orthopedics* 1992;15:855–859.
4. Ogilvie-Harris DJ, Schemitsch E. Arthroscopy of the elbow for removal of loose bodies. *Arthroscopy* 1993;9:5–8.
5. O'Driscoll SW, Morrey BF. Arthroscopy of the elbow. In: Morrey BF, ed. *The elbow and its disorders*, 2nd ed. Philadelphia: WB Saunders; 1993:120–130.
6. Carson WG Jr, Meyers JF. Diagnostic arthroscopy of the elbow: Supine position surgical technique, arthroscopic and portal anatomy. In: McGinty JB, Caspari RB, Jackson RW, et al., eds. *Operative arthroscopy*, 2nd ed. Philadelphia: Lippincott-Raven; 1996:851–868.
7. Andrews JR, Craven WM. Lesions of the posterior compartment of the elbow. *Clin Sports Med* 1991;10:637–652.
8. Turek SL. The elbow. In: *Orthopaedics: Principles and their application*. Philadelphia: Lippincott; 1984:967–984.
9. Andrews JR, McKenzie PJ. Surgical techniques "supine" with arthroscopic surgical treatment of elbow pathology. In: McGinty JB, Caspari RB, Jackson RW, et al., eds. *Operative arthroscopy*, 2nd ed. Philadelphia: Lippincott-Raven, 1996:877–885.
10. Jackson DW, Silvino N, Reiman P. Osteochondritis in the female gymnast's elbow. *Arthroscopy* 1989;5:129–136.
11. Ruch DS, Poehling GG. Arthroscopic treatment of Panner's disease. *Clin Sports Med* 1991;10:629–636.
12. Shaughnessy WJ, Bianco AJ. Osteochondritis dissecans. In: Morrey BF, ed. *The elbow and its disorders*, 2nd ed. Philadelphia: WB Saunders; 1993:282–287.
13. Morrey BF. Loose bodies. In: Morrey BF, ed. *The elbow and its disorders*, 2nd ed. Philadelphia: WB Saunders; 1993:860–871.

14. Singer KM, Roy SP. Osteochondrosis of the humeral capitellum. *Am J Sports Med* 1984;12:351–360.
15. O'Driscoll SW, Morrey BF. Arthroscopy of the elbow: A critical review. *Orthop Trans* 1990;14:258–259.
16. O'Driscoll SW, Morrey BF. Arthroscopy of the elbow: Diagnostic and therapeutic benefits and hazards. *J Bone Joint Surg* 1992;74A:84–94.
17. Pope TL Jr, Siegel DB, Poehling GG, Chen MYM. Imaging of the elbow. In: McGinty JB, Caspari RB, Jackson RW, et al., eds. *Operative arthroscopy*, 2nd ed. Philadelphia: Lippincott-Raven; 1996:829–849.
18. Fritz RC, Stoller DW. The elbow. In: Stoller DW, ed. Magnetic resonance imaging in orthopaedics & sports medicine. Philadelphia: Lippincott-Raven; 1997:803–812.
19. Timmerman LA, Andrews JR. Histology of arthroscopic anatomy of the ulnar collateral ligament of the elbow. *Am J Sports Med* 1994;22:667–673.
20. Field LD, Callaway GH, O'Brien SJ, et al. Arthroscopic assessment of the medial collateral ligament complex of the elbow. *Am J Sports Med* 1995;23:396–400.
21. Field LD, Altchek DW. Evaluation of the arthroscopic valgus instability test of the elbow. *Am J Sports Med* 1996;24:177–181.

CHAPTER 17

Arthroscopic Treatment of Ankylosis of the Elbow

Felix H. Savoie III, Larry D. Field, and Charles W. Hartzog Jr.

INTRODUCTION

Arthroscopy of the elbow joint has become a well-accepted surgical procedure. To perform this technique, the surgeon must have a thorough knowledge of elbow anatomy and the proper indications for surgery. Recent advances in elbow arthroscopy have allowed expansion of these indications. Certain types of elbow ankylosis or flexion contracture are now amenable to arthroscopic as well as to open treatment. We present the arthroscopic treatment of ankylosis of the elbow, focusing on the development of posttraumatic arthrofibrosis, surgical technique, and treatment precautions.

ETIOLOGY

Any loss of motion sufficient to cause functional limitations is termed an elbow contracture or arthrofibrosis. Fractures, dislocations, arthritic conditions, burns, and various cerebral injuries can lead to arthrofibrosis.[1–6] These conditions may be grouped into intrinsic, extrinsic, and peripheral causes. Intrinsic causes have an intra-articular origin, such as fractures, bone spurs, loose bodies, and synovitis. Extrinsic causes include capsular contracture, flexor–extensor muscle damage, collateral ligament scarring, heterotopic bone, and skin contractures. Head injury, cerebral palsy, and neuromuscular dysfunction are examples of peripheral causes. Before treating the patient who has an ankylosed elbow, the examining physician should evaluate all potential causes. Contractures resulting from peripheral causes must be treated differently from those resulting from intrinsic causes. The neurovascular structures must always be evaluated carefully for potential involvement in the contracture process.

INCIDENCE

Elbow stiffness impairs hand function significantly, with a 50% loss of elbow motion resulting in nearly an 80% loss of upper extremity function.[7] Although the true incidence of elbow flexion contracture is unknown, researchers have reported that it affects nearly 5% of elbows after traumatic injury.[7] In 1972, Mohan[8] published the results of 200 cases of posttraumatic elbow arthrofibrosis. Supracondylar, T-condylar, and condylar fractures composed 20% of these injuries; dislocations, 20%; radial head fractures, 10%; and fracture–dislocation, 38%. The risk of developing posttraumatic arthrofibrosis is directly related to the severity of the initial trauma. Cooney[9] believed that the most important factor in the development of elbow stiffness was the degree of the initial intra-articular involvement. However, he noted that the degree of periosteal stripping and length of immobilization were additional risk factors.

PATHOGENESIS OF POSTTRAUMATIC ARTHROFIBROSIS

Posttraumatic arthrofibrosis of the elbow results from soft-tissue trauma, hemarthrosis, and the patient's reaction to pain.[10] Elbow trauma can cause tearing and contusion of the periarticular soft tissues, including the joint capsule.[7–10] The patient often holds the injured elbow in a flexed position to reduce pain from the resulting hemarthrosis. A fibrous tissue response can be stimulated within the hematoma and damaged muscle tissues. The formation of fibrous tissue can lead to ectopic bone formation or myositis ossificans.[11] Overaggressive physical therapy during the rehabilitation process may further exacerbate these injuries. A cycle of pain, swelling, motion limitations, and subsequent contracture can result.

Collateral ligament injury often contributes significantly to elbow flexion contracture.[10,12–14] These ligaments can develop a primary fibrosis due to the initial injury or a secondary fibrosis due to subsequent immobilization and scar formation. Significant injury to the elbow joint often damaged the joint capsule and the adjacent brachialis muscle. The resultant capsular hypertrophy and fibrotic reaction can contribute to elbow ankylosis and are particularly common in association with elbow fracture–dislocations.[15–17]

Intrinsic causes also can lead to mechanical limitations of elbow motion. Intra-articular lesions can occur as a result of fractures, osteochondral lesions, or other articular incongruencies. In the lateral portion of the elbow joint, these abnormalities are commonly due to residual deformity in the radial head following a radial head fracture or due to an injury to the capitellum. A significant incidence of elbow flexion contracture has been noted following a type I radial head fracture.[18,19] It is thought that this flexion contracture is due to the combination of radial head incongruency and significant soft-tissue trauma from the initial injury.

Mild injuries to the coronoid or olecranon can produce significant stiffness secondary to the increased incongruity of the medial portion of the elbow joint. Any bony fracture or loose body within the olecranon fossa can restrict elbow extension, and posterior pericapsular fibrosis can limit elbow flexion.

The specific mechanism of injury often dictates which structures are involved in the posttraumatic arthrofibrotic process.[20,21] Therefore, knowing how the initial injury occurred is helpful when planning treatment for these patients. Additionally, combined injuries of the elbow can lead to a multifaceted etiology of the contracture secondary to involvement of various structures.

TREATMENT INDICATIONS AND CONTRAINDICATIONS

In 1981, Morrey et al.[22] determined that 90% of the typical activities of daily living could be performed within a functional arc of motion of 30° to 130° of flexion. However, they did not include sports and work activities in this determination. Certain occupations and activities (e.g., shoe tying, personal hygiene) require more than 30° of elbow extension. We believe that treatment, therefore, is indicated for patients who have flexion contractures of more than 30° and for patients whose occupations or lifestyle requires more than 30° of elbow extension. Certain patients who have lesser degrees of flexion contracture, yet have symptoms of intra-articular pathologic lesions (e.g., pain, popping, locking), may be candidates for surgical treatment.

Surgeons have used various nonoperative modalities, including physical therapy, manipulation, and static and dynamic splinting, to treat the arthrofibrotic elbow.[9,23,24] These nonoperative measures can be used successfully particularly in cases of acute contracture, which is caused by periarticular soft-tissue injury and in cases without significant intra-articular involvement. Therefore, the treating physician should use nonoperative treatment for a minimum of 3 months before considering surgery to treat these patients.

Various surgical procedures have been developed for treatment of the ankylosed elbow.[24,25–30] These techniques employ soft-tissue releases with or without bony procedures. They may be performed arthroscopically, through a limited open incision, or through an extensive open technique. Arthroscopic surgery can be used to treat contractures with intrinsic or extrinsic causes.

Contraindications to arthroscopic surgery include altered neurovascular anatomy of the elbow joint (i.e., ulnar nerve transposition) or certain extra-articular deformities in which neurovascular structures are entrapped. Certain conditions that produce extensive scar tissue in this area (anteriorly displaced radial head fractures or dislocations) are contraindications to arthroscopic release of elbow contracture. Arthroscopic management of this condition is contraindicated if the surgeon has limited experience using arthroscopy to treat elbow conditions. Treatment of this condition can be extremely difficult, and the surgeon must have extensive arthroscopic experience to achieve successful results.[31]

SURGICAL TECHNIQUE

When performing arthroscopic surgical release of elbow flexion contracture, the surgeon uses a 4.5-mm arthroscope, shaver, and standard camera and video recording equipment. The patient is placed in the prone position. The patient's arm is elevated with a 4-in. block on a standard arm board that is oriented parallel to the operating room table (Fig. 17.1). This placement maintains the elbow in a flexed position with adequate mobility and portal access. A proximal tourniquet is used and typically is inflated to 250 mm Hg after exsanguination of the extremity. The arm is prepared and draped. Coban material is used to wrap the forearm distal to the elbow to decrease fluid extravasation into the forearm compartments during arthroscopy. The surgeon examines the elbow of the anesthetized patient, testing range of motion in neutral rotation, pronation, and supination.

Next, the elbow joint is insufflated with normal saline solution through a soft-spot portal, which is in the trian-

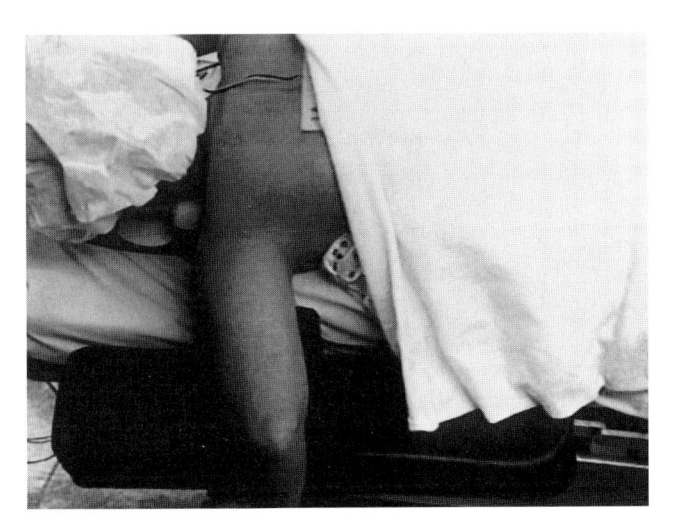

FIGURE 17.1. The patient is placed in the prone position for elbow arthroscopy. Note that the arm board is oriented parallel to the operating room table, with the elbow elevated on a 4-in. padded block to allow ease of access to portal sites.

gular area formed posteriorly by the palpable epicondyle, radial head, and ulna. A proximal medial portal is established 2 cm proximal to the medial epicondyle and anterior to the medial intermuscular septum. Incisions for portals are kept superficial to avoid injury to the underlying cutaneous nerves. The surgeon can use a blunt trocar to palpate the intermuscular septum; he or she directs it anterior to the septum, through muscular layers, and into the elbow joint capsule. We prefer to enter the joint with this blunt trocar, but we occasionally need a sharp trocar to penetrate the thickened, fibrotic joint capsule. The surgeon positions the arthroscope through this proximal medial portal and evaluates the anterior compartment.

A proximal anterolateral portal is the second portal established. We prefer to establish this portal using an outside-in technique with a spinal needle, but the surgeon may need to use an inside-out technique with a Wissinger rod in patients who have significant scarring in the lateral portion of the elbow. The surgeon must know the location of the posterior interosseous nerve during lateral portal placement. This portal should be placed just superior to the capitellum to ensure the safety of the nerve. After positioning a cannula within the proximal anterolateral portal, the surgeon can use it as a working portal to remove inflamed soft tissues and adhesions from the anterior aspect of the radiocapitellar joint and coronoid process. Debridement is performed with the patient's arm pronated and supinated to allow adequate visualization of the anterior radiocapitellar joint.

The surgeon performs an anterior capsulectomy next. With the arthroscope positioned in the proximal medial portal and a full-radius shaver placed in the proximal anterolateral portal, he or she releases the anterior capsule from its proximal humeral insertion. This release begins at approximately the mid-sagittal plane of the humerus and moves laterally until capsular release has been effected from the mid-portion of the humerus to the lateral intermuscular septum (Fig. 17.2). The proximal 1 to 2 cm of capsule are excised to prevent recurrent scarring. Using switching sticks, the surgeon switches portals so that the arthroscope is positioned in the proximal anterolateral portal and the shaver is placed through the proximal medial portal (Fig. 17.3). Then anterior capsular excision is completed from the mid-portion of the humerus to the medial intermuscular septum (Fig. 17.4). Extension beyond the insertion of the septum into the medial humeral cortex should be avoided because of the risk of injuring the ulnar nerve.

Upon completion of release, the muscle fibers of the brachialis should be visible from the medial septum to the lateral septum in the area of proximal capsular insertion (Figs. 17.2 and 17.4). Capsular release is completed when the anterior capsular structures are no longer tight, a posterior block to extension has been encountered, or brachialis fibers are directly visible from medial to lateral along the anterior humeral cortex.

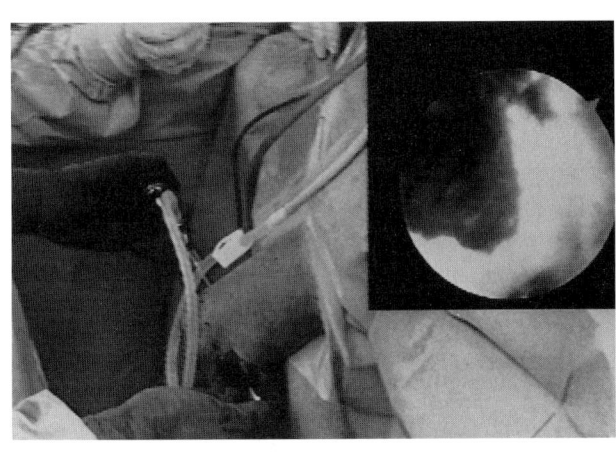

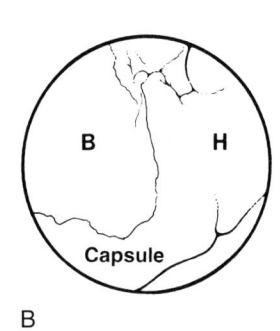

FIGURE 17.2. Arthroscopic view of the completed lateral portion of an anterior capsular release. The arthroscope is positioned within the proximal medial portal, and a working cannula is positioned through the proximal anterolateral portal. The arthroscopic inset shows the humeral cortex on right, the released capsule is located inferiorly, and the brachialis fibers are in the upper left quadrant. (A) Exterior and arthroscopic views. (B) Line drawing. B, brachialis fibers; H, humerus.

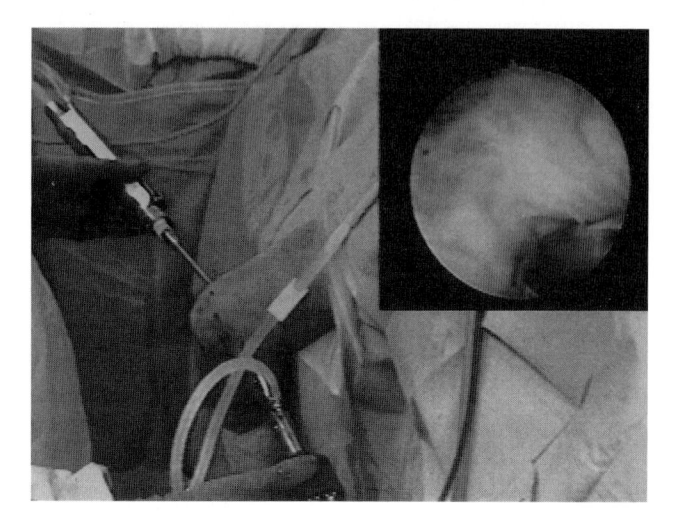

FIGURE 17.3. Arthroscopic view of the elbow before the surgeon begins the proximal medial portion of an anterior capsular release. The arthroscope is positioned within the proximal anterolateral portal, and the shaver is positioned through the proximal medial portal. In the arthroscopic inset, note the thickened, fibrotic anterior capsule adherent to the medial humeral cortex. The capsule is in the upper right quadrant, the humeral cortex is on the left, and the shaver blade is in the lower right quadrant.

During the anterior capsular release, the surgeon must maintain the shaver blade in close contact with the anterior aspect of the humerus at all times and must confirm that the arthroscope and shaver are within the elbow joint. Failure to observe these principles can lead to injury of the surrounding neurovascular structures.

After completing the anterior capsular release, the surgeon can remove the instrumentation from the anterior portion of the joint and can use one of the anterior portals for inflow. Posterolateral and posterocentral portals are established. The arthroscope is initially positioned through the posterolateral portal with a full-radius resector positioned through the posterocentral portal. Any adhesion or scar tissue within the olecranon fossa is removed. Next, bony spurs on the olecranon can be debrided with a burr or notchplasty blade. The surgeon continues to excise these osteophytes until he or she can move the patient's elbow into full extension (Fig. 17.5). The surgeon must remove all osteophytes from the medial and lateral aspects of the olecranon. Posterior capsular adhesions can be debrided from the posterior-superior portion of the elbow joint. Debridement of these adhesions between the triceps tendon and the posterior humerus should allow increased elbow flexion.

When the debridement of the posterior aspect of the joint is complete, the surgeon addresses the lateral and medial gutters. With the arthroscope in the posterocentral portal and the shaver in the posterolateral portal, he or she excises adhesions from the proximal to the distal portion of the lateral gutter. A straight lateral or soft-spot portal may be needed to complete debridement of the posterior radiocapitellar joint, the posterior radioulnar joint, or a prominent posterolateral plica (Figs. 17.6 and 17.7). Debridement of the medial gutter is performed with the arthroscope positioned within the posterolateral portal and the shaver positioned within the posterocentral portal. A fully hooded shaver should be used during this portion of the debridement to prevent ulnar nerve injury.

Persistent bony block to extension after debridement of the olecranon fossa and excision of olecranon osteophytes is an indication for an olecranon fossa fenestration. At the suggestion of Outerbridge, Kashiwagi originally described fenestration of the olecranon fossa, or the Outerbridge–Kashiwagi (O–K) procedure.[32] The thickened bone between the coronoid and olecranon fossa, which contributes to impingement and a reduction in elbow motion, is resected through an arthrotomy. A drill is used to fenestrate the floor of the olecranon fossa, providing a communication between the olecranon and the coronoid fossa. This opening is widened to produce a window that is approximately 1.5 cm in diameter, which

FIGURE 17.4. Arthroscopic view of the completed medial portion of an anterior capsular release. The humeral cortex is in the upper left quadrant, the released capsule is located inferiorly, and brachialis fibers are on the right. (A) Arthroscopic view. (B) Line drawing. H, humerus; B, brachialis fibers.

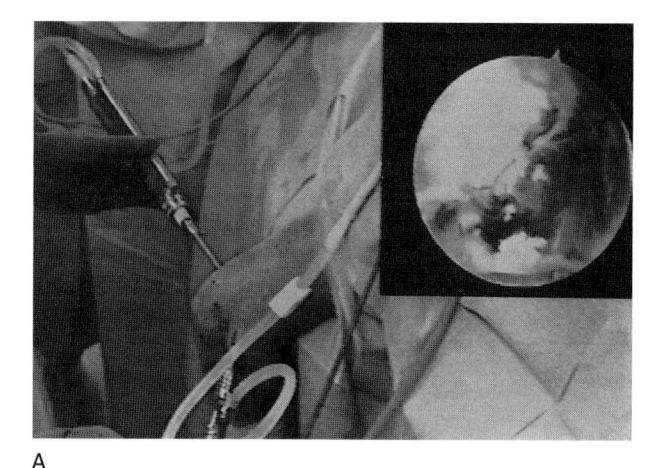

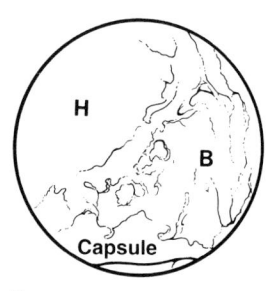

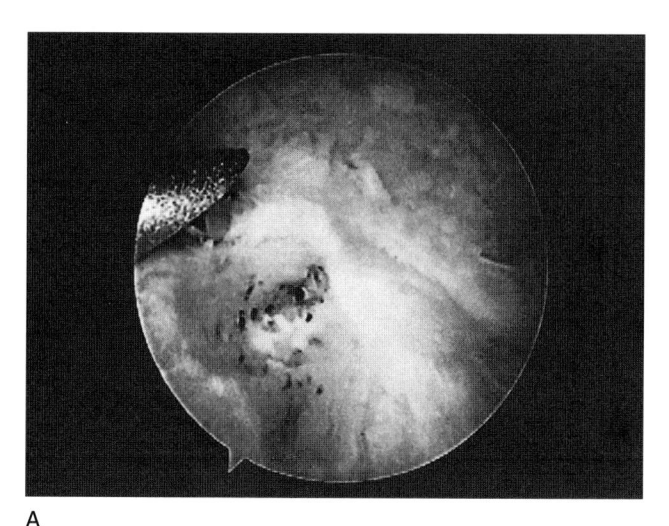

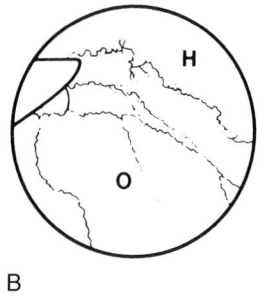

FIGURE 17.5. Arthroscopic view of excision of a prominent olecranon osteophyte. The arthroscope is positioned within the posterolateral portal, and the shaver is positioned posterocentrally. The abraded olecranon is in the inferior half of this view, and the distal humerus is located superiorly. (A) Arthroscopic view. (B) Line drawing. H, humerus; O, olecranon.

corresponds to the original shape and size of the olecranon fossa.

Open ulnohumeral arthroplasty as Morrey[33] described is a modification of Kashiwagi's O–K procedure. By working through the humeral fenestration, Morrey performed an open osteotomy of the olecranon tip and removal of loose bodies from the olecranon fossa, and he excised coronoid process osteophytes and removed anterior loose bodies by working through the humeral fenestration. Morrey also used an approach that elevated the medial triceps insertion, rather than split the triceps tendon as Kashiwagi described.

We perform a variation of Morrey's and Kashiwagi's techniques.[33] We use the arthroscope to create a fenestration without an arthrotomy. In our technique, while visualizing through a posterolateral portal, the surgeon places a 5-mm drill bit in the center of the olecranon fossa through the posterocentral portal. He or she drills from back to front at an angle toward the center of the coronoid fossa to connect the olecranon fossa with the coronoid fossa (see Fig. 18.7). The intersection of the long axis of the humerus with the inflow cannula positioned in the anterior portal provides a guide for proper orientation of the drill. After assessing the location and depth of this channel connecting the two fossae, the surgeon uses an aggressive arthroscopic shaver to enlarge the hole until full flexion and extension can be achieved. This enlargement requires that a concentric hole be established in the olecranon fossa (see Fig. 18.8). If orientation or other technical considerations make arthroscopic fenestration difficult or impossible, the surgeon should be willing to perform an open fenestration of the olecranon fossa instead. A Cloward drill should be available in case this procedure becomes necessary. In addition, a mini-fluoroscopic unit is valuable not only in assessing the position and adequacy of arthroscopic olecranon fossa fenestration, but also in the evaluation of an arthroscopic radial head excision.

At the completion of the procedure, the surgeon inserts drains for postoperative decompression of the joint. The lateral soft-spot portal is sutured; the remaining portals are left open. After the surgeon makes a final determination of range of motion, sterile bandages are applied. A soft-tissue dressing is applied before the patient is extubated.

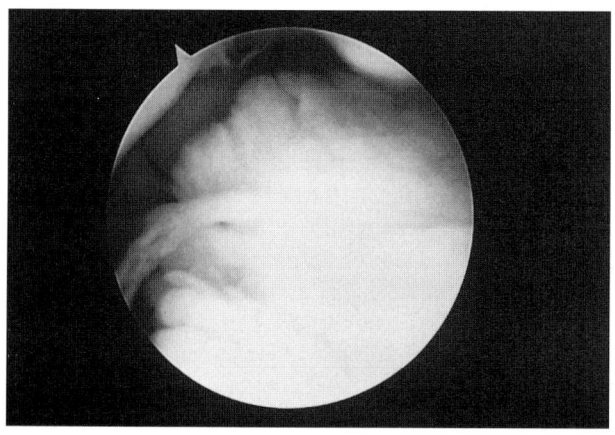

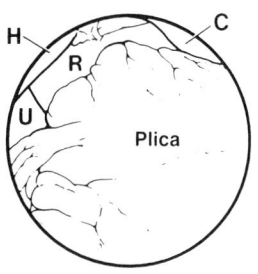

FIGURE 17.6. Arthroscopic view of a prominent, fibrotic posterolateral plica. The arthroscope is positioned within the posterocentral portal with visualization from posterior to anterior along the posterolateral gutter. The radial head can be visualized just beyond the plica, which occupies most of this view. (A) Arthroscopic view. (B) Line drawing. H, humerus; R, radial head; C, capitellum; U, ulna.

FIGURE 17.7. Arthroscopic view after excision of fibrotic posterolateral plica. The radial head can now be well visualized in the center of view. The capitellum is located superiorly, and the proximal radioulnar joint is in the lower left quadrant. (A) Arthroscopic view. (B) Line drawing. C, capitellum; R, radial head.

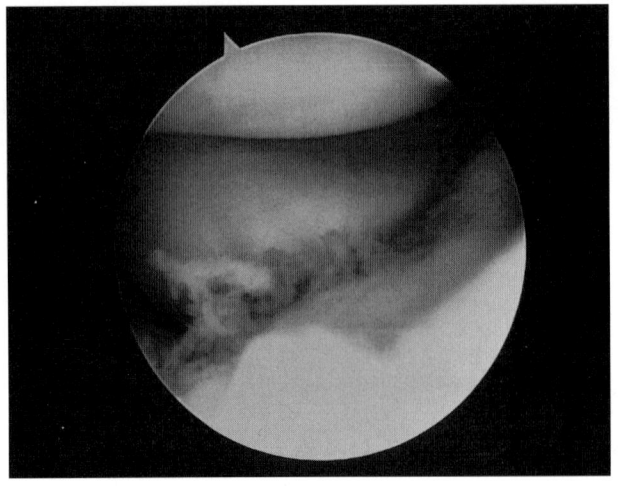

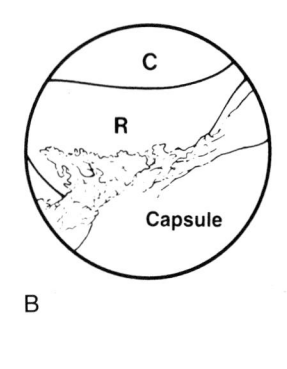

POSTOPERATIVE MANAGEMENT

Continuous passive motion (CPM) is begun in the recovery room and continued until the patient is discharged.[27,34] The patient remains in the hospital for 2 to 3 days to receive active physical therapy three times each day. Upon discharge, an aggressive active and passive physical therapy program is maintained, with static splinting or CPM used at night and during rest. Night splinting (or CPM) may be discontinued 3 weeks after surgery if the patient has maintained adequate range of motion in the elbow. Active and passive physical therapy are continued daily or twice daily for 6 weeks after surgery. Patients whose jobs require moderate or heavy use of the extremity can return to work when they can perform their duties without pain (approximately 8 weeks). Others can return within a few days. Patients who lose motion within the first 3 weeks after surgery are hospitalized to have gentle manipulation performed again. The standard postoperative protocol is then reinitiated.

PRECAUTIONS

The risks to the neurovascular structures are increased during arthroscopic surgery secondary to previous injury and scarring with neurovascular involvement. The surgeon must have a thorough understanding of the pathogenesis of the contracture and of how it alters the anatomy. When the elbow joint is contracted, it may not distend normally with insufflation, and neurovascular structures may not be displaced safely from the elbow joint. The anterior neurovascular structures (e.g., median nerve, brachial artery) should be protected proximally by the brachialis muscle. Despite previous surgical procedures or injury, the medial epicondyle and medial intermuscular septum typically are preserved. These structures can serve as a guide to the initial entrance to the elbow joint through a proximal medial portal.

Protecting the ulnar nerve is of utmost importance during medial portal placement. The surgeon establishes the proximal medial portal only after adequately identifying the medial intermuscular septum. During debridement of the medial gutter, the surgeon must be careful. Release of adhesions within this area should be accomplished with a hooded non-end-cutting shaver so that the covered portion of the blade is always directed toward the ulnar nerve and the open shaver face is directed toward the elbow joint. If the ulnar nerve is displaced posteromedially due to an adherent capsule or extensive olecranon deformity, it is at increased risk of injury when the surgeon creates the posterocentral portal. Therefore, the surgeon must direct the cannula into the olecranon fossa and avoid medial displacement that can injure the ulnar nerve.

Trauma or contracture involving the lateral structures of the elbow can cause capsular hypertrophy in this area and subsequently can bind the posterior interosseous nerve. Proximal anterolateral portal placement with the inside-out technique decreases the risk of posterior interosseous nerve injury. If the posterior interosseous nerve is tethered when it is adjacent to the anterior joint capsule in the distal portion of the elbow, it is at increased risk of injury during anterior debridement. The bound nerve is at increased risk for stretch injury or transection during the procedure. Lateral capsular excision, therefore, should remain proximal to the radiocapitellar joint, avoiding the inferior aspect of the anterolateral joint capsule to minimize risk to the posterior interosseous nerve.

During the anterior capsular release, the surgeon must remember the relationship of the capsule and the brachialis muscle to the anterior neurovascular structures. The brachialis muscle separates the anterior capsule from the median nerve and brachial artery. The surgeon performs arthroscopic release and capsular excision within the joint only until brachialis muscle fibers are visible. Shaver blades and cutting instruments are maintained in close proximity to the humerus at all times to avoid straying anteriorly and damaging these neurovascular structures.

RESULTS

Many authors have reported acceptable results with open surgical release of the arthrofibrotic elbow.[25,29,35,36] However, the procedure has advantages that include increased soft-tissue trauma and postoperative scarring of the capsule and anterior structures. These conditions add to the risk of recurrent contracture, and they increase the time interval before aggressive physical therapy programs can be initiated. Completely evaluating and addressing the intra-articular pathologic lesions during these open techniques is difficult without considerable added dissection.

In contrast to open surgical release, the arthroscopic technique allows the surgeon to completely evaluate and treat intra-articular pathologic lesions. Debridement of intra-articular adhesions not only increases the range of motion, but also helps to decrease the pain associated with arthroscopic release. The decreased surgical trauma and postoperative scarring reduce the risk of recurrent contracture and allow for early aggressive physical therapy.

The results of arthroscopic capsular release for ankylosis of the elbow are equal to or better than the results of open procedures. In 1994, Byrd[19] reported his results of arthroscopic treatment for arthrofibrosis after type I radial head fractures. His patients gained an average of 30° of extension (from 41° to 11°) and 14° of flexion (from 124° to 138°). He also noted that pain significantly diminished in his patients.

The senior author's (FHS) experience with arthroscopic release for arthrofibrosis of the elbow has continued since the initial report by Jones and Savoie.[30] Currently, 53 capsular releases have been performed in 53 patients. The average preoperative range of motion of these patients was 46° of extension to 96° of flexion. Postoperative motion averaged 5° of extension to 138° of flexion, representing a 41° improvement in extension and a 42° improvement in flexion. The patients also had significant increases in pronation (from 75° to 82°) and supination (from 47° to 86°). The procedure failed in two of our patients. One patient underwent another arthroscopic capsular excision with continued aggressive physical therapy, but did not maintain normal range of motion despite obtaining normal motion at the time of surgery. Range of motion at final follow-up was 0° of extension to 100° of flexion, and the patient had no further surgical intervention. The other failure occurred in a patient who was unable to comply with postoperative rehabilitation due to personal conflicts. Although this person's range of motion improved significantly, from a fixed 90° of flexion contracture to a range of motion of 45° of extension to 100° of flexion, with marked decrease in pain, we consider this procedure a failure because the patient had significant limitations of motion. The only significant complication in this series was a previously reported posterior interosseous nerve disruption.[30]

SUMMARY

Arthroscopic capsular release of the ankylosed elbow is a distinct advance in the management of elbow pathologic lesions. The ability to evaluate and treat intra-articular pathologic lesions and extrinsic capsular and collateral ligament contracture with arthroscopy offers significant advantages over open techniques. The advantages of limited skin incisions, limited soft-tissue dissection, and increased visualization allow better definition of the lesions and treatment directed specifically at involved structures. They also allow the patient to begin and maintain an aggressive physical therapy program immediately after surgery, decreasing the risk of anterior scarring and recurrent contracture.

Arthroscopic capsular release is a technically demanding procedure that should be attempted only by surgeons with extensive experience using arthroscopic surgery of the elbow. Meticulous attention to detail is required. However, with proper patient selection and surgical technique, excellent results can be expected.

REFERENCES

1. Protzman RR. Dislocation of the elbow joint. *J Bone Joint Surg* 1978;60A:539–541.
2. Bede WB, Lefebvre AR, Rosman MA. Fracture of the medial humeral epicondyle in children. *Can J Surg* 1975;18:137–142.
3. Saito T, Koshino T, Okamoto R, Horiuchi S. Radial synovectomy with muscle release for the rheumatoid elbow. *Acta Orthop Scan* 1986;57:71–73.
4. Huang TT, Blackwell SJ, Lewis SR. Ten years of experience in managing patients with burn contractures of the axilla, elbow, wrist, and knee joints. *Plast Reconstr Surg* 1978;61:70–76.
5. Sherk HH. Treatment of severe rigid contractures of cerebral palsied upper limbs. *Clin Orthop* 1977;125:151–155.
6. Freehafer A. Flexion and supination deformities of the elbow in tetraplegics. *Paraplegia* 1977;15:221–225.
7. Søjbjerg JO. The stiff elbow. *Acta Orthop Scand* 1996;67:626–631.
8. Mohan K. Myositis ossificans traumatica of the elbow. *Int Surg* 1972;57:475–478.
9. Cooney WP. Contractures of the elbow. In: Morrey BF, ed. *The elbow and its disorders*. Philadelphia: WB Saunders; 1993:464–475.
10. Tucker K. Some aspects of post-traumatic elbow stiffness. *Injury* 1977;9:216.
11. Thorndike A Jr. Myositis ossificans traumatica. *J Bone Joint Surg* 1940;22:315–323.

12. Buxton St JD. Ossification in the ligaments of the elbow joint. *J Bone Joint Surg* 1938;20:709–714.
13. Gutierre LS. A contribution to the study of the limiting factors of elbow extension. *Acta Anat* 1964;56:146.
14. Morrey BF, An KN. Articular and ligamentous contributions to the stability of the elbow joint. *Am J Sports Med* 1983;11: 315–319.
15. Wheeler D, Linscheid RL. Fracture–dislocations of the elbow. *Clin Orthop* 1967;50:95–106.
16. Linscheid RL, Wheeler D. Elbow dislocations. *JAMA* 1965; 194:1171–1176.
17. Silva JF. The problems relating to old dislocations and the restriction on elbow movement. *Acta Orthop Belg* 1975;41:399–411.
18. Jones GS, Geissler WB. Complications associated with nondisplaced radial head fractures. *Orthop Trans* 1993;17(2):438.
19. Byrd JW. Elbow arthroscopy for arthrofibrosis after type I radial head fractures. *Arthroscopy* 1994;10:162–165.
20. Roberts PH. Dislocation of the elbow. *Br J Surg* 1969;56: 806–815.
21. Thompson HC III, Garcia A. Myositis ossificans: Aftermath of elbow injuries. *Clin Orthop* 1967;50:129–134.
22. Morrey BF, Askew LJ, Chao EY. A biomechanical study of normal functional elbow motion. *J Bone Joint Surg* 1981;63A: 872–877.
23. Green DP, McCoy H. Turnbuckle orthotic correction of elbow-flexion contractures after acute injuries. *J Bone Joint Surg* 1979;61A:1092–1095.
24. Morrey BF. Post-traumatic contracture of the elbow. Operative treatment, including distraction arthroplasty. *J Bone Joint Surg* 1990;72A:601–618.
25. Urbaniak JR, Hansen PE, Beissinger SF, Aitken MS. Correction of post-traumatic flexion contracture of the elbow by anterior capsulotomy. *J Bone Joint Surg* 1985;67A:1160–1164.
26. Itoh Y, Saegusa K, Ishiguro T, Horiuchi Y, Sasaki T, Uchinishi K. Operation for the stiff elbow. *Int Orthop* 1989;13:263–268.
27. Gates HS III, Sullivan FL, Urbaniak JR. Anterior capsulotomy and continuous passive motion in the treatment of post-traumatic flexion contracture of the elbow. A prospective study. *J Bone Joint Surg* 1992;74A:1229–1234.
28. Redden JF, Stanley D. Arthroscopic fenestration of the olecranon fossa in the treatment of osteoarthritis of the elbow. *Arthroscopy* 1993;9:14–16.
29. Søjbjerg JO, Kjærsgaard-Andersen P, Johanssen HV, Sneppen O. Release of the stiff elbow followed by continuous passive motion and indomethacin treatment. *J Shoulder Elbow Surg* 1995;4:S20.
30. Jones GS, Savoie FH III. Arthroscopic capsular release of flexion contractures (arthrofibrosis) of the elbow. *Arthroscopy* 1993; 9:277–283.
31. Savoie FH, Field LD. *Arthroscopy of the elbow*. New York: Churchill Livingstone; 1996.
32. Kashiwagi D. Articular changes of the osteoarthritic elbow, especially about the fossa olecrani. *J Jap Orthop Assoc* 1978; 52:1367–1382.
33. Morrey BF. Primary degenerative arthritis of the elbow: Treatment by ulnohumeral arthroplasty. *J Bone Joint Surg* 1992; 74B:409–413.
34. Breen TF, Gelberman RH, Ackerman GN. Elbow flexion contractures: Treatment by anterior release and continuous passive motion. *J Hand Surg* 1988;13B:286–287.
35. Husband JB, Hastings H II. The lateral approach for operative release of post-traumatic contracture of the elbow. *J Bone Joint Surg* 1990;72A:1353–1358.
36. Tsuge K, Mizuseki T. Debridement arthroplasty for advanced primary osteoarthritis of the elbow: Results of a new technique used for 29 elbows. *J Bone Joint Surg* 1994;76B:641–646.

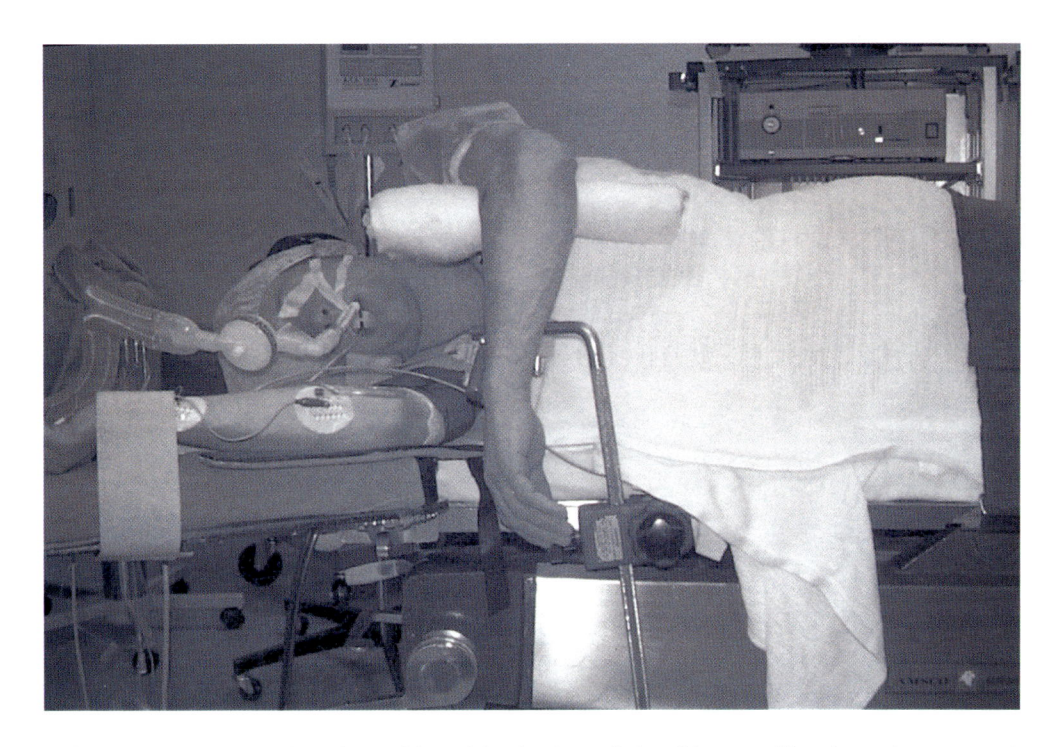

FIGURE 15.1. The patient is positioned in the lateral decubitus position for arthroscopy. A tourniquet is placed on the arm. The arm hangs free over a padded bolster with the elbow flexed to 90°.

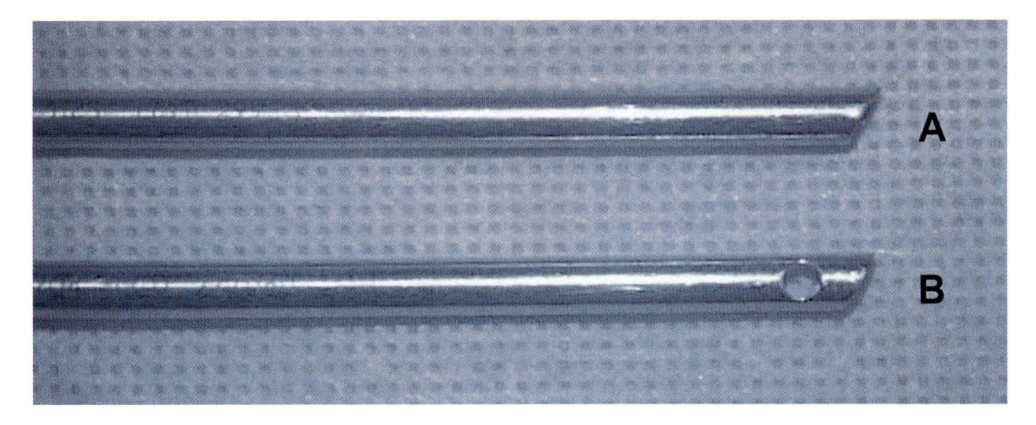

FIGURE 15.2. (A) The arthroscopic cannula should have no side fenestrations. (B) Side fenestrations allow extracapsular fluid extravasation.

FIGURE 15.3. The radiocapitellar joint is the initial landmark in the lateral aspect of the anterior compartment. The capitellum is visualized with elbow flexion and extension. A portion of the concave articular surface of the radial head usually can be seen.

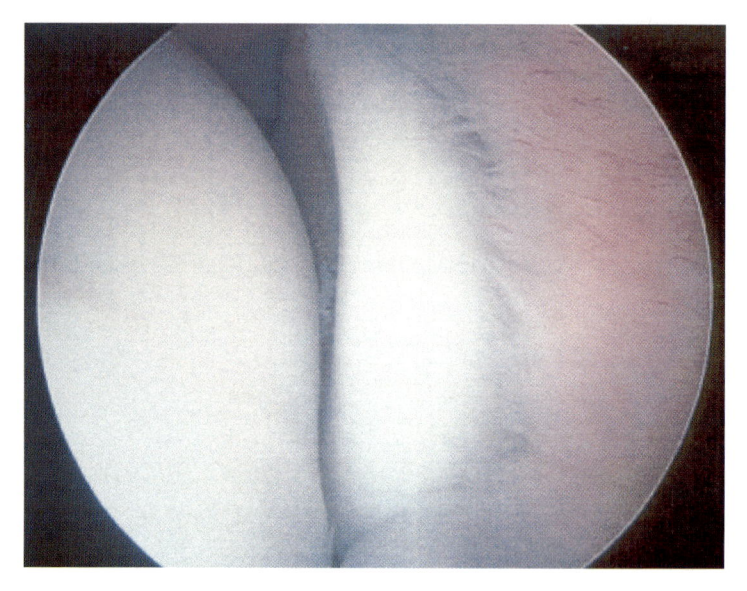

FIGURE 15.4. The proximal radioulnar joint is visualized as the arthroscope is withdrawn (arrows). The surgeon can view the marginal circumference of the radial head by taking the arm from pronation to supination (*).

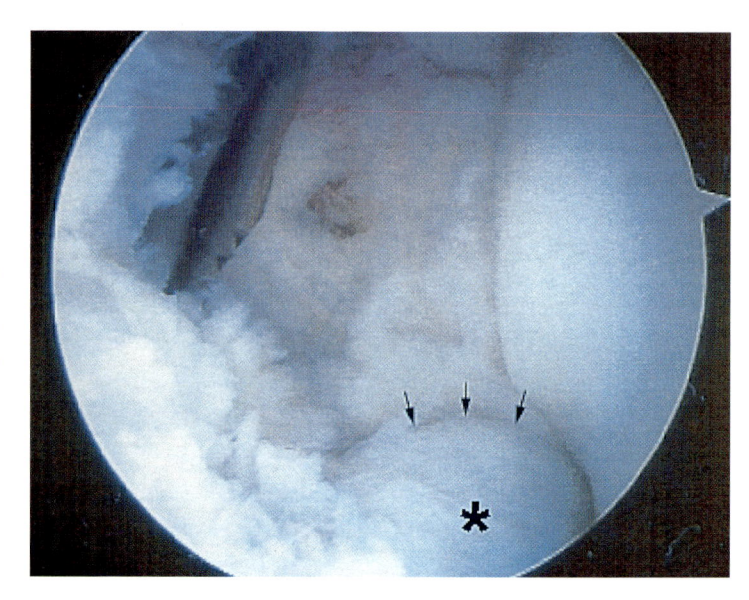

FIGURE 15.5. The initial landmark in the medial aspect of the anterior compartment is the ulnohumeral articulation. The coronoid process (*) should be inspected for osteophytes, and the articulation between the coronoid fossa and trochlea should be examined. Extension of the elbow allows visualization of a portion of the trochlear articular surface.

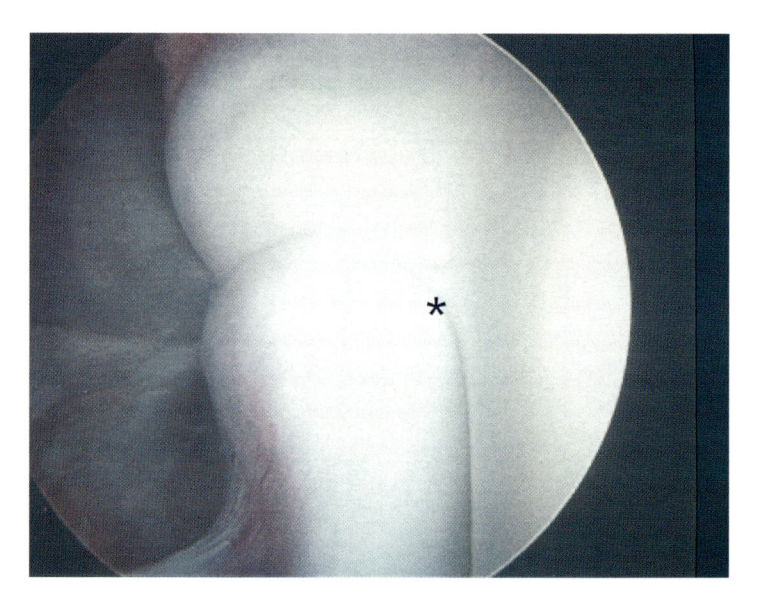

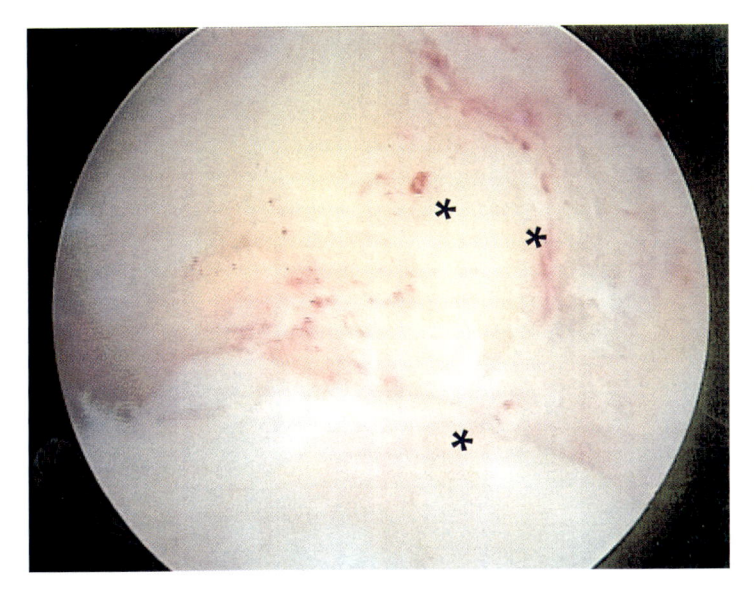

FIGURE 15.6. The articulation between the olecranon process (*) and the trochlea is visualized in the posterior compartment. The articular surface of the posterior aspect of the trochlea is best visualized in flexion. With the elbow in extension, the articulation between the olecranon and the olecranon fossa (**) is assessed.

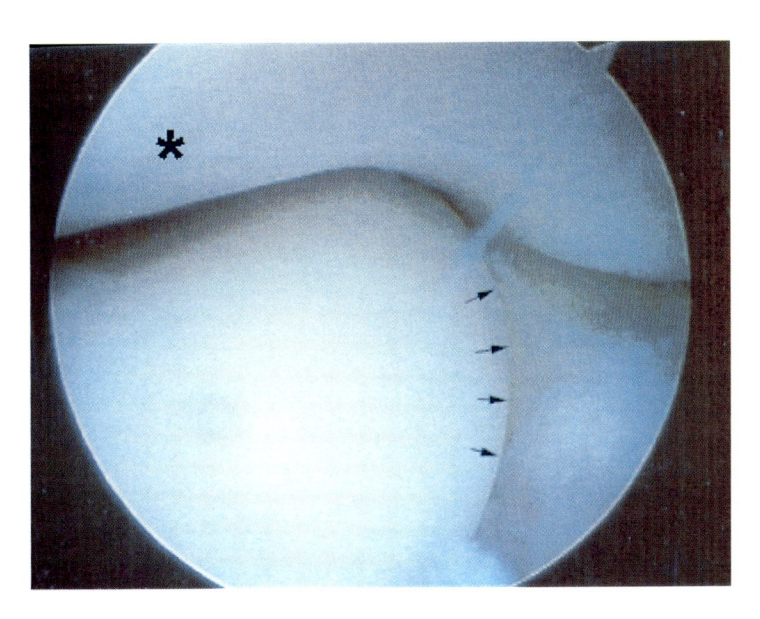

FIGURE 15.7. The inferior portion of the capitellum (*) and inferior aspect of the proximal radioulnar joint (arrows) are best visualized from the direct lateral (soft spot) portal.

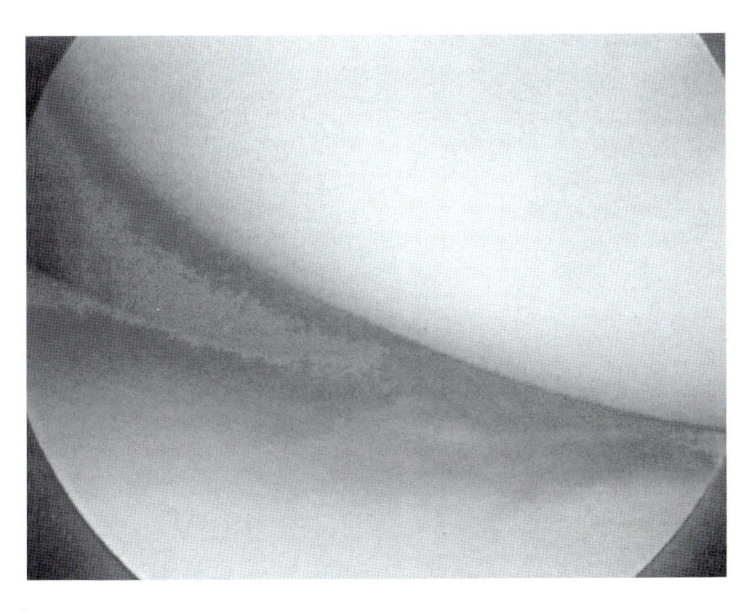

FIGURE 15.8. In a patient who has posterolateral rotary instability, the ulna rotates away from the distal humerus when the forearm is in forced supination. This rotation is visualized well from the direct lateral portal.

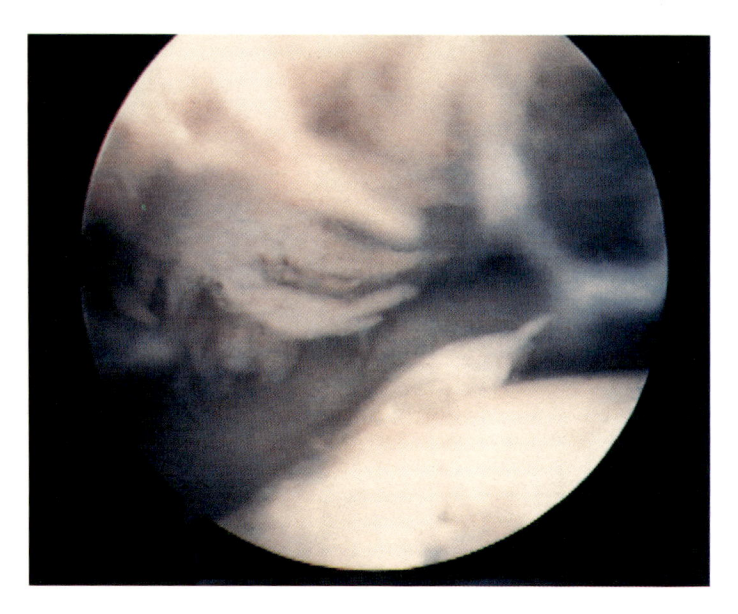

FIGURE 16.1. Arthroscopic appearance, as viewed from anterolateral portal, of osteochondritis dissecans. Fragmentation of articular cartilage from the capitellum is seen in the bottom half of the field of view. Above, synovitis is prevalent.

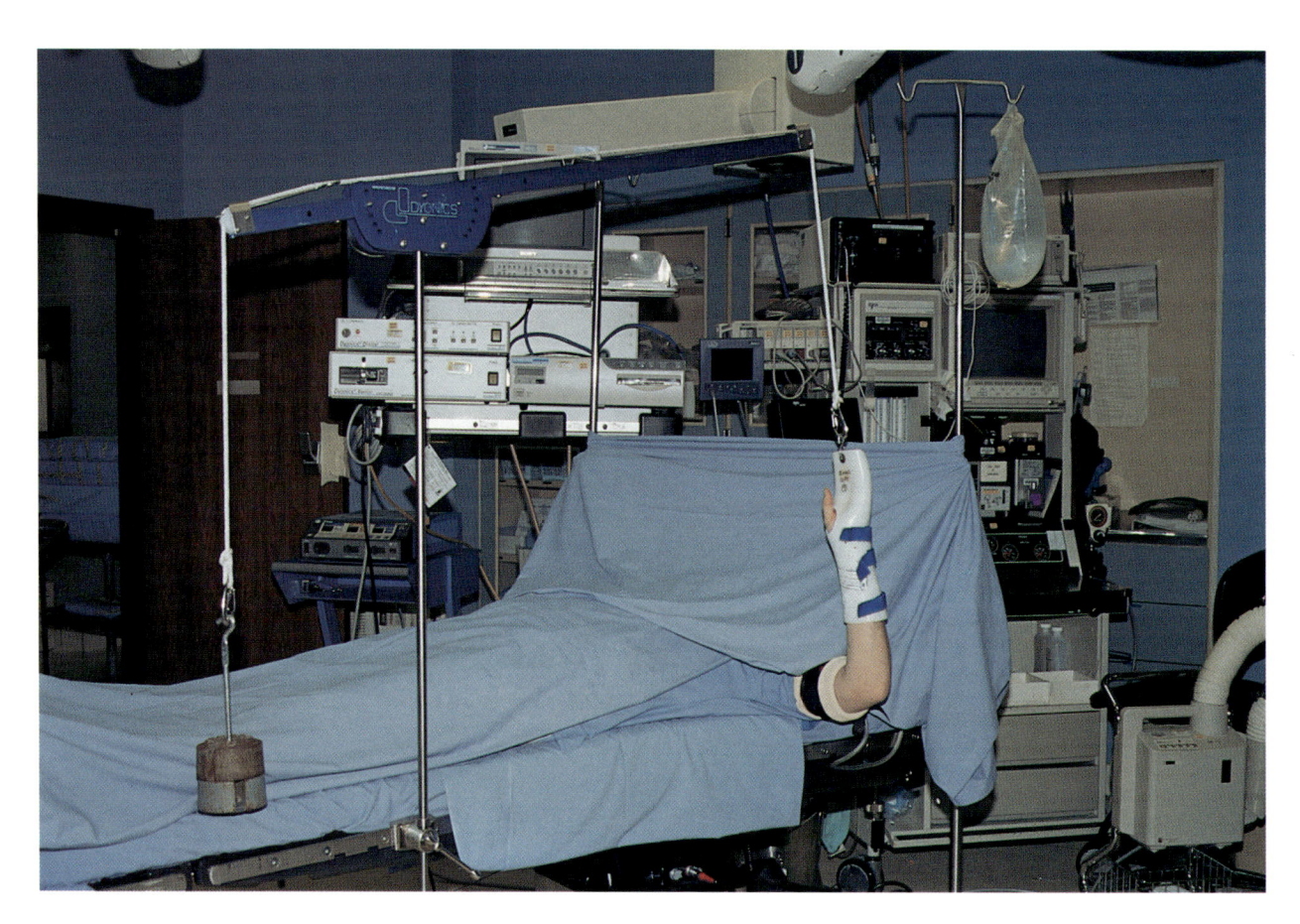

FIGURE 16.3. Operating room setup and patient positioning. The patient's arm is suspended with 10 lb of traction in 90° of flexion.

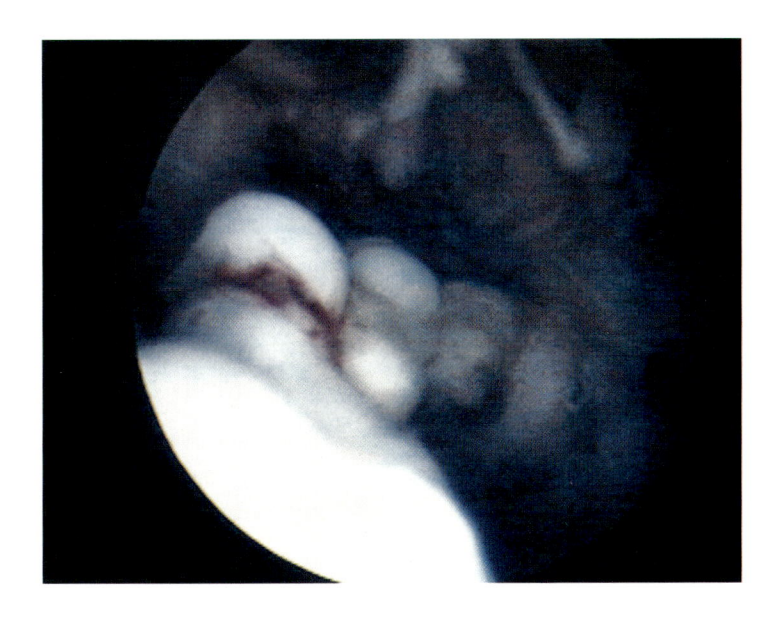

FIGURE 16.4. Small osteochondral loose bodies adherent to synovium in the anteromedial aspect of the elbow as viewed from the anterolateral portal.

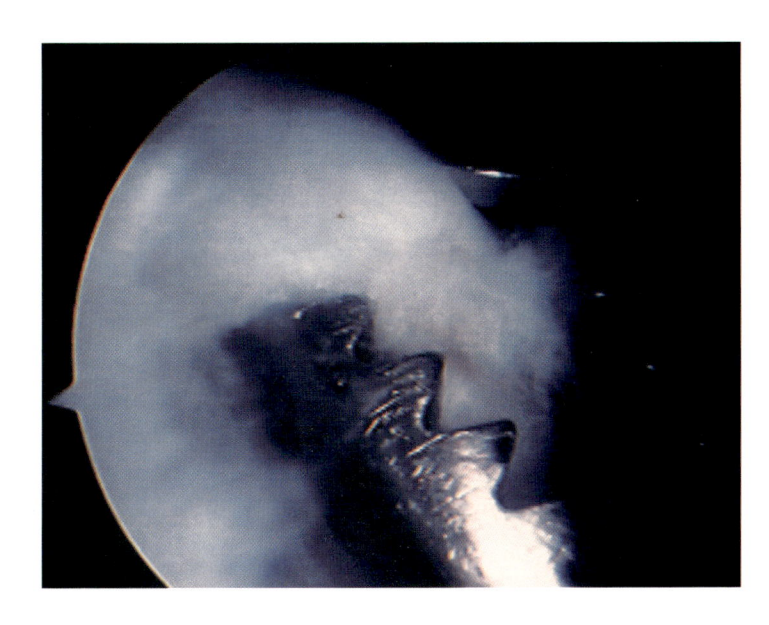

FIGURE 16.5. Removal of large loose body using a grasping forceps.

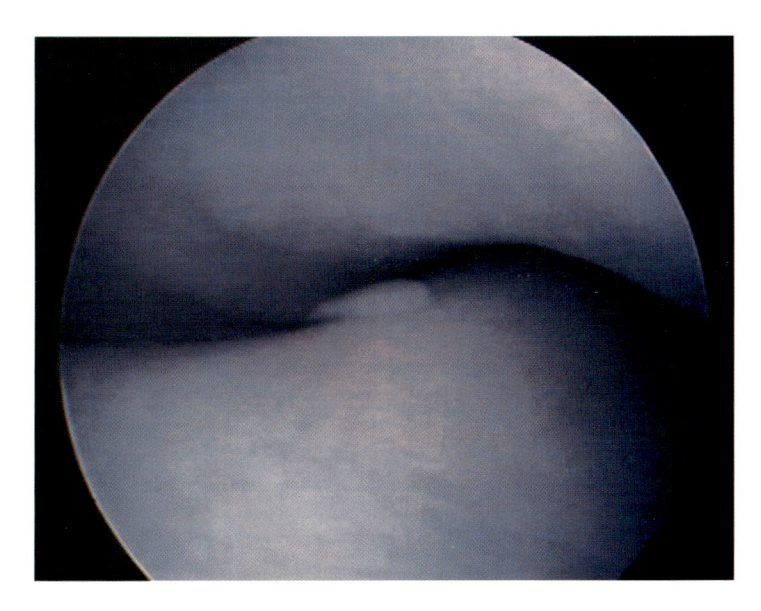

FIGURE 16.6. Small loose body in the ulnohumeral joint as viewed through the posterolateral portal.

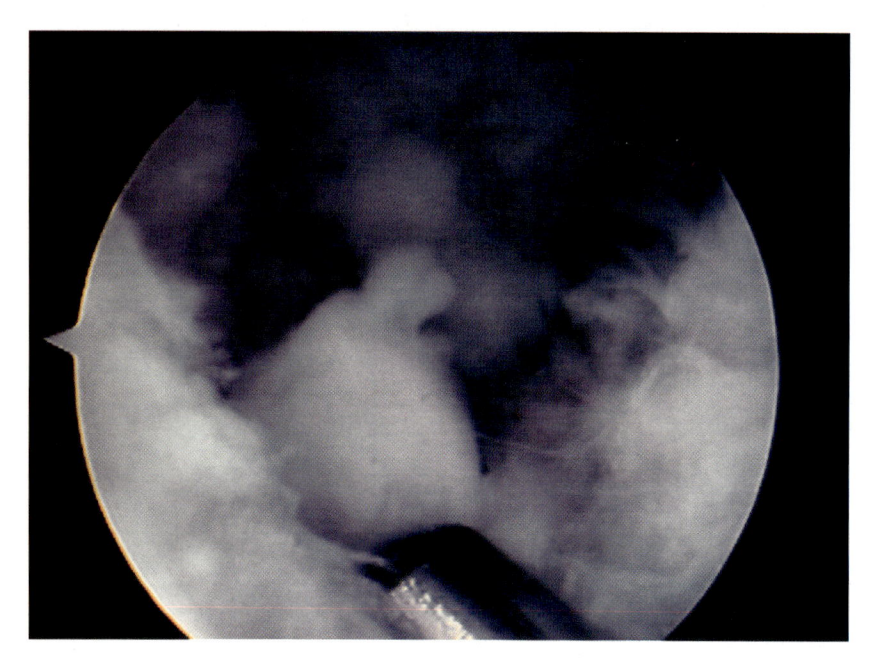

FIGURE 16.7. Large loose body in the posterior compartment as viewed from the posterolateral portal.

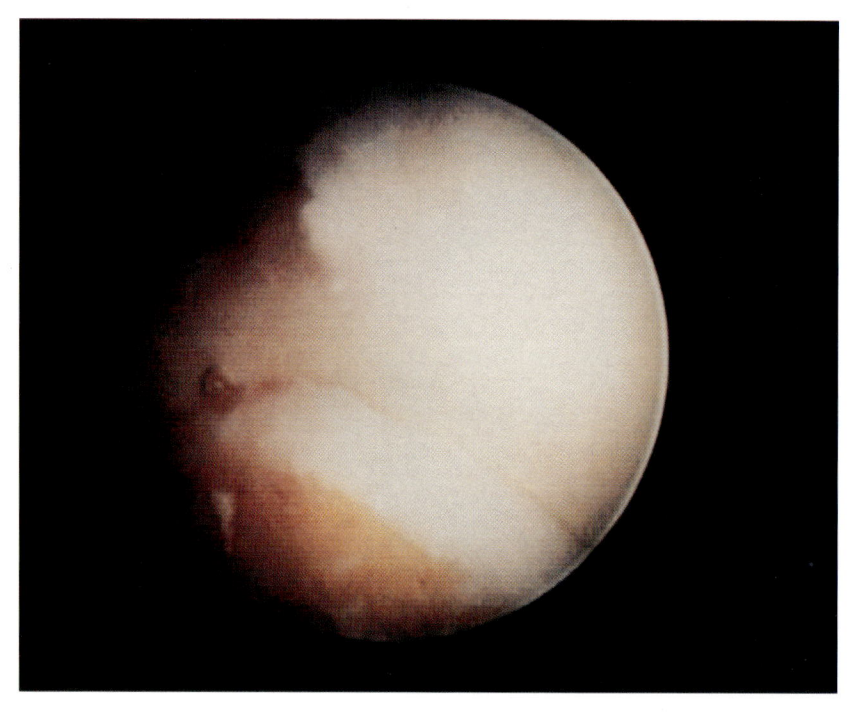

FIGURE 16.8. Posteromedial osteophyte in the elbow of a throwing athlete as viewed from the posterolateral portal.

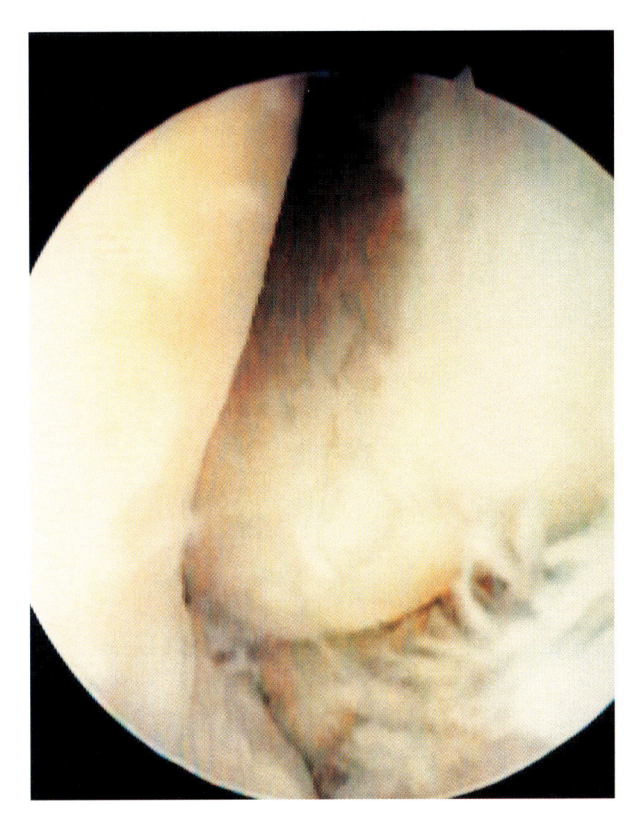

FIGURE 18.4. An arthroscopic photograph of the radiocapitellar joint as viewed from the proximal anteromedial portal.

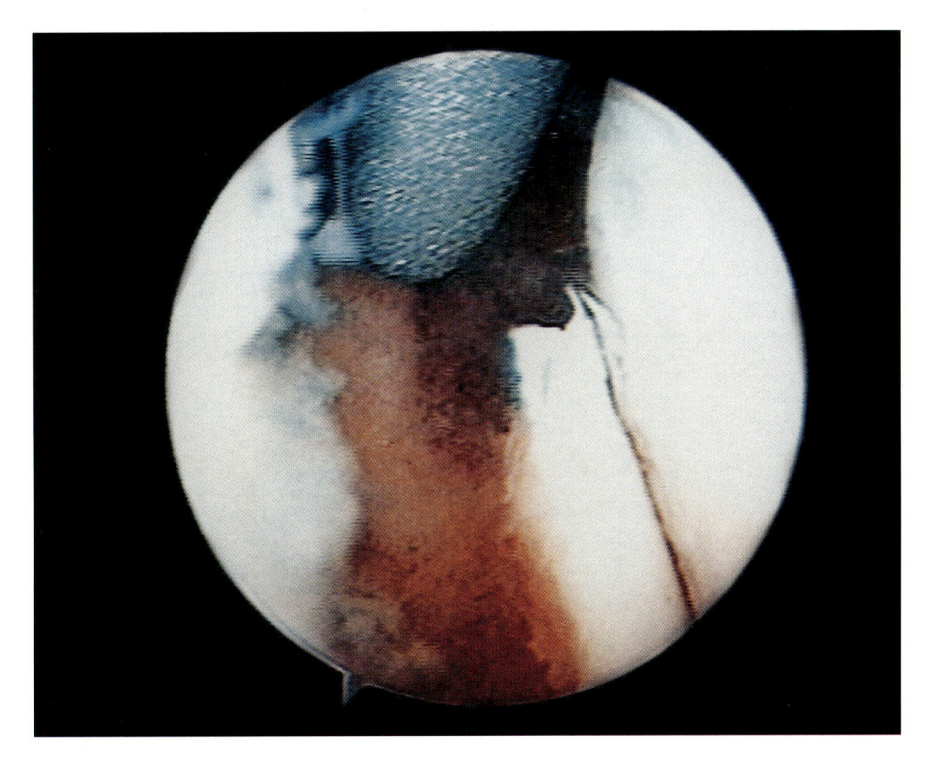

FIGURE 18.5. While supinating and pronating the forearm, the surgeon accomplishes progressive removal of the radial head.

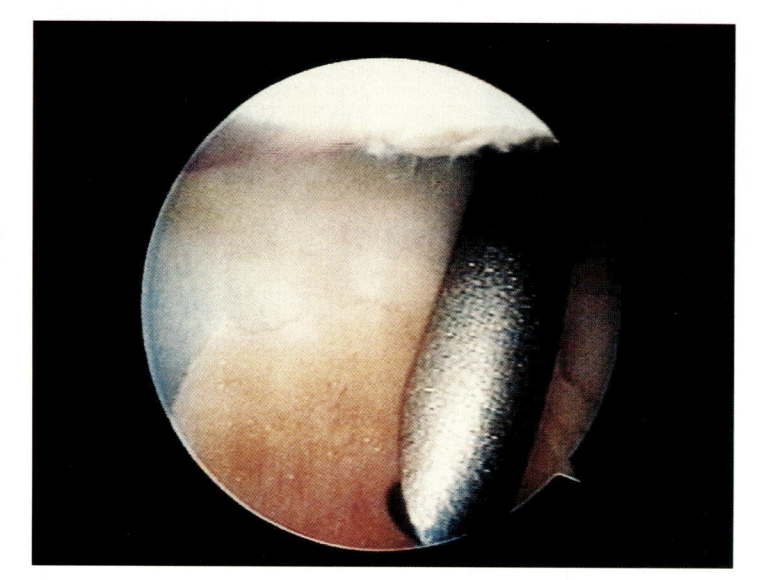

FIGURE 18.6. While visualizing the joint through the anteromedial portal, the surgeon uses the direct lateral, or soft spot, portal to complete radial head excision.

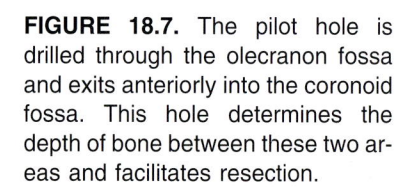

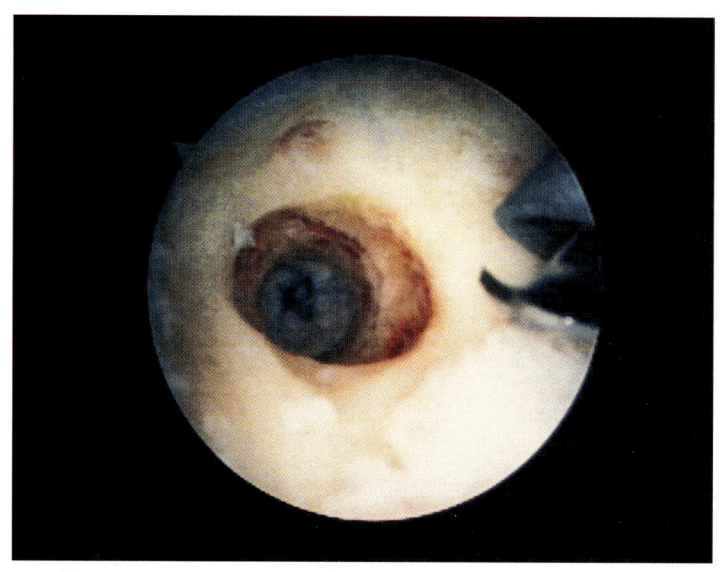

FIGURE 18.7. The pilot hole is drilled through the olecranon fossa and exits anteriorly into the coronoid fossa. This hole determines the depth of bone between these two areas and facilitates resection.

FIGURE 18.8. The previously made drill hole is enlarged until it can accommodate the coronoid in flexion and the olecranon in extension. The hole can be extended until the medial and lateral columns of the distal humerus are encountered.

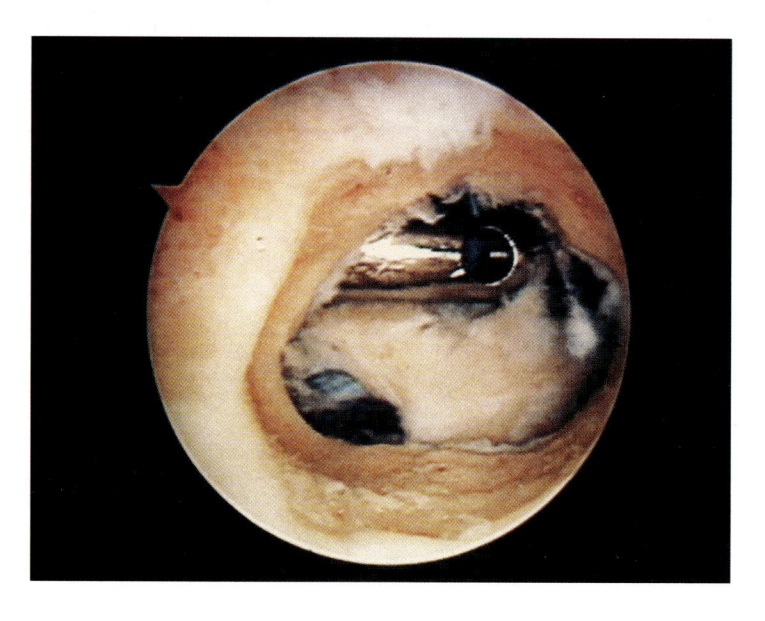

CHAPTER 18

Arthroscopic Radial Head Resection

Larry D. Field and Felix H. Savoie III

INTRODUCTION

The role of the arthroscope in the management of elbow disorders continues to evolve. Advances in instrumentation and technique have expanded the indications for arthroscopic treatment. When indicated, radial head excision can be accomplished using an arthroscopic technique. Degeneration of the radiocapitellar joint that occurs following radial head fracture, in the presence of chronic valgus or posterolateral rotatory instability or following long-standing primary or inflammatory arthritis, often can be managed with arthroscopic surgery. Arthroscopic radial head excision offers several potential advantages. The ability to evaluate thoroughly and completely the anterior and posterior compartments of the elbow without an extensive arthrotomy minimizes the soft-tissue disruption, postoperative scarring, and capsular contracture. Arthroscopic excision preserves the capsule, annular ligament, and radial ulnohumeral ligament in their normal state. General arthroscopic techniques, such as lavage, debridement, spur excision, and synovectomy, also can be employed effectively at the time of radial head excision.

HISTORY

The signs and symptoms associated with radiocapitellar or proximal radioulnar joint degeneration are recognized easily sometimes, but often coexist with other elbow problems. Isolated radiocapitellar joint degeneration can occur subsequent to a radial head fracture. Even minimally displaced radial head fractures can result in persistent, significant symptoms. Malunited radial head fractures predispose the elbow not only to radiocapitellar joint degeneration, but also to proximal radioulnar joint changes. More often, symptoms of degeneration in the radiocapitellar joint constitute only a small part of the overall elbow symptom complex that often is seen in systemic illnesses, such as rheumatoid arthritis with progressive synovitis and joint destruction. Likewise, chronic valgus instability of the elbow in overhead athletes (i.e., athletes who participate in sports involving overhead motions) causes not only radiocapitellar joint degeneration, but also posteromedial gutter symptoms and osteophyte formation. Radiocapitellar joint degeneration that results from primary osteoarthritis can lead to symptoms, but the pain associated with ulnohumeral joint arthritic changes often dominates this clinical picture.

Patients who have symptoms of radiocapitellar joint degeneration generally report pain and loss of motion. Extremes of forearm rotation also cause pain. In our experience, maximal pronation causes greater pain than maximal supination, presumably due to some proximal migration of the radius in pronation. With pronation, ulnar variance becomes progressively more positive, thereby increasing the radiocapitellar compression load. Application of an axial load on the forearm combined with passive supination and pronation might aid the examiner in differentiating lateral epicondylitis from degenerative changes in the radiocapitellar joint as the source of pain in the lateral portion of the elbow. This test compresses the radiocapitellar joint and often causes pain when articular degeneration is responsible for symptoms, but it usually does not exacerbate lateral epicondylitis.

Some loss of motion can be detected when significant radiocapitellar joint degeneration is present. Again, isolated radiocapitellar joint changes are rare and usually are associated either with generalized degenerative changes resulting from osteoarthritis or with systemic disease. Loss of 30° or more of elbow extension is not uncommon and is seen more often than significant loss of elbow flexion. Loss of supination and pronation generally is mild except in advanced radiocapitellar joint degeneration. Conversely, posttraumatic radiocapitellar joint arthritis secondary to radial head malunion can cause extensive loss of forearm rotation. Motion that is lost as a result of an unrecognized or inadequately treated mechanical block due to radial head displacement generally does not improve over time. Such articular incongruity often leads to progressive degenerative changes and an increase in symptoms.

Patients who have radiocapitellar joint changes generally report activity-related pain and swelling in the elbow. Pain usually is centered near the lateral and posterolateral aspects of the elbow joint, but finding the exact location of the pain is difficult sometimes. Difficulty finding the location of the pain occurs particularly in radiocapitellar joint arthritis secondary to chronic valgus instability, because significant posteromedial gutter changes are common. Progressive degeneration of the elbow joint also can lead to loose-body formation in patients who have clinical and radiographic evidence of radiocapitellar arthritis, which can cause symptoms of locking, catching, and popping.

CLINICAL ANATOMY

The palpable radial head is located 1 cm distal to the lateral epicondyle, which is palpated easily and serves as an important landmark. The radial head is cylindrical in shape and has a central concavity to accommodate the convex capitellum. It articulates with the capitellum and is aligned concentrically in all radiographic planes. The radial head also articulates with the proximal ulna at the lesser sigmoid fossa; the annular ligament secures this articulation. The radial neck forms a 15° angle relative to the shaft in the area of the radial tuberosity. This radiocapitellar joint alignment allows approximately 150° of flexion and 160° of forearm rotation.[1-3]

Articular cartilage covers approximately 80% of the radial head's circumference. Palpating the radial head while passively rotating the forearm through supination and pronation can help the examiner to identify this structure. In addition, the radial tuberosity is just distal to the radial head, and the examiner can best palpate it with the patient's forearm in maximal pronation. Another important structure in the vicinity of the radiocapitellar joint is the posterolateral gutter. The examiner can best identify an intra-articular effusion in this area because of the thin capsule and absence of muscular coverage. Likewise, a normally occurring plica can become thickened and symptomatic as a result of radiocapitellar joint degeneration and osteophyte formation. If arthroscopic or open excision is carried out to treat radiocapitellar joint degeneration, the thickened and symptomatic plica might need to be excised as well.

The lateral collateral ligament complex is another important anatomic structure in the vicinity of the radiocapitellar joint. This complex comprises the radial collateral ligament, the lateral ulnar collateral ligament (UCL), the accessory lateral collateral ligament, and the annular ligament (Fig. 18.1).[4,5] This fan-shaped ligamentous complex originates from the lateral epicondyle and inserts onto the radial head, annular ligament, and margins of the anterior and posterior lesser sigmoid notch. The lateral UCL and the accessory lateral collateral ligament insert on the ulna at the crista musculi supinatoris just distal to the sigmoid notch. An understanding of the role of this lateral collateral ligament complex is important in assessing radiocapitellar joint stability. We have identified a number of patients in whom significant radiocapitellar joint degeneration has occurred secondary to chronic posterolateral rotatory instability. Recognition of this instability pattern is important in treating this condition.

The radiocapitellar joint serves as an important secondary restraint to valgus stress. The anterior bundle of the medial UCL serves as the primary restraint to valgus stress.[6-14] However, in the presence of an incompetent or disrupted anterior bundle, the radiocapitellar joint limits valgus opening. This increased radiocapitellar compression clinically is important, particularly in overhead-throwing athletes. Abnormal stresses on the articular surface lead to injury and degenerative changes with osteophyte formation that also can produce symptoms in the medial portion of the elbow. Pain in the lateral portion of the elbow can result from both radiocapitellar joint degeneration and asynchronous firing of the wrist extensor musculature. Glousman and colleagues[15] compared electromyographic data from a group of medial-UCL-insufficient pitchers with data from a group of uninjured pitchers and demonstrated that the extensor carpi radialis brevis and longus muscles showed greater activity in the injured pitchers. This increased activity not only might contribute to further joint injury through its asynchronous

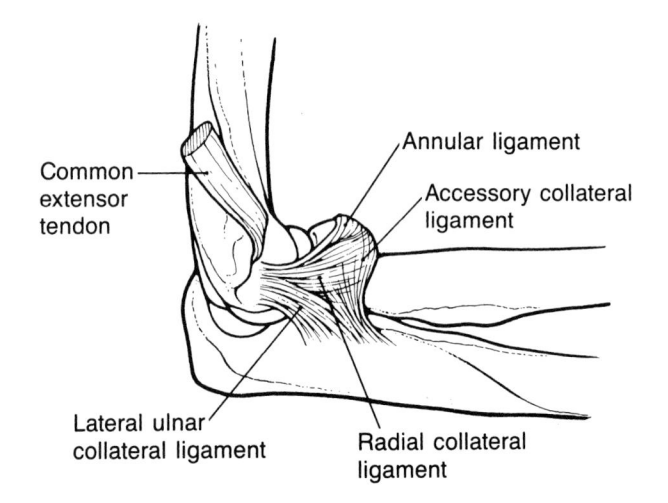

FIGURE 18.1. Components of the lateral collateral ligament complex of the elbow.

action, but also might predispose overhead athletes to lateral epicondylitis.

Normal axial loading results in the transmission of 60% of the force across the elbow joint through the radiocapitellar joint, depending on the position of the joint in its arc of motion.[16] Experimentally, the greatest force across the radiocapitellar joint occurs with the elbow in extension and the forearm in pronation.[17] This arm position accounts for most radial head fractures, because patients generally fall onto an outstretched, pronated upper extremity. Forearm pronation results in proximal migration of the radius that increases the radiocapitellar compression force.[18]

PHYSICAL EXAMINATION

Some patients who have symptomatic radiocapitellar joint changes demonstrate loss of motion and crepitation. As stated earlier, loss of 30° or more of extension is not uncommon; significant loss of elbow flexion occurs less commonly. Variable amounts of forearm rotation loss are seen at clinical examination and depend to a great extent on the cause of the radiocapitellar joint degeneration. Radial head malunion with mechanical block usually demonstrates moderate (from 30° to 60°) to severe (more than 60°) loss of forearm rotation, but radiocapitellar joint degeneration that occurs secondary to primary osteoarthritis generally results in milder (less than 30°) loss. Palpation of the lateral elbow generally causes pain in the area of the radiocapitellar joint, and the examiner often can appreciate palpable, or even audible, crepitation. Full pronation maximizes the compressive load at the radiocapitellar joint and usually causes the greatest pain. Physical examination also demonstrates tenderness in the area of the posterolateral gutter. An effusion often can be appreciated in the posterolateral aspect of the elbow joint. In addition, progressive degeneration of the radiocapitellar joint with widening and osteophyte formation can cause impingement of a normal capsular thickening or plica in the posterolateral gutter. This impingement can lead to thickening of the plica with subsequent inflammation, catching, and painful popping. Careful palpation in the posterolateral gutter can demonstrate this thickening, and range of motion sometimes can reproduce the symptoms of catching.

An important aspect of the examination in overhead athletes is a careful evaluation for valgus instability. Repetitive valgus stress can lead to recurrent microtraumatic injury to the medial UCL that ultimately results in its failure. This type of injury significantly increases the compression load on the radiocapitellar joint and within the posteromedial gutter. Careful palpation of the medial structures and localization of the points of maximal tenderness are important in identifying medial UCL injury and in differentiating it from other common causes of medial elbow pain, such as medial epicondylitis, ulnar neuritis, and ulnohumeral arthritis. However, these conditions commonly occur in association with chronic medial UCL insufficiency.

Most cases of radiocapitellar joint degeneration occur in conjunction with other changes in and around the elbow. Radiocapitellar joint degeneration occurs commonly in patients who have rheumatoid arthritis and frequently is the cause of the symptoms. These patients also have pain and swelling attributable to synovitis and progressive articular destruction of the elbow joint. Likewise, osteoarthritis of the elbow joint leads to symptoms in the ulnohumeral joint due to articular degeneration and osteophyte formation and due to radiocapitellar joint pain. These generalized elbow changes make the physical examination important, because the examiner must accurately characterize and assess the relative contribution that each of these changes makes in the overall elbow symptom complex. Simply excising the radial head may not adequately treat the elbow condition when other significant underlying problems, such as valgus instability or synovitis, are present.

Standard anteroposterior and lateral radiographs generally allow the examiner to assess accurately the radiocapitellar joint (Fig. 18.2). Significant radiocapitellar joint narrowing and osteophyte formation generally are seen. Careful evaluation of the radiographs for loose bodies is important especially when symptoms suggest their presence. Radiographs also can allow the examiner to assess accurately the size and extent of coronoid process and olecranon process osteophytes. In addition, the examiner can appreciate the thickness of the olecranon fossa on the lateral radiograph. This bone, which is normally from 2 to 4 mm thick, often increases to as much as 1 cm thick with progressive degenerative changes. The thickness of this olecranon fossa is important when the

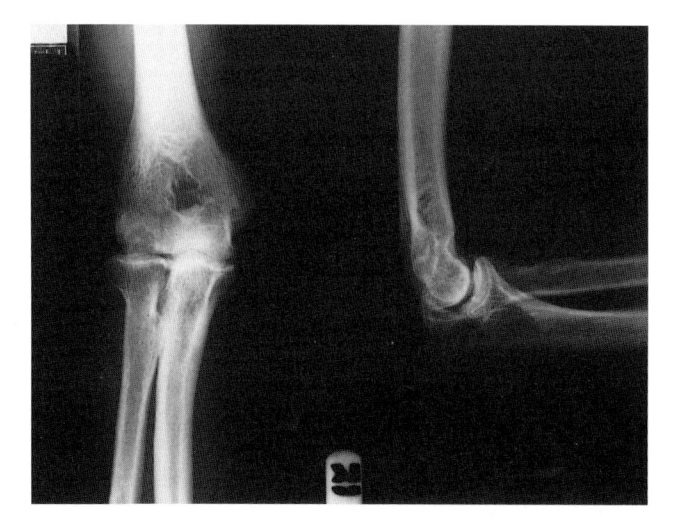

FIGURE 18.2. An anteroposterior and lateral radiograph of a patient who has significant radiocapitellar joint degeneration.

surgeon considers arthroscopic or open fenestration of it. Determining the size and orientation of the radial head also is important when the surgeon plans to excise the radial head, because marked deformity of the head with distortion of anatomic landmarks is a relative contraindication to arthroscopic excision.

NONOPERATIVE TREATMENT

Symptomatic radiocapitellar joint or proximal radioulnar joint degeneration often can be treated without surgery.[19] Nonsteroidal anti-inflammatory medications, along with the judicious use of intra-articular corticosteroid injections, can reduce or even eliminate symptoms. A gentle range-of-motion exercise program can benefit the patient as well. Likewise, appropriate management of any underlying condition, such as rheumatoid arthritis, is important. Splinting the elbow at night or splinting the elbow in a relaxed position also can decrease symptoms. Hinged elbow braces can be helpful in the treatment of patients who have instability.

Some radial head fractures that occur in conjunction with radiocapitellar joint degeneration can be treated without surgery. Important factors to consider at the time of injury include a concurrent elbow dislocation, disruption of the medial UCL, and the radial head fracture pattern itself. Significantly displaced radial head fractures should be treated with surgery by open reduction and internal fixation or primary excision. Minimally displaced radial head fractures that do not demonstrate a mechanical block to forearm rotation are best treated without surgery. However, persistent symptoms of radiocapitellar joint degeneration and loss of motion in the elbow are not uncommon following even minimally displaced radial head fractures. Therefore, the clinician must emphasize the early restoration of elbow motion and forearm rotation to minimize elbow stiffness. Even so, articular cartilage flaps, chondromalacia, and arthritis occasionally do occur and can lead to persistent symptoms despite early, aggressive range-of-motion exercises.

OPERATIVE TREATMENT

Indications

Arthroscopic excision of the radial head is an effective technique, and it has several potential advantages over open excision. Arthroscopic evaluation of the anterior and posterior compartments allows for identification of loose bodies, effective debridement, osteophyte excision, and synovectomy at the time of radial head excision without an arthrotomy. Disruption of the lateral collateral ligament complex at the time of arthrotomy occasionally leads to persistent postoperative symptoms of pain and instability; therefore, incision through this ligamentous complex is undesirable unless necessary. Arthroscopic evaluation of the anterior and posterior compartments of the elbow joint also allows for a more thorough assessment than the assessment possible through the limited arthrotomy that generally is carried out to accomplish open radial head excision. In fact, even an extended Kocher approach with release of the lateral collateral ligament complex and dislocation of the elbow joint still allows for only limited access to the most medial recesses of the ulnohumeral joint. In addition, an arthrotomy increases the soft-tissue disruption about an elbow that already has sustained significant injury or loss of motion and possibly can adversely affect postoperative motion. Immediate motion is allowed following evaluation and treatment using arthroscopic surgery, but is not allowed following radial head excision and debridement accomplished using an extended arthrotomy, because the latter technique generally necessitates some period of immobilization while ligaments and other soft tissues heal.

Arthroscopic radial head excision is indicated (1) as a treatment for primary degenerative changes; (2) as a treatment for posttraumatic radiocapitellar joint changes without significant deformity of the radial head or radiocapitellar joint; (3) as a treatment modality in conjunction with arthroscopic synovectomy when symptomatic radiocapitellar joint symptoms, such as in rheumatoid arthritis, exist; (4) as a treatment alternative in patients who have chronic symptoms associated with osteochondritis dissecans of the capitellum after bone growth maturity has occurred; and (5) as a component of the operative management of patients who have generalized elbow degeneration and are not candidates for total elbow arthroplasty. Radiocapitellar arthritis can occur in isolation, such as following a radial head fracture, but is seen more often in conjunction with more global elbow degenerative changes or systemic illness. Loose bodies also can cause progressive degeneration of the elbow. In the presence of such generalized elbow problems, arthroscopic surgery is particularly valuable as a tool to evaluate and treat the ulnohumeral articulation at the time of radial head excision without an extended lateral arthrotomy or combined medial and lateral arthrotomies.

Patients who have radiocapitellar degeneration and who have an underlying systemic illness, such as rheumatoid arthritis, present a difficult clinical problem. Elbow synovectomy and debridement is an effective method of managing rheumatoid arthritis in patients at certain stages of their disease process.[20] Several classification schemes for rheumatoid arthritis have been suggested.[20] The Hospital for Special Surgery's classification for rheumatoid arthritis uses clinical and radiographic criteria to define the degree, or level, of joint involvement.[20] Grade I disease indicates only a mild to moderate degree of synovitis and no radiographic changes, and it is managed with aspirin or nonsteroidal anti-inflammatory medications. Grade II disease indicates a recalcitrant synovitis that generally cannot be managed with aspirin and requires intermittent arthrocentesis and intra-articular injections of corticosteroids. Radiographs show minimal architectural changes. Grade IIIA disease indicates an unremitting, active synovitis with variable signs of articular joint damage. Grade IIIB disease indicates extensive articular damage and subchondral bone loss and ligamentous instability. Grade IV disease indicates gross destruction and loss of normal architectural landmarks. In addition, gross instability generally is seen.

The surgeon can use synovectomy and debridement to effectively treat grade II disease. Patients who have this degree of the disease have uncontrolled synovitis of the elbow joint with pain and limitation of function. They often demonstrate symptoms attributable to radiocapitellar joint degeneration. Generally, no extensive joint or ligamentous destruction exists. Synovectomy should be performed before gross joint destruction occurs, rather than after the more destructive grade III level of disease has occurred. Although a synovectomy with the removal of the radial head can be performed through a lateral arthrotomy of the elbow joint, we prefer to perform arthroscopic synovectomy accompanied by arthroscopic radial head excision. The arthroscope is an excellent tool that allows for nearly complete elbow synovectomy and for minimally invasive radial head excision. Neither the open nor arthroscopic technique can enable the surgeon to remove all the synovium, but this arthroscopic subtotal synovectomy has proved extremely useful.

Radiocapitellar joint degeneration resulting from primary osteoarthritis of the elbow can cause symptoms. Advanced degenerative arthritis can be diagnosed based on the patient's history, physical examination, and classic radiographic findings. Such patients often present with an insidious onset and history of progressive loss of motion. Some pain is present, but often does not lead these patients to seek medical attention. More commonly, they present when their loss of motion becomes a significant functional impairment, which is generally when the loss of extension exceeds 30°.[19] However, presentation based on loss of extension is variable and is highly dependent on the activity level of the patient. These patients sometimes report symptoms of locking and catching, which are compatible with loose bodies in the elbow.

Some patients who have advanced degenerative arthritis of the elbow improve with initiation of an exercise program combined with nonsteroidal anti-inflammatory medications. However, they usually present when the disease process is advanced, making these interventions often inadequate. For example, this treatment is inadequate when the patient reports not only pain and loss of motion, but also symptoms compatible with the presence of loose bodies. In the past, management options for the arthritic elbow were limited to a medication and bracing program, open debridement, or elbow replacement surgery. Although each of these options can provide significant relief, the advent of arthroscopic surgery has introduced a new option for patients. Arthroscopic radial head excision combined with arthroscopic debridement, loose-body removal, and osteophyte excision can significantly improve a patient's postoperative function.[19] In addition, encouraged by the results of open fenestration (Outerbridge–Kashiwagi procedure) and ulnohumeral arthroplasty, we have developed an arthroscopic approach to the debridement of these elbows. Our systematic approach combines synovectomy, arthroscopic debridement, osteophyte removal, radial head excision, and olecranon fossa fenestration with the known advantages of arthroscopic surgery, providing an excellent method for managing the arthritic elbow.

Another indication for arthroscopic radial head excision includes posttraumatic radiocapitellar joint arthritis. Malunited radial head fractures can lead to significant loss of elbow flexion and extension, as well as forearm rotation. Degeneration of the radiocapitellar joint, as well as the proximal radioulnar joint, commonly is seen. Arthroscopic surgery is a valuable tool in such cases, because it not only allows for effective radial head excision, but also provides an opportunity to evaluate the elbow joint to rule out loose bodies and symptomatic cartilage flaps. However, marked deformity of the radial head that penetrates or is scarred to the anterior capsule is a contraindication to arthroscopic excision unless the posterior interosseous nerve is isolated. Because of the extreme proximity of the radial nerve and its branches to the radial head, particularly when capsular contracture and scarring around the radial head have occurred, arthroscopic radial head excision puts the nerve at risk for injury. If the surgeon attempts arthroscopic radial head excision for a malunited radial head fracture, he or she should be willing to abandon the arthroscopic procedure in favor of a formal arthrotomy when any difficulty is encountered.

Another posttraumatic cause of radiocapitellar joint degeneration occurs in the presence of chronic valgus instability. Increased radiocapitellar joint loading is seen in overhead athletes who have chronic disruption of the medial UCL (Fig. 18.3). The radiocapitellar joint serves as an important secondary restraint to valgus opening when the medial UCL is not functional. Over time, radiocapitellar joint degeneration and posteromedial gutter impingement with secondary osteophyte formation occur. Athletes who have persistent symptoms of radiocapitellar joint degeneration that is unresponsive to nonoperative measures may require arthroscopic debridement, osteophyte excision, removal of any loose bodies, and arthroscopic radial head excision.

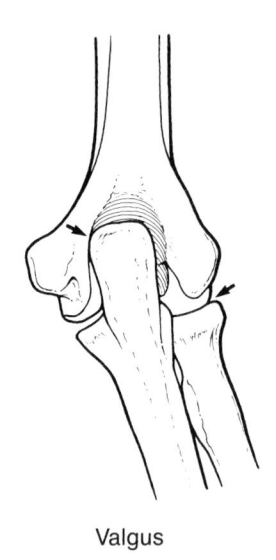

FIGURE 18.3. Valgus overload of the elbow can cause posteromedial impaction of the olecranon within its fossa and increased radiocapitellar joint loading (arrows).

Contraindications

Several factors must be considered before deciding to perform arthroscopic radial head excision. The examiner must evaluate each patient for the appropriateness of arthroscopic excision of the radial head based on the history, physical examination, and radiographic findings. Some radial head excisions are best accomplished using a standard arthrotomy because arthroscopic excision of the radial head might not be possible or might expose the patient to an increased risk of complications. Some contraindications to arthroscopic radial head excision include the following: (1) moderate to severe radial head deformity following fracture malunion, particularly when soft-tissue elbow contractures accompany it, because of the extreme proximity of the radial nerve to the radial head; (2) inadequate visualization of anatomic landmarks or lack of technical expertise in this arthroscopic technique; and (3) the need to use a lateral arthrotomy for treatment, such as when excision of large amounts of ectopic bone is required, or for placement of an elbow distraction devise.

Arthroscopic radial head excision is a technically demanding procedure and requires much experience with arthroscopic surgery of the elbow. If problems arise during the procedure, the surgeon should be willing to abandon arthroscopic surgery and to perform an arthrotomy instead to accomplish radial head excision, along with any additional procedures necessary. Orientation can be difficult to maintain in elbows that have significant bony deformity, soft-tissue scarring, or contracture. Failure to adequately visualize the joint and the arthroscopic instruments not only will lead to an inadequately performed procedure, but also will increase the risk of neurovascular injury. A well-performed radial head excision, capsular release, and debridement carried out through an extended arthrotomy is always preferable to a poorly performed arthroscopic procedure.

Operative Technique

When following proper technique and paying attention to detail, the surgeon can accomplish arthroscopic radial head excision with minimal complications. To ensure safe and effective arthroscopic radial head excision, the surgeon must visualize the arthroscopic instruments at all times and must maintain proper orientation with identified anatomic landmarks. Significant scarring, loss of motion, and bony deformity usually are present in these elbows, making arthroscopic maneuverability and orientation sometimes difficult. Nevertheless, the advantages of arthroscopic surgery for radial head excision make its use desirable.

We prefer the prone or lateral decubitus position for patients undergoing arthroscopic radial head excision. These positions allow for excellent access to the posterior portion of the elbow joint; access to the posterolateral gutter is imperative to completing the procedure. Excision of the radial head should be carried out only after a thorough arthroscopic evaluation of the entire anterior and posterior portions of the elbow joint.

Following placement of the patient in the prone or lateral decubitus position, the surgeon preps and drapes the extremity and leaves it free. A tourniquet is placed on the arm before it is sterilized and draped, but is not used routinely unless untoward bleeding is encountered. The arthroscopic procedure always should start with insufflation of the joint through the direct lateral portal. Approximately 25 mL of normal saline is generally instilled, but the surgeon must take care not to overdistend the joint, because capsular rupture can occur easily. The surgeon first establishes a proximal anterolateral portal, as Field et al.[21] described, that is positioned 2 cm proximal and 1 cm anterior to the lateral epicondyle. This portal has been shown to be much farther from the radial nerve and its branches than more distal portals.[21] Maximizing the distance from the radial nerve is particularly important in patients who have posttraumatic radiocapitellar joint degeneration, because scarring and contracture of the capsule might bind the radial nerve and its branches, minimizing the positive effect that distention of the joint can provide. The surgeon establishes all portals by pulling the skin under a knife and using a hemostat to dissect down to the level of the capsule.

Alternatively, the surgeon can first establish a proximal anteromedial portal. He or she evaluates the coronoid, trochlea, and coronoid fossa with the arthroscope in either the proximal anterolateral or proximal antero-

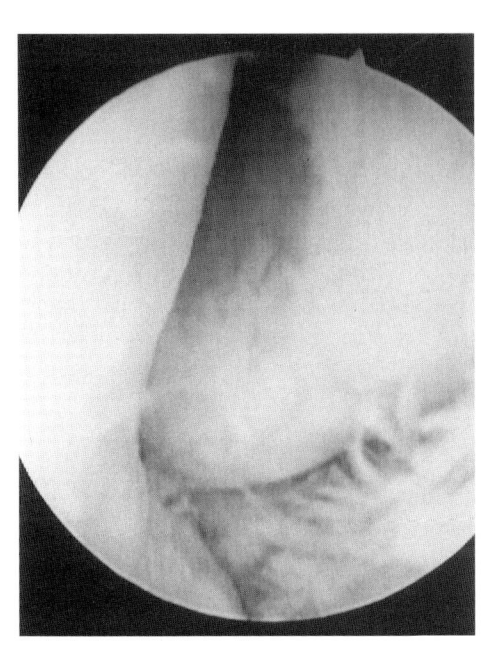

FIGURE 18.4. An arthroscopic photograph of the radiocapitellar joint as viewed from the proximal anteromedial portal.

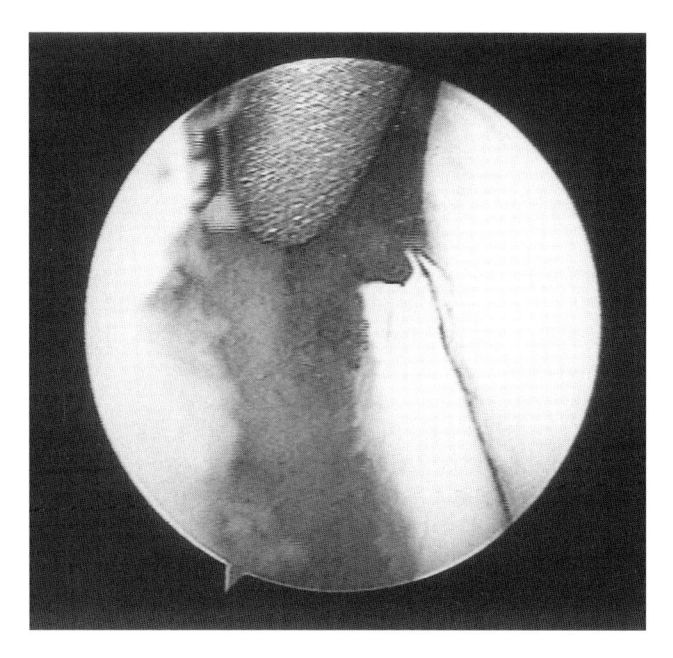

FIGURE 18.5. While supinating and pronating the forearm, the surgeon accomplishes progressive removal of the radial head.

medial portal. Instrumentation is carried out through the other portal. Using a motorized burr, the surgeon excises coronoid spurs and deepens the coronoid fossa as necessary. Thorough evaluation for loose bodies is carried out in the anterior compartment.

The surgeon finishes the evaluation of the anterior compartment by viewing the radial head and capitellum through the proximal anteromedial portal. To completely evaluate the capitellum, he or she carefully examines the radiocapitellar joint and flexes and extends the elbow (Fig. 18.4). Pronation and supination of the forearm allow for adequate evaluation of and maximal access to the radial head. Radial head and capitellar spurs are excised through the anterolateral portal. If the surgeon needs to excise the radial head as well, he or she continues to pronate and supinate the forearm until all the exposed radial head has been excised through the proximal anterolateral portal (Fig. 18.5).

Almost always some residual radial head persists. While continuing to visualize through the anteromedial portal, the surgeon completes radial head excision by placing the arthroscopic shaver through the direct lateral, or soft spot, portal. The remaining radial head then can be excised from back to front using a cutting block technique, with medial and lateral sweeps of the arthroscopic shaver (Fig. 18.6). The forearm is pronated and supinated to ensure complete resection of the radial head. The resection is continued until full pronation and supination can be achieved and no radiocapitellar impingement occurs through a normal flexion and extension arc of motion. The surgeon should pay particular attention to the radiocapitellar joint while the forearm is in full prona-

tion, because maximal pronation narrows the radiocapitellar joint interval and puts the radial neck at risk for impingement on the capitellum.

In certain cases, radiocapitellar joint degeneration is seen without significant proximal radioulnar joint degeneration. This type of degeneration occurs in certain cases of radial head fractures, capitellum fractures, and osteochondritis dissecans of the capitellum. If the proxi-

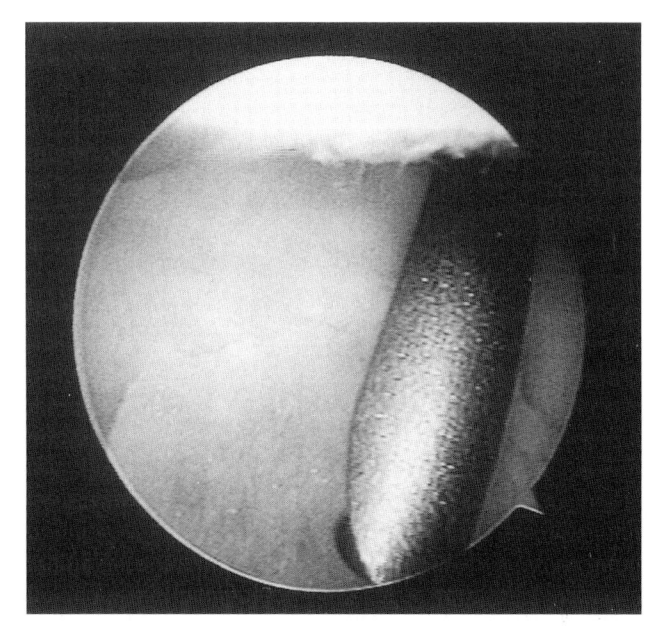

FIGURE 18.6. While visualizing the joint through the anteromedial portal, the surgeon uses the direct lateral, or soft spot, portal to complete radial head excision.

mal radioulnar joint appears normal at the time of arthroscopic evaluation, the surgeon should consider a limited radial head excision that maintains some of the most distal aspect of the proximal radioulnar joint articulation. Retention of the most distal aspect of the radial head is reasonable as long as significant radiocapitellar joint space is maintained under direct arthroscopic visualization through a range of motion.

After debriding the anterior compartment and excising the radial head, the surgeon evaluates the posterior compartment. An inflow cannula is maintained using either the anteromedial or anterolateral portal. The arthroscope then is inserted into a proximal posterolateral portal. Through this portal site, the surgeon can evaluate the posterolateral gutter and confirm adequate radial head excision. If present, a symptomatic posterolateral plica can be excised through the direct lateral portal. In addition, posterolateral gutter osteophytes can be removed under direct visualization. Next, the surgeon can establish a posterocentral portal, can debride the olecranon fossa, and can remove any olecranon osteophytes. Visualization of the posterolateral and posteromedial gutters also allows for the identification and removal of any loose bodies. Full range of motion confirms the adequacy of the olecranon osteophyte excision and olecranon fossa debridement. If the surgeon sees persistent impingement in the olecranon fossa near full elbow extension, he or she can accomplish an arthroscopic ulnohumeral arthroplasty as well.

Persistent bony block to extension after debridement of the olecranon fossa and excision of olecranon osteophytes is an indication for an olecranon fossa fenestration. At the suggestion of Outerbridge, Kashiwagi originally described fenestration of the olecranon fossa, or the Outerbridge–Kashiwagi (O–K) procedure.[20] The thickened bone between the coronoid and olecranon fossa, which contributes to impingement and a reduction in elbow motion, is resected through an arthrotomy. A drill is used to fenestrate the floor of the olecranon fossa, providing a communication between the olecranon and the coronoid fossa. This opening is widened to produce a window that is approximately 1.5 cm in diameter, which corresponds to the original shape and size of the olecranon fossa.

Open ulnohumeral arthroplasty as Morrey[19] described is a modification of Kashiwagi's O–K procedure. By working through the humeral fenestration, Morrey performed an open osteotomy of the olecranon tip and removal of loose bodies from the olecranon fossa, and he excised coronoid process osteophytes and removed anterior loose bodies by working through the humeral fenestration. Morrey also used an approach that elevated the medial triceps insertion, rather than split the triceps tendon as Kashiwagi described.

We perform a variation of Morrey's and Kashiwagi's techniques.[19] We use the arthroscope to create a fenestration without an arthrotomy. In our technique, while visualizing through a posterolateral portal, the surgeon places a 5-mm drill bit in the center of the olecranon fossa through the posterocentral portal. He or she drills from back to front at an angle toward the center of the coronoid fossa to connect the olecranon fossa with the coronoid fossa (Fig. 18.7). The intersection of the long axis of the humerus with the inflow cannula positioned in the anterior portal provides a guide for proper orientation of the drill. After assessing the location and depth of this channel connecting the two fossae, the surgeon uses an aggressive arthroscopic shaver to enlarge the hole until full flexion and extension can be achieved. This enlargement requires that a concentric hole be established in the olecranon fossa (Fig. 18.8). If orientation or other technical considerations make arthroscopic fenestration difficult or impossible, the surgeon should be willing to perform an open fenestration of the olecranon fossa instead. A Cloward drill should be available in case this procedure becomes necessary. In addition, a minifluoroscopic unit is valuable not only in assessing the position and adequacy of arthroscopic olecranon fossa fenestration, but also in the evaluation of an arthroscopic radial head excision.

Patients undergoing arthroscopic debridement and radial head excision generally are discharged from the hospital on the same day as their surgery. If extensive arthroscopic removal of osteophytes and arthroscopic olecranon fossa fenestration are carried out, a suction drain usually is placed intra-articularly, and the patient must stay in the hospital overnight. In either case, immediate

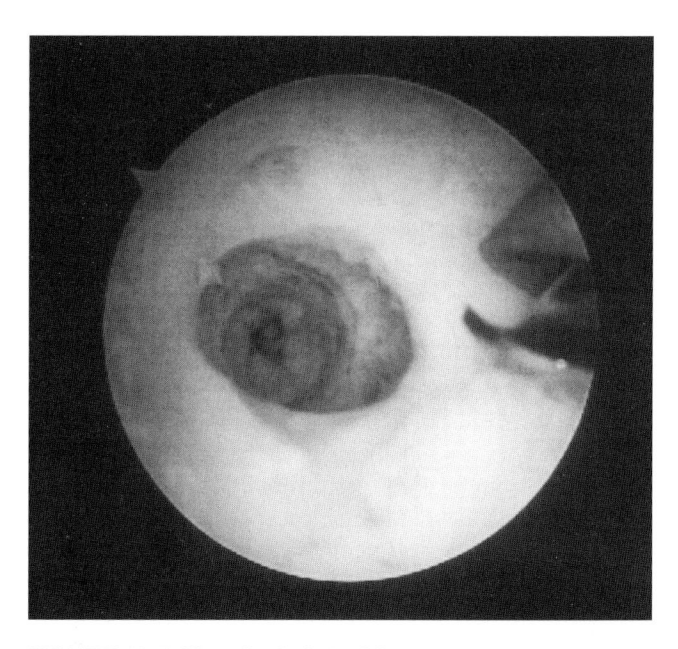

FIGURE 18.7. The pilot hole is drilled through the olecranon fossa and exits anteriorly into the coronoid fossa. This hole determines the depth of bone between these two areas and facilitates resection.

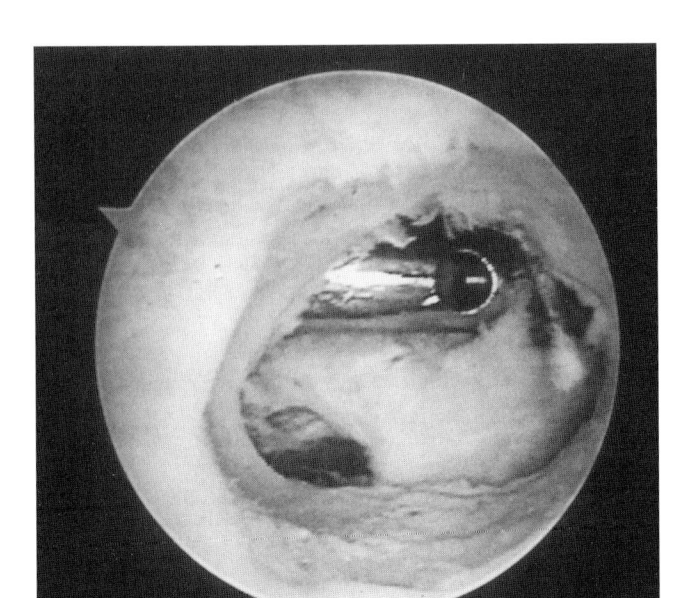

FIGURE 18.8. The previously made drill hole is enlarged until it can accommodate the coronoid in flexion and the olecranon in extension. The hole can be extended until the medial and lateral columns of the distal humerus are encountered.

motion is allowed and encouraged, and no specific limitations or restrictions are given. Most patients return to normal activities within 2 months after surgery. An organized physical therapy regimen helps the patient to recover motion, particularly when significant loss of motion was present before surgery.

Patients who have radiocapitellar joint changes sufficient to require radial head excision generally have accompanying intra-articular problems. These problems commonly include degenerative changes in the ulnohumeral joint, accompanied by coronoid process and olecranon process osteophytes and posterolateral and posteromedial gutter osteophytes. Loose bodies often are seen in this clinical situation and should be searched for extensively in both the anterior and posterior compartments. In addition, patients who have radiocapitellar joint degeneration sometimes develop a symptomatic posterolateral plica. This normal thickening of the posterolateral capsule sometimes becomes fibrosed in the presence of long-standing inflammatory changes in and around the radiocapitellar joint.

This thickened and fibrotic plica becomes symptomatic when it is impinged on the posterolateral bony structures during movement through a range of motion. This impingement can result in pain, swelling, and tenderness in the area of the posterolateral elbow joint, along with symptoms of popping, clicking, and catching. Recurrent irritation of the plica by impingement on the bony structures creates a cycle of injury, inflammation, and fibrosis. If the patient demonstrates findings compatible with a symptomatic posterolateral plica, he or she can have arthroscopic excision or release of the plica during the arthroscopic radial head excision.

RESULTS

We have performed arthroscopic radial head excision routinely since 1990. Other arthroscopic procedures generally are required at the time of radial head excision including synovectomy, loose-body removal, osteophyte excision, and olecranon fossa fenestration. Arthroscopic treatment in such patients has proved effective and has a low complication rate for this sometimes complex clinical condition. We reviewed the results of 37 patients following arthroscopic radial head excision. Results in 34 of the 37 patients were successful. An unsuccessful result in one patient was caused by continued loss of motion and pain despite radiographic evidence of adequate radial head excision. An unsuccessful result in another patient was due to development of significant wrist pain and loss of motion following radial head excision; the patient ultimately needed radial head replacement surgery to eliminate radioulnar instability. The third patient who had an unsuccessful result had arthrofibrosis and posterolateral rotatory instability and regained motion after surgery. However, the patient subsequently developed recurrent symptoms in the lateral portion of the elbow and needed additional surgery.

We also reviewed the results of 24 consecutive patients who had arthroscopic olecranon fossa fenestration with or without arthroscopic radial head excision. Average preoperative flexion was 90°, and the average loss of extension was 40°. Average postoperative flexion was 139°, and average extension was 8°. All patients were reexamined from 2 to 5 years after surgery, and the results in 23 of the 24 patients were considered successful. The one patient in the series who had an unsuccessful result initially was satisfied with the outcome; however, the patient subsequently developed significant rheumatoid arthritic changes in the ulnohumeral joint and eventually needed total elbow arthroplasty.

The arthroscopic management of elbow arthritis has proved effective in our experience. When the surgeon uses proper indications and technique, he or she can achieve a high success rate. Careful attention to detail and maintenance of intra-articular orientation provide reproducible results with a low complication rate.

COMPLICATIONS

The most serious potential complication from arthroscopic radial head excision is injury to the radial nerve or its branches. The risk of nerve injury is particularly high when moderate to severe deformity of the radial head is present following a malunited fracture. Such fractures often lead to capsular contracture in the proximity of the radial head, with scarring of the radial head in some cases. This capsular contracture tethers the radial nerve, making arthroscopic release of the soft-tissue scarring about the radial head a risky intervention because of the potential for nerve damage. Even in untraumatized patients, the posterior interosseous nerve lies directly on the distal anterior portion of the capsule in the area of the radial head. Patients who have severe radial head deformities are best treated using arthrotomy with isolation of the posterior interosseous nerve.

Another potential complication with arthroscopic radial head excision and elbow debridement centers on the ability to excise adequately either the radial head or elbow osteophytes. An inadequately performed excision or joint debridement results in persistent elbow pain and loss of motion. If the surgeon has inadequate visualization or maneuverability of the arthroscopic instruments, he or she should abandon arthroscopic surgery and carry out an arthrotomy with open radial head excision and elbow joint debridement.

SUMMARY

Arthroscopic excision of the radial head has several potential advantages. Removal of intra-articular debris and thickened synovium can decrease symptoms and temporarily retard progression of the arthritic process. Removal of bone spurs and loose bodies also can provide transient relief of symptoms and improved postoperative function. Accomplishing all these procedures without an extensive elbow arthrotomy allows the patient to participate immediately in range-of-motion and strengthening exercises and minimizes postoperative scarring.

The surgical technique for arthroscopic radial head excision and associated procedures is a demanding technical intervention and requires the skill of an experienced arthroscopic surgeon. However, careful attention to the described surgical technique, as well as a thorough knowledge of elbow anatomy, should minimize these complications. Finally, the surgeon needs to be prepared to abandon the arthroscopic approach in favor of a standard arthrotomy when technical considerations or visualization become less than adequate.

REFERENCES

1. *Grant's atlas of anatomy*, 6th ed. Basmajian JV, ed. Baltimore: Williams & Wilkins; 1980:362–369.
2. Morrey BF, Chao EY. Passive motion of the elbow joint: A biomechanical analysis. *J Bone Joint Surg* 1976;58A:501–508.
3. Youm Y, Dryer RF, Thambyrajah K, et al. Biomechanical analyses of forearm pronation–supination and elbow flexion–extension. *J Biomech* 1979;12:245–255.
4. Martin BF. The annular ligament of the superior radio-ulnar joint. *J Anat* 1958;59:473–482.
5. Morrey BF, An KN. Articular and ligamentous contributions to the stability of the elbow joint. *Am J Sports Med* 1983;11:315–319.
6. Field LD, Altchek DW. Evaluation of the arthroscopic valgus instability test of the elbow. *Am J Sports Med* 1996;24:177–181.
7. Hotchkiss RN, Weiland AJ. Valgus stability of the elbow. *J Orthop Res* 1987;5:372–377.
8. Morrey BF. Applied anatomy and biomechanics of the elbow joint. *Instr Course Lect* 1986;35:59–68.
9. Morrey BF, An KN. Functional anatomy of the ligaments of the elbow. *Clin Orthop* 1985;201:84–90.
10. Morrey BF, Tanaka S, An KN. Valgus stability of the elbow: A definition of primary and secondary constraints. *Clin Orthop* 1991;265:187–195.
11. Regan WD, Korinek SL, Morrey BF, et al. Biomechanical study of ligaments around the elbow joint. *Clin Orthop* 1991;271:170–179.
12. Schwab GH, Bennett JB, Woods GW, et al. Biomechanics of elbow instability: The role of the medial collateral ligament. *Clin Orthop* 1980;146:42–52.
13. Søjbjerg JO, Ovesen J, Nielsen S. Experimental elbow instability after transection of the medial collateral ligament. *Clin Orthop* 1987;218:186–190.
14. Timmerman LA, Schwartz ML, Andrews JR. Preoperative evaluation of the ulnar collateral ligament by magnetic resonance imaging and computed tomography arthrography. Evaluation in 25 baseball players with surgical confirmation. *Am J Sports Med* 1994;22:26–31.
15. Glousman RE, Barron J, Jobe FW, et al. An electromyographic analysis of the elbow in normal and injured pitchers with medial collateral ligament insufficiency. *Am J Sports Med* 1992;20:311–317.
16. Morrey BF, An KN, Stormont TJ. Force transmission through the radial head. *J Bone Joint Surg* 1988;70A:250–256.
17. An KN, Hui FC, Morrey BF, et al. Muscles across the elbow joint: A biomechanical analysis. *J Biomech* 1981;14:659–669.
18. Palmer AK, Glisson RR, Werner FW. Ulnar variance determination. *J Hand Surg* 1982;7:376–379.
19. Morrey BF. Primary degenerative arthritis of the elbow: Treatment by ulnohumeral arthroplasty. *J Bone Joint Surg* 1992;74B:409–413.
20. Kashiwagi D. Intraarticular changes of the osteoarthritic elbow, especially about the fossa olecrani. *J Jap Orthop Assoc* 1978;52:1367–1382.
21. Field LD, Altchek DW, Warren RF, et al. Arthroscopic anatomy of the lateral elbow: A comparison of three portals. *Arthroscopy* 1994;10:602–607.

CHAPTER 19

Problem Fractures of the Distal Humerus

Arnold-Peter C. Weiss and Hill Hastings II

INTRODUCTION

Intra-articular fractures of the distal humerus present special problems with regard to their assessment and treatment. These fractures often include significant intra-articular or periarticular bone comminution, poor bone quality, significant soft-tissue injury, and rotatory deformities that the surgeon must address with a clear, concise treatment protocol to obtain optimal results (Fig. 19.1).

In his classic work of 1811, Desault[1] was the first to emphasize the importance of alignment of intra-articular distal humeral fractures in obtaining optimal functional results. Unfortunately, nearly two centuries of advances in orthopedic surgery have not made these fractures significantly easier to treat. Treatment of intra-articular fractures of the distal humerus requires careful preoperative planning, a step-by-step operative approach, and, in most cases, stable internal fixation of the fracture fragments.[2-5] Although some severely comminuted distal fractures of the humerus are treated most appropriately with closed fixation methods,[6-10] we believe that, almost without exception, all displaced intra-articular fractures of the distal humerus require open reduction and internal fixation. In this chapter, we address the principles involved in treating the most problematic intra-articular and extra-articular fractures of the distal humerus and place special attention on operative technique.

ANATOMY

Three major components of the distal humerus provide structural stability: the medial column, the lateral column, and the articular trochlea. Because of the presence of the olecranon fossa in the distal humerus, this region forms a triangle from a mechanical strength standpoint; the base is the articular trochlea, and the other two sides are the medial and lateral columns (Fig. 19.2). With any fracture of the distal humerus, reconstruction of all three mechanical components of this triangle is essential for successful fracture fixation.

The radiocapitellar joint contributes less significantly than the trochlea to the mechanical aspects of intra-articular reconstruction. When reconstructing a difficult distal humeral fracture, the surgeon must pay attention to this joint, because it imparts mechanical stability to the arm as it approaches extension, involves an articulation important in hand function, and contributes to axial load sharing, with up to 40% of the total elbow joint forces traversing the radiocapitellar joint.[11] However, reconstruction of this joint should be seen as an adjunct to the main stabilizing components of the elbow that require initial internal fixation.

GENERAL PRINCIPLES OF TREATMENT IN PROBLEM FRACTURES

Regardless of the specific type of fracture pattern presented or the characteristics that contribute to difficult treatment, the surgeon must follow specific principles of treatment to eliminate complications. When treating a particular fracture by open reduction and internal fixation, rather than by alternative methods (e.g., closed reduction in casting or olecranon pin traction), the most important factor in attaining and maintaining a good postoperative result is stable fixation of the fracture fragments.

Numerous classification systems have been proposed

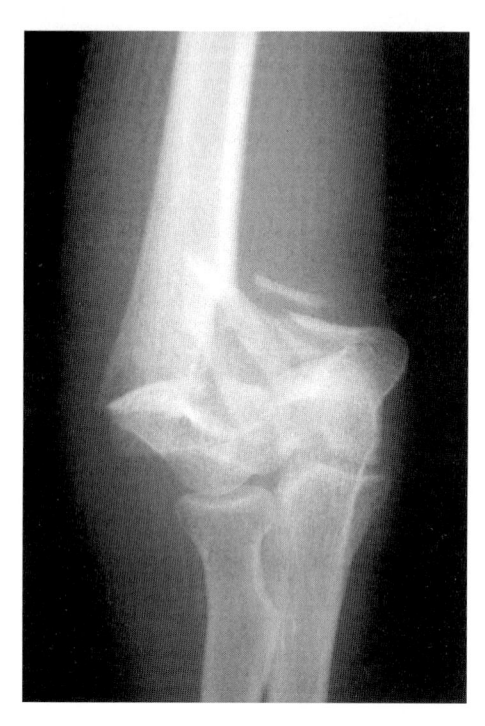

FIGURE 19.1. Anteroposterior radiograph of a comminuted AO C3 fracture.

for fractures of the distal humerus.[12–16] Each system has its merits and considers these fractures from somewhat different views. With several fracture patterns, surgeons have particular difficulty choosing and maintaining operative fixation. Müller et al. of the Swiss AO group proposed a classification scheme that involves nine subtypes of fracture and that mainly is based on the anatomic location of the fracture fragments[12,14] (Fig. 19.3). Although the classification considers fracture comminution, it does not consider fracture pattern orientation or mechanism of injury.[12,14] Despite this drawback, their classification system provides a useful means to describe the types of fractures that are particularly difficult to treat surgically and to get good to excellent functional results.

Any fracture pattern involving comminution of the distal humeral cortex with or without intra-articular extension imparts significant difficulty in obtaining appropriate alignment, operative fixation, and maintenance of reduction during early postoperative range of motion. Using the AO classification scheme, these fracture patterns are represented as A3, C2, and C3 that involve supracondylar and columnar comminution. In addition, C3 includes intra-articular comminution at the trochlear level. If the patient is elderly and has significant osteoporotic bone, any of the articular fractures in the AO classification, that is, the previously mentioned fracture groups as well as B1 through C1, pose significant difficulties mainly with obtaining rigid internal fixation intraoperatively because of the lack of bone-screw interface strength. Very low or shearing intra-articular fractures of the distal humerus, which generally involve a transverse fracture through or just above the trochlea, that do not

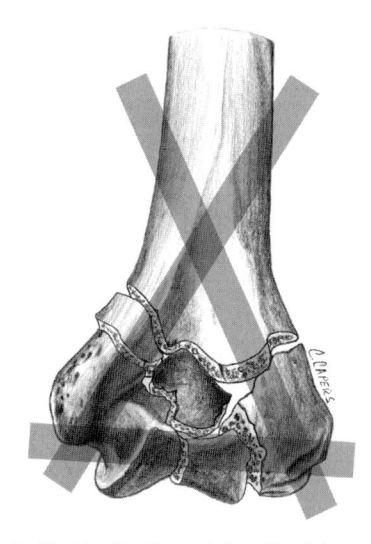

FIGURE 19.2. Stable fixation of the distal humerus requires restoring all three elements of the triangular construct: the lateral column, the medial column, and the trochlea and capitellum.

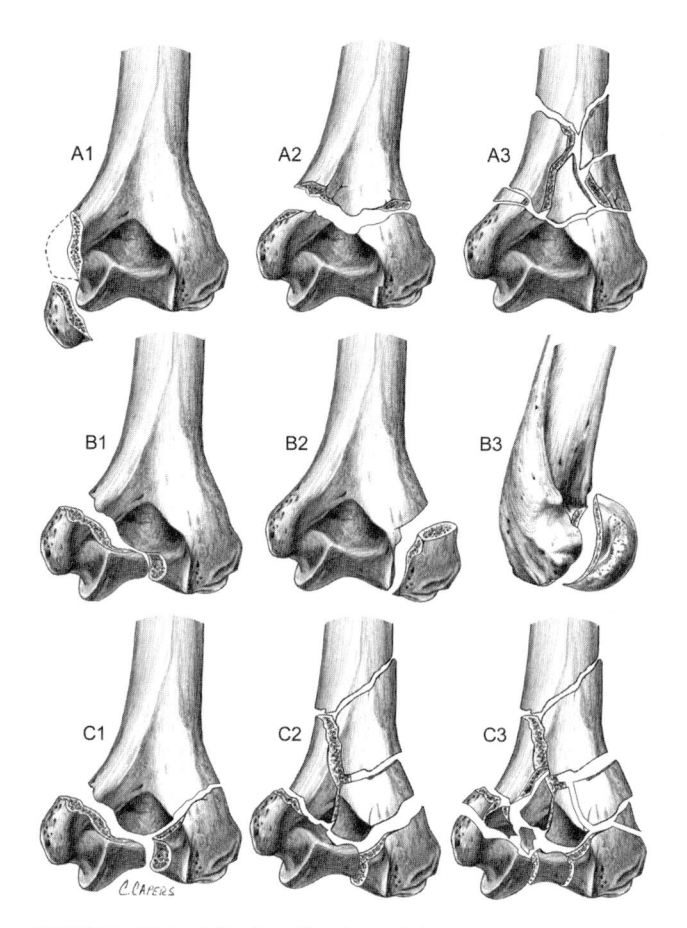

FIGURE 19.3. AO classification of fractures of the distal humerus.

fall into a specific AO group classification present significant problems as well (Fig. 19.4). The surgeon cannot obtain rigid distal fixation in the high torque forces that occur postoperatively with range of motion, because the fracture line is so near the axis of rotation to the elbow. If the surgeon approaches these problem fractures in the step-by-step operative approach presented in this chapter, their treatment can be simplified greatly.

Radiographs

Before beginning an operative procedure to treat any fracture of the distal humerus, the surgeon should visualize clearly the fracture fragments and their relative anatomy. The surgeon must obtain anteroposterior (AP) and lateral radiographs of the distal humerus as one entity and, of lesser importance, of the proximal forearm unit as another entity. In and of themselves, AP and lateral radiographs of the elbow joint do not provide adequate visualization of the fracture pattern, because the patient cannot fully extend the arm at the elbow joint. Flexing the patient's elbow joint to 40° when obtaining the AP radiograph of the humerus moves the olecranon out of the fossa and allows better humeral visualization (Fig. 19.5). Obliquely ori-

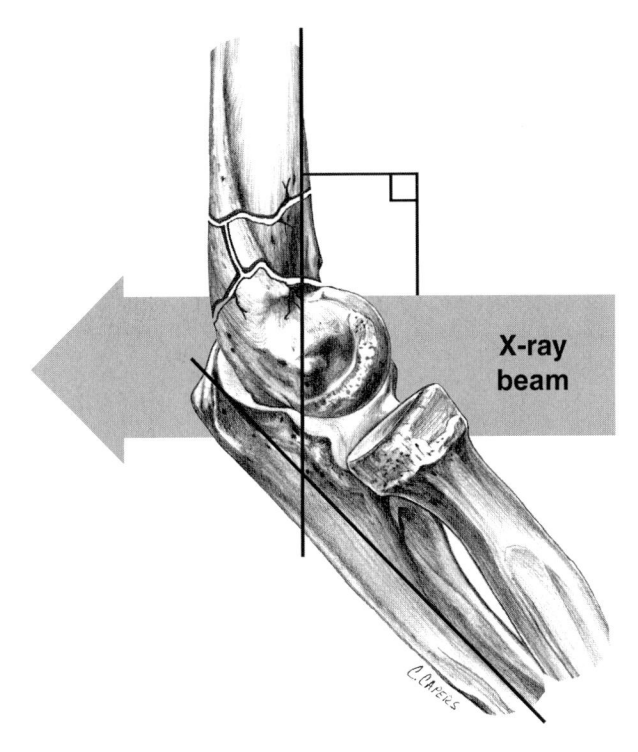

FIGURE 19.5. Correct positioning of the elbow in 40° of flexion for an AP radiograph of the distal humerus.

ented radiographs often uncover hidden fragments or provide better definition of known fragments. Occasionally, we have found the use of computed tomography or trispiral tomography scans of the distal humerus to be helpful in further defining the size, number, and displacement of fracture fragments. Traction radiographic views taken intraoperatively can significantly simplify identification of what further steps may be needed to obtain appropriate fracture alignment (Fig. 19.6).

If the fracture fragments are of a sufficient size, making templates of each of the fragments and trying to piece together the fracture preoperatively can help the surgeon to predict what type of problems may be found at surgery. The surgeon frequently can make this prediction by tracing the fracture fragments with onion skin paper or with a translucent radiographic film, cutting out the traced fragments, and planning the reduction preoperatively.

Patient Positioning

We have found that placing the patient in the lateral decubitus position with an arm holder under the brachium provides easier access to the posterior aspect of the elbow (Fig. 19.7). This position allows the arm to be rotated freely and places the distal humerus in an orientation consistent with the views often seen in anatomic drawings. Although it imparts more anesthetic ventila-

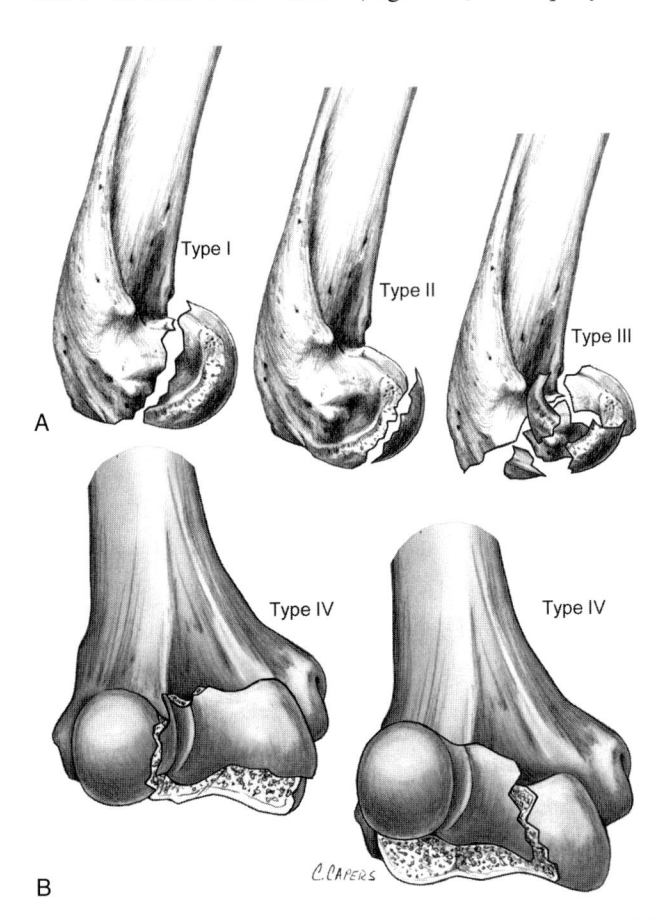

FIGURE 19.4. (A) Three types of capitellar fractures and (B) one type each of shearing intra-articular trochlear and capitellar fracture as described by McKee et al.[20]

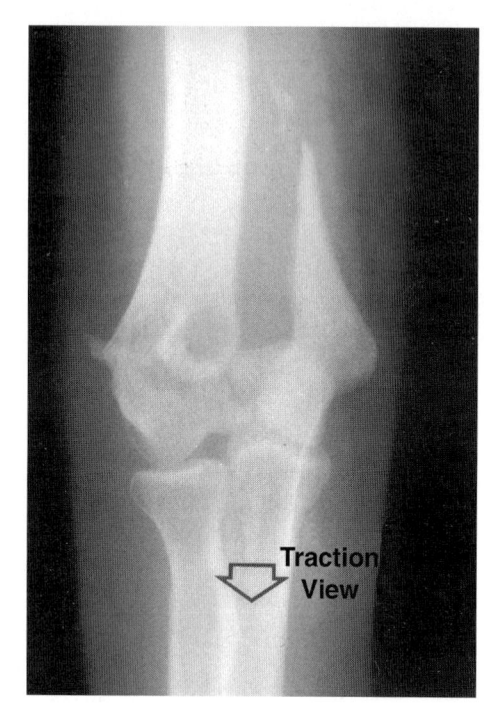

FIGURE 19.6. Traction radiographic views help to separate overriding fragments and assist the surgeon in preoperative planning.

tory compromise, placing the patient in the prone position is a suitable alternative.

Surgical Approach

We use the straight midline posterior surgical approach, passing slightly lateral to the elbow. If any portion of the distal humeral fracture involves intra-articular comminution, we prefer to use a chevron olecranon osteotomy. This method affords excellent visualization of the intra-articular component and allows for proximal extension if unexpected supracondylar comminution or fracture lines warrant increased mobilization.[17] In cases of a simple noncomminuted fracture above the distal olecranon fossa or simple intra-articular involvement, we use the posteromedial approach that Bryan and Morrey[18] described. However, note that this does not afford the same mobility in manipulating fracture fragments as olecranon osteotomy affords. Therefore, if the fracture above the olecranon fossa involves comminution that might require significant manipulation, we still favor an olecranon osteotomy, because it allows appropriate anatomical alignment to be addressed more easily.

Immediately after appropriate exposure, the ulnar nerve should be isolated and decompressed so that its position can be monitored during fracture manipulation. As mentioned earlier, we prefer the chevron intra-articular osteotomy. We use two Kirschner wires (K-wires) in a tension-band technique because of the increased resistance to rotational forces that both the chevron orientation and multiple fixation points of the K-wires provide. When accomplishing the osteotomy, the surgeon should use the thinnest possible saw blade and appropriate irrigation to maintain low bone temperature; he or she should saw partially through the olecranon and use osteotomes to complete the crack through the cartilage. Using the saw to complete the osteotomy puts the cartilage at risk of damage, because the articular surface of the olecranon rides in an articular "valley" of the trochlea. Therefore, we toggle the saw back and forth from the medial side to cut laterally and from the lateral side to cut medially, and we accomplish the final breakthrough with a thin osteotome.

The chevron should be fashioned so that its apex points distally, providing for a more stable osteotomized fragment (Fig. 19.8). Because the osteotomy involves violating the olecranon articular surface, particular care should be taken in placing it in the "void" region. This area, which is just distal to the mid-articular level, is where the synovial membrane inserts; it is relatively void of cartilage and is stress load shielded during normal elbow mechanics. Therefore, any slight incongruities during osteotomy repair fall in a region where some tolerance exists.

We repair the osteotomy using two parallel 1.6-mm K-wires drilled proximal to distal from the fragment to the anterior cortex just distal to the beginning of the olecranon metaphyseal flare (Fig. 19.9). Although predrilling is mandatory in any straight-type olecranon osteotomy, we have not found it essential to predrill these K-wires in a chevron osteotomy. If the surgeon chooses to predrill the chevron osteotomy, he or she should not include the anterior cortex; drilling this region for the first time during definitive K-wire placement imparts a better interference fit between wires and cortex.

For tension banding, a 16-gauge needle is passed parallel to the olecranon articular surface and perpendicular to the ulnar shaft underneath the triceps tendon, "hug-

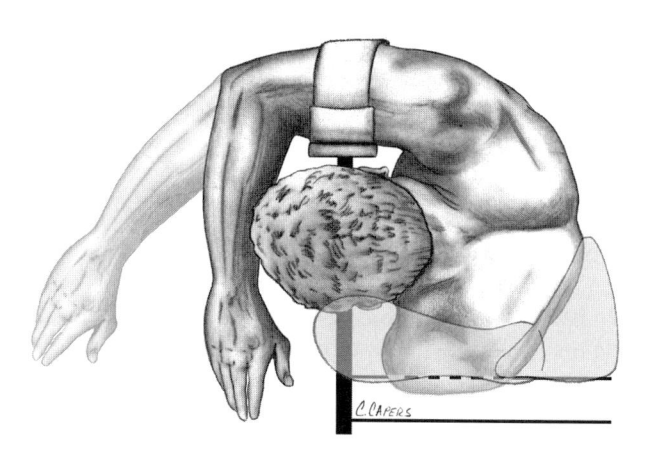

FIGURE 19.7. Lateral decubitus positioning for comparative exposure of the distal humerus.

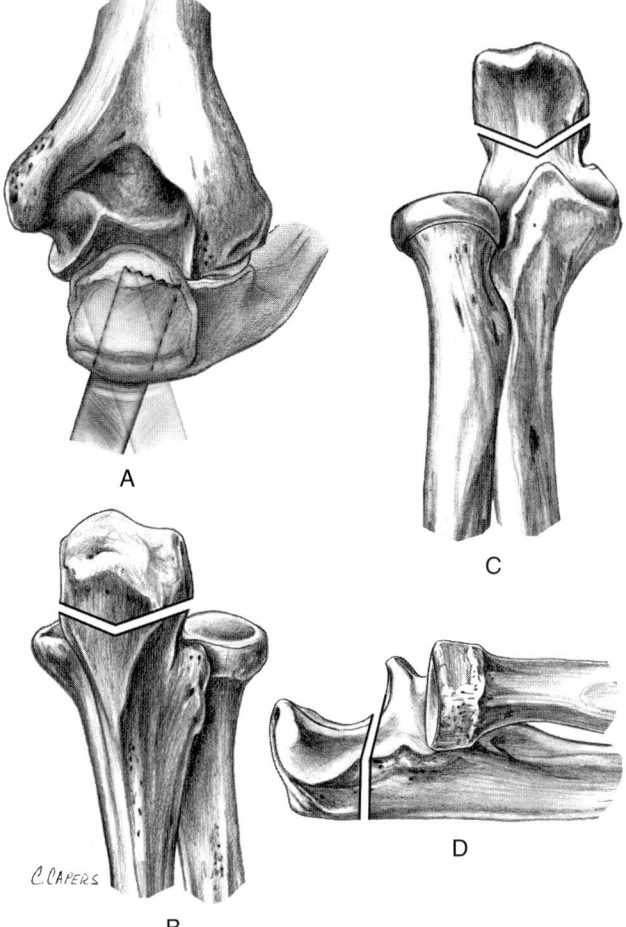

FIGURE 19.8. Chevron osteotomy maximizes bone surface for healing with morphology adding to stability. (A) posterior view of humerus and ulna (note angle of saw blade with elbow in flexion); (B) posterior view; (C) anterior view; and (D) lateral view after the osteotomy (adapted from Hastings H, Engles DR, *Hand clinics* 1997;13:703).

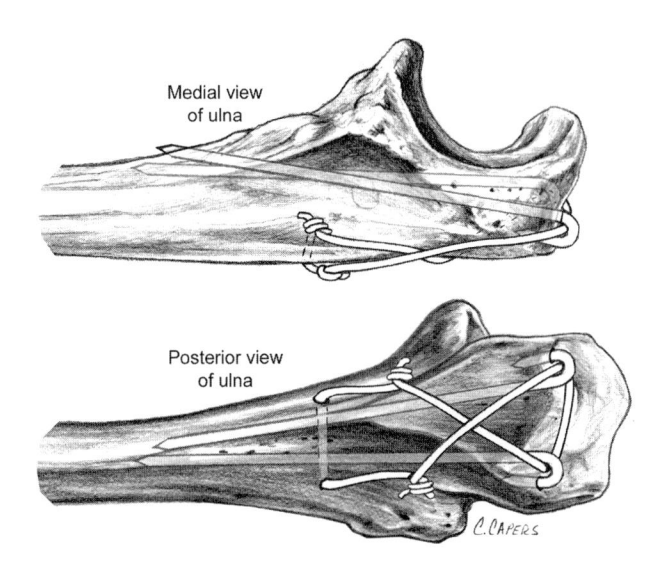

FIGURE 19.9. Tension-band fixation of chevron osteotomy of the olecranon.

ging" bone. A 1-mm stainless steel wire is passed through the needle; then the needle is withdrawn. A distal transverse hole is drilled in the ulna so that the osteotomy lies midway between the olecranon tip and the transverse drill hole. The wire is passed through the holes in a figure-of-eight fashion. The surgeon double-twists the wire to obtain even osteotomy compression mechanics when tightening the wire.

Order of Fracture Assembly

With few exceptions, the order of approach to fixation of distal humeral fractures requires initial stable fixation of the trochlea (i.e., joint), using appropriate bone grafting with K-wire and screw fixation when necessary. After reducing and stabilizing the intra-articular components, the surgeon should approach both the lateral and medial columns. In general, one of the two columns has large enough fracture fragments that, with appropriate keying, or locking in, of one of these fragments, the surgeon can judge the original length of the distal humerus, as well as its orientation. In these cases, we prefer to initially fix the column with the largest fragments to establish alignment and then to reconstruct the column with smaller fragments, which usually involves some bone grafting from the iliac crest.

Choosing and Positioning Plates

Plate and screw fixation of the fracture fragments remains the mainstay of appropriate treatment today. In general, only the lateral and medial columns can be reconstructed with plates. The plate type generally used in the fixation of distal humeral fractures is a 3.5-mm reconstruction plate. Another type of plate designed specifically for distal humeral fractures is a Y-type configuration placed in an inverted fashion. We have found the Y-plate difficult to use and too malleable. Additionally, the Y-plate provides less mechanical stability than two separate 3.5-mm reconstruction plates placed in a perpendicular plane to each other.

Multiplanar fixation gives this region significant extra stability, which is required for early mobilization of the elbow. Therefore, we generally have used single malleable reconstruction plates (one along each column), attempting to place these plates in noncollinear planes and, preferably, at a 90° angle to one another. The plate on the lateral column most often is placed posteriorly and extended low, covering the posterior aspect of the capitellum (Fig. 19.10). Screws through the plate can lag any fracture fragment oblique to the coronal plane. The plate on the medial column generally is placed medially, imparts a multiplanar reconstruction, and allows for medial to lateral lag-screw fixation of any fragment oblique to the sagittal plane.

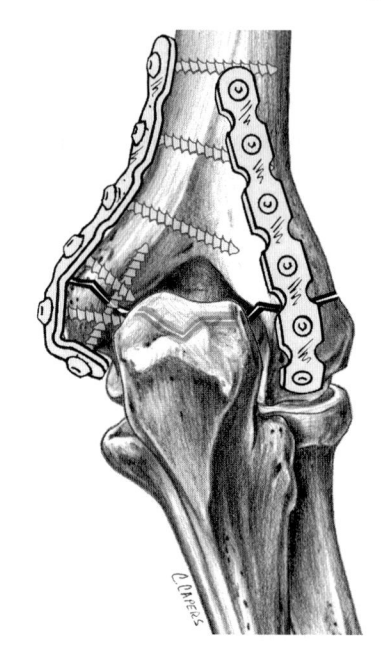

FIGURE 19.10. Orthagonal plating of the distal humerus.

Bone Graft

Obtaining and using appropriate cancellous bone graft from the iliac crest is an important technique and should be used without hesitation when the surgeon is confronted with either osteoporotic fractures or fractures that involve significant comminution of either the trochlea or column. Using cancellous bone graft or a corticocancellous bone block for subchondral bone grafting of any trochlear defects can impart significant mechanical resistance to compression, which is essential when fixing the two columns together by a lag-screw technique. Frequently, in the highly comminuted column fractures, the surgeon finds devascularized bone of small size and replaces it more appropriately by autogenous bone graft. As a secondary consideration, bone grafting imparts a higher propensity for the fracture fragments to heal, especially when an eggshell type of cortical bone is present.

However, the surgeon always must be cognizant of the olecranon fossa and must ensure that this area is constantly maintained free of obstruction so that no bony block occurs during normal elbow motion. We have used iliac crest exclusively as a donor site for cancellous bone. We prefer to use the anterior crest; however, if insufficient anterior graft is available or if the patient previously had the anterior crest harvested, we can easily approach the posterior crest, because the lateral decubitus position of the patient allows equal access.

Handling of the Ulnar Nerve

In all patients, we decompress the ulnar nerve regardless of whether a preoperative ulnar neuropathy exists. Unless hardware considerations dictate otherwise, the nerve is only decompressed and not transposed anteriorly. Anterior transposition is performed only when low placement of a medial plate is required around the medial epicondyle or when undue tension or instability of the nerve is noted after completion of the reconstruction.

Mobilization

Significantly improved long-term functional results, which are the most important end results of any fracture fixation, have been demonstrated with early range of motion after complicated fracture repair.[16] Early mobilization of the elbow not only reduces periarticular adhesions and soft tissue scar formation, but, in severely comminuted intra-articular fractures, it can provide a *form molding* for appropriate cartilage repair or fibrocartilage formation. If appropriate fixation can be obtained, early continuous passive motion is an excellent treatment option after surgery.[19] In the short term, this modality reduces overall postoperative pain and improves long-term functional range of motion.

GUIDELINES FOR TREATMENT SPECIFIC PROBLEM FRACTURES

Significant Comminution

Significant comminution of a distal humeral fracture remains the single most important challenge and impediment to an appropriate operative repair. Intra-articular comminution not only presents a problem in restoring anatomic fracture fragment alignment, but also jeopardizes postoperative stability and the early range of motion that needs to be initiated. Extra-articular comminution, mainly involving that of the lateral or medial columns, also requires careful, appropriate fixation so that the mechanical axis of rotation about the elbow is maintained.

If the intra-articular fracture component involves just a single fracture line and no significant comminution, the surgeon uses preliminary fracture reduction forceps instead of K-wires to maintain provisional reduction and secures definitive fixation by placing a cancellous screw in a lag-type fashion. Generally, the surgeon has no difficulty obtaining appropriate intra-articular compression (Fig. 19.11). Occasionally, drilling the lagged fragment from the fracture line outward before placing the screw is easier and allows precise placement of the screw in the exact center of the distal articular fragment.

The second phase of operative fixation involves placing the repaired distal intra-articular unit onto the proximal humeral shaft. This step of repair can be just as difficult as the first step because of the need to obtain appropriate alignment of the articular unit with regard to the humeral shaft. As stated earlier, one of the two

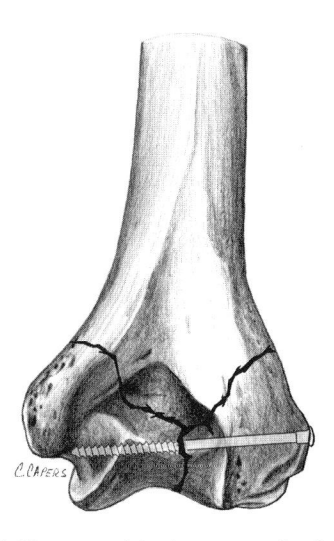

FIGURE 19.11. Transcondylar lag-screw fixation across non-comminuted trochlear fracture.

columns is less comminuted and can be reconstructed anatomically from three or less fragments to provide orientation and alignment of the reconstructed distal humeral articular fragment. In this case, provisional fixation of the column is obtained using clamps or K-wires; then the distal unit is affixed to the proximal humeral shaft using distal to proximal crossed K-wires. The other column then can be pieced together or, if too much comminution exists, can be adequately bone grafted.

In some instances of trochlear comminution, fixing one condyle back to its column, reducing the other condyle, and evaluating the trochlear relationship provide the easiest approach. Bone graft and trochlear fixation are accomplished last. Despite severe comminution, cartilage surfaces invariably show the true contours.

If significant intra-articular comminution is present, the surgeon should approach initial reduction of the joint surfaces with multiple K-wires for preliminary fixation. In this case, placing at least one, if not two, screws across the comminuted segment is always preferable; however, the screws used generally should not be lag screws, because of the significant intra-articular comminution and the possibility of compression resulting in inappropriate narrowing of the intra-articular trochlear component. Use of 3.5- or 4.5-mm cannulated screws allows for predictable placement over the provisional fixation guide pins. Autogenous bone graft should be used liberally and should be packed densely in all voids with intra-articular trochlear comminution. If corticocancellous compression-resistant bone graft can be obtained and the intra-articular component can be well filled, a lag screw can be used for compression against the bone graft; however, a fine balance must be maintained between the compression from the lag effect and the relatively soft intra-articular substance against which it is compressing (Fig. 19.12). The surgeon should place multiple screws in as many fracture fragments as possible. If some of the provisional K-wires appear to afford additional stability to small fracture fragments or to fragments that cannot be fixed easily using screws through the plates or single screws, they are left in place, and they are cut, turned, and hammered into the cortex of the distal humerus. The surgeon must remember that the 3.5-mm cortical and 4.0-mm cancellous screws are limited in length to 50 mm. If a long screw is required, then the 4.5-mm cortical screw should be used.

A significant problem arises when both columns of the distal humerus are comminuted significantly and cannot be reconstructed with any assurance of the intra-articular component alignment relative to the shaft. In this case, the surgeon must make a best guess of the alignment of the distal component to the proximal component. The 15° angle between a line connecting the trochlea to the capitellum and a line perpendicular to the long axis of the humeral shaft and the 40° anterior angulation of the trochlea and capitellar complex relative to the humeral shaft must be re-created for fixation purposes when aligning the two main components. Occasionally, if the arc of comminution of the distal humerus is significant (greater than 1 cm in width), although relatively short in length, the two main components of the fracture can be compressed (i.e., shortening of the humerus), rather than reduced at their original length relationship. The 15° carrying angle and 40° anterior angulation of the distal humeral component should be maintained even if the humerus is shortened. In general, we try to re-create an appropriate length relationship, but we have found that humeral shortening of 3 cm or less rarely causes any demonstrable postoperative deficiency in function.

The use of a cannulated screw system may aid in reducing overall operative time, because the surgeon can obtain provisional fixation using the threaded guide pins for these screws and can place the screws in appropriate position without removing the K-wire. The use of cannulated screws is appropriate in fixation of the intra-articular fracture components, as well as in the fixation of widely separated cortical fragments. One difficulty with using this system is that the guide wires bend relatively easily during drilling, so the surgeon should use a low axial pressure, high-speed drilling method when placing the guide pins. Whether cannulated screws significantly add to the fixation techniques of distal humeral fractures remains to be seen, but they do present an attractive alternative.

Low Fractures

A low fracture of the distal humerus—most often a transverse fracture through or just above the trochlea—is also frequently difficult to treat effectively. Even without significant comminution, these fractures afford little bony purchase for appropriate internal fixation distally and re-

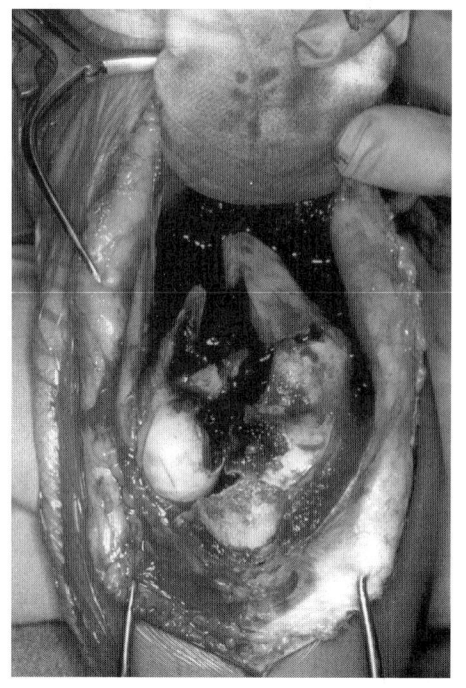

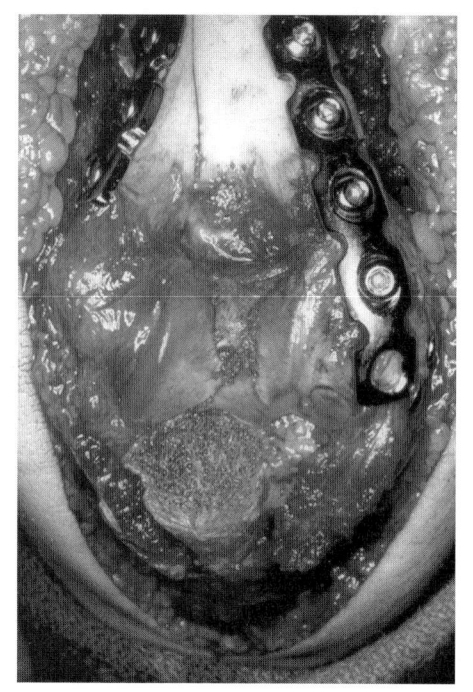

FIGURE 19.12. (A) AO C3 fracture with comminution of trochlea visualized posteriorly after olecranon osteotomy (shoulder above, olecranon below). (B) Same view after fracture reduction with plating. Note that substance loss below cartilage surface of central trochlea has been densely packed with cancellous bone. (C) AP (left) and lateral (right) radiographs after reconstruction (from Hastings H, Engles DR, *Hand clinics* 1997;13:703).

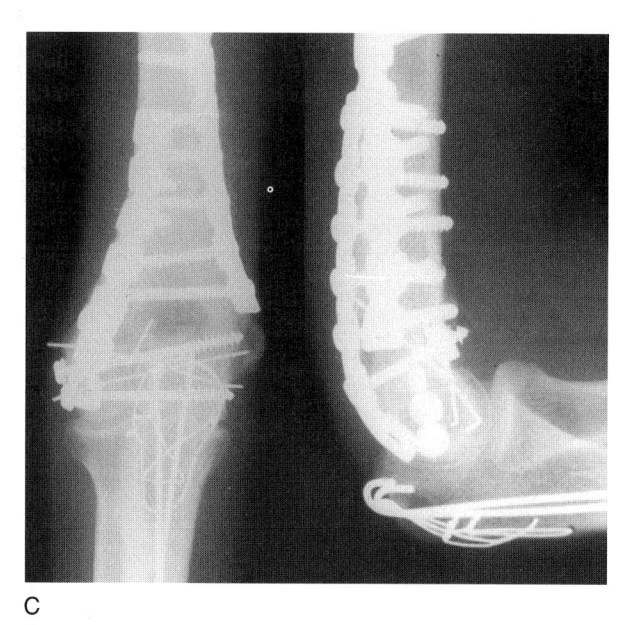

quire special techniques for appropriate fixation so that early postoperative range of motion can be initiated. In general, fractures that occur below the transverse axis and run through the distal olecranon fossa have little distal bony support for internal fixation.

When treating a very low fracture, medial and lateral plates are used to maximize the number of screws in the distal fragment. The medial plate is wrapped around the medial epicondyle, thereby "grabbing" it for additional fixation. In this case, an ulnar nerve transposition is necessary to prevent hardware impingement on the nerve. The surgeon can obtain additional fixation by passing a screw from the last distal hole of the wrapped plate in an oblique proximal fashion to the lateral supracondylar cortex (Fig. 19.13). This method can add significant stability to the distal fragment.

Another technique that can be used in the low fracture patterns is oblique bilateral K-wire tension banding. The

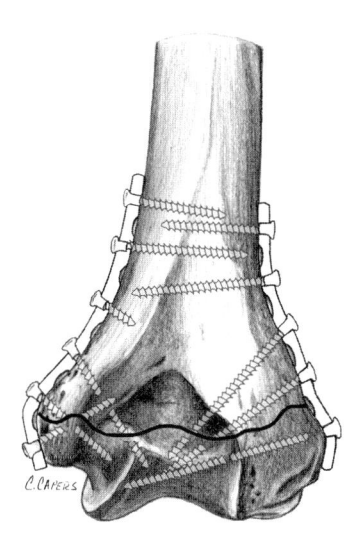

FIGURE 19.13. Low transcondylar fractures are best fixed with medial and lateral plates that maximize the number of screws that can be used to obtain purchase in the distal articular fragment.

K-wires are passed distal to proximal in the same fashion as in the initial preliminary reduction. Next, the K-wires are passed to the supracondylar cortical columns with a tension-band wire tightened on both K-wires, maintaining reduction of the low fracture fragment.

If excellent bone stock is present, a third option for fixation of the low fracture patterns is a blade plate. This method affords excellent distal fixation. However, it allows little room for error in placement of the plate, and it requires appropriate bending of the plate before fixation so that the distal fragment is aligned anatomically relative to the proximal humeral shaft.

Intra-articular Shear Fractures of the Trochlea

Shearing forces can produce a coronal shear fracture involving the trochlea and, at times, a portion of the capitellum.[20] Proper reduction and fixation of this fracture and an olecranon osteotomy are difficult through a triceps-preserving approach, because the procedures require an approach to both the anterior and the posterior trochlea. A proper exposure can be accomplished through an extended Kocher incision. The terminal triceps insertion is detached, and the anconeus and triceps are reflected medially. The entire common extensor origin and lateral collateral–annular ligament complex is released subperiosteally off the distal humerus. The anterior capsule is incised. This allows the elbow to be dislocated, hinging on the medial structures. Reduction usually requires supporting bone graft. Fixation is accomplished either through reabsorbable Kirshner wires or buried headless screws (Fig. 19.14).

Osteoporotic Bone

Distal humeral fractures are not uncommon in elderly people, who frequently slip and fall on an outstretched

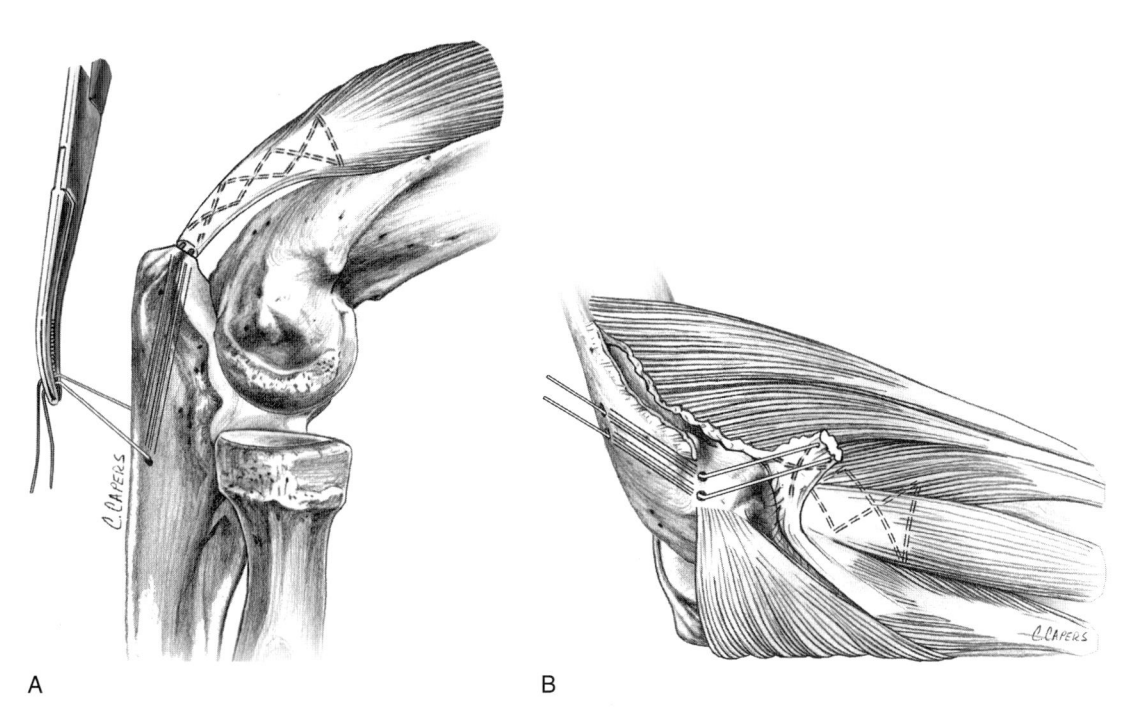

FIGURE 19.14. (A) Reconstruction of the triceps is accomplished with no. 5 braided nylon suture passed through drill holes. (B) Repair of the common extensor origin and lateral collateral–annular ligament complex is accomplished with no. 5 braided nylon passed through drill holes centered over the axis of motion, brought out, and tied posteriorly.

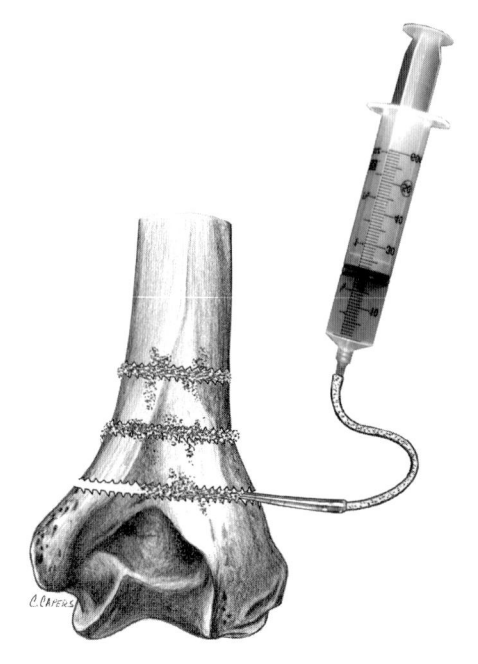

FIGURE 19.15. Polymethyl methacrylate bone cement augmentation of screw fixation.

arm. Osteoporotic bone, which is often present in this patient population, is another characteristic of these fractures that must be assessed preoperatively to plan for the appropriate fixation technique and for the possible need for more aggressive fracture–fragment buttressing using bone raft or bone cement. Adequately assessing the degree of comminution and the anatomical orientation of the fracture lines on preoperative radiographs is frequently difficult in these types of fractures.

When working with osteoporotic bone in any fracture, the surgeon initially should consider autogenous bone grafting to increase stable fixation of the plate and screw complex. However, if insufficient bone graft is available or if other circumstances prevent its use, the administration of polymethyl methacrylate bone cement with screw fixation can provide excellent postoperative stability (Fig. 19.15). This technique is best used sparingly so that healing of the distal humerus is not impeded. After reduction of the cortical components and provisional plate placement, all the appropriate cortical holes through the bicolumnar plates are drilled, measured for depth, and tapped, and the appropriate length screws are placed. Next, the surgeon removes these screws, injects the holes with cement, and quickly reinserts the screws before the cement hardens. This technique affords excellent stability in the osteoporotic bone of elderly people in whom rigid fixation is essential for appropriate healing purposes, but it has more limited applications in younger nonosteoporotic patients.

In older patients with low fractures and multiple comminuted fragments, stable fixation may not be achievable. In such patients with lower physical demands, the fragmented distal condyles are excised and the elbow is reconstructed by a semiconstrained implant arthroplasty (Fig. 19.16).

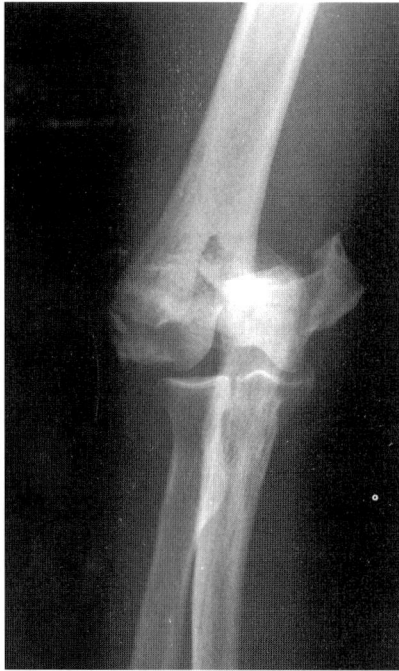

FIGURE 19.16. (A) This elderly woman with osteoporosis sustained an AO C3 fracture with severe comminution of the lateral condyle. (B) Function was restored with a semiconstrained implant arthroplasty (from Hastings H, Engles DR, *Hand clinics* 1997;13:703).

Soft Tissue

Radiographs of a distal humeral fracture do not reveal an important component of their operative treatment: soft-tissue management. Large open fractures accompanied by significant degloved or avulsed skin can leave large areas of articular cartilage poorly vascularized, exposed, and in need of aggressive debridement and coverage. Fixation of any fracture involving significant soft-tissue injury should be combined with early surgical coverage of the open defect. If at all possible, soft-tissue coverage should be undertaken concurrently or, at the latest, within several days of operative fracture fixation.

A nontensioned closure of the soft tissue surrounding the elbow joint is essential in obtaining long-term soft-tissue coverage and eliminating possible necrosis of any skin region. Local means should be used whenever possible to accomplish a soft-tissue closure without tension. If this closure cannot be accomplished without difficulty, distant means or even free-tissue transfers should be used.

The simplest method of local wound coverage at the elbow for small defects involves skin transposition from proximal to distal, with secondary skin grafting of the proximal defect.[21] Although a somewhat more involved procedure, lateral and medial defects at the epicondyles can be covered using fasciocutaneous flaps based on the radius and ulna, respectively.[22]

When extensive tissue loss is encountered, local muscle rotation flaps, such as the brachioradialis flap, can provide significant coverage with relatively little morbidity.[23] More distant myocutaneous flaps, such as lateral arm or radial forearm flaps, can provide excellent coverage as well.[24] Occasionally, wound coverage can be accomplished only by distant means with free muscle microvascular transfer from several donor areas. The elbow is rich in vascular collateral blood supply, so it is easily amenable to microvascular anastomoses.[25]

POSTOPERATIVE CONSIDERATIONS

An intraoperative assessment of the range of motion should be undertaken after rigid internal fixation of the fracture components, appropriate bone grafting, or use of bone cement in the patient who has osteoporotic bone. This assessment is important to ensure that the posterior olecranon fossa is free of obstruction and that the surgeon has obtained appropriate alignment of the fracture fragments, with the elbow following a normal arc of motion. Additionally, an intraoperative assessment of the range of motion aids the postoperative rehabilitation and provides physical therapists with information about what goals can be expected for the patient's motion.

We believe that, before closing the wound, the surgeon always should release the upper extremity tourniquet and should undertake adequate hemostasis with irrigation of the operative site. If the patient will begin early postoperative range-of-motion exercises or a continuous passive motion regimen, this practice is essential to prevent significant postoperative bleeding, resulting in soft-tissue compromise or hematoma. Hematoma leads to swelling that compromises motion and places additional demands on the internal fixation; therefore, a hemovac drain is placed in the postoperative wound. A light, compressive, bulky dressing should be placed along the entire length of the upper extremity.[26,27]

If rigid internal fixation has been achieved, immediate continuous passive motion is indicated. We believe that early continuous passive motion, which one of several commercially available machines can provide, can significantly reduce overall postoperative pain when active motion is initiated and potentially can aid in fibrocartilaginous remodeling of fracture surfaces. Our regimen involves placing the patient's upper extremity in a continuous passive motion machine in the recovery room, maintaining this motion continuously in the recovery room, and maintaining this motion continuously through the range-of-motion measure postoperatively, only interrupting this regimen if significant postoperative bleeding occurs through the hemovac drain. Active range of motion from four to six times each day is initiated as soon as the patient is able to tolerate these exercises (generally, from 2 to 4 days after surgery).

SUMMARY

Intra-articular fractures of the distal humerus require the surgeon to pay careful attention to detail for optimal functional results. Preoperative planning with AP and lateral radiographs of both the distal humerus and forearm should be used to plan the appropriate surgical approach and to assess the quality of bone stock. The use of oblique radiographs and computed tomography scans of the distal humerus can aid in further defining the fracture pattern and degree of comminution.

Surgical exposure of the fracture is simplified by draping the patient so that the arm is free and can be maneuvered easily. In most cases involving intra-articular comminution, an olecranon osteotomy provides the best exposure of the joint surfaces. We recommend a chevron osteotomy placed through the relative "void" region of the olecranon, with closure using a tension-band technique. Simple fracture patterns are surgically treated through a Bryan–Morrey approach.

After adequate surgical visualization of the fracture fragments, treatment efforts should center on reconstruction of the stabilizing components of the distal humerus (i.e., lateral column, medial column, and trochlea). Rigid internal fixation, even in patients who have osteoporotic and highly comminuted bone, remains the pivotal principle to functional rehabilitation of the elbow after surgery. Requirements for fixation are the use of 3.5-mm reconstruction plates along the columns in a multiplanar fashion after provisional K-wire fixation, the use of the appropriate lag-screw technique to stabilize individual fracture fragments, and the liberal use of bone grafting for areas of comminution. Advanced techniques using selective bone cement application, tension banding in an oblique plane, and plate wrapping of the fracture fragments might be needed in the most complicated fractures.

Following fracture fixation, a nontensioned closure of the surgical wound is essential to provide a stable, vascular bed for tissue healing and to permit early range-of-motion exercises. If the need for advanced tissue coverage techniques is required for such a closure, these techniques should be performed concurrently or, at the latest, within several days of fracture fixation. We have found that the use of continuous passive motion postoperatively helps to reduce overall pain levels when active exercises are begun. This modality has the additional benefit of providing a molding to the highly comminuted intra-articular fracture.

Adherence to these standard principles of fracture fixation and a step-by-step operative approach to even the most problematic fractures provides a predictable framework for early postoperative rehabilitation.

REFERENCES

1. Desault PJ. *A treatise on fractures, luxatins and other affections of the bones*. Bichat X, ed. Caldwell C, trans. Philadelphia: Kimber and Conrad; 1811.
2. Bryan RS, Bickel WH. "T" condylar fractures of distal humerus. *J Trauma* 1971;11:830–835.
3. Helfet DL, Schmeling GJ. Bicondylar intra-articular fractures of the distal humerus in adults. *Clin Orthop* 1993;292:26–36.
4. Jupiter JB, Neff U, Holzach P, et al. Intercondylar fractures of the humerus. An operative approach. *J Bone Joint Surg* 1985;67A:226–239.
5. Jupiter JB, Mehne DK. Fractures of the dostal humerus. *Orthopedics* 1992;15:825–833.
6. Brown RF, Morgan RG. Intercondylar T-shaped fractures of the humerus. Results in ten cases treated by early mobilisation. *J Bone Joint Surg* 1971;53B:425–428.
7. Dowden JW. The classic: The principle of early active movement in treating fractures of the upper extremity. *Clin Orthop* 1980;146:4–8.
8. Eastwood WJ. The T-shaped fracture of the lower end of the humerus. *J Bone Joint Surg* 1937;19:364–369.
9. Hitzrot JM. Fractures of the lower end of the humerus in adults. *Surg Clin North Am* 1932;12:291–304.
10. Reich RS. Treatment of intercondylar fractures of the elbow by means of traction. *J Bone Joint Surg* 1936;18:997–1004.
11. Halls AA, Travill R. Transmission of pressures across the elbow joint. *Anat Reconst* 1964;150:243–247.
12. Heim U, Pfeiffer KM. *Small fragment set manual. Technique recommended by the ASIF group* (ASIF: Swiss Association for Study of Internal Fixation), 2nd ed. New York: Springer-Verlag; 1982.
13. Johansson H, Olerud S. Operative treatment of intercondylar fractures of the humerus. *J Trauma* 1971;11:836–843.
14. Müller ME, Allgower M, Schneider R, et al. *Manual of internal fixation. Techniques recommended by the AO group*, 3rd ed. New York: Springer-Verlag; 1991.
15. Riseborough EJ, Radin EL. Intercondylar T fractures of the humerus in the adult. A comparison of operative and nonoperative treatment in twenty-nine cases. *J Bone Joint Surg* 1969;51A:130–141.
16. Shetty S. Surgical treatment of T and Y fractures of the distal humerus. *Injury* 1983;14:345–348.
17. Tubiana R, McCullough CJ, Masquelet AC. *An atlas of surgical exposures of the upper extremity*. London: Martin Dunitz; 1990.
18. Bryan RS, Morrey BF. Extensive posterior exposure of the elbow: A triceps-sparing approach. *Clin Orthop* 1982;166:188–192.
19. Salter RB, Simmonds DF, Malcolm BW, et al. The biological effect of continuous passive motion on the healing of full-thickness defects in articular cartilage. An experimental investigation in the rabbit. *J Bone Joint Surg* 1980;62A:1232–1251.
20. McKee MD, Jupiter JB, Bamberger HB. Coronal shear fractures of the distal end of the humerus. *J Bone Joint Surg* 1996:78A:49–54.
21. Hentz VR, Pearl RM, Kaplan EN. Use of medial upper arm skin as an arterialised flap. *Hand* 1980;12:241–247.
22. Lamberty BG, Cormack GC. Fasciocutaneous flaps. *Clin Plast Surg* 1990;17:713–726.
23. Lai MF, Krishna BV, Pelly AD. The brachioradialis myocutaneous flap. *Br J Plast Surg* 1981;34:431–434.
24. Soutar DS, Tanner NS. The radial arm forearm flap in the management of soft tissue injuries of the hand. *Br J Plast Surg* 1984;37:18–26.
25. Godina M. Early microsurgical reconstruction of complex trauma of the extremities. *Plast Reconstr Surg* 1986;78:285–292.
26. Cassebaum WH. Operative treatment of T and Y fractures of the lower end of the humerus. *Am J Surg* 1952;83:265–270.
27. Horne G. Supracondylar fractures of the humerus in adults. *J Trauma* 1980;20:71–74.

CHAPTER 20

Radial Head Fractures

Frances Sharpe and Stuart H. Kuschner

INTRODUCTION

In 1926, Cutler stated that the lack of uniformity in the treatment and results of radial head fractures makes these fractures interesting and in need of further investigation, especially "because of their importance to patients, entailing, as they not infrequently do, permanent disabling injury to the elbow joint."[1] Certainly, progress has been made toward a better understanding of the treatment of these injuries; however, their management is still both difficult and controversial.

The treatment of radial head fractures has developed over the years and has employed various techniques and fixation methods. In their review, Schwartz and Young[2] summarized the treatment of radial head fractures up to 1932. Until that time, treatment entailed various methods of closed reduction and immobilization, instead of partial or total radial head excision. Neuwirth in 1942 and Mason and Shutkin in 1943 were some of the first advocates of early active motion after treatment of radial head fractures.[3,4] In 1941, Speed introduced a radial head prosthesis that used a ferrule cap; in 1953, Cherry suggested using an acrylic spacer for the prosthesis.[5,6] In the late 1960s, Swanson began using Silastic radial head spacers.[7,8] Subsequently, various metallic spacers have been reintroduced. Harrington and Tountas began using titanium prostheses in the late 1960s and repeated their results in 1980.[9] Open reduction and internal fixation, with the exception of suture fixation of large fragments, was rarely seen until the late 1960s and early 1970s. In 1979, Odenheimer and Harvey cited the good results with anatomical reduction and internal fixation of radial head fractures reported earlier by French and German authors.[10] They reported excellent results in their two cases and subsequently it has been an area of active interest.

Over the past 15 years, much controversy has arisen over the treatment of fractures of the radial head since the introduction of open reduction and stable internal fixation in the late 1970s. In addition, pitfalls associated with radial head excision, as well as better recognition of concomitant injuries leading to later elbow instability or dysfunction at the wrist, have drawn attention to the management of radial head fractures. Improvements in implants for fixation of small fracture fragments have made preservation of the head more technically feasible. In addition, more interest has focused on the design and indications for using radial head prostheses.

Authors have reported that the incidence of radial head and neck fractures is between 3% and 30% of elbow fractures.[11–15] In most series, the minimally displaced or nondisplaced fractures (Mason type I fractures) represent from 40% to 60% of the fracture types seen. The remainder are equally divided between the displaced marginal fractures and comminuted fractures.[16–19] Fractures of the radial head are most commonly seen in adults, with the greatest incidence occurring in patients between the ages of 30 to 60 years old.[1,20,21] The high incidence of elbow injuries that accompanies radial head fractures is important to recognize too. The most common injury is posterior elbow dislocation, which has been estimated to be between 10% and 30% of accompanying injuries.[14,15,20,21]

In this chapter, we discuss the diagnosis of various types of radial head fractures and the appropriate treatment methods for each type. Our discussion covers the clinical anatomy, mechanism of injury, diagnosis, review of treatment, and the authors' preferred techniques.

CLINICAL ANATOMY

The radial head has two primary functions: (1) load transfer from the hand and wrist to the distal humerus, longitudinally stabilizing the hand and wrist during grip and loading activities; and (2) secondary restraint to valgus stress at the elbow.

The radial head is a disc-shaped structure that is approximately 3.5 mm thick. Its articular surface with the capitellum is ovoid in shape; that is, it is longer in the anteroposterior than coronal plane (approximately 2.5 cm by 2.2 cm).[22] The head is placed eccentrically relative to the central axis of the smaller-diameter neck, leaving the anterolateral aspect of the head relatively unsupported by subchondral bone. The subchondral support consists of longitudinal columns of dense cancellous bone. This architecture is important in fracture patterns that are observed clinically.[4,23] Both the capitellar surface and the circumference of the head are covered in articular cartilage. The circumferential cartilage narrows laterally, because this area does not articulate with the lesser sigmoid notch of the ulna and is therefore a useful area for placing internal fixation.

The radial head is reciprocally curved with the capitellum. However, Mason stated that in the unloaded forearm the radial head does not contact the capitellum except at extremes of flexion.[16] The circumference of the head is held tightly in the lesser sigmoid notch of the ulna. Pronation and supination occur over an arc of 160° to 170°,[4,16,22] corresponding to a 320° arc of the articular circumference of the head. However, in a cadaver study, Smith and Hotchkiss found only a 250° arc on the articular surface that contacted the lesser sigmoid notch.[24] Thus, fractures of the radial head occurring within the arc of rotation necessarily would interfere with pronation and supination. This involvement of the arc of rotation is also the basis of Mason's distinction between type I and II fractures in his classification system.[16]

The ligamentous anatomy is important to elbow stability, and this fact is apparent in the discussion of complex radial head fractures, which occur in combination with ligamentous disruptions about the elbow, and in the consideration of radial head excision. The annular ligament, reinforced by the quadrate ligament, holds the radial head in the lesser sigmoid notch.[22] Soft-tissue constraints contribute both to the longitudinal and the varus–valgus stability of the elbow. In their work, Morrey et al., Schwab et al., and Tullos et al. identified the medial collateral ligament, especially its anterior fibers, as the primary stabilizer to valgus stress at the elbow and identified the radial head as a secondary stabilizer.[25–30] They act in this way in both flexion and extension. The radial head, in part, provides longitudinal stability. However, again, ligamentous contributions of the interosseous membrane and triangulofibrocartilage complex play an important role, with the central portion of the interosseous membrane as the most important contributor to stability.[31] This ligamentous stability allows radial head excision without leading to significant cubitus valgus or proximal migration of the radius. Thus, the ligamentous integrity about the elbow and forearm must be assessed carefully.

Finally, vascular supply to the radial head should be considered. Avascular necrosis is rarely seen in the radial head, despite the fact that many of the fracture fragments are stripped completely of soft-tissue attachments and that many fractures are reduced and provisionally stabilized entirely ex vivo. However, when a fracture is treated with internal fixation rather than excision, the blood supply is a concern. In injection studies, Girard et al. found several contributions to the blood supply of the radial head, including the branches of the recurrent radial artery, the first collateral vessel of the ulnar artery, and a periosteal network arising from the pericervical anastomotic ring.[32] They found the most important zone was from the dorsolateral periosteal layer at the dorsolateral aspect of the neck. Consideration should be given to soft-tissue stripping, especially with regard to dorsolateral fragments.

MECHANISM OF INJURY

In several early articles, authors attributed radial head fractures to both direct and indirect mechanisms, with a preponderance of articles describing direct blows to the radial head as a cause of fracture.[1,17,33] However, more recently, authors of several clinical and laboratory studies have favored an indirect mechanism involving a fall onto the partially extended, pronated forearm as the predominant mechanism of radial head fracture.[4,13,27,34] Amis and Miller re-created elbow fractures in a cadaver model under various loading conditions, including both direct and indirect loads.[34] They found that all radial head fractures were produced through indirect forces that simulated falls onto the outstretched arm with the elbow between 0° to 80° of flexion. Higher-energy loads produced commensurate elbow dislocations in 6 of 12 specimens. In his clinical findings, Bakalim showed a high percentage of marginal fractures in the anterolateral quadrant of the head; these findings support the theory that the indirect mechanism of injury involves the pronated forearm.[35] Further support of the indirect mechanism of injury comes from the frequent findings of fibrillation or laceration of the articular portion of the capitellar cartilage.[11,33,36,37] A direct blow to the radial head can cause fracture, but is considered an unusual mechanism of injury.

CLINICAL FINDINGS

Physical findings depend on the severity of injury. Typically, swelling occurs about the elbow and often is localized to the lateral side of the elbow. Hemarthrosis of the elbow may be visible because of the loss of the bony landmarks at the triangular region, which the lateral epicondyle, olecranon, and radial head define, on the lateral side of the elbow. The effusion or hemarthrosis also can be palpated as a bogginess in this area. The patient usually holds his or her arm in a position of flexion and midpronation. The patient has localized tenderness to palpation about the radial head. Range of motion is guarded and painful when the patient attempts pronation or supination. The examiner should carefully assess the arm for medial tenderness at the elbow, as well as for tenderness and swelling at the wrist and along the interosseous membrane. Morrey stated that, in his experience, tenderness at the distal radioulnar joint was the most sensitive measure of longitudinal instability.[38] Neurologic injury in an isolated fracture of the radial head is rare; however, the relatively high incidence of associated injuries to the elbow with a radial head fracture warrants a careful neurologic examination.

RADIOGRAPHIC EXAMINATION

Standard anteroposterior and lateral radiographs are used in the initial evaluation of the elbow. In nondisplaced fractures, the fracture line may be difficult to see initially. However, the presence of a hemarthrosis, which displacement of the posterior fat pad indicates,[39] and the physical findings of localized tenderness about the radial head indicate radial head fracture.

The examiner also should carefully evaluate radiographs for signs of injury to the capitellum. Fracture fragments proximal to the radial head or within the radiocapitellar joint strongly suggest a fracture of the capitellum. Further information may be obtained from additional views, such as oblique and radial head–capitellum views. The radial head–capitellum view (see Fig. 3.3) is taken with the elbow in the lateral position (i.e., elbow flexed to 90°, humeral condyles located in the same plane and positioned perpendicular to the film plate, and thumb pointed upward with the forearm supinated). The beam is projected at 45° to the forearm and centered over the radial head. This view removes the overlapping shadows of the olecranon and trochlea and provides an unimpaired view of the capitellum and radial head.[40–42]

Tomography or computed tomography scanning can be useful in defining fracture fragments when considering open reduction and internal fixation. The role of magnetic resonance imaging is seldom discussed, but it can help the examiner view the injury when he or she suspects disruption of the interosseous membrane, but cannot confirm it on clinical examination.

CLASSIFICATION SYSTEMS

Classification systems not only provide guidelines for treatment and prognosis, but also provide a common language for comparing outcomes among different treatments and different observers. The most commonly used classification system[43,44] is a modified version of the system that Mason proposed in 1954.[16] Before the publication of Mason's classification system, several authors used their own classification systems; most of these systems are adequately similar to allow comparison between studies.[1,11,36,45] Mason classified radial head fractures into three types: (1) type I, fissure fracture or marginal fracture without displacement (Fig. 20.1); (2) type II, marginal sector fracture with displacement (Fig. 20.2); and (3) type III, comminuted fractures involving the entire head (Fig. 20.3). Mason emphasized two related features of the fractures as important in determining treatment, but neither of these features is included in his classification system. The first feature is the involvement of more than 25% of the circumference of the head, which

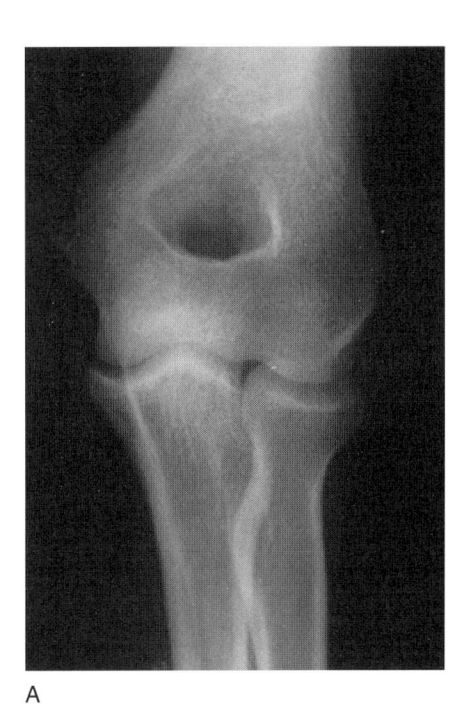

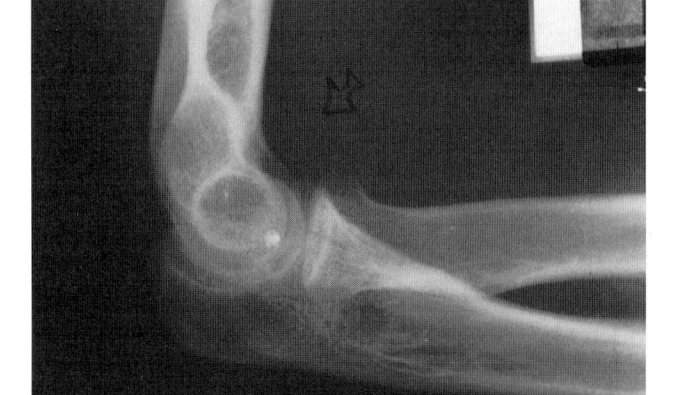

FIGURE 20.1. (A) Anteroposterior and (B) lateral views of a Mason type I fracture. In this patient, the fracture is best seen in the lateral radiographic view. In addition, the lateral view demonstrates distension of the joint capsule and displacement of the anterior fat pad (arrow).

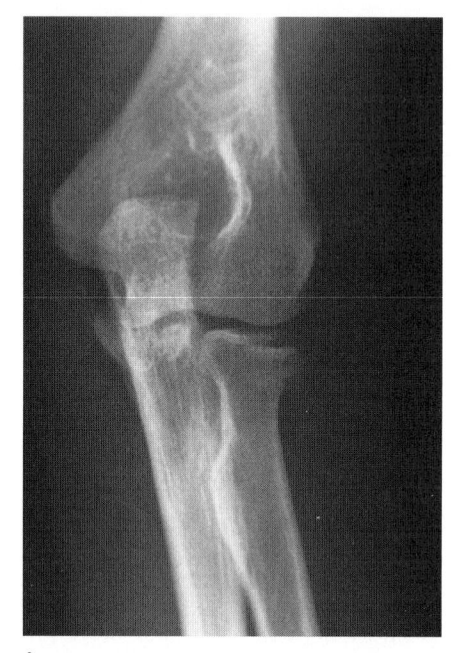

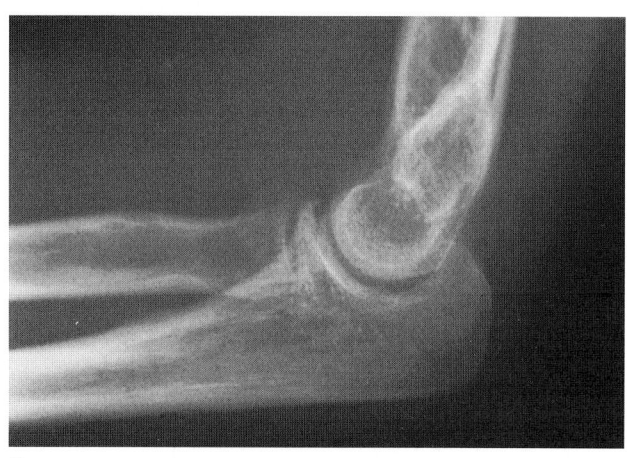

ers[14,21,36] recognized the association of radial head fractures with concomitant injuries about the elbow, especially posterior dislocation, and proposed adding this fracture as a type IV injury.

Mason's classification system has several shortcomings. As stated, although Mason emphasized the importance of a mechanical block to motion in recommending treatment, he did not include it in his classification system. Furthermore, he did not include complex injuries about the elbow that were associated with ligamentous disruption. Finally, a review of inter- and intra-observer error in the use of Mason's system demonstrated only necessarily articulates in the sigmoid notch. The second feature is the presence of a mechanical block to motion. In his own series, Mason recognized 8 of 20 type II fractures as "borderline cases."[16] He considered these fractures as bordering on the need for operative treatment. They met the criterion of involving more than 25% of the articular surface; however, the amount of deformity in the articular surface was small and judged unlikely to interfere with joint motion. McLaughlin proposed further criteria to help to describe the type II fractures, using more than 3 mm of displacement or 30° of angulation to define these borderline fractures.[43] Johnston[44] and oth-

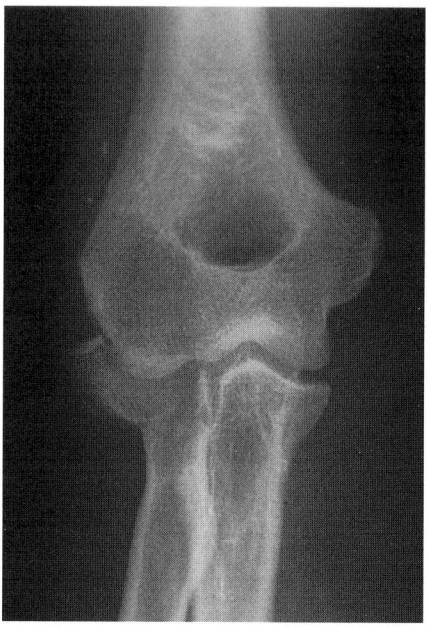

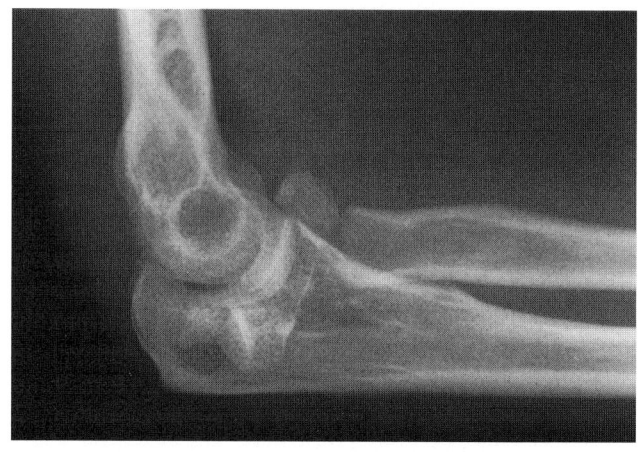

FIGURE 20.2. (A) Anteroposterior and (B) lateral radiographic views show that this displaced marginal fracture, or Mason type II fracture, involves less than 25% of the circumference of the head. If no mechanical block to rotation is found, the fracture may be treated nonoperatively.

FIGURE 20.3. (A) Anteroposterior and (B) lateral radiographic views show that this comminuted, or Mason type III, fracture involves the entire radial head. Although radiographs do not always demonstrate the degree of comminution, these fragments appear amenable to open reduction and internal fixation.

a 60% to 65% interobserver agreement in classifying fractures.[46] Despite its shortcomings, the modified Mason classification remains the most commonly used classification system. More complex systems add little to improve treatment recommendations or interobserver reliability.

REVIEW OF TREATMENT AND RESULTS

Selection of a treatment method requires consideration of the fracture type, the patient's activity level and general health, and the presence or absence of associated injuries.

Type I Fractures

Surgeons generally agree that type I fractures are best treated nonoperatively.[1,3,4,11,16,37,38,47,48] Various periods of immobilization have been recommended, ranging from as short a time period as the patient can tolerate it[3] to up to 3 weeks.[23,49,50] Additionally, authors have advocated various positions of immobilization, ranging from full pronation[51] to full supination.[11] Both Thompson[47] and Unsworth-White et al.[52] compared splinting the elbow in 90° of flexion with splinting in full extension. Thompson found a slight decrease in flexion contracture and an insignificant decrease in rotation when he used full-extension splinting. Two of eleven patients treated with 90° flexion splinting had a greater than 10° loss of extension. None of the nine patients treated with extension splinting had more than a 10° loss of extension. Unsworth-White et al. more strongly advocate splinting in full extension, reporting a loss of more than 10° of extension in 21% of patients splinted in 90° of flexion compared with no loss in the patients splinted in full extension.

Several authors have evaluated the role of aspiration with or without the injection of lidocaine.[18,23,36,47,51,53] Wagner advocated the use of aspiration of the hematoma, followed by an intra-articular injection of lidocaine to allow examination of joint range of motion and to evaluate the elbow for a mechanical block or persistent click.[18] Others have advocated aspiration alone or in combination with an anesthetic for pain relief, especially in the presence of a tense hemarthrosis. Holdsworth et al.[53] conducted a randomized study of patients who were treated with and without aspiration. These researchers found that patients treated with aspiration had better range of motion earlier, but their long-term outcome was unchanged. They concluded that aspiration was a safe procedure that afforded early pain relief and allowed the patient to begin active range of motion, which they believed should be the initial treatment for radial head fractures. There have been no reports of joint sepsis following aspiration and injection for radial head fractures.

The results of treatment in type I fractures are generally good, with most authors reporting 75% or 85% good to excellent results. Some patients have residual loss of extension, but the loss is rarely more than 10°. For most patients, the loss does not represent any functional loss. Occasional aching at the elbow is not uncommon, especially with a change in the weather. This fracture type rarely results in significant loss of motion or severe residual pain.

Type II Fractures

A variety of treatments has been recommended for marginal fractures with displacement.[10,14–16,19,38,48,54] These fractures can be treated nonoperatively or operatively. Nonoperative treatment is similar to that recommended for type I fractures. Operative treatment options include open reduction and internal fixation, excision of the displaced fragment, and complete radial head excision. The use of a radial head prosthesis following excision has been described; however, this option usually is reserved for complex fractures involving associated injuries about the elbow and forearm.[7,9,55]

In early studies, several authors advocated nonoperative treatment, with most authors recommending a longer period of immobilization than the period recommended for the nondisplaced or minimally displaced fractures. Late excision was recommended if satisfactory results were not obtained with closed management.[4,23] Others advocated partial or total excision of the displaced fragment.[14,15] Watson-Jones[14] and Wilson[15] advocated partial excision if less than one-third of the radial head was involved and advocated complete excision if more than one-third was involved. In his classification, Mason used the amount of involvement of the radial head as an important criterion for recommending treatment.[16] If more than one-fourth of the articular circumference of the radial head was involved, he recommended complete excision. He believed that a fracture with less involvement of the articular circumference could be managed nonoperatively.

Currently, most authors agree that not all displaced marginal fractures require internal fixation.[38,48] Rather, fractures that are displaced and present a mechanical block to motion should be treated with open reduction and internal fixation. Although authors occasionally mention suture fixation of large, displaced fracture fragments,[11] Odenheimer and Harvey were the first to discuss open reduction and stable internal fixation in the English-language literature.[10] Since then, many others have advocated fixing displaced marginal fractures with various methods of fixation, including Herbert screws (Zimmer; Warsaw, Indiana),[56,57] small and minifragment screws and plates (Synthes; Paoli, Pennsylvania),[58–60] and Kirschner-wire fixation.[10,61] Yuan-Zhang et al. reported the results in 34 patients who had a large, displaced, marginal fracture and who were treated with closed reduction and percutaneous pinning of their fracture.[61] When performing internal fixation, the surgeon must consider whether he or she can achieve stable internal fixation. If the surgeon cannot achieve fixation, then he or she probably should excise the radial head instead of leaving poorly stabilized fragments that will require prolonged immobilization to maintain reduction.

Although not widely used, two additional techniques of fixation have been described in Europe, but have not been reported in the United States. The first technique involves the use of bioabsorbable polyglycolide pins for radial head fracture fixation. Most reports on this method come from Finland[62–64] and Germany.[65] Based on the functional scoring system of Morrey et al., researchers report results comparable with results of fixation with metallic implants.[64] Absorbable implants do not require later removal; however, the rate of implant removal following metallic fixation already is low, and the cost of the absorbable implant is high. Also, absorbable implants sometimes form sterile abscesses; however, Pelto et al. state that the incidence of this problem has decreased since the introduction of a new generation of polyglycolide rods.[64]

The second technique, first described in a dog model, involves the use of a fibrin adhesive glue.[66] With this technique, the surgeon used a two-component system of fibrinogen catalyzed by thrombin that provided a glue strength of 135 kg/cm.^{2} A subsequent clinical trial undertaken in Spain reported the results in 15 patients.[67] Although the researchers presented scant results, they showed that the outcome at 2 years was similar to other methods of fixation and showed that no fracture displacement was seen. The disadvantages of this technique appear to be a limited population for whom this method can be used, a somewhat longer period of immobilization, and the use of human plasma extract in manufacturing the components of the sealant.[67]

Type III Fractures

Most authors advocate complete excision for isolated type III radial head fractures and report good results with this treatment.[13,16,17,27,68–71] Most authors believe that acute excision is better than delayed excision.[14,17,38] However, this belief generally seems to be founded on low numbers of patients who had a delayed excision. Based on a somewhat larger population, Adler and Shaftan found as good or better results with delayed excision than with acute excision.[54] Radial head replacement has been proposed for type III fractures; however, most authors believe this option should be used only for complex injuries about the elbow.[38,48] Internal fixation of type III fractures has been reported; however, this option is reserved for fractures with good bone quality and relatively large fragments.[56,59,72] Authors also have advocated nonoperative treatment.[4,19,54] Weseley et al. stated that only widely displaced comminuted fractures should be treated operatively,[19] and Adler and Shaftau stated that they obtained better results with nonoperative treatment.[54]

Results of Treatment for Type II and Type III Fractures

Direct comparison of the results of one study with the results of another is difficult, because treatment and outcome measures vary from one study to another. Several authors have stated that equally important to the type of treatment used are other parameters, such as severity of initial injury, patient motivation and compliance, and presence of associated injuries.[19,35,54] Perhaps the most important determinant of satisfactory outcome is the early initiation of active range of motion. Bakalim believed that early range of motion "molds the radial head" in the early phases of healing and produces secondary congruence of displaced fractures.[35,54]

Nonoperative Treatment

Good or excellent results have been reported with closed treatment in type II fractures.[19,35,49] For this reason, most current authors recommend evaluating the elbow for the presence of a mechanical block or instability before recommending operative treatment in the management of type II fractures.[38,49,73] Authors also have reported good results after nonoperative treatment of type III fractures.[19,35,54,74] These fractures usually are comminuted without wide displacement. An important point is that in all studies reporting good results with nonoperative treatment the surgeon initiated a program of active range of motion early in the course of treatment.

Partial Excision

Partial excision for the treatment of displaced fracture fragments has been described primarily only in early literature.[13,17,20] Based on findings of several authors, this method of treatment currently is not recommended.[13,15,17,18,75] Nonetheless, Carstam reported the results of 33 partial excisions in 33 patients (which is the largest report to date).[20] Of those patients, 75% obtained overall good or excellent results. Results were better when more than two-thirds of the radial head was left intact. Using this selection criterion, many of these patients may have done equally well with nonoperative treatment.

Open Reduction and Internal Fixation

The results achieved with open reduction and internal fixation appear to be independent of the type of fixation used. Fixation of type II fractures results in an overall better outcome than fixation of type III fractures, which would be expected because of the difference in severity of the initial injury. Authors of most series report good or excellent results of fixation of all type II fractures, with patients reporting little or no pain. Loss of extension ranges from 0° to 5°, and loss of rotation ranges from 0° to 15°.[56–58,72,76]

In most series of isolated type III fractures treated with internal fixation, authors report good or excellent results, with an average loss of extension ranging from 3° to 14° and a loss of rotation of 20°.[58,59,72] Patients report only occasional mild to moderate pain, which usually occurs after heavy labor. King et al. reported the results in 19 patients with 20 radial head fractures treated with open reduction and internal fixation.[76] Thirteen of the patients with 14 fractures were available for follow-up. Several of these (11 of 20) had associated injuries of the elbow, but the results were not listed separately for this group. The results of treatment in type II fractures (8 of 14) were excellent, but the results in type III fractures (6 of 14) were not as good, giving an overall fair outcome. In two of these six patients, an anatomic reduction could not be achieved at the time of surgery. In two patients, the reduction was lost postoperatively. The poor outcomes in this group were seen only in patients who had loss of reduction or initial nonanatomic reduction. The results of this study emphasize the importance of obtaining both an anatomic reduction and stable internal fixation. If these goals cannot be achieved, these injuries are better treated with early excision.

Radial Head Excision

The literature includes several long-term studies of outcome following radial head excision, with a follow-up ranging from 15 to 30 years.[12,16,27,68–71,77,78] Seventy percent to 80% of patients in these studies had an overall good or excellent result, with most patients returning to their previous occupation. Wagner found that residual symptoms at the elbow were most correlated with loss of motion and predominately with loss of complete extension.[18] Seventy percent to 85% of patients regained full range of motion, and the remainder of patients was limited primarily in extension.[16,17,19,69] Strength testing about the elbow in flexion, extension, pronation, and supination demonstrated a decrease in strength of between 5% and 20%; rotational strength was affected more than flexion. Grip strength decreased by 15% to 20%.[27,68] In most series, the carrying angle increased typically by 7° to 10°. Although most patients were asymptomatic, intermittent ulnar nerve symptoms could occur.[20,68,70] The average proximal radial migration ranged from 2 to 3 mm, with asymptomatic subluxation found at the distal radioulnar joint in up to 65% of patients. An estimated 5% of patients reported symptoms at the wrist, but these symptoms seldom were so severe that they had to be treated. Degenerative changes at the distal radioulnar joint could be seen on radiographs, but radiographic changes did not correlate well with symptoms.[68,69]

Delayed Excision

The results reported for type II and III fractures treated with delayed excision have been comparable. Most authors have advocated early excision; however, this preference appears largely based on a small number of patients and anecdotal experience.[13,17,36] Gaston et al. believed that the radial head should be excised within 24 hours of injury to assure a good functional result.[36] Murray stated that patients undergoing acute excision had better results than patients treated with delayed excision.[13] Radin and Riseborough strongly advocated acute excision based on poor functional results in four patients who had delayed excision.[17] A more recently published study of a larger population suggests improved range of motion and strength with primary excision.[79]

Other authors have advocated delayed excision. Charnley believed that excision should be delayed to allow soft-tissue healing, thus minimizing problems of proximal radial migration or cubitus valgus.[75] Adler and Shaftan found no difference in results when comparing patients treated with acute excision and patients treated with delayed excision.[54] Based on their experience of better results in nonoperatively managed patients, they recommended an 8-week trial of nonoperative management before excising the radial head. Finally, Broberg and Morrey evaluated the results of delayed excision in 21 patients at an average follow-up of 15 years.[80] Most patients had a clinically significant decrease in pain scores and improvement in range of motion, with 77% of patients achieving a good or excellent result. They did not advocate routine treatment with delayed excision, but it certainly is a viable treatment alternative.

Complex Injuries

Morrey suggested that radial head fractures associated with concomitant injuries about the elbow should be classified as complex injuries.[38,81] The treatment of these injuries is often more dependent on the associated injury than on the fracture pattern of the radial head. Many patterns of associated injury have been reported in the literature.[9,44,82–89] The most common associated injury is posterior elbow dislocation, which occurs in approximately 10% of patients.[21,36,38,44,81]

Based on the frequency of occurrence of elbow dislocation and its notably poorer prognosis, Johnston recommended a separate category for this injury within the Mason classification system, describing it as a type IV injury.[44] Regardless of the method used to treat this injury, the fracture carries a poorer prognosis with higher pain scores and greater loss of motion in flexion and rotation than other elbow fractures. In several series, authors noted that the average loss of extension was 20°. A higher incidence of heterotopic ossification is also seen with these injuries.[82,86,87]

Further concerns with these injuries are related to elbow stability. Often, an elbow dislocation is accompanied by an injury to the medial ligaments, which normally function as the primary restraint to valgus stress at the elbow. When combined with a radial head fracture, both the primary and secondary restraints are lost. In this situation, most authors recommend attempted retention of the radial head. If the head cannot be preserved, it should be replaced with a prosthesis.

Radial Head Prostheses

Routine use of a radial head prosthesis following a radial head excision is not recommended, but the prosthesis plays a useful role in the treatment of complex injuries about the elbow. For example, it can be useful in the treatment of an active young adult who has had a radial head excision for an isolated radial head fracture.

Morrey et al. compared their results in patients who had a Silastic radial head prostheses with the results in a previous series of patients who had radial head excision.[90] They found no advantage and some disadvantages with the routine use of the Silastic head. These disadvantages included dislocation and breakage of the prosthesis, silicone synovitis, and the necessity for another operation in 24% of their patients. They did recognize its usefulness in patients who had complex injuries and instability following radial head excision. They later recommended that when the Silastic radial head is used it should be removed after 6 months to prevent the development of silicone synovitis.[91–93]

More recently, authors of several biomechanical studies have demonstrated the inability of silicone implants to resist proximal migration and valgus loads.[94–96] They have further studied the use of metallic radial head replacements and have found better re-creation of resistance to axial and valgus loads. Recent clinical studies also have focused on the use of metallic radial head replacements.[9,55,94,97] Harrington and Tountas[9] reported the results of metallic radial head replacement in 17 patients who had radial head fractures associated with gross instability of the elbow. They obtained 14 good or excellent results with the use of a titanium implant. They emphasized, as did Morrey et al.,[90] that they do not recommend radial head replacement following routine radial head excision. However, they achieved good functional results when using the prosthesis to treat these complex injuries.

Radial Head Fractures and Longitudinal Instability

Acute

Acute longitudinal instability with disruption of the interosseous membrane and of the distal radioulnar joint associated with radial head fractures is an uncommon, but problematic, injury. Although Brockman first reported two cases of disability at the wrist associated with radial head excision, it was not clear from the report whether this was a missed acute injury to the interosseous membrane or a chronic development.[98] In 1946, Curr and Coe first described acute distal radioulnar joint dislocation associated with radial head fractures.[99] However, after Peter Essex-Lopresti described the injury in 1951, his name became synonymous with this injury.[100] Tearing of the interosseous membrane has been confirmed subsequently by direct inspection[101,102] and by magnetic resonance imaging.[31]

Treatment of acutely diagnosed longitudinal instability has not changed significantly since 1951 when Essex-Lopresti recommended attempted preservation of the radial head or, in cases in which the head cannot be reconstructed, the use of a prosthetic replacement.[100] In fractures amenable to open reduction, rigid internal fixation restores radial length and obviates future problems associated with implant failure. Severely comminuted fractures requiring radial head excision can be treated with a radial head prosthesis. Metallic implants that do not require removal later should be used; otherwise, the interosseous membrane may not heal with adequate mechanical integrity despite months of protection. This phenomenon was described by Knight et al., who reported the case of a patient with 1 cm of radial shortening following removal of a metallic prosthesis.[55] The dislocation at the distal radioulnar joint is treated with closed reduction in supination with or without supplemental, temporary percutaneous pinning. This position is maintained with a cast or splint from 4 to 6 weeks.[103] Some authors have suggested repair of the triangulofibrocartilage complex or distal ligamentous constraints, but this repair remains controversial.[38,104] In the presence of an irreducible dislocation, soft-tissue repair may have a role, but this role is rare in the acute setting. Additionally, Hotchkiss et al. and Rabinowitz et al. found that the interosseous membrane, and not the distal ligaments, is the most critical structure for preventing proximal migration of the radius.[31,105,106]

Edwards and Jupiter reported on seven patients who had Essex-Lopresti injuries treated between 5 days and 10 weeks after injury.[103] Two patients were treated with rigid internal fixation; four, with Silastic radial head replacement; and one, who refused further surgery, with radial head excision. Results were based on the 100-point scale that Morrey described.[107] The two patients treated with early internal fixation and the one patient treated with an early Silastic head spacer achieved excellent results. The three patients treated with Silastic radial head spacers between 4 and 10 weeks after injury achieved only fair or good results. Whether the results reflect the timing or the type of surgery is unclear.

Chronic

Chronic proximal migration of the radius has been reported following nonoperative treatment of radial head fractures[98] and following radial head resection.[27,70,71,90,108] Researchers evaluating proximal migration have found an average of 2 to 3 mm of proximal migration (range, 0 to 10 mm) at the distal radioulnar joint on long-term follow-up. None of these researchers has found a correlation between wrist symptoms and radiographic findings.[17,27,68,69,71] Morrey suggested that the chronic proximal migration may represent a spectrum of injury to the interosseous membrane and distal ligaments that occurs at the time of injury.[38] It also may represent a gradual attenuation of the interosseous membrane over time as a response to repeated axial loading in the absence of the buttressing of the radial head against the capitellum.

Although most chronic proximal migration is small and asymptomatic, even greater translation has not correlated consistently with symptoms at the wrist.[27,68,109] However, Taylor and O'Connor reported the results in 58 patients at an average follow-up of 7.5 years after radial head excision and found a higher incidence of symptomatic proximal migration than the incidence in other series.[110] They reported a 50% incidence of wrist symptoms, typically consisting of wrist weakness with or without stiffness and mild to moderate wrist pain. They believed that these symptoms correlated with the level of activity, rather than with the degree of proximal migration.

Treatment of symptomatic proximal migration remains controversial. Swanson et al. recommended the use of a Silastic radial head prosthesis to salvage failed radial head excisions.[8] They reported the results in 12 patients who had Silastic radial head replacement between 1 and 20 years after radial head excision. All patients had decreased wrist pain, and most patients had decreased elbow pain and improved elbow range of motion. Other authors have found the treatment more problematic.[82,103,108] Sowa et al. presented eight patients who had symptomatic proximal migration; each patient was treated with a different surgical procedure.[108] These different treatments included those described by Darrach, Bower, and Suave-Kapandji; step-cut shortening osteotomy of the ulna; Silastic radial head replacement; and radioulnar synostosis that creates a one-bone forearm. Wrist pain recurred in all patients except the patient who had radioulnar synostosis. Although Sowa et al.[108] found persistent proximal migration following ulnar shortening, Morrey currently recommends ulnar shortening for symptomatic proximal migration and has not reported problems with persistent wrist pain or further shortening.[38] He recommends that the amount of ulnar shortening should be based on the amount of radial shortening that has occurred. Although he states that any method of shortening is acceptable, he prefers a step-cut shortening osteotomy of the ulna. Edwards and Jupiter also had success with a shortening osteotomy of the ulna in chronic cases in which radial length could not be restored.[103]

ARTHROSCOPIC TREATMENT

The role of arthroscopy has not yet been defined in the treatment of acute fractures. Byrd described arthroscopic intervention for the treatment of arthrofibrosis following nonoperative treatment of type I Mason fractures.[111] He reported his results in five patients treated with arthroscopic debridement. These patients had an average of 65% improvement in the arc of motion, with nearly equal gains in flexion and extension.

Arthroscopic radial head resection for posttraumatic arthritis was also described in 1994.[112] Menth-Chiari et al. describe their technique using proximal medial, anterolateral, and midlateral portals.[113] They did not report the number of patients in their series or their long-term outcome, but they stated that no complications occurred. Certainly, the greatest concern with this procedure is injury to the neurovascular structures, particularly the radial and posterior interosseous nerves.[114] Contributing to this risk is the potential distortion of normal anatomy related to the injury.

COMPLICATIONS

Complications of nonoperative management of radial head fractures include loss of range of motion, residual pain, and radiographic degenerative arthritis at the elbow. Heterotopic ossification also may occur, but this problem is associated most often with more severe injuries and concomitant soft-tissue injuries.

In addition to these risks, operative treatment additionally involves risk of injury to the posterior interosseous nerve. This nerve injury has been reported in as many as 7% of patients.[115] Usually, the injury is a neuropraxia that resolves in time. Operative treatment also carries a higher risk of heterotopic ossification than nonoperative treatment carries. Risks specific to internal fixation include fracture nonunion, avascular necrosis, implant failure, and prominent or painful hardware. However, these complications rarely occur.[58,72,115] Complications specific to radial head excision already have been discussed and include cubitus valgus with tardy ulnar nerve palsy, proximal radial migration, loss of grip strength, and radiographic degenerative changes at the wrist and elbow.[27,68–70,116]

The most common complications with the use of a radial head prosthesis are the problems associated with silicone synovitis and resultant erosive changes of the capitellum.[91,93] Implant loosening rarely has been reported with the use of metallic radial head prostheses.[55]

AUTHORS' PREFERRED TECHNIQUE

Type I Fractures

Patients who have a type I fracture are evaluated for the presence of a hemarthrosis and their ability to move their elbow through an active range of motion. Patients who present with either a tense hemarthrosis or significant pain with active range of motion are treated with joint aspiration, followed by an injection of a local anesthetic. Patients who do not have a significant hemarthrosis and who can move their elbow through an active range of motion do not need joint aspiration. A sling or splint is applied for a short period that usually lasts no longer than 1 week. We recommend that the patient continue to use the splint or sling for an additional week when he or she is at work or out in the community. However, the patient should frequently remove the splint throughout the day to do active range-of-motion exercises, including flexion, extension, and rotation exercises. These exercises should be started no later than 7 days after the injury. Supervised physical therapy is not necessary unless the patient is not showing improvement. The physician monitors the fracture for displacement at 5 to 7 days after the injury and after the patient begins active range-of-motion exercises. The physician should advise the patient that, although an uncommon occurrence, this fracture can displace.

Type II and Type III Fractures

The surgeon first evaluates type II fractures for the presence of a mechanical block to motion or a grinding sensation when the patient's elbow is taken through flexion, extension, and rotation. In the absence of a mechanical block or grinding, the surgeon treats type II fractures in the same manner as type I fractures. Radiographs are taken and followed closely during the first 2 weeks after injury to monitor the fracture for displacement. In the presence of a mechanical block to motion, we prefer to use open reduction and internal fixation to treat young patients or patients who place high demands on their elbow. We use the same technique for the treatment of both type II and type III fractures, which are amenable to stable internal fixation. For both type II and III fractures, we reserve the option of radial head excision if stable and accurate reduction cannot be achieved.

With the patient under anesthesia, the surgeon first evaluates the elbow for stability, especially for valgus stability and longitudinal stability. For uncomplicated fractures, we use the posterolateral (Kocher) approach to access the radial head. The skin incision is placed over the lateral epicondyle and extended distally over the radial head. The interval between the anconeus and the extensor carpi ulnaris is more easily identified distally. This interval is opened, and the extensor carpi ulnaris is elevated and reflected anteriorly. The underlying capsule and lateral ligamentous complex are exposed. The ulnar collateral portion of the lateral ligamentous complex is identified, and the capsular incision is placed anterior to it. Fracture lines that extend into the neck require more distal exposure, and the surgeon can divide the annular ligament. At this level, the posterior interosseous nerve is at risk for injury. Pronation of the forearm helps to move the nerve medially and away from the operative field; however, the nerve moves closer to the edge of the supinator and the posterior border of the radius as the dissection is continued distally. The more immediate risk to the nerve stems from the use of Hohmann retractors, which are placed for exposure. The surgeon must remain subperiosteal with the retractors and must not use excessive force while retracting.

The joint is irrigated, and the fracture site is cleaned of hematoma. The surgeon should evaluate the fracture for comminution, loose fragments without soft-tissue attachment, and injury to the capitellum. The very small, loose fragments from either the radial head or capitellum are removed. The fracture fragments are reduced and provisionally stabilized with 0.045 and 0.035 Kirschner wires. Fractures involving only the radial head can be fixed with either the Herbert miniscrew set or minifragment screws. If possible, the screws should be placed in the "safe-zone."[24,117] This area encompasses an arc of about 100°. With the patient's forearm in a neutral position, the surgeon centers the arc on the lateral aspect of the radial head. This portion of the radial head does not articulate with the sigmoid notch. If this zone cannot be used because of the fracture pattern, the Herbert miniscrews or the low-profile minifragment screws should be used with the radial head buried below the surface of the cartilage (Fig. 20.4). The standard lag-screw technique involving overdrilling of the proximal cortex should be used with caution, because it can cause further fragmentation of small pieces. The technique is seldom required, provided that the fragments are tapped while held in compression. Fractures that extend into the radial neck require plate stabilization. The 2.0- or 2.7-mm L or T plates provide stabilization. Soyer et al. recently described optimal plate position as directly lateral with the forearm in neutral rotation. They also described functional deficits related to a more anterior or posterior application.[118]

Once stabilized, the elbow should be taken through the complete arc of rotation. This rotation should be done in several positions of flexion. The surgeon should evaluate the reduction for any mechanical blocks to motion or grinding. Mechanical blocks can represent unreduced or

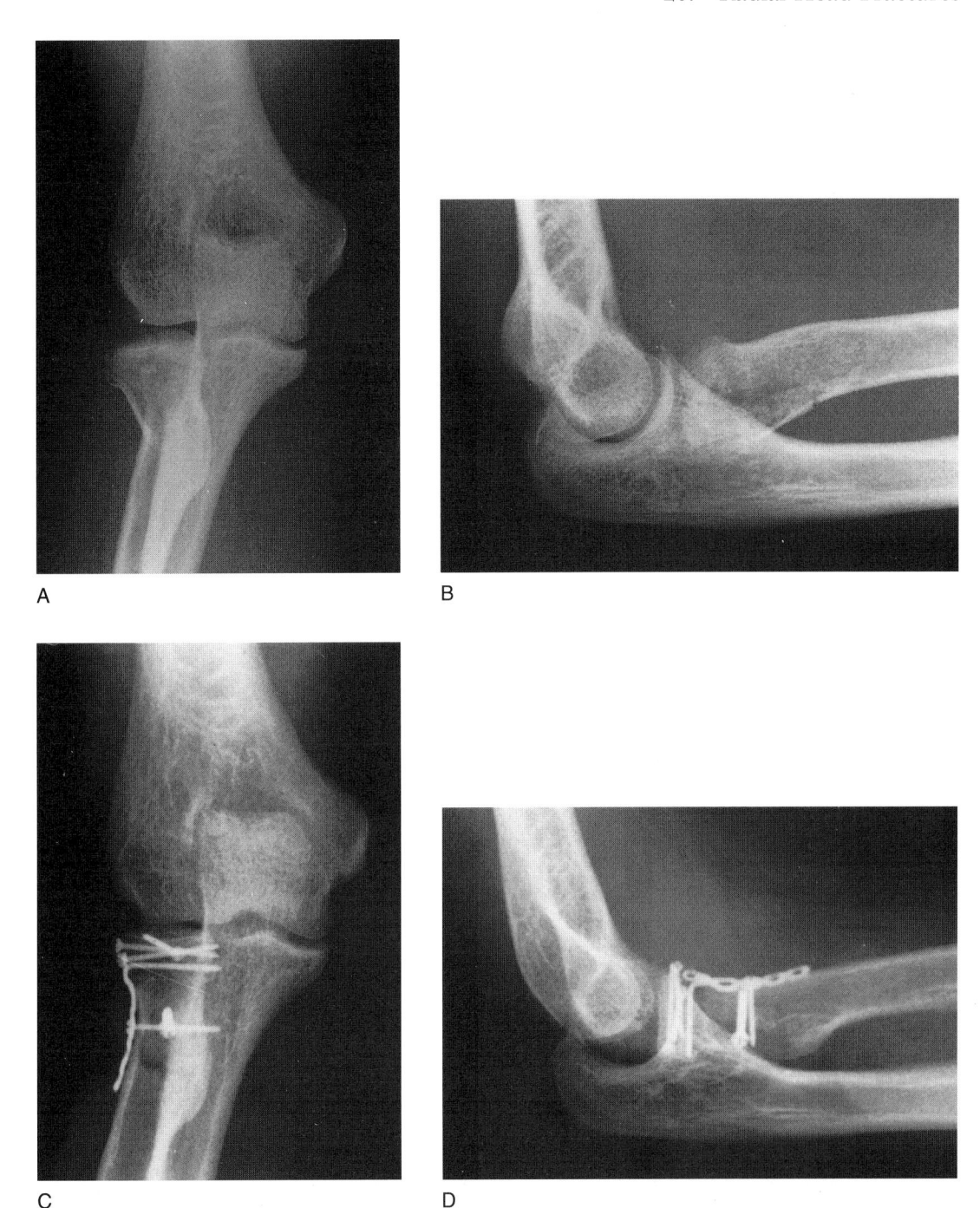

FIGURE 20.4. This fracture had more comminution than the examiner anticipated from the initial (A) anteroposterior and (B) lateral radiographic views. It was still amenable to internal fixation. The fracture line extended into the radial neck, which the surgeon stabilized by a screw and the miniblade plate. Postoperative (C) anteroposterior and (D) lateral radiographic views.

loose fragments or can represent improper placement of implants. The capsule is closed, and an intra-articular drain is used as necessary. Provided that the lateral ligament complex is left intact, the annular ligament does not have to be closed separately. If disrupted, the complex is repaired with nonabsorbable sutures placed through drill holes in the lateral epicondyle. The interval between the anconeus and the extensor carpi ulnaris is closed with an absorbable suture. The patient's upper extremity is splinted in full extension in a bulky dressing. This dressing is removed 3 days after surgery, and gentle active range of motion is initiated. The patient continues splinting the elbow at night for comfort for up to 2 weeks.

We use the same approach for radial head excision. The annular ligament is left intact, and the radial head is excised just below the metaphyseal flare. We carefully excise all fragments and check the radiographs during surgery to assure that the excision is complete. The elbow is taken through a range of motion to assure the absence of a mechanical block to motion, and elbow stability is assessed carefully with valgus and longitudinal stresses. The patient begins active range-of-motion exercises 3 to 5 days after surgery.

Complex Fractures

Treatment of complex fractures is based on the associated injury. Associated fractures are stabilized according to the fracture type. We stabilize capitellar fracture fragments of sufficient size and excise fragments that are too small for stable fixation. When possible, we preserve the

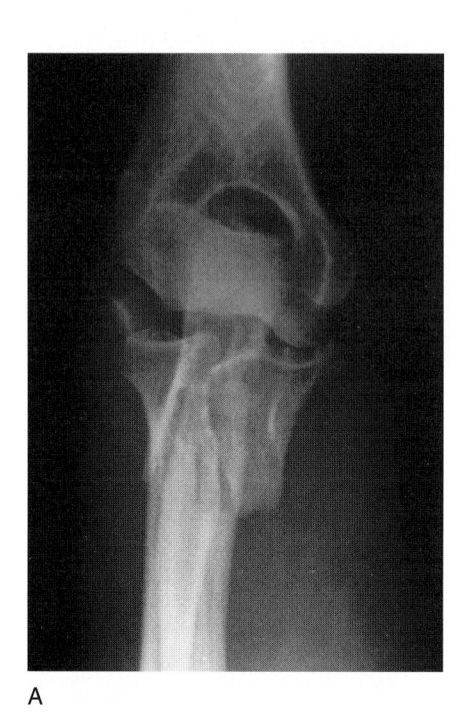

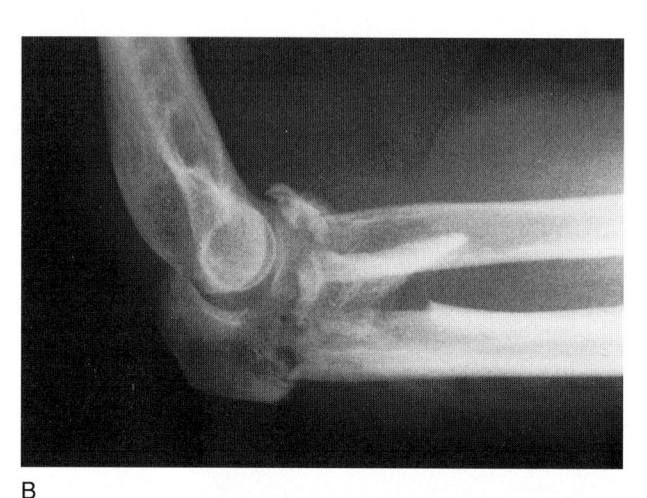

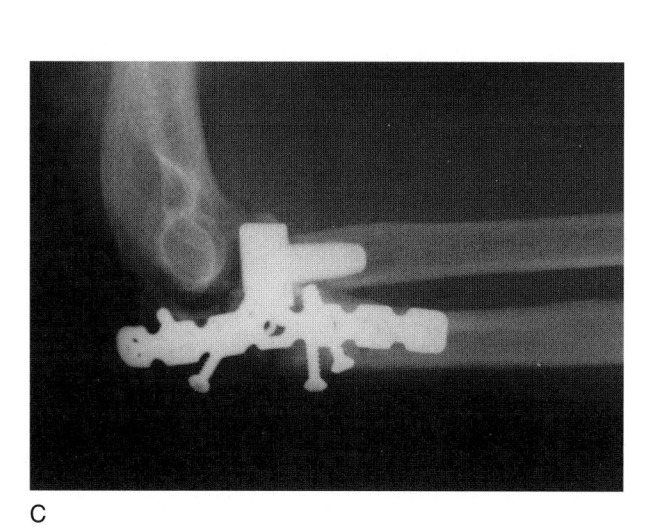

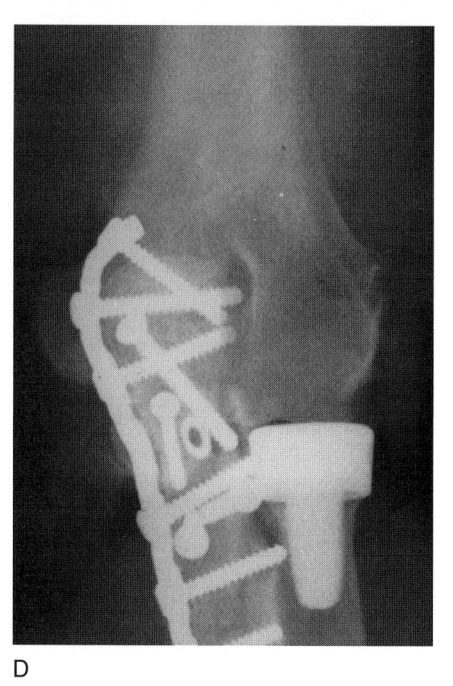

FIGURE 20.5. (A) Anteroposterior and (B) lateral radiographic views show a complex fracture dislocation. The radial head could not be salvaged, and the elbow was grossly unstable. Use of the radial head implant improved stability. The surgeon obtained additional stability by repairing the coronoid process with a washer and suture. (C and D) Postoperative radiographic views.

radial head. In the presence of valgus instability, we use a hinged elbow orthosis to protect the fixation. The preferred orthosis has both medial and lateral hinges to provide additional stability.

A radial head prosthesis is used if the elbow is unstable and the radial head has been excised. We use a titanium radial head that does not require subsequent removal. The stem design on this prosthesis is relatively wide compared with the medullary canal. Often, this procedure involves opening the medullary canal with a drill or burr in order to seat the prosthesis. We do not routinely repair the medial collateral ligament. However, when instability persists, repair of the medial collateral ligament or fixation of the coronoid process may be necessary to prevent another dislocation (Fig. 20.5).

In patients who have acute longitudinal instability (i.e., Essex-Lopresti injuries), we attempt to preserve the radial head with internal fixation. Again, if the head cannot be preserved, it can be replaced with a titanium prosthesis. The distal radioulnar joint is reduced by supination. We supplement reduction with percutaneous Kirschner-wire fixation of the distal radioulnar joint and maintain this position for a minimum of 4 weeks. A removable splint or hinged elbow orthosis that allows free flexion and extension, but prohibits rotation, is used to control the elbow. Patients begin active flexion and extension exercises 3 to 5 days after surgery and begin rotation exercises when the Kirshner wires are removed at 4 to 6 weeks.

CONCLUSION

The treatment of radial head fractures remains controversial and difficult. Despite appropriate treatment, the outcome may still be unsatisfactory if the patient has residual stiffness and discomfort at the elbow. Because it is critical to the outcome of all treatment methods, early range of motion should be emphasized. When operative treatment is indicated, a procedure that allows early range of motion should be chosen. If stable fixation cannot be achieved, it is often better to proceed with radial head excision. Currently, the use of a radial head prosthesis is best limited to complex fractures with associated longitudinal instability and possibly in younger patients with high functional demands. The role of arthroscopy in managing these fractures has yet to be defined. Caution is emphasized with particular regard to neurologic injury.

REFERENCES

1. Cutler C. Fractures of the head and neck of the radius. *Ann Surg* 1926;8:267–278.
2. Schwartz RP, Young F. Treatment of fractures of the head and neck of the radius and slipped radial epiphysis in children. *Surg Gynecol Obstet* 1933;57:528–537.
3. Neuwirth AA. Nonsplinting treatment of fractures of the elbow joint. *JAMA* 1942;118:971–972.
4. Mason JA, Shutkin NM. Immediate active motion treatment of fractures of the head and neck of the radius. *Surg Gynecol Obstet* 1943;76:731–737.
5. Speed K. Ferrule caps for the head of the radius. *Surg Gynecol Obstet* 1941;73:845–850.
6. Cherry JC. Use of acrylic prosthesis in the treatment of fractures of the head of the radius. *J Bone Joint Surg* 1953;35B:70–71.
7. Swanson AB. Synovectomy of the elbow and implant replacement of radial head. In: *Flexible implant resection arthroplasty in the hand and extremities*. St. Louis: CV Mosby Co., 1973:265–275.
8. Swanson A, Jaeger S, La Rochelle D. Comminuted fractures of the radial head. The role of silicone-implant replacement arthroplasty. *J Bone Joint Surg* 1981;63A:1039–1049.
9. Harrington IJ, Tountas AA. Replacement of the radial head in the treatment of unstable elbow fractures. *Injury* 1981;12:405–412.
10. Odenheimer K, Harvey JP Jr. Internal fixation of fracture of the head of the radius. Two case reports. *J Bone Joint Surg* 1979;61A:785–787.
11. Bohrer J. Fractures of the head and neck of the radius. *Ann Surg* 1933;97:204–208.
12. Hein B. Fractures of the head of the radius. An analysis of 52 cases with special reference to disabilities. *Indust Med* 1937;6:529–532.
13. Murray R. Fractures of the head and neck of the radius. *Br J Surg* 1940;28:106–118.
14. Watson-Jones R. Discussion of minor injuries of the elbow joint. *Proc Roy Soc Med* 1930;23:323–327.
15. Wilson P. Fractures and dislocations in the region of the elbow. *Surg Gynecol Obstet* 1933;56:335–359.
16. Mason M. Some observations on fractures of the head of the radius with a review of one hundred cases. *Br J Surg* 1954;42:123–132.
17. Radin EL, Riseborough EJ. Fractures of the radial head. A review of eighty-eight cases and analysis of the indications for excision of the radial head and non-operative treatment. *J Bone Joint Surg* 1966;48A:1055–1064.
18. Wagner C. Fractures of the head of the radius. *Am J Surg* 1955;80:911–918.
19. Weseley MS, Barenfeld PA, Eisenstein AL. Closed treatment of isolated radial head fractures. *J Trauma* 1983;23:36–39.
20. Carstam N. Operative treatment of fractures of the head and neck of the radius. *Acta Orthop Scand* 1950;19:502–526.
21. Conn J, Wade PA. Injuries of the elbow: A ten year review. *J Trauma* 1961;1:248–268.
22. Spinner M, Kaplan EB. The quadrate ligament of the elbow—Its relationship to the stability of the proximal radio-ulnar joint. *Acta Orthop Scand* 1970;41:632–647.
23. Jacobs JE, Kernodle HB. Fractures of the head of the radius. *J Bone Joint Surg* 1946;28:616–622.
24. Smith GR, Hotchkiss RN. Radial head and neck fractures: Anatomic guidelines for proper placement of internal fixation. *J Shoulder Elbow Surg* 1996;5:113–117.
25. Morrey BF, An KN. Articular and ligamentous contributions to the stability of the elbow joint. *Am J Sports Med* 1983;11:315–319.
26. Morrey BF, An KN. Functional anatomy of the ligaments of the elbow. *Clin Orthop* 1985;201:84–90.
27. Morrey BF, Chao EY, Hui FC. Biomechanical study of the

elbow following excision of the radial head. *J Bone Joint Surg* 1979;61A:63–68.
28. Morrey BF, Tanaka S, An KN. Valgus stability of the elbow. A definition of primary and secondary restraints. *Clin Orthop* 1991;265:187–195.
29. Schwab GH, Bennett JB, Woods GW, et al. Biomechanics of elbow instability: The role of the medial collateral ligament. *Clin Orthop* 1980;146:42–52.
30. Tullos HS, Bennett J, Shepard D, et al. Adult elbow dislocations: Mechanism of instability. *Instr Course Lect* 1986;35:69–82.
31. Hotchkiss R. Injuries to the interosseous ligament of the forearm. *Hand Clin* 1994;10:391–398.
32. Girard JY, Rogez JM, Robert R, et al. Vascularisation of the head of the radius in the adult. *Surg Radiol Anat* 1995;17:41–45.
33. Flemming C. Fractures of the head of the radius. *Proc Royal Soc Med* 1932;25:1011–1015.
34. Amis AA, Miller JH. The mechanisms of elbow fractures: An investigation using impact tests in vitro. *Injury* 1995;26:163–168.
35. Bakalim G. Fractures of radial head and their treatment. *Acta Orthop Scand* 1970;41:320–331.
36. Gaston SR, Smith FM, Baab OD. Adult injuries of the radial head and neck. Importance of time element in treatment. *Am J Surg* 1949;78:631–635.
37. Key A. Treatment of fractures of the head and neck of the radius. *JAMA* 1931;96:101–104.
38. Morrey BF. Current concepts in the treatment of fractures of the radial head, the olecranon, and the coronoid. *J Bone Joint Surg* 1995;77A:316–327.
39. Bledsoe R, Izenstark J. Displacement of fat pads in disease and injury of the elbow. *Radiology* 1959;73:717–724.
40. Greenspan A, Norman A, Rosen H. Radial head–capitellum view in elbow trauma: Clinical application and radiographic–anatomic correlation. *Am J Radiol* 1984;143:355–359.
41. Grundy A, Murphy G, Barker A, et al. The value of the radial head–capitellum view in radial head trauma. *Br J Radiol* 1985;58:965–967.
42. Hall-Craggs MA, Shorvon PJ, Chapman M. Assessment of the radial head-capitellum view and the dorsal fat-pad sign in acute elbow trauma. *Am J Radiol* 1985;145:607–609.
43. McLaughlin H. Fracture of the head of the radius. In: *Trauma*. Philadelphia: WB Saunders, 1959:221–225.
44. Johnston G. A follow-up of one hundred cases of fractures of the head of the radius with a review of the literature. *Ulster Med J* 1962;31:51–56.
45. Speed K. Fracture of the head of the radius. *Am J Surg* 1924;38:157–159
46. Morgan SJ, Groshen SL, Itamura JM, et al. Reliability evaluation of classifying radial head fractures by the system of Mason. *Bull Hosp Joint Dis* 1997;56:95–98.
47. Thompson JD. Comparison of flexion versus extension splinting in the treatment of Mason type I radial head and neck fractures. *J Orthop Trauma* 1988;2:117–119.
48. Hotchkiss R. Displaced fractures of the radial head: Internal fixation or excision? *J Am Acad Orthop Surg* 1997;5:1–10.
49. Mathur N, Sharma CS. Fracture of the head of the radius treated by elbow cast. *Acta Orthop Scand* 1984;55:567–568.
50. Sever J. Fractures of the radius. A study of end-results. *JAMA* 1925;84:1551–1555.
51. Quigley T. Aspiration of the elbow joint in the treatment of fractures of the head of the radius. *N Engl J Med* 1949;240:915–916.
52. Unsworth-White J, Koka R, Churchill M, et al. The nonoperative management of radial head fractures: A randomized trial of three treatments. *Injury* 1994;25:165–167.
53. Holdsworth BJ, Clement DA, Rothwell PN: Fractures of the radial head—the benefit of aspiration: A prospective controlled trial. *Injury* 1987;18:44–47.
54. Adler JB, Shaftan GW. Radial head fractures, is excision necessary? *J Trauma* 1964;4:115–136.
55. Knight DJ, Rymaszewski LA, Amis AA, et al. Primary replacement of the fractured radial head with a metal prosthesis. *J Bone Joint Surg* 1993;75B:572–576.
56. Bunker TD, Newman JH. The Herbert differential pitch bone screw in displaced radial head fractures. *Injury* 1985;16:621–624.
57. Pearce MS, Gallannaugh SC. Mason type II radial head fractures fixed with Herbert bone screws. *J Royal Soc Med* 1996;89:340P–344P.
58. Esser RD, Davis S, Taavao T. Fractures of the radial head treated by internal fixation: Late results in 26 cases. *J Orthop Trauma* 1995;9:318–323.
59. Sanders RA, French HG. Open reduction and internal fixation of comminuted radial head fractures. *Am J Sports Med* 1986;14:130–135.
60. Shmueli G, Herold HZ. Compression screwing of displaced fractures of the head of the radius. *J Bone Joint Surg* 1981;63B:535–538.
61. Yuan-Zhang M, Zheng-Shong C, Chun-bo S, et al. Treatment of radial head split fracture. *Chinese Med J* 1987;100:831–834.
62. Bostman O. Economic considerations on avoiding implant removals after fracture fixation by using absorbable devices. *Scand J Soc Med* 1994;22:41–45.
63. Hirvensalo E, Bostman O, Rokkanen P. Absorbable polyglycolide pins in fixation of displaced fractures of the radial head. *Arch Orthop Trauma Surg* 1990;109:258–261.
64. Pelto K, Hirvensalo E, Bostman O, et al. Treatment of radial head fractures with absorbable polyglycolide pins: A study on the security of the fixation in 38 cases. *J Orthop Trauma* 1994;8:94–98.
65. Jahn R, Diederichs D, Friedrich B. Resorbierbare Implantate und Ihre Anwendung am Beispiel der Radiuskoepfchenfraktur. *Aktuelle Traumatol* 1989;19:281–286.
66. Meyers MH, Herron M. A fibrin adhesive seal for the repair of osteochondral fracture fragments. *Clin Orthop* 1984;182:258–263.
67. Arce AA, Garin DM, Garcia VM, et al. Treatment of radial head fractures using a fibrin adhesive seal. A review of 15 cases. *J Bone Joint Surg* 1995;77B:422–424.
68. Coleman DA, Blair WF, Shurr D. Resection of the radial head for fracture of the radial head. Long-term follow-up of seventeen cases. *J Bone Joint Surg* 1987;69A:385–392.
69. Goldberg I, Peylan J, Yosipovitch Z. Late results of excision of the radial head for an isolated closed fracture. *J Bone Joint Surg* 1986;68A:675–679.
70. Postacchini F, Morace GB. Radial head fracture treated by resection. Long-term results. *Italian J Orthop Traumatol* 1992;18:323–330.
71. Stephen IB. Excision of the radial head after closed fracture. *Acta Orthop Scand* 1981;52:409–412.

72. Geel CW, Palmer AK, Ruedi T, et al. Internal fixation of proximal radial head fractures. *J Orthop Trauma* 1990;4: 270–274.
73. Kanlic E, Perry CR. Indications and technique of open reduction and internal fixation of radial head fractures. *Orthopedics* 1992;15:837–842.
74. Vertongen P. Displaced fractures of the radial head. *J Bone Joint Surg* 1961;43B:191–192.
75. Charnley J. *The closed treatment of common fractures.* Edinburgh: Livingstone; 1950.
76. King GJ, Evans DC, Kellam JF. Open reduction and internal fixation of radial head fractures. *J Orthop Trauma* 1991;5: 21–28.
77. King BB. Resection of the radial head and neck. An end-result study of thirteen cases. *J Bone Joint Surg* 1939;21:839–857.
78. Janssen RP, Vegter J. Resection of the radial head after Mason type-III fractures of the elbow: follow-up at 16–30 years. *J Bone Joint Surg* 1998;80B:231–233.
79. Fuchs S, Chylarecki C. Do functional deficits result from radial head resection? *J Shoulder Elbow Surg* 1999;8:247–251.
80. Broberg MA, Morrey BF. Results of delayed excision of the radial head after fracture. *J Bone Joint Surg* 1986;68A:669–674.
81. Broberg MA, Morrey BF. Results of treatment of fracture–dislocations of the elbow. *Clin Orthop* 1987;216:109–119.
82. Davidson PA, Moseley JB Jr, Tullos HS. Radial head fracture. A potentially complex injury. *Clin Orthop* 1993;297: 224–230.
83. Dee R, Hindes R, Silverberg S. "Ratchet-type" marginal fracture of the radial head with locked anterior dislocation. A case report. *Clin Orthop* 1991;265:196–199.
84. Geissler WB, Freeland A. Radial head fracture associated with elbow dislocation. *Orthopedics* 1992;15:874–877.
85. Hendel D, Halperin N. Fracture of the radial head and capitellum humeri with rupture of the medial collateral ligament of the elbow. *Injury* 1982;14:98–99.
86. Josefsson PO, Gentz CF, Johnell O, et al. Dislocations of the elbow and intraarticular fractures. *Clin Orthop* 1989;246: 126–130.
87. Perry CR, Tessier JE. Open reduction and internal fixation of radial head fractures associated with olecranon fracture or dislocation. *J Orthop Trauma* 1987;1:36–42.
88. Rodriguez-Merchan EC. Controversies on the treatment of irreducible elbow dislocations with an associated nonsalvageable radial head fracture. *J Orthop Trauma* 1995;9:341–344.
89. Ward WG, Nunley JA. Concomitant fractures of the capitellum and radial head. *J Orthop Trauma* 1988;2:110–116.
90. Morrey BF, Askew L, Chao EY. Silastic prosthetic replacement for the radial head. *J Bone Joint Surg* 1981;63A:454–458.
91. Gordon M, Bullough PG. Synovial and osseous inflammation in failed silicone-rubber prostheses. *J Bone Joint Surg* 1982;64A:574–580.
92. Mayhall WS, Tiley FT, Paluska DJ. Fracture of Silastic radial-head prosthesis. Case report. *J Bone Joint Surg* 1981; 63A:459–460.
93. Vanderwilde RS, Morrey BF, Melberg MW, et al. Inflammatory arthritis after failure of silicone rubber replacement of the radial head. *J Bone Joint Surg* 1994;76B:78–81.
94. Gupta GG, Lucas G, Hahn DL. Biomechanical and computer analysis of radial head prostheses. *J Shoulder Elbow Surg* 1997;6:37–48.
95. Pribyl CR, Kester MA, Cook SD, et al. The effect of the radial head and prosthetic radial head replacement on resisting valgus stress at the elbow. *Orthopedics* 1986;9:723–726.
96. Sellman DC, Seitz WH Jr, Postak PD, et al. Reconstructive strategies for radioulnar dissociation: A biomechanical study. *J Orthop Trauma* 1995;9:516–522.
97. Nonnenmacher J, Schurch B. Fractures of the radial head and lesions of the lower radius and ulna in the adult: The importance of the prosthesis in resection [Fre]. *Ann Chir Main* 1987;6(2):123–130.
98. Brockman E. Two cases of disability at the wrist-joint following excision of the head of the radius. *Proc Roy Soc Med* 1930;24:904–905.
99. Curr J, Coe W. Dislocation of the inferior radio-ulnar joint. *Br J Surg* 1946;34:74–77.
100. Essex-Lopresti P. Fractures of the radial head with distal radio-ulnar dislocation. Report of two cases. *J Bone Joint Surg* 1951;33B:244–247.
101. Eglseder WA, Hay M. Combined Essex-Lopresti and radial shaft fractures: Case report. *J Trauma* 1993;34:310–312.
102. Khurana JS, Kattapuram SV, Becker S, et al. Galleazzi injury with an associated fracture of the radial head. *Clin Orthop* 1988;234:70–71.
103. Edwards GS Jr, Jupiter JB. Radial head fractures with acute distal radioulnar dislocation. Essex-Lopresti revisited. *Clin Orthop* 1988;234:61–69.
104. Trousdale RT, Amadio PC, Cooney WP, et al. Radio-ulnar dissociation: A review of twenty cases. *J Bone Joint Surg* 1992;74A:1486–1497.
105. Hotchkiss RN, An KN, Sowa DT, et al. An anatomic and mechanical study of the interosseous membrane of the forearm: Pathomechanics of proximal migration of the radius. *J Hand Surg* 1989;14A:256–261.
106. Rabinowitz RS, Light TR, Havey RM, et al. The role of the interosseous membrane and triangular fibrocartilage complex in forearm stability. *J Hand Surg* 1994;19A:385–393.
107. Morrey BF. Functional evaluation of the elbow. In: Morrey BF. *The elbow and its disorders*. Philadelphia: WB Saunders; 1985:73–91.
108. Sowa DT, Hotchkiss RN, Weiland AJ. Symptomatic proximal translation of the radius following radial head resection. *Clin Orthop* 1995;317:106–113.
109. Mackay I, Fitzgerald B, Miller JH. Silastic replacement of the head of the radius in trauma. *J Bone Joint Surg* 1979; 61B:494–497.
110. Taylor TKF, O'Connor BT. The effect upon the inferior radio-ulnar joint of excision of the head of the radius in adults. *J Bone Joint Surg* 1964;46B:83–88.
111. Byrd JW. Elbow arthroscopy for arthrofibrosis after type I radial head fractures. *Arthroscopy* 1994;10:162–165.
112. Lo IK, King GJ. Arthroscopic radial head excision. *Arthroscopy* 1994;10:689–692.
113. Menth-Chiari WA, Poehling GG, Ruch DS. Arthroscopic resection of the radial head. *Arthroscopy* 1999;15:226–230.
114. Rodeo SA, Forster RA, Weiland AJ. Neurological compli-

cations due to arthroscopy. *J Bone Joint Surg* 1993;75A:917–926.
115. Wallenbock E, Plecko M. Komplikationen nach Operativer Versorgung von RadiusKoepfchenfrakturen. *Unfallchirurgie* 1992;18:339–343.
116. Sutro CJ, Sutro WH. Fractures of the radial head in adults with the complication "cubitus valgus." *Bull Hosp Joint Dis Orthop Inst* 1985;45:65–73.
117. Caputo AE, Mazzocca AD, Santoro VM. The nonarticulating portion of the radial head: anatomic and clinical correlations for internal fixation. *J Hand Surg* 1998;23A:1082–1090.
118. Soyer AD, Nowotarski PJ, Kelso TB, Mighell MA. Optimal position for plate fixation of complex fractures of the proximal radius: a cadaver study. *J Orthop Trauma* 1998;12:291–293.

CHAPTER 21

Supracondylar Fractures of the Humerus in Children

W. David Bruce and Hugh P. Brown

INTRODUCTION

Supracondylar fractures of the humerus are the second most common type of fracture in children (16.6%).[1–4] The fracture usually occurs secondary to a fall from a height with most (29%) occurring after a fall from playground equipment.[3] Children are prone to this injury because of their physiologic ligamentous laxity and because of the weak metaphyseal bone of the distal humerus, coupled with the thin metaphyseal bone between the coronoid and olecranon fossa. The impact from a fall onto the outstretched hand causes the elbow to hyperextend. This hyperextension causes the olecranon to concentrate most of the force at the supracondylar region of the humerus, and the axial force is converted to a bending force, resulting in an extension-type supracondylar fracture. The extension-type fracture represents 96% to 98% of supracondylar fractures.[2,3,5,6]

The flexion-type fracture is usually the result of a fall on the olecranon with the elbow flexed, a mechanism that flexes the distal humerus at the fracture site. This type of fracture represents 2% to 4% of supracondylar fractures.[2,3,5,6]

Fractures about the child's elbow can be challenging to treat. However, if the treating physician has a thorough understanding of the anatomy and adheres to surgical principles, he or she can expect good to excellent outcomes. In this chapter, we focus on the clinical presentation and operative treatment of extension-type supracondylar fractures of the humerus in children, and we briefly discuss the flexion-type fractures.

CLINICAL ANATOMY

The ossification of the distal humerus progresses with age. The surgeon needs to understand the age at which the ossification centers appear and the centers' relationships so that he or she does not overlook fractures that occur through these nonossified structures.[7] The ossification and fusion of these structures is discussed in Chapter 1.[8]

The distal humerus is unique. A 1-mm wafer of bone that is flanked by larger medial and lateral columns forms the distal metaphysis. This thin bone separates the anterior coronoid fossa from the posterior olecranon fossa. When rotation occurs with a fracture in this region, the only area of fracture contact is this thin bone. Therefore, rotational deformity after reduction is poorly tolerated, offers little stability to the fracture, and often results in loss of reduction, with resultant angular deformity (Fig. 21.1).[9] Dameron and Green likened holding a reduction with rotational deformity of the supracondylar humerus to balancing two knives on one another.[10,11] A near anatomic reduction is essential to prevent this unsatisfactory result.

CLINICAL PRESENTATION

Typically, the child is brought to the emergency department after a fall on an outstretched hand. With extension-type fractures, the child often holds his or her elbow in an extended position. The examiner should evaluate the entire involved extremity, because concomitant injury to

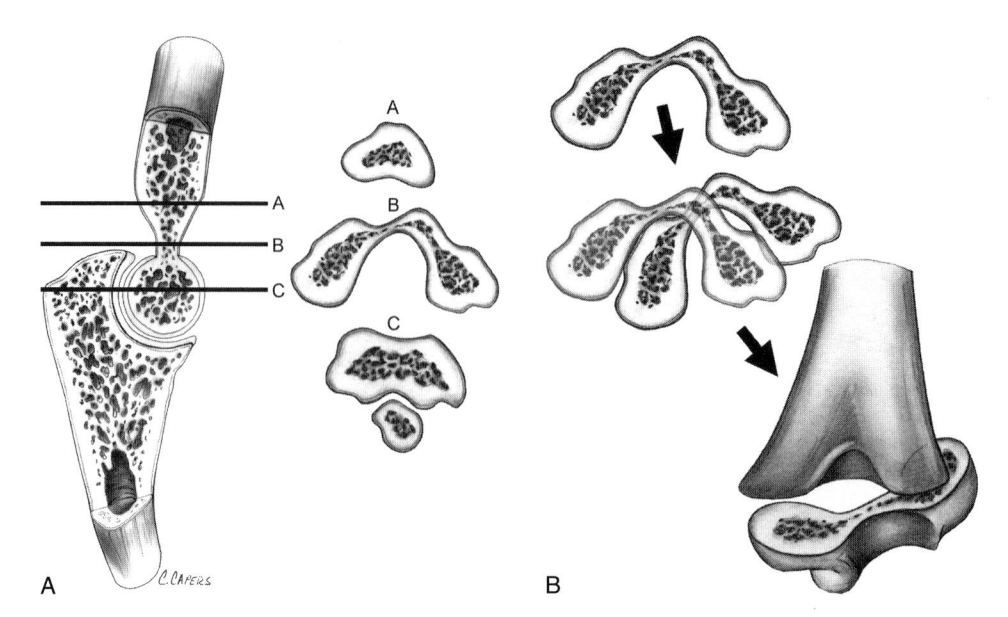

FIGURE 21.1. (A) Cross-section of the distal humerus through different levels of the supracondylar region. (B) Cross-sectional depiction of fracture through the supracondylar region of the humerus demonstrating lack of fracture stability when rotatation persists. Persistent fracture rotation can result in cubitus varus (redrawn with permission[9]).

other osseous structures, that is, distal forearm and proximal humerus, can occur. Swelling and skin punctures should be noted. A thorough neurovascular examination should be performed, and, if signs of ischemia are seen, the elbow should be gently flexed to 30° and reevaluated. Radiographs should be obtained with the elbow immobilized in a radiolucent temporary splint.

RADIOGRAPHIC EXAMINATION

Good anteroposterior (AP) and lateral radiographs are necessary to evaluate the child's elbow. At times, it is useful to apply longitudinal traction during the radiographic examination so that details of the fracture are not obscured.

Many different radiographic lines and angles can be used to aid in diagnosis and reduction of supracondylar fractures. The examiner, however, should not rely on just one of these tools, and he or she should always make use clinically and radiographically of the uninvolved extremity when questions arise. As originally described, Baumann's angle is created by the intersection of a line drawn parallel to the physis of the capitellum and a line drawn perpendicular to the humeral longitudinal axis as seen on an AP radiograph[4,12–14] (Fig. 21.2). Most researchers now describe this angle as the intersection of a line drawn parallel to the physis of the capitellum and a line formed by the longitudinal axis of the humerus (the humerocapitellar angle).[14] The modified Baumann's angle averages 72° (range, 64° to 81°) for normal individuals[14,15] (see Fig. 21.2). A change of 5° in the Baumann's angle usually results in a 2° change in carrying angle.[15] Comparison views of the uninvolved elbow are helpful to establish the normal angles. Some authors question the reliability of the Baumann's angle secondary to unappreciated rotational deformity.[13,14]

The ulnohumeral angle also provides a radiographic carrying angle. On an AP view, the intersection of a line drawn longitudinally along the humerus and a line drawn

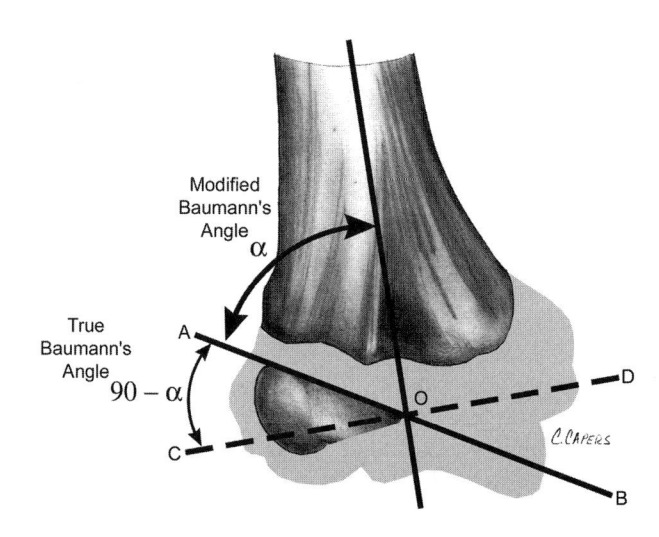

FIGURE 21.2. Baumann's angle and modified Baumann's angle. The modified Baumann's angle averages 72° (range, 64° to 81°) for normal individuals.

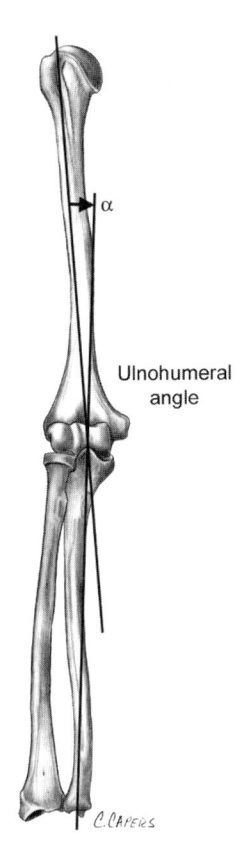

FIGURE 21.3. Ulnohumeral angle is a radiographic angle that corresponds to the anatomic carrying angle.

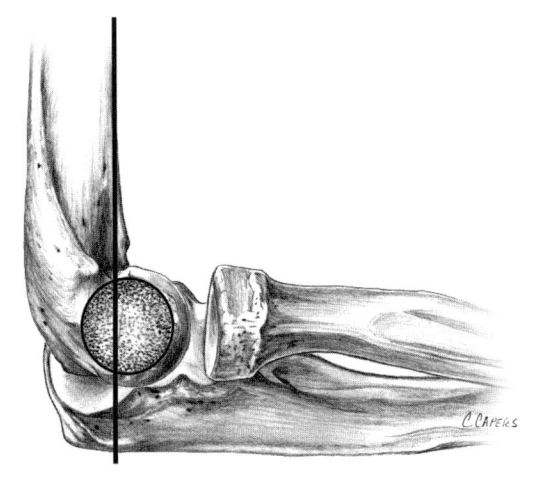

FIGURE 21.4. Anterior humeral line normally passes through the center of the ossific nucleus of the capitellum. Extension fractures cause the line to be anterior and flexion fractures cause the line to be posterior to the center of the nucleus.

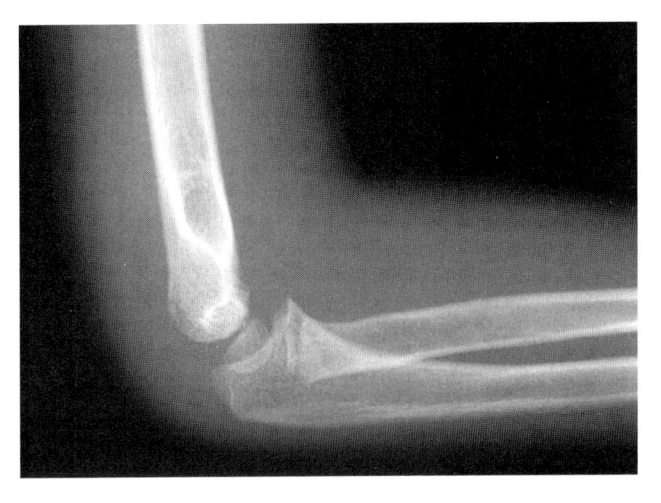

FIGURE 21.5. A crescent sign, created by an overlapping capitellum and olecranon, can be seen on this lateral radiographic view of an elbow with cubitus varus.

longitudinally along the ulna forms the angle (Fig. 21.3). This angle varies widely and, as with the clinical carrying angle, should be compared with the angle in the uninvolved elbow.

The anterior humeral line, as seen on the lateral view, is drawn along the anterior cortex of the humerus (Fig. 21.4). It should pass through the center of the ossified capitellum. The examiner should suspect extension fractures when the anterior humeral line is anterior to the center of the capitellum and should suspect flexion fractures when the line falls posterior to the capitellum's center.[5,11] The normal physis of the capitellum, as seen on the lateral view, is thicker posteriorly and should not be confused with a fracture.[5]

The crescent sign is produced on the true lateral radiograph when a varus deformity has occurred and the proximal ulna overlies the capitellum, resulting in a double density in this region (Fig. 21.5).[4,5,11]

Fat pads, which can be seen on a lateral view, exist anteriorly and posteriorly within the capsule of the distal humerus. Nondisplaced fractures in this region often only result in distention of these pads with hematoma.

The examiner needs to use all available resources when evaluating the child's elbow. These lines and angles can help the surgeon to evaluate an injury and reduce a fracture.[16] However, radiographs should never outweigh the results of the clinical examination. After treatment, comparing the carrying angles of the involved and uninvolved elbows is the most helpful way to evaluate the adequacy of reduction of the pinned elbow.

VASCULAR AND NERVE INJURY

The elbow has a rich vascular supply with a substantial collateral circulation. Permanent vascular compromise occurs in only 1% of supracondylar fractures.[11] The brachialis muscle protects the brachial artery from injury. However, if the fracture is displaced significantly, the anterior spike of the proximal humerus can tear the brachi-

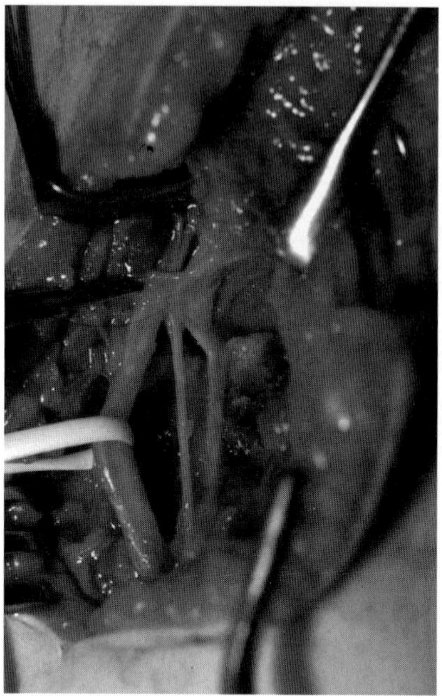

FIGURE 21.6. Type IIIB fracture with median nerve neuropraxia and complete disruption of the brachial artery treated with elbow reduction and pinning and reverse vein grafting of the brachial artery.

alis muscle and compromise the brachial artery, either by kinking the artery or by tearing it secondarily to the distal vascular tether from the supratrochlear artery (Fig. 21.6). The child's hand often has good perfusion due to the collateral circulation even with complete occlusion or complete tear of the brachial artery.[11,17–24]

The incidence of nerve injury due to a supracondylar fracture ranges from 5% to 19%.[11,25–29] The anterior interosseous nerve is the most commonly injured nerve from extension-type supracondylar fractures.[5,10,27,30] This injury is probably caused by a tethering effect from the deep head of the pronator teres. The radial, median, and ulnar nerves, in that order, are involved less often than the anterior interosseous nerve.[5,11,27,30] Median nerve injuries are associated with posterolaterally displaced fractures.[30] Ulnar nerve injuries are associated with flexion-type supracondylar fractures.[14] The surgeon needs to recognize the nerve injury before the reduction, because noniatrogenic nerve injuries demonstrate spontaneous recovery in 86% to 100% of children as late as 5 months after injury.[11,25,30] Injuries caused by fracture reduction or pinning may need to be explored.

CLASSIFICATION

Many authors have classified extension-type supracondylar fractures.[12,31] Gartland described the most uni-

TABLE 21.1. *Classification of extension supracondylar humerus fractures*

Type	Description	Treatment
IA	Nondisplaced	Immobilization at 90°, long-arm splint for 3 to 4 weeks
IB	Medial compression <3° to 4° side-to-side difference	Immobilization at 90°, long-arm splint with slight forearm pronation
	>3° to 4° side-to-side difference	Closed reduction and percutaneous pinning versus ORIF
IIA	Anterior angulation, posterior hinge intact <20°	Immobilization at 90°, long-arm splint for 3 to 4 weeks
	>20°	Closed reduction with or without percutaneous pinning
IIB	Anterior angulation with rotation	Closed reduction and percutaneous pinning
IIIA	Complete displacement with loss of any intact cortex posteromedial displacement	Closed reduction and percutaneous pinning versus ORIF
IIIB	Complete displacement with loss of any intact cortex posterolateral displacement	Closed reduction and percutaneous pinning versus ORIF

ORIF, open reduction internal fixation.

versally accepted system, which is a modification of the Holmberg system.[3,4,11,12,31,32] We use a modification of the Gartland classification for the following description (Table 21.1).[3] The type IA fracture is nondisplaced (Fig. 21.7). The diagnosis is made by clinical examination; that is, a fracture is present unless proved otherwise. Usually, the patient exhibits tenderness over the distal medial and lateral condyles. The radiographs often exhibit a posterior fat pad sign and a hint of cortical disruption anteriorly. The type IB fracture is minimally displaced with medial compression (Fig. 21.8). Careful examination using the carrying angle and radiographic angles with which the examiner is comfortable helps with accurate classification and treatment of the fracture.[16,33] Researchers once thought that growth disturbances in this region produced late cubitus varus, but most authors now recognize that, if cubitus varus occurs, it existed at the time of treatment and was either unrecognized or misdiagnosed.[4,11,33–37]

The type IIA fracture (Fig. 21.9) demonstrates an extension-type fracture with the posterior cortex intact and

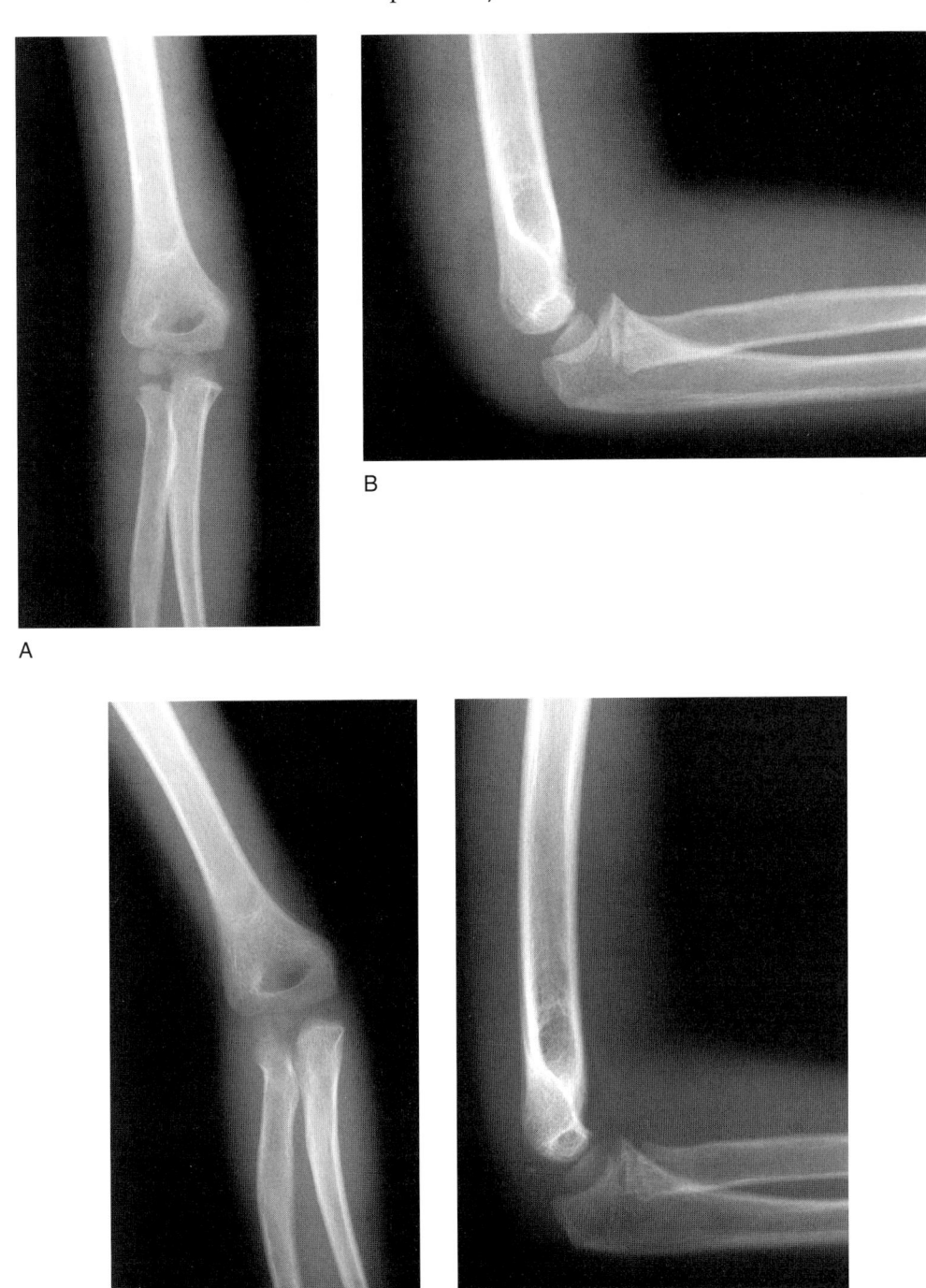

FIGURE 21.7. (A) Anteroposterior and (B) lateral radiographic views of a type IA fracture. (Note fat pad sign on lateral view.) (C) Anteroposterior and (D) lateral views at 3 weeks after splint immobilization. Healing is indicated by new periosteal bone.

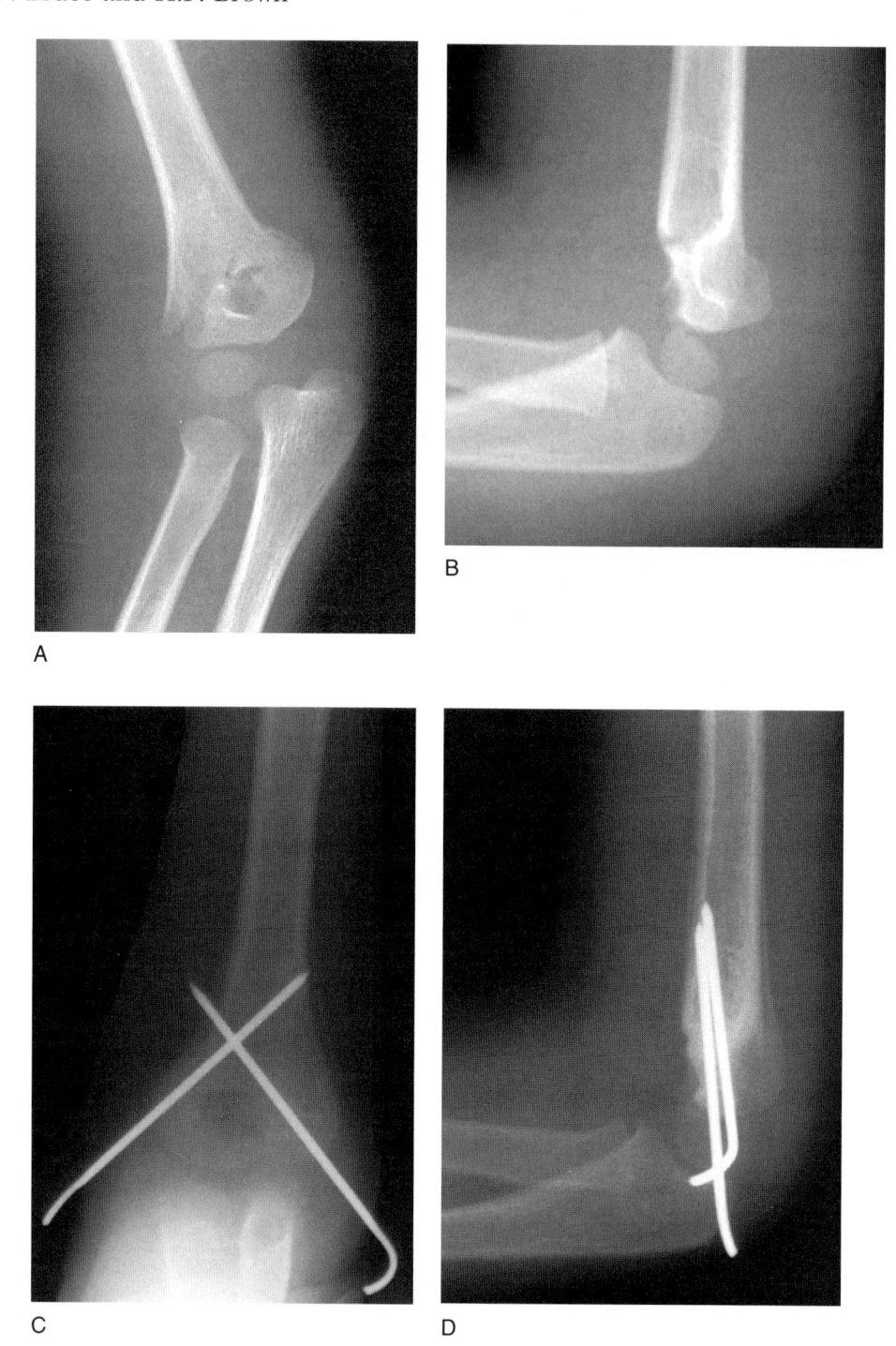

FIGURE 21.8. (A) Anteroposterior and (B) lateral radiographic views of a type IB fracture exhibiting medial compression. (C) Anteroposterior and (D) lateral views at 3 weeks after closed reduction with percutaneous pinning. Healing is indicated by new periosteal bone.

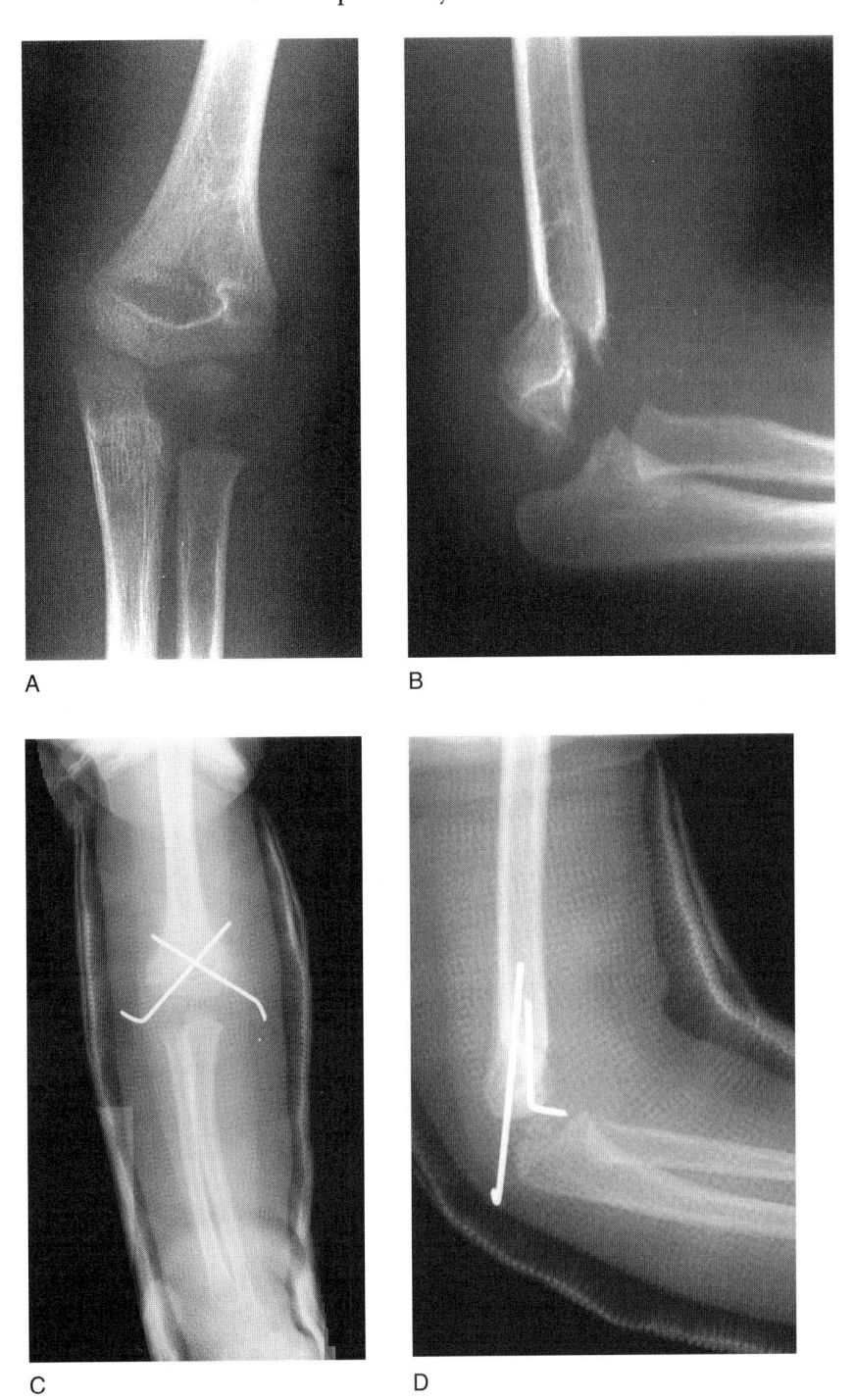

FIGURE 21.9. (A) Anteroposterior and (B) lateral radiographic views of a type IIA fracture exhibiting 20° anterior angulation necessitating closed reduction and pinning. (C) Anteroposterior and (D) lateral views at 3 weeks postinjury show healing.

acting as a hinge. This fracture is best viewed on the lateral radiograph, with an angular deformity apex anterior showing extension of the normal humeral–capitellar relationship. The type IIB fracture (Fig. 21.10) exhibits a posterior hinge with an intact posterior cortex and exhibits rotation (usually medial).

The type III fracture demonstrates complete displacement with loss of any intact cortex. Typically, the fracture is displaced posteromedially (70%) and is classified as type IIIA (Fig. 21.11).[3] Posterolateral displacement is seen less often and is classified as type IIIB (Fig. 21.12).

TREATMENT OPTIONS

Nonoperative Treatment

Closed Reduction and External Immobilization

The most common nonoperative treatment technique employs fracture manipulation and reduction. The physician corrects rotation, medial or lateral displacement, and extension by closed means. After reduction, the elbow is flexed to approximately 120°, and the forearm is pronated in patients who have a medially displaced fracture. To maintain reduction of most type III fractures, the elbow

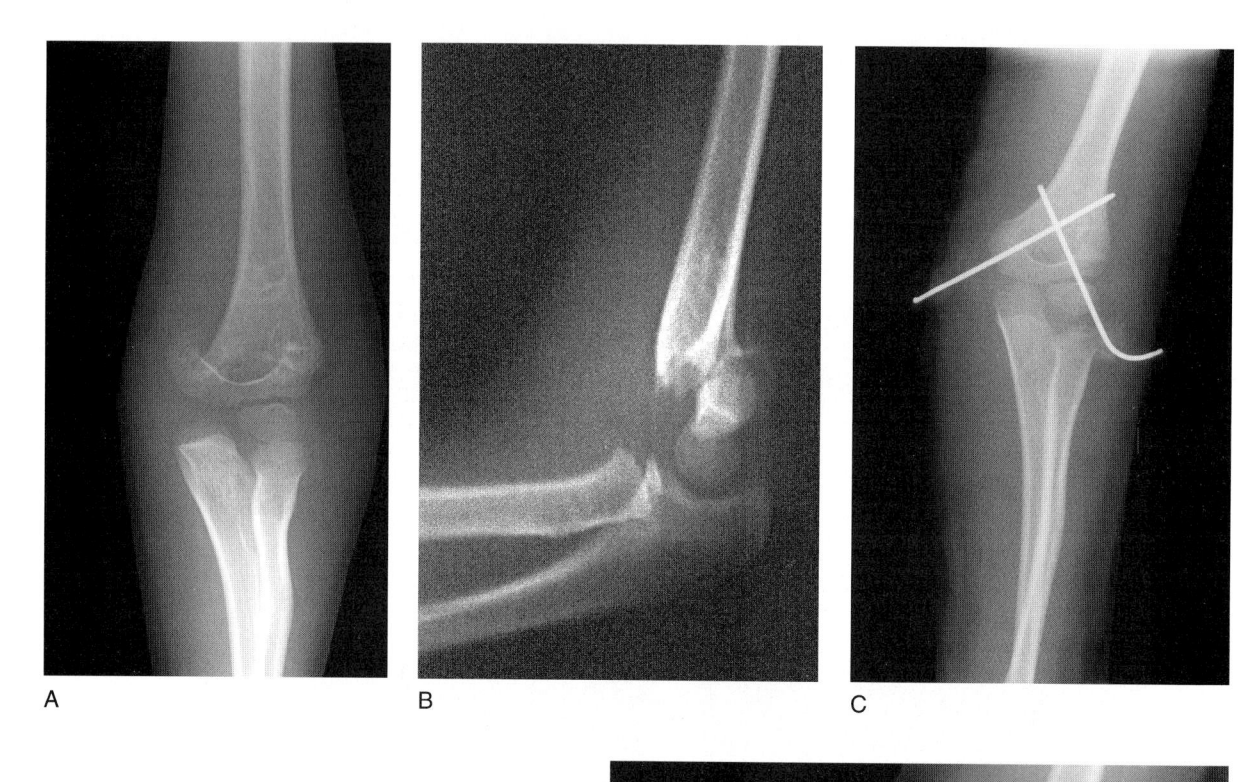

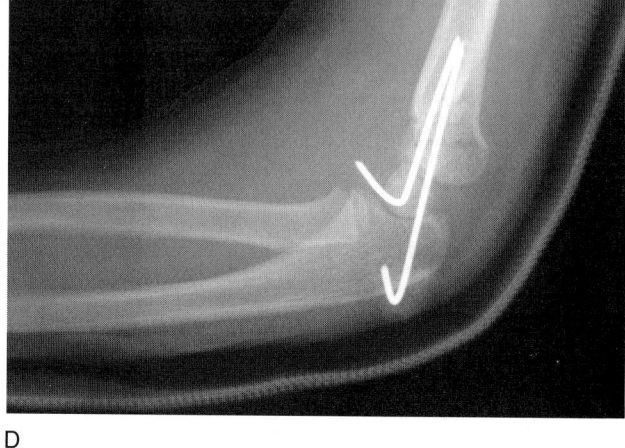

FIGURE 21.10. (A) Anteroposterior and (B) lateral radiographic views of a type IIB fracture shows angulation and medial compression. (C) Anteroposterior and (D) lateral views at 2 weeks postinjury show early healing.

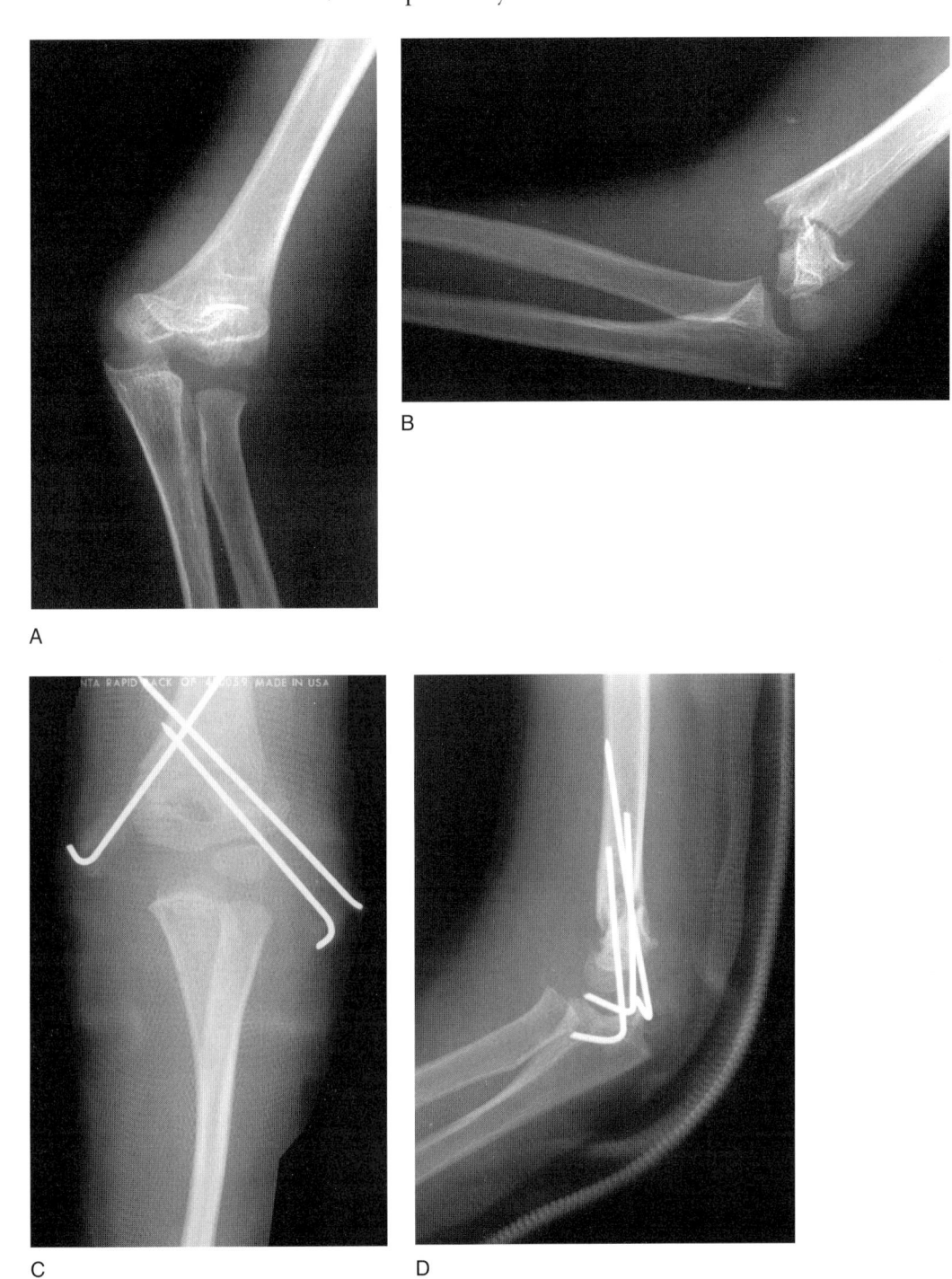

FIGURE 21.11. (A) Anteroposterior and (B) lateral radiographic views of a type IIIA fracture with posteromedial displacement. (C) Anteroposterior and (D) lateral views show three pins used to stabilize the fracture.

must be flexed to 120°. If less flexion is used, the reported risk of loss of reduction is 86%.[4,11,12] However, flexing the elbow to 120° greatly increases the risk of vascular compromise and resultant Volkman ischemia.[11,12] Given the risks of ischemia and loss of reduction associated with closed reduction and casting, many orthopedists choose to treat the fracture operatively.

Traction

Dunlop described the use of straight skin traction with the elbow in extension, and he later advised the use of elbow flexion with forearm skin traction.[38] Other authors recommend using a Kirschner wire (K-wire) placed transversely through the olecranon and placing traction about

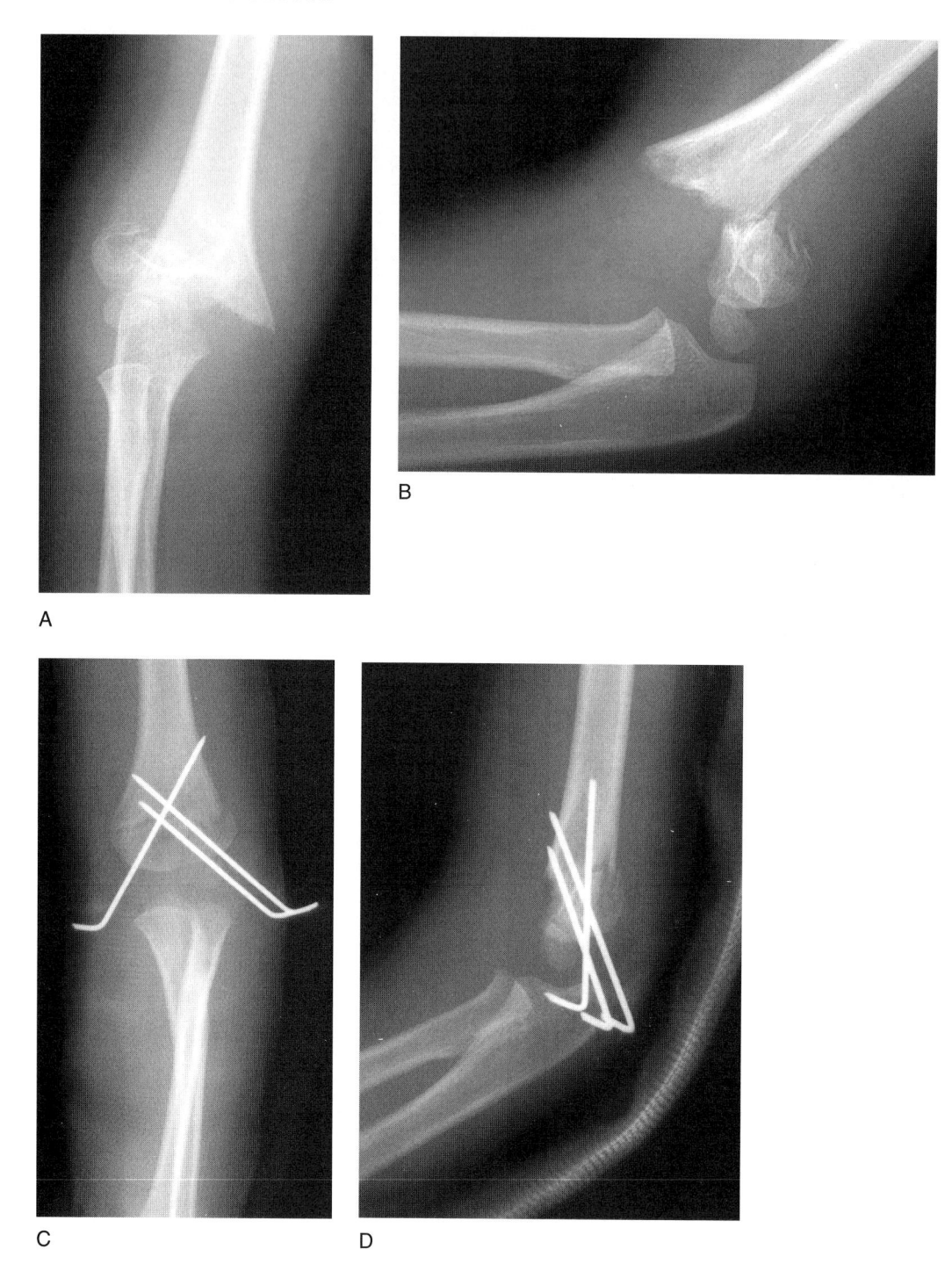

FIGURE 21.12. (A) Anteroposterior and (B) lateral radiographic views of a type IIIB fracture with posterolateral displacement associated with median nerve and brachial artery injury. (C) Anteroposterior and (D) lateral views after closed reduction. Three pins were used to aid stability.

the wire with the elbow flexed.[39,40] Bosanquet and Middleton used Thomas splints as a form of traction.[41] Palmar et al. and Worlock and Colton described the placement of an olecranon screw for traction.[42,43] Physicians have used these forms of treatment when they could not obtain an adequate closed reduction or when severe soft-tissue swelling was present.[43–45] The incidence of malunion associated with the use of traction is reported to be as high as 33%.[4] The process of traction is labor intensive, and, because it requires long hospital stays, it is expensive. Given the variability of results, this form of treatment is reserved for special cases, and we do not advocate its use as the primary treatment.

Operative Treatment

Closed Reduction and Percutaneous Pinning

Currently, the most widely accepted form of treatment for displaced or angulated supracondylar fractures of the humerus, types IB, IIA and IIB, and IIIA and IIIB, is closed reduction and percutaneous pinning.[1,3,4,11,12,25,27,28,44,46–53] Flynn and coworkers popularized the Swenson's technique of closed reduction and pinning in the management of supracondylar fractures.[49] Pirone and associates showed that closed reduction and percutaneous pinning offer superior results to closed reduction and external immobilization, traction, and open reduction and internal fixation.[28] However, a successful outcome depends on a near anatomic reduction, followed by adequate pin placement for stability. An advantage of treating supracondylar fractures by this method instead of by closed reduction and external immobilization includes the ability to hold the elbow splinted in a less flexed position (usually 70° to 90°), thus decreasing the risk of Volkmann's ischemia.[5,11,54] The procedure is relatively noninvasive and allows for accurate intraoperative assessment of radiographs and the carrying angle with the elbow extended. Range of motion in the elbow after this treatment is superior to range of motion in elbows treated with open reduction and internal fixation. The disadvantages include the risk of pin tract infection and iatrogenic nerve injury (most commonly, the ulnar nerve).[25,27,30,51,55]

Authors have reported iatrogenic ulnar nerve injury as a complication of using closed reduction and percutaneous pinning.[25,27,54] Hennrikus et al. reported a 2% rate of iatrogenic ulnar nerve injury while pinning the medial column;[27] these ulnar nerve deficits resolved spontaneously at an average of 62 days. Similarly, Brown and Zinar had a 1.8% incidence of iatrogenic ulnar nerve palsy in 162 patients with displaced supracondylar fractures.[25] The symptoms completely resolved at an average of 5 months. Lyons et al. found a 5% rate of ulnar nerve palsy after reduction of 375 supracondylar fractures[54] and complete resolution of the nerve palsy by an average of 18 weeks after reduction. Furthermore, in those cases of iatrogenic nerve palsy, they recommended not exploring the nerve and advocated leaving the medial pin in place. (One of their poor results occurred in a patient who had the medial pin removed, resulting in instability and late cubitus varus.) The medial pin should be removed if it is positioned in the ulnar notch.

Diligent use of fluoroscopy during reduction and palpation of the ulnar nerve and medial epicondyle lessen the risk of ulnar nerve injury during placement of the medial pin.[25,51,55] The surgeon also can reduce these risks with accurate reduction and pin placement and with removal of the pins 3 weeks after surgery. Recently, good results have been achieved with absorbable pins, but a risk of loss of reduction from pin breakage has been reported.[46]

Open Reduction

The use of open reduction is necessary for fractures that cannot be reduced by closed means. It also is applied as treatment for open fractures and for fractures with a concomitant vascular injury. The posterior approach has fallen out of favor secondary to a reported loss of elbow extension.[5,11,39] In 1972, Carcassonne et al. reported good to excellent results in 39 of 40 patients in whom they used an anteromedial approach and pinned each condyle.[39,56] Weiland and coworkers advocated using a lateral approach and pinning and using medial pinning through a small second incision.[53] Danielsson and Pettersson recommended a medial approach and pinning through a small lateral incision.[57] Archibald et al. and Childress advocated using a medial approach for reduction and using a transolecranon pin for fixation.[39,58] Archibald et al. reported 79% good to excellent results in 34 fractures treated with this method.[39] However, five of the fractures had a change in carrying angle of more than 10°.

Some surgeons use open reduction for the primary treatment of uncomplicated type III fractures.[4,59] They cite the advantages of hematoma evacuation; reduction in edema; direct, accurate fracture reduction; and exploration of arterial and nerve injuries. They acknowledge, however, that the technique carries an increased risk of infection, creates an unsightly scar, and leads to a high incidence of loss of motion.

We usually reserve open reduction for patients who have open fractures, concomitant arterial injury, suspected nerve entrapment, and irreducible fractures. The medial approach has a lower reported rate of motion loss than other approaches, and it is advocated for open reduction when necessary.[4,11,39]

PREFERRED TREATMENT OF EXTENSION-TYPE FRACTURES

The preferred treatment for type IA fractures is a long-arm splint or cast with the elbow flexed to 90° for 3 weeks (see Fig 21.7). At 3 weeks, the presence of callus confirms clinical suspicion of a fracture. Immobilization usually can be removed at 3 weeks, and the patient can begin unprotected motion.

When diagnosing a type IB fracture, the examiner must determine the patient's appropriate carrying angle.[33] If the examiner cannot make this determination because of the patient's pain and guarding, he or she should assess it with the patient under general anesthesia and should treat the fracture at that time. The fracture should be reduced, and most fractures should be pinned if the examiner diagnoses medial compression and notes that the side-to-side difference in the carrying angle or its radiographic equivalent is more than 3° to 4°.[47] Typically, two 0.062 lateral pins suffice for this fracture type, but some authors believe that one medial and one lateral pin are more reliable, even when an isolated medial compression-type fracture is present[33] (see Fig. 21.8). Many authors believe that pronation of the forearm at the time of splinting lessens the risk of cubitus varus.[5,11,47] Theories supporting the use of pronation include an intact posteromedial periosteal hinge becoming taut with pronation and the wrist extensors and the brachioradialis becoming taut in pronation, resulting in closure of the lateral column.[5,11,47] Regardless of the theory, pronation of the forearm should be used when medial displacement is present.

After reducing the fracture, the examiner should place the patient's elbow in a long-arm splint; a long-arm cast should not be used because it affords little room for acute swelling. The elbow is flexed to no more than 90°, and the forearm is pronated slightly. The radial pulse and amount of swelling determine the amount of flexion that should be used.[19] Radiographs with the arm splinted are taken 1 week after treatment to assure that the reduction is maintained. The splint is removed 3 weeks after treatment, and radiographs are obtained. Three to four weeks is usually adequate for healing. If sufficient healing is demonstrated at 3 to 4 weeks, the pins are removed, and unprotected motion is begun at this time. Activities should be restricted for 2 to 3 more weeks to allow adequate healing once the immobilization has been removed.

Management of type IIA fractures consists of elbow immobilization for 3 weeks for fractures with less than 20° of angulation.[11,60] If the fracture shows more than 20° of angulation, a closed reduction should be performed. Some authors reduce this fracture without pinning and immobilize the elbow in approximately 90° of flexion for 3 weeks. As do others, we believe that reducing this fracture and stabilizing it with percutaneous pins is a more reliable technique[12] (see Fig. 21.9). The management is similar to that described for the type IB fracture.

Type IIB fractures are treated with reduction and placement of percutaneous pins (see Fig. 21.10). Using radiographs of the patient's elbow in a splint, the examiner evaluates the elbow 1 week after treatment to assure that reduction is maintained. The splint immobilization is continued for a total of 3 weeks, at which time a radiograph is taken with the elbow out of the splint. If healing is apparent on the radiographs, the pins are removed, and the patient is allowed unprotected motion with restricted activities for 2 additional weeks.

Type III fractures can be challenging to treat and should be addressed only by a surgeon with experience and comfort in handling the irreducible fracture and the open reduction. As with all supracondylar fractures, a thorough neurovascular examination should be performed before and after reduction. While under anesthesia, the patient should undergo semi-urgent closed reduction of the fracture along with percutaneous pinning (one medial and one lateral pin) (see Figs. 21.11 and 21.12). However, Iyengar and associates found no clinical differences in treatment and outcome when patients with displaced fractures had their treatment delayed for an average of 15.5 hours.[61]

Zionts et al. showed a significant difference in the torsional strength of different pinning configurations.[62] Cross-pinning (i.e., placing one pin medially and one pin laterally) provided the greatest control and resistance to torsion and exhibited ten times more torsional control of the fracture than did two parallel lateral pins (Fig. 21.13). This cross-pinning technique demonstrated 30% more torque resistance than did three lateral pins, which offered the second greatest torque resistance. It is imperative to correct any rotation that is seen during the radiographic and clinical examinations, because this fracture has a high propensity for cubitus varus deformity. After pinning, the fracture is managed like a type II fracture.

The type III supracondylar fracture is more likely than the type II fracture to be irreducible, because the proxi-

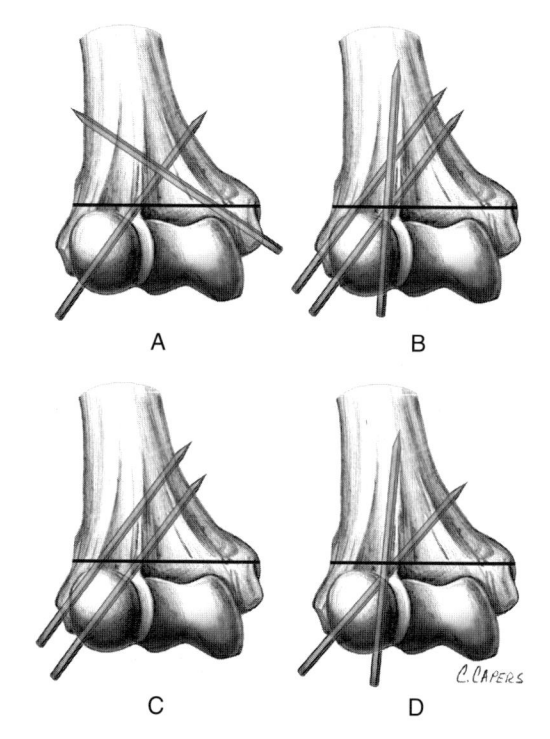

FIGURE 21.13. The four configurations of pins. (A) Medial and lateral crossed pins; (B) three lateral pins; (C) two lateral parallel pins; and (D) two lateral crossed pins (redrawn with permission[62]). Maximum stability is provided by (A).

mal fragment can buttonhole the brachialis muscle, and, with a reduction maneuver, the muscle becomes entrapped in the fracture site.[63–65] The type III fracture is more likely than a type II fracture to be an open fracture; open fractures should be managed with irrigation, debridement, open reduction, and either internal fixation or pinning.[66] Compared with the type II fracture, the type III fracture shows a higher propensity for associated neurovascular injury, which is discussed later.

OPERATIVE TECHNIQUE

Closed Reduction and Percutaneous Pinning

Closed reduction and percutaneous pinning of supracondylar fractures of the humerus should be performed with the patient under general anesthesia with complete muscle relaxation. Having either a second surgeon or a skilled physician's assistant to help to reduce and pin these fractures is helpful and probably necessary. The patient is placed supine on a radiolucent table with the affected arm abducted and the shoulder positioned at the edge of the operating table. Anesthesia personnel should be positioned so that they can help with under-the-drape countertraction and control of the patient's airway. The receiver on the fluoroscopy unit can be brought in under the table or from the side and can be used as the arm board for pinning the elbow (Fig. 21.14). Alternatively, a formal radiolucent arm board can be used, but we have found that using the fluoroscopy receiver is easier. Take care to not drape yourself out of the field; use only one folded towel around the patient's arm at shoulder level and a single extremity drape. To allow better access for reduction, use a sterile tourniquet. The surgeon and operating personnel should wear protective lead gowns.

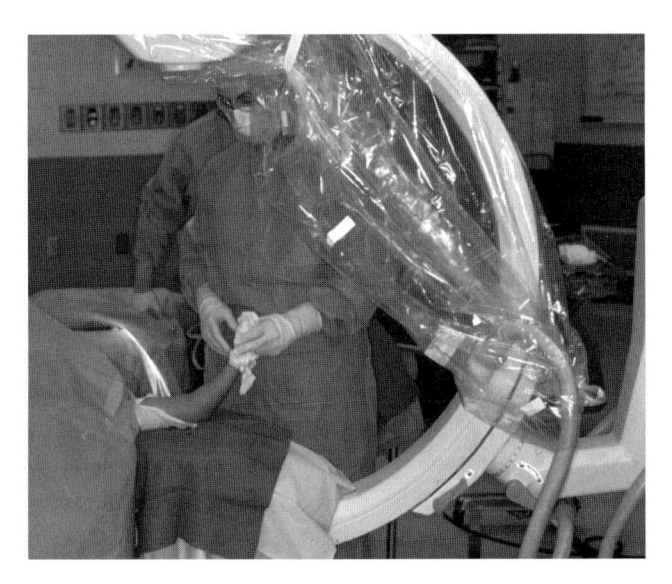

FIGURE 21.14. The receiver on the fluoroscopy unit is used as the arm table with the patient in the supine position.

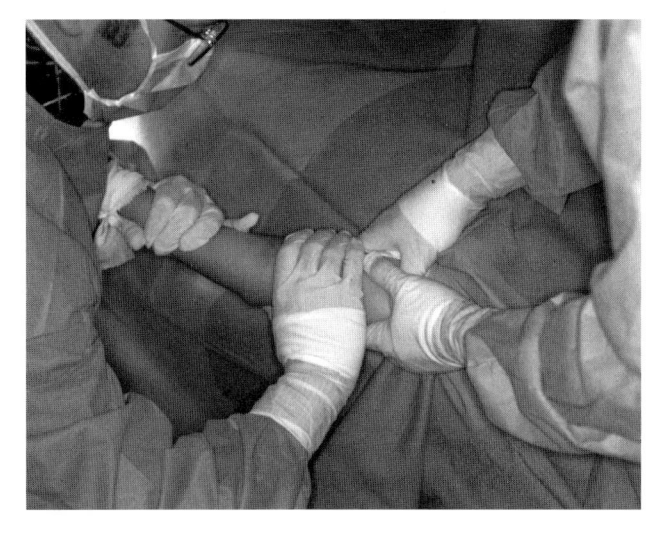

FIGURE 21.15. The reduction is accomplished with the aid of a knowledgeable assistant.

After sterile preparation and draping, the fracture is reduced. With the elbow in extension, the medial or lateral displacement is corrected. For posteriorly displaced fractures, the elbow is maintained in extension, and the posterior cortices of the proximal and distal fragments are engaged by distal traction and by a posterior force on the proximal fragment coupled with an anterior force on the distal fragment. After engaging the posterior cortices, the surgeon flexes the elbow gradually while forcing the distal fragment forward with his or her thumb placed on the posterior portion of this fragment just proximal to the olecranon tip (Fig. 21.15). Maintaining pressure posteriorly prevents loss of reduction of the posterior cortical hinge. The elbow is hyperflexed up to 140°, and the fracture should hinge on the posterior cortices and reduce.

Fluoroscopic views are taken to assess the reduction. The surgeon must keep the patient's elbow flexed to at least 120° to maintain the reduction until pinning takes place. An AP Jones view is obtained by maintaining the elbow in maximal flexion, by placing the receiver on the posterior aspect of the distal humerus, and by directing the tube 90° to the longitudinal axis of the humerus or perpendicular to the humeral shaft (Fig. 21.16). This view is helpful, but shows significant bone-over-bone artifact. We have found it more helpful to take the same view with 15° to 20° of internal and external rotation, thus obtaining oblique views that allow for independent determination of both the medial and lateral column reductions while maintaining elbow flexion. These views also enable the surgeon to assess residual medial or lateral impaction, which should be corrected.

Next, a lateral radiograph is obtained either by moving the fluoroscopy unit for a lateral projection or by externally rotating the humerus with careful maintenance of elbow flexion. Internal rotation can displace the fracture secondary to the internal rotatory instability that most of-

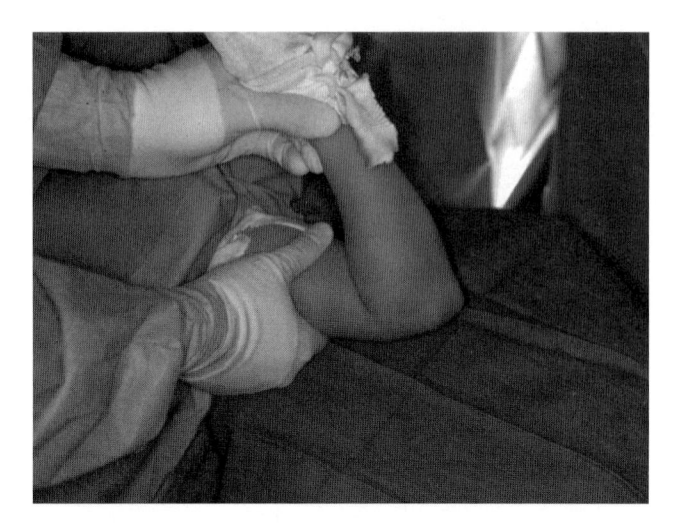

FIGURE 21.16. An anteroposterior Jones view is taken under fluoroscopy.

ten is found with supracondylar fractures. The lateral radiograph should show reduction of the anterior and posterior cortices. If a difference in width is seen between the proximal fragment at the level of the fracture and the distal fragment, then a rotational deformity persists and should be reduced. As described earlier, the crescent sign implies residual cubitus varus; 3° to 4° of residual clinical or radiographic angular deformity is the most deformity that is acceptable.[47] Near anatomic reduction is the minimal acceptable reduction.

After reducing the fracture and restoring near anatomic position, the surgeon pins the elbow beginning with the lateral side (Fig. 21.17). He or she palpates the lateral condyle and joint line while maintaining fracture reduction through elbow hyperflexion. A 0.062-in. K-wire is advanced percutaneously from the lateral condyle at the level of the lateral edge of the capitellum across the distal humeral physis and the fracture site in a superomedial direction. The pin should engage the opposite cortex and should penetrate just outside the outermost cortical bone. If two lateral pins are sufficient to stabilize the fracture, then the second parallel pin is placed laterally at the level of the lateral condyle. Zionts and coworkers showed that parallel placement of two lateral pins provided significantly more torsional control of the fracture than did divergent placement (see Fig. 21.13).[62] In fractures that are inherently unstable, such as the type III fractures, one medial and one lateral crossing pin are recommended. After placing the lateral pin, the elbow is gradually extended to around 70°, which allows the ulnar nerve to fall away from the anterior portion of the ulnar groove. The medial epicondyle and the ulnar nerve are palpated. If swelling does not allow palpation, a small 5- to 10-mm incision is made over the medial epicondyle, and hemostats are used to spread the soft tissue longitudinally over the medial epicondyle. This should allow palpation of the epicondyle and accurate placement of the medial pin. The pin is advanced through the center of the medial epicondyle, is advanced across the fracture, and is directed superolaterally into the opposite cortex of the humerus.

After placing both pins, the surgeon can extend the elbow and evaluate reduction by fluoroscopy (Fig. 21.18). The crossed K-wires should cross above the level of the fracture, because they control rotation better at this level than at the level of the fracture site.[62] The fracture should be stable with the pins placed as described. The pins are cut and bent 90° at a level 1 cm from the skin surface, and they are left protruding from the skin (Fig. 21.19). The bend prevents proximal migration of the pin. We believe that leaving the pins protruding from the skin makes postoperative management easier, because it enables pin removal in the office setting.

With the reduction and pinning completed, the surgeon immobilizes the elbow in a posterior splint with the elbow flexed 70° to 90° as dictated by the radial pulse.[11,54]

FIGURE 21.17. The K-wire is inserted by palpating the condyles and using fluoroscopy.

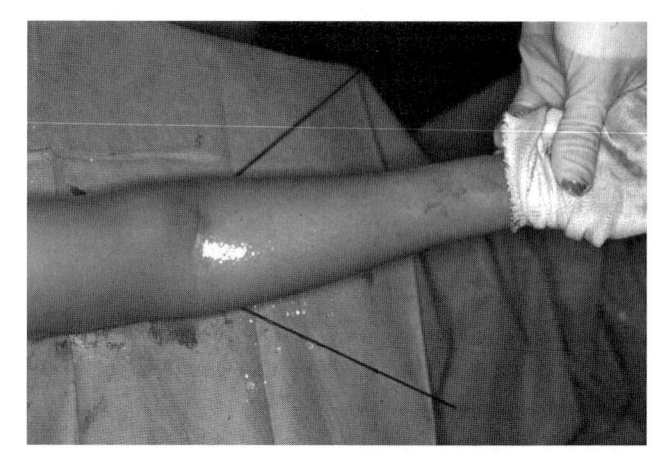

FIGURE 21.18. With both wires in place, the fracture should be stable. The elbow is extended and the carrying angle is observed along with the reduction and the radiographic ulnohumeral angle.

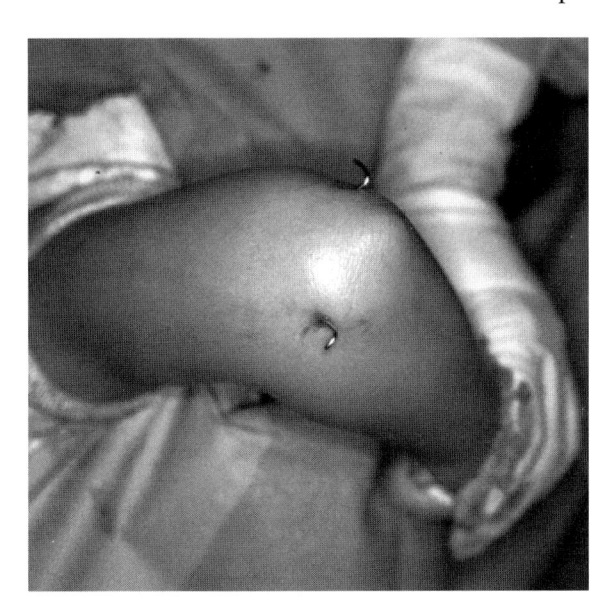

FIGURE 21.19. The pins are left to protrude at skin level and are bent to prevent migration and to allow removal.

A thorough neurovascular examination should be performed as soon as the patient is no longer under general anesthesia. The patient should be observed in the hospital for 24 hours after reduction. Postoperative management follows as described previously. If the reduction is not satisfactory or if the pins are not in good position, the surgeon should reduce and pin the fracture again.

If an adequate reduction is impossible, the brachialis muscle may be entrapped.[64] Archibeck et al. reported that 20 of their 152 study patients had irreducible extension-type supracondylar fractures.[63] Brachialis muscle interposition caused 90% of the irreducible fractures. The authors described a reliable technique (15 of 16 patients) for closed removal of the brachialis muscle interposition. The technique involves milking the anterior arm muscle mass, beginning at the shoulder and moving down to the elbow, by applying thumb pressure over the lateral edge of the anterior compartment muscles. They reported that release of the entrapped muscle is heralded by a palpable or audible pop and increased fracture mobility.

If the surgeon cannot accomplish a closed reduction, then he or she should perform an open reduction. Although both medial and lateral approaches can be used, the medial approach and percutaneous pinning are preferred, because this method has lower reported rates of range of motion loss and avascular necrosis.[4,11,38]

Open Reduction and Internal Fixation

Open reduction is used for fractures that cannot be reduced satisfactorily by closed means (e.g., open fracture) and for fractures with entrapped nerves or limb ischemia.

If the surgeon suspects vascular compromise, he or she should employ the help of a hand surgeon or vascular surgeon to accomplish an anterior approach. We prefer the medial approach for irreducible fractures without concomitant vascular insult. An incision is made medially over the elbow.[67] The ulnar nerve is identified and protected. Usually, the fracture has stripped much of the periosteum, and little deep dissection is necessary. No more than 1 mm of periosteum should be stripped from the distal fragment because stripping more can lead to avascular necrosis. The surgeon carefully removes entrapped tissue (usually the brachialis muscle and possibly the brachial artery or median nerve) from the fracture site. Next, the fracture is reduced and pinned similarly to the closed pinning technique. The medial exposure can be extended transversely across the antecubital fossa to allow exposure of the brachial artery and median nerve. If the surgeon cannot obtain a near anatomic reduction through the medial approach, he or she may need to use a small lateral exposure.[56] The surgeon must not retract or expose the posterior column on the lateral side, because the vascular supply to the distal fragment might be compromised. Postoperative care after this procedure follows the same approach as care after closed reduction and internal fixation described previously.

COMPLICATIONS

Neurologic Injury

Neural injuries occur in 5% to 19% of the displaced supracondylar fractures of the humerus.[25–28] Brown and Zinar showed an 11% rate of traumatic nerve injury and a 3% rate of iatrogenic nerve injury associated with 162 displaced supracondylar fractures of the humerus.[25] They also showed spontaneous, complete resolution of the traumatic nerve palsy in all patients by 6 months after surgery (average, 2.3 months). Similarly, all iatrogenic nerve palsies resolved spontaneously by 6 months (average, 5 months). As stated, the anterior interosseous nerve is injured most often, followed, in order, by the radial, median, and ulnar nerves. Posterolateral displacement is highly associated with median nerve and brachial artery injury.[30] Posteromedial displacement more often has an associated radial nerve injury.[29,30] The neurovascular examination before fracture reduction is important because, during reduction, a nerve (especially the median nerve) can become entrapped in the fracture site. If a nerve palsy is present after reduction and an anatomic reduction is not possible, the physician should suspect nerve entrapment and should explore it. Because most nerve palsies (nearly 100%) resolve spontaneously, routine exploration for nerve palsy is not recommended.[26,27,54,55] Electromyography is recommended for patients who do not exhibit return of nerve function by 6 months. Exploration is recommended for injuries that do not spontaneously recover by 6 months and that demonstrate no electromyographical recovery.[54,55]

Vascular Injury

Many authors have addressed vascular injury, but this topic remains controversial.[21,22] Vascular insufficiency is reported in 3% to 12% of displaced supracondylar fractures.[11,18,22,24,68] Fortunately, less than 1% have a significant risk of sequelae from vascular compromise.[53] To diagnose vascular insufficiency, the surgeon can use arteriography, magnetic resonance angiography, Doppler ultrasonography, or exploration.[18,20,21,23,24] Significant debate concerning the use of any diagnostic tool has occurred as a result of several reports that show use of these tools does not change the final treatment.[17,20,21]

Little debate exists regarding initial management of the pulseless, ischemic hand associated with a supracondylar fracture. Emergent reduction and pinning should be performed with the patient under general anesthesia, and a vascular or hand surgeon should be consulted for the possibility of vascular exploration and repair.[11,18,21,23,24] After the reduction, the surgeon should reassess the vascular status. He or she may note return of pulses and no signs of ischemia, absent pulses and no signs of ischemia, or absent pulses and an ischemic hand. The patient who has return of pulses and no signs of ischemia after reduction and pinning should have his or her elbow splinted with less than 90° of flexion and should be monitored for the next 48 hours. The patient's caregiver should be educated about the complications of the injury and about the signs of ischemia so that treatment is not delayed if a late vascular insult occurs.

To treat the patient who has absent pulses and signs of ischemia after reduction, the surgeon should do an emergent exploration and repair of the vascular injury with the help of a vascular or hand surgeon (Fig. 21.20). Usually, either a complete tear or intimal injury is found and repaired with excision and reverse vein interposition grafting (Fig. 21.6). If the compartments of the forearm are not soft or the compartment pressure is 30 mm Hg or more, fasciotomies should be performed.[5,11] The fasciotomy should release the volar superficial and deep compartments; the extensor compartment is rarely involved.

The treatment of patients who have absent or diminished pulses after reduction and have little or no signs of ischemia is controversial. Arteriography may be helpful in these patients. Authors who disagree with the use of arteriography believe that, in the absence of ischemia, the brachial artery should not be explored, and thus it does not need to be studied.[21,22] Sabharwal et al. found that "early revascularization of a pulseless, otherwise well-perfused hand in children with type III supracondylar fractures, although technically feasible and safe, has a high rate of asymptomatic reocclusion and residual stenoses of the brachial artery."[23] Furthermore, they stated, "It appears that had the vascular reconstruction not been done, collateral circulation would have been adequate to maintain a viable extremity."

Shaw et al. found that 17 of 143 patients with type III supracondylar fractures had signs of vascular impairment.[22] Thirteen of these 17 patients had a normal vascular examination after emergent closed reduction and pinning. One of the four remaining patients had an absent radial pulse with no signs of ischemia; this patient was observed without exploration of the artery. The other three patients underwent exploration and repair of the brachial artery. At final follow-up, no signs of ischemia or claudication were seen in any of their 143 patients. The authors recommended diligent examination and observation, rather than arteriography, for patients who have absent pulses and no signs of ischemia. Any signs of ischemia, especially significant pain with passive motion of the forearm musculature, should be explored emergently, and fasciotomies should be performed. Diligent observation and appropriate treatment should reduce the risk of Volkmann's ischemia.

Cubitus Varus

Cubitus varus is one of the most common complications of supracondylar fractures of the humerus[11,34–36,50,69,70] (Fig. 21.21). Researchers once thought it resulted from an overgrowth of the lateral column following the supracondylar fracture that was similar to the overgrowth occurring after lateral condylar fractures.[4] Most authors now agree that cubitus varus after a supracondylar fracture results from poor reduction or loss of reduction.[4,36,69] The malunion of the fracture occurs in three planes: internal rotation in the horizontal plane, medial rotation in the coronal plane, and extension in the sagittal plane.[34] Cubitus varus is reported as a complication in 9% to 58%

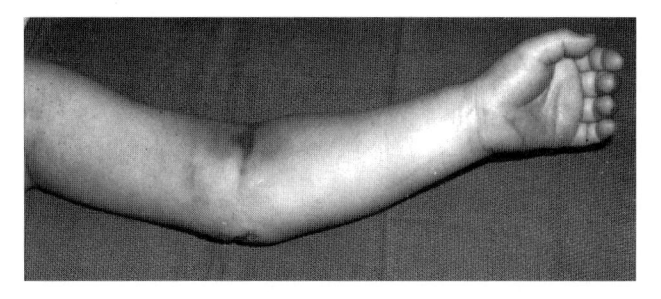

FIGURE 21.20. This patient had a type III fracture with median nerve and brachial artery injury and associated ischemic hand. Note skin bruise and pucker associated with severe fracture and brachial artery injury.

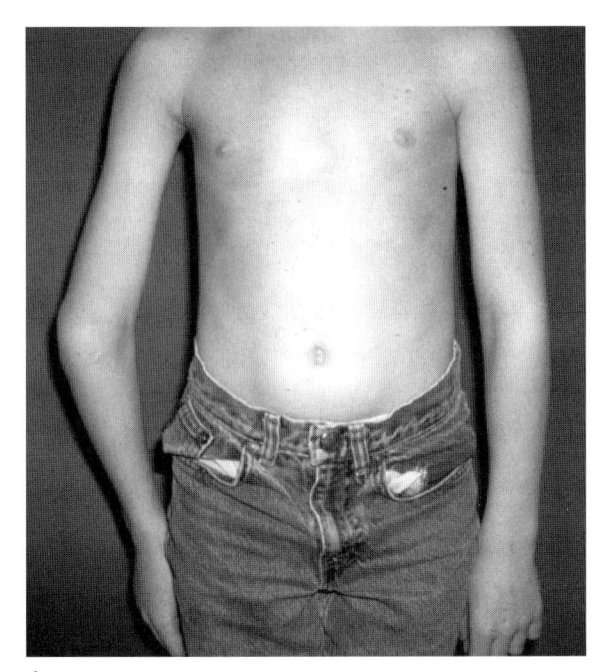

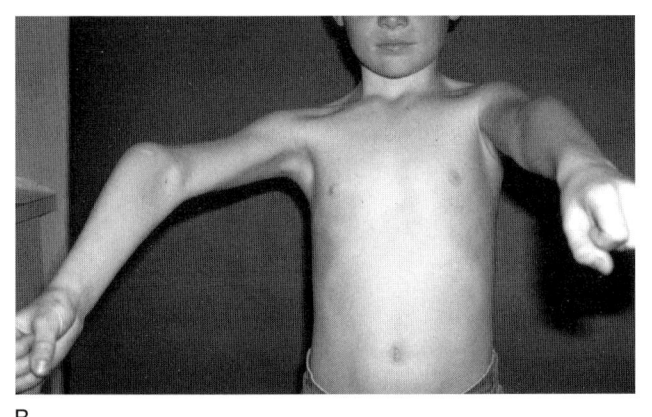

FIGURE 21.21. (A) This 9-year-old patient with cubitus varus sustained a supracondylar fracture at age 6. (B) Patient has 35° of varus and 45° of inward rotation.

of supracondylar fractures of the humerus.[11,36,69] Recently, newer techniques of anatomic reduction and percutaneous pinning have reduced the rate of cubitus varus to around 3%.[5,28]

Cubitus varus is reported as only a cosmetic deformity, but we and other authors believe that the deformity can be more problematic.[69–71] Patients who have cubitus varus often can have difficulty participating in throwing sports, push-ups, and swimming. Recently, Davids and associates reported an increased incidence of lateral condylar fracture resulting from poor biomechanical alignment of the distal humerus with cubitus varus[69] (Fig. 21.22). Cubitus varus should be approached carefully with the family and patient. Often, the patient exhibits little or no limitation and only has a problem with cosmesis.

Early reports have shown poor results with osteotomies to correct cubitus varus. Ippolito et al. reported a 45% rate of poor results in patients who had a supracondylar osteotomy to treat cubitus varus and who were followed for an average of 23 years.[35] Newer techniques have increased the reported good results, and many techniques produce 80% to 94% good to excellent results.[34,36,37,70] Barrett et al. reported 94% good to excellent results using a lateral closing wedge osteotomy.[34] Levine et al. have reported similar improved outcomes for supracondylar osteotomies stabilized with a lateral external fixator.[36] Several types of osteotomy can be used, such as lateral closing wedge, medial opening wedge, step-cut lateral wedge, and dome osteotomies.

We believe that patients do not tolerate significant cubitus varus and internal rotation as well as much of the literature indicates. Activities that require the hand to be positioned in the extremes of external rotation about the shoulder are impossible. However, if a patient has no activity-related problems, the osteotomy is discouraged. If a significant cosmetic deformity exists or if the deformity limits the patient's activities, an osteotomy should be considered.

We prefer to use a posterior triceps-splitting or a lateral approach. Reference pins are placed laterally in the proximal and distal fragments to assure that the osteotomy has accomplished the planned correction. The surgeon performs either a dome or lateral closing wedge osteotomy just above the olecranon fossa. All planes of deformity correction are completed when the pins are brought parallel. After correcting the deformity, we prefer to use crossed percutaneous K-wires in a manner similar to pinning a supracondylar fracture (Fig. 21.23). Preoperative planning through comparative range of motion aids in determining the necessary planes of correction. It is tempting to correct only the deformity of the coronal plane varus and disregard the extension and internal rotation. We believe that some of the internal rotation should be corrected to improve the patient's hand position with the shoulder in maximum external rotation. If the surgeon makes equal limb cuts laterally for the osteotomy, he or she can reduce the often reported risk of a prominent lateral condyle.

FLEXION-TYPE FRACTURES

As noted, flexion-type fractures represent only 2% to 4% of supracondylar humeral fractures.[6] Classification of these fractures is based on a modification of Gartland's classification of extension-type fractures.[4] Type I fractures are nondisplaced. Type II fractures are angulated or rotated with an intact anterior hinge. Type III fractures are

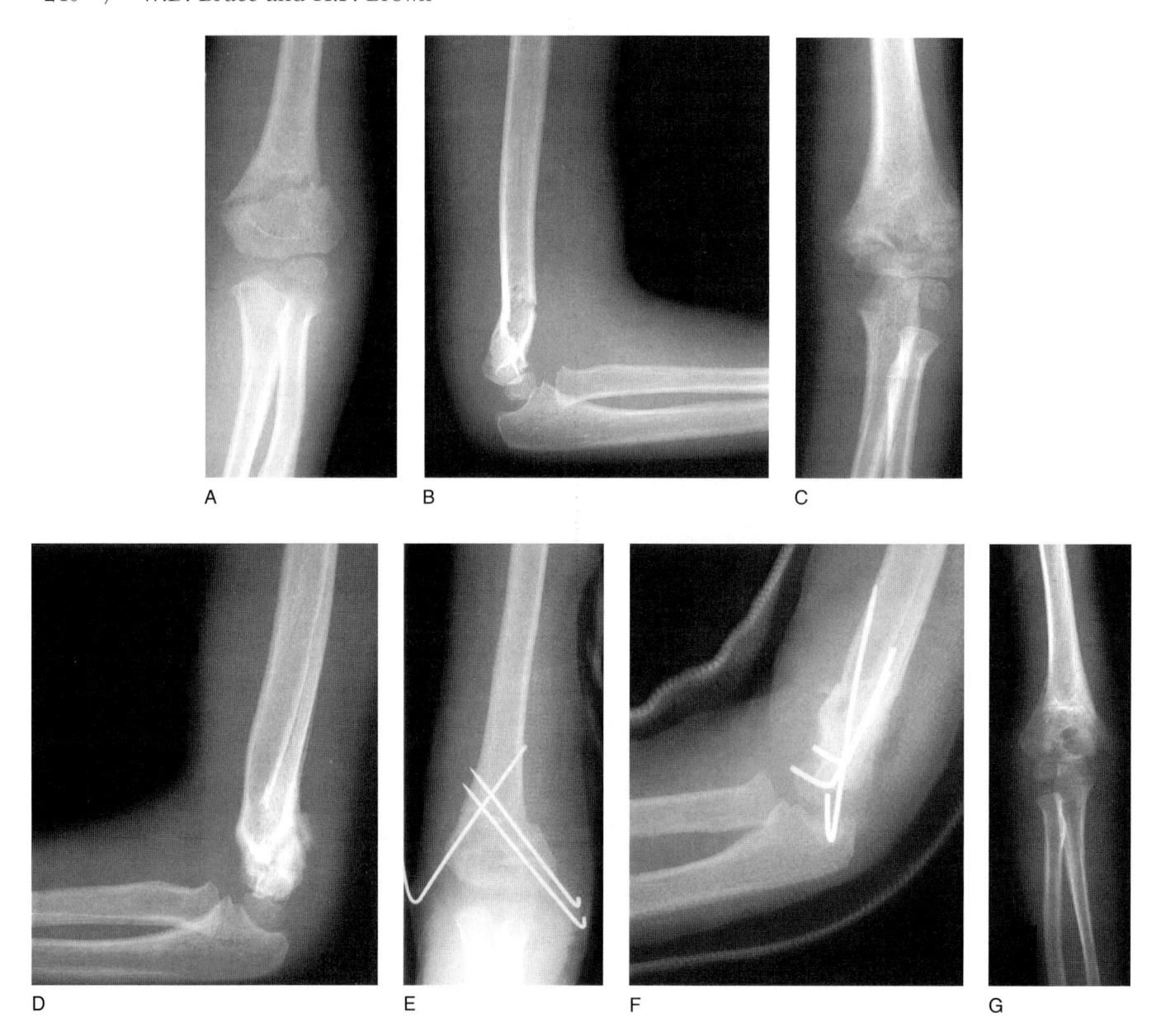

FIGURE 21.22. (A) Anteroposterior and (B) lateral radiographic views of a type IIA fracture with 20° of anterior angulation was treated closed without pinning. (C) Anteroposterior and (D) lateral radiographic views of the same patient 18 months later. The patient has cubitus varus and and a resultant reinjury, a fracture of the lateral condyle. (E) Anteroposterior and (F) lateral postoperative radiographic views after a lateral closing wedge osteotomy with restoration of carrying angle and normal rotation. (G) Anteroposterior radiographic view at 2 months after surgery.

displaced anteriorly with an absence of any normal cortical contact (Fig. 21.24). The flexion-type fracture that is severely displaced can buttonhole the triceps muscle.[4,6]

Flexion-type supracondylar fractures have a higher association with ulnar nerve injury.[6,30] Management of these fractures is much the same as the management of extension-type fractures, except that the elbow is immobilized in extension because the fracture is more stable in this position.[4] Otherwise, nondisplaced fractures are splinted. Angulated or displaced fractures are reduced and percutaneously pinned (see Fig. 21.24). The displaced flexion supracondylar fracture more often requires open reduction than its extension counterpart. Good results have been reported for flexion-type supracondylar fractures treated in this manner; however, cubitus varus is a known complication.[6]

CONCLUSION

Fractures about the elbow in children can be very difficult to diagnose and repair. As with all fractures, man-

21: Supracondylar Fractures of the Humerus in Childen / 241

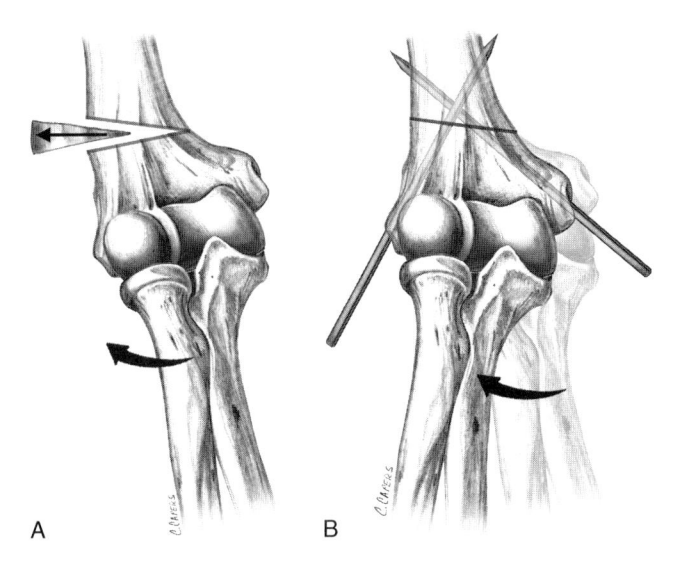

FIGURE 21.23. (A) Lateral closing wedge osteotomy for cubitus varus. Making the limbs of the osteotomy cut equal in length decreases lateral condyle prominence. The osteotomy can also be rotated to reduce the extremity's internal rotation. (B) Pinning of the osteotomy is similar to the pinning of a supracondylar fracture.

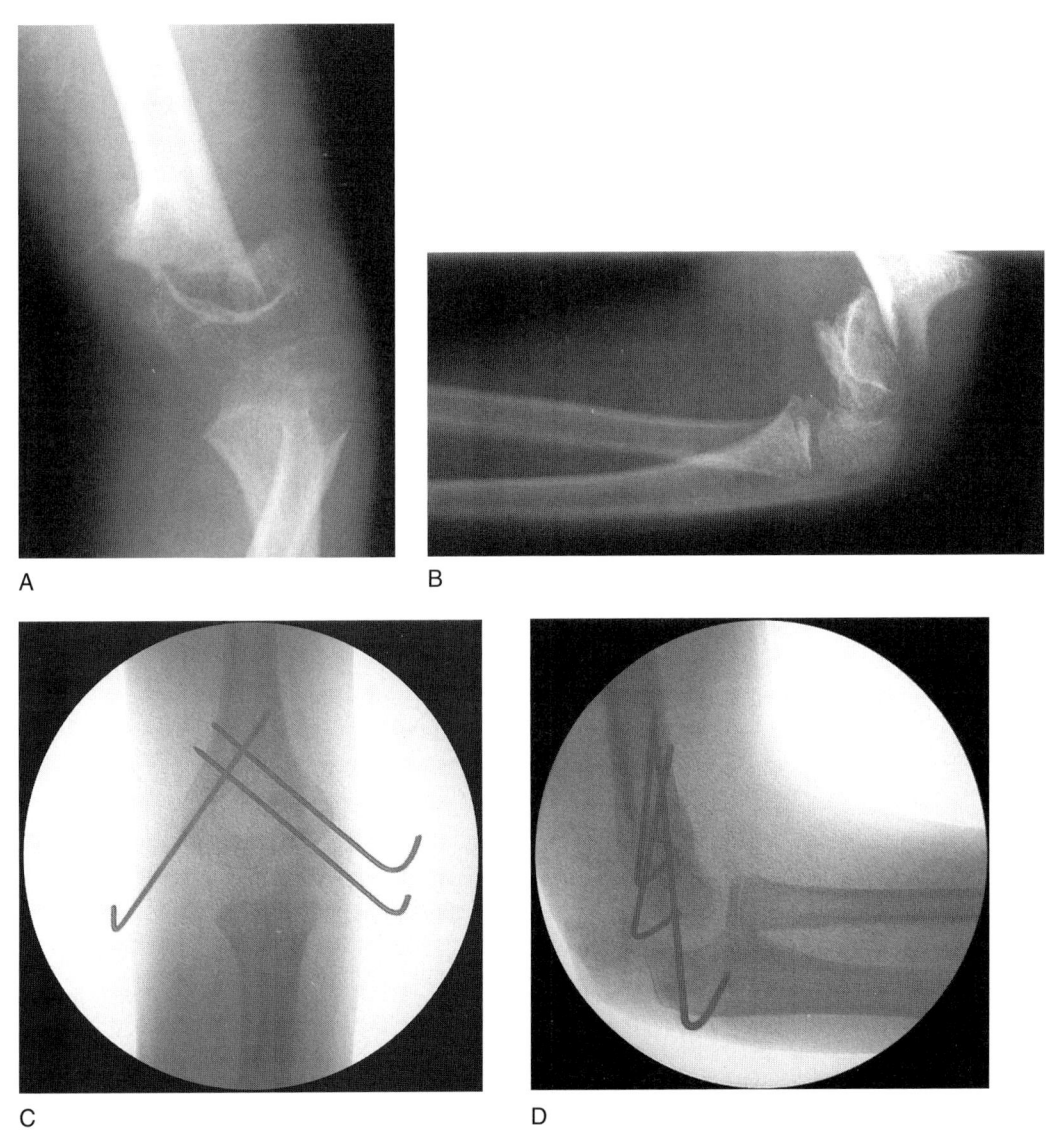

FIGURE 21.24. (A) Anteroposterior and (B) lateral radiographic views of an 8-year-old patient with a type III flexion fracture of the humerus. (C) Anteroposterior and (D) lateral postoperative radiographic views of the same patient after open reduction and pinning. At surgery, the triceps muscle was found to be buttonholed by the proximal fragment.

agement directed toward anatomic reduction should relieve stresses about the elbow and the stresses felt by the surgeon. We have found the approaches presented here to be successful in the management of pediatric elbow fractures.

REFERENCES

1. Cheng JCY, Lam TP, Shen WY. Closed reduction and percutaneous pinning for type III displaced supracondylar fractures of the humerus in children. *J Orthop Trauma* 1995;9:511–515.
2. Farnsworth CL, Silva PD, Mubarak SJ. Etiology of supracondylar humerus fractures. *J Pediatr Orthop* 1998;18:38–42.
3. Mubarak SJ, Davids JR. Closed reduction and percutaneous pinning of supracondylar fractures of the distal humerus in the child. In: Morrey BF, ed. *The elbow*. New York: Raven Press; 1994:37–51.
4. Wilkins KE, ed. *Operative management of upper extremity fractures in children*. Rosemont, IL: American Academy of Orthopaedic Surgeons; 1994:75–86.
5. Canale ST. Fractures and dislocations in children. In: Canale ST, ed. *Campbell's Operative Orthopaedics*, 9th ed. St. Louis MO: CV Mosby-Yearbook; 1998:2363–2536.
6. Williamson DM, Cole WG. Flexion supracondylar fractures of the humerus in children: Treatment by manipulation and extension cast. *Injury* 1991;22:451–455.
7. Yates C, Sullivan JA. Arthrographic diagnosis of elbow injuries in children. *J Pediatr Orthop* 1987;7:54–60.
8. Haraldsson S. On osteochondrosis deformans juvenilis capituli humeri including investigation of intra-osseous vasculature in distal humerus. *Acta Orthop Scand* (Suppl) 38, 1959.
9. Smith JT, Morrissy RT. Preventing complications of supracondylar fractures in children. *Complications orthop* 1989;4:135–146.
10. Dameron TB. Transverse fractures of the distal humerus in children. *Instr Course Lect* 1981;30:224–235.
11. Green NE. Fractures and dislocations about the elbow. In Green NE, ed. *Skeletal trauma in children*. Philadelphia: WB Saunders Co.; 1994:213–256.
12. Kasser JA. Percutaneous pinning of supracondylar fractures of the humerus. *Instr Course Lect* 1992;41:385–390.
13. Mohammad S, Rymaszewski LA, Runciman J. The Baumann angle in supracondylar fractures of the distal humerus in children. *J Pediatr Orthop* 1999;19:65–69.
14. Williamson DM, Coates CJ, Miller RK, et al. Normal characteristics of the Baumann (humerocapitellar) angle: An aid in assessment of supracondylar fractures. *J Pediatr Orthop* 1992;12:636–639.
15. Worlock P. Supracondylar fractures of the humerus. Assessment of cubitus varus by the Baumann angle. *J Bone Joint Surg* 1986;68B:755–757.
16. Kissoon N, Galpin R, Gayle M, et al. Evaluation of the role of comparison radiographs in the diagnosis of traumatic elbow injuries. *J Pediatr Orthop* 1995;15:449–453.
17. Clement DA. Assessment of a treatment plan for managing acute vascular complications associated with supracondylar fractures of the humerus in children. *J Pediatr Orthop* 1990;10:97–100.
18. Copley LA, Dormans JP, Davidson RS. Vascular injuries and their sequelae in pediatric supracondylar humeral fractures: Toward a goal of prevention. *J Pediatr Orthop* 1996;16:99–103.
19. Mapes RC, Hennrikus WL. The effect of elbow position on the radial pulse measured by Doppler ultrasonography after surgical treatment of supracondylar elbow fractures in children. *J Pediatr Orthop* 1998;18:441–444.
20. Schoenecker PL, Delgado E, Rotman M, et al. Pulseless arm in association with totally displaced supracondylar fracture. *J Orthop Trauma* 1996;10:410–415.
21. Shaw BA. Letter to the editor. *J Pediatr Orthop* 1998;18:273.
22. Shaw BA, Kasser JR, Emans JB, et al. Management of vascular injuries in displaced supracondylar humerus fractures without arteriography. *J Orthop Trauma* 1990;4:25–29.
23. Sabharwal S, Tredwell SJ, Beauchamp RD, et al. Management of pulseless pink hand in pediatric supracondylar fractures of humerus. *J Pediatr Orthop* 1997;17:303–310.
24. Vasli LR. Diagnosis of vascular injury in children with supracondylar fractures of the humerus. *Injury* 1988;19:11–13.
25. Brown IC, Zinar DM. Traumatic and iatrogenic neurological complications after supracondylar humerus fractures in children. *J Pediatr Orthop* 1995;15:440–443.
26. Culp RW, Osterman AL, Davidson RS, et al. Neural injuries associated with supracondylar fractures of the humerus in children. *J Bone Joint Surg* 1990;72A:1211–1215.
27. Hennrikus WL, O'Brien T, Champa J, et al. Neurologic complications stemming from displaced supracondylar fractures and from the treatment of these fractures in children. *Orthop Trans* 1993;16:818.
28. Pirone AM, Graham HK, Krajbich, JI. Management of displaced extension-type supracondylar fractures of the humerus in children. *J Bone Joint Surg* 1988;70A:641–649.
29. Sairyo K, Henmi T, Kanematsu Y, et al. Radial nerve palsy associated with slightly angulated pediatric supracondylar humerus fracture. *J Orthop Trauma* 1997;11:227–229.
30. Campbell CC, Waters PM, Emans JB, et al. Neurovascular injury and displacement in type III supracondylar humerus fractures. *J Pediatr Orthop* 1995;15:47–52.
31. Holmberg L. Fractures of distal end of the humerus in children. *Acta Chir Scand* 1945;92 Suppl 103:1–69.
32. Gartland JJ. Management of supracondylar fractures of the humerus in children. *Surg Gynecol Obstet* 1959;109:145–154.
33. De Boeck H, De Smet P, Penders W, et al. Supracondylar elbow fractures with impaction of the medial condyle in children. *J Pediatr Orthop* 1995;15:444–448.
34. Barrett IR, Bellemore MC, Kwon Y-M. Cosmetic results of supracondylar osteotomy for correction of cubitus varus. *J Pediatr Orthop* 1998;18:445–447.
35. Ippolito E, Moneta MR, D'Arrigo C. Post-traumatic cubitus varus: Long-term follow-up of corrective supracondylar humeral osteotomy in children. *J Bone Joint Surg* 1990;72A:757–765.
36. Levine MJ, Horn, BD, Pizzutillo PD. Treatment of posttraumatic cubitus varus in the pediatric population with humeral osteotomy and external fixation. *J Pediatr Orthop* 1996;16:597–601.
37. Wong HK, Balasubramaniam P. Humeral torsional deformity after supracondylar osteotomy for cubitus varus: Its influence on the postosteotomy carrying angle. *J Pediatr Orthop* 1992;12:490–493.

38. Dunlop J. Transcondylar fractures of the humerus in childhood. *J Bone Joint Surg* 1939;21:59–73.
39. Archibald DAA, Roberts JA, Smith MGH. Transarticular fixation for severely displaced supracondylar fractures in children. *J Bone Joint Surg* 1991;73B:147–149.
40. Smith FM. Kirschner wire traction in the elbow and upper arm injuries. *Am J Surg* 1947;74:770–787.
41. Bosanquet JS, and Middleton RW. The reduction of supracondylar fractures of the humerus in children treated by traction-in-extension: a review of 18 cases. *Injury* 1983;14:373–380.
42. Palmar EE, Niemann KMW, Vesely D, Armstrong JH. Supracondylar fractures of the humerus in children. *J Bone Joint Surg* 1978;60A:653–656.
43. Worlock PH, Colton C. Severely displaced supracondylar fractures of the humerus in children: A simple method of treatment. *J Pediatr Orthop* 1987;7:49–53.
44. Alburger PD, Weidner PL, Betz RR. Supracondylar fractures of the humerus in children. *J Pediatr Orthop* 1992;12:16–19.
45. Rodriguez-Merchan EC. Letter to the editor. *J Pediatr Orthop* 1997;17:127.
46. Böstman O, Mäkelä EA, Södergård J, et al. Absorbable polyglycolide pins in internal fixation of fractures in children. *J Pediatr Orthop* 1993;13:242–245.
47. Boyd DW, Aronson DD. Supracondylar fractures of the humerus: A prospective study of percutaneous pinning. *J Pediatr Orthop* 1992;12:789–794.
48. Cramer KE, Devito DP, Green NE. Comparison of closed reduction and percutaneous pinning versus open reduction and percutaneous pinning in displaced supracondylar fractures of the humerus in children. *J Orthop Trauma* 1992;6:407–412.
49. Flynn JL, Matthews JG, and Benoit, RL. Blind pinning of displaced supracondylar fractures of the humerus in children. Sixteen years experience with long-term follow-up. *J Bone Joint Surg* 1974;56A:263–272.
50. Mehserle WL, Meehan PL. Treatment of the displaced supracondylar fracture of the humerus (type III) with closed reduction and percutaneous cross-pin fixation. *J Pediatr Orthop* 1991;11:705–711.
51. Rasool MN. Ulnar nerve injury after K-wire fixation of supracondylar humerus fractures in children. *J Pediatr Orthop* 1998;18:686–690.
52. Topping RE, Blanco JS, Davis TJ. Clinical evaluation of crossed-pin versus lateral-pin fixation in displaced supracondylar humerus fractures. *J Pediatr Orthop* 1995;15:435–439.
53. Weiland AJ, Meyer S, Tolo VT, et al. Surgical treatment of displaced supracondylar fractures of the humerus in children: analysis of fifty-two cases followed up for five to fifteen years. *J Bone Joint Surg* 1978;60A:657–661.
54. Lyons JP, Ashley E, Hoffer MM. Ulnar nerve palsies after percutaneous cross-pinning of supracondylar fractures in children's elbows. *J Pediatr Orthop* 1998;18:43–45.
55. Royce RO, Dutkowsky JP, Kasser JR, et al. Neurologic complications after K-wire fixation of supracondylar humerus fractures in children. *J Pediatr Orthop* 1991;11:191–194.
56. Carcassonne M, Bergoin M, Hornung H. Results of operative treatment of severe supracondylar fractures of the elbow in children. *J Pediatr Surg* 1972;7:676–679.
57. Danielsson L, Pettersson H. Open reduction and pin fixation of severely displaced supracondylar fractures of the humerus in children. *Acta Orthop Scand* 1980;51:249–255.
58. Childress HM. Transarticular pin fixation in supracondylar fractures at the elbow in children. *J Bone Joint Surg* 1972;54A:1548–1552.
59. Sibly TF, Briggs PJ, Gibson MJ. Supracondylar fractures of the humerus in childhood: Range of movement following the posterior approach to open reduction. *Injury* 1991;22:456–458.
60. Walløe A, Egund N, Eikelund L. Supracondylar fracture of the humerus in children: Review of closed and open reduction leading to a proposal for treatment. *Injury* 1985;16:296–299.
61. Iyengar SR, Hoffinger SA, Townsend DR. Early versus delayed reduction and pinning of type III displaced supracondylar fractures of the humerus in children: A comparative study. *J Orthop Trauma* 1999;13:51–55.
62. Zionts LE, McKellop HA, Hathaway R. Torsional strength of pin configurations used to fix supracondylar fractures of the humerus in children. *J Bone Joint Surg* 1994;76A:253–256.
63. Archibeck MJ, Scott SM, Peters CL. Brachialis muscle entrapment in displaced supracondylar humerus fractures: A technique of closed reduction and report of initial results. *J Pediatr Orthop* 1997;17:298–302.
64. Peters CL, Scott SM, Stevens PM. Closed reduction and percutaneous pinning of displaced supracondylar humerus fractures in children: Description of a new closed reduction technique for fractures with brachialis muscle entrapment. *J Orthop Trauma* 1995;9:430–434.
65. Thomas AP. Entrapment of the proximal fragment of supracondylar fractures. *J Bone Joint Surg* 1990;72B:321–322.
66. Haasbeek JF, Cole WG. Open fractures of the arm in children. *J Bone Joint Surg* 1995;77B:576–581.
67. Hoppenfeld S, deBoer P. *Surgical exposures in orthopaedics*, 2nd ed. Philadelphia: JB Lippincott Co., 1994:83–116.
68. Garbuz DS, Leitch K, Wright JG. The treatment of supracondylar fractures in children with an absent radial pulse. *J Pediatr Orthop* 1996;16:594–596.
69. Davids JR, Maguire MF, Mubarak SJ, et al. Lateral condylar fracture of the humerus following posttraumatic cubitus varus. *J Pediatr Orthop* 1994;14:466–470.
70. Usui M, Ishii S, Miyano S, et al. Three-dimensional corrective osteotomy for treatment of cubitus varus after supracondylar fracture of the humerus in children. *J Shoulder Elbow Surg* 1995;4:17–22.
71. Fujioka H, Nakabayashi Y, Hirata S, et al. Analysis of tardy ulnar nerve palsy associated with cubitus varus deformity after a supracondylar fracture of the humerus: A report of four cases. *J Orthop Trauma* 1995;9:435–440.

CHAPTER 22

Pediatric Lateral Condylar Fractures

Michael Ehrlich and Donna Pacicca

INTRODUCTION

Fractures of the lateral condylar physis are common childhood injuries; they represent 16.9% of distal humeral fractures and 54.2% of distal humeral physeal fractures in children.[1] These fractures occur most commonly between 3 and 14 years of age, with a peak incidence from 6 to 10 years of age.[2]

In this chapter, we present the clinical anatomy, physical examination, nonoperative and operative treatments, and complications associated with lateral condylar fractures. Our discussion of operative treatment focuses on the appropriate methods for addressing acute, semi-acute, and chronic fractures.

CLINICAL ANATOMY

The bones that form the elbow ossify at different times over an 11-year period after birth. Remembering the mnemonic CRMTOL (capitellum, radial head, medial epicondyle, trochlea, olecranon, and lateral epicondyle) can help the examiner recall the order of ossification in the elbow joint. The ossific nucleus of the lateral condyle (capitellum) appears between ages 18 months and 2 years; the radial head, around age 4; and the medial epicondyle, at age 5. The other ossification centers appear thereafter in 2-year increments. The ossified trochlea appears at age 7; the olecranon, at age 9; and the lateral epicondyle, at age 11.

Remember that the lateral condylar physis differs from the lateral epicondyle. Although they are located adjacent to each other, they ossify at different times. The lateral epicondyle does not ossify until a child is approximately 11 years of age; therefore, the examining physician cannot diagnose a lateral epicondylar fracture on radiographs in a patient younger than about 10 years of age. A fracture in the lateral portion of the distal humerus in a child younger than 10 years of age probably affects the lateral condyle.

The medial edge of the capitellar ossific nucleus extends to the mid-portion of the joint surface, meeting with the lateral edge of the trochlea. On a lateral radiograph, the capitellar physis appears wider posteriorly.[1] Because of this appearance, lateral condylar fractures may not be recognized.

The mechanism of injury in a lateral condylar fracture is a varus stress to an extended elbow with the forearm supinated. Jakob et al. used a cadaveric model to demonstrate this mechanism.[3] The fracture line begins at the lateral aspect of the distal metaphysis and traverses obliquely and medially through the physis. Depending on the force of energy, the fracture may hinge on the articular cartilage or may enter the joint at the lateral trochlea. As Jakob et al. demonstrated, a valgus stress applied after the fracture is sustained can disrupt the cartilaginous hinge and cause rotation and lateral displacement of the fracture fragment.

Milch devised a classification scheme for lateral condylar fractures based on the location of the fracture line.[4] The Milch type I fracture line extends through the ossific nucleus and exits at the radiocapitellar groove (Fig. 22.1A). This type is considered rare. The type II fracture line extends around the entire physis and exits through the trochlear notch (Fig. 22.1B).

The Salter–Harris classification orders physeal fractures. A type II fracture runs through the calcified zone of the metaphysis and avulses a fragment of bone. A type IV fracture extends from the bone of the metaphysis, through the physis, and into the bone of the epiphysis. Significant debate has risen over whether these fractures should all be considered type IV by the Salter–Harris classification or whether fractures with lines extending through the trochlear notch should be considered Salter–

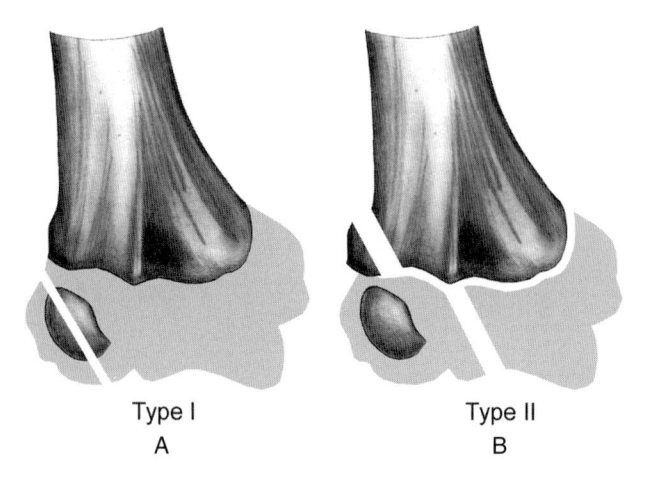

FIGURE 22.1. Milch classification. (A) The Milch type I fracture line, which is rare, splits the capitellar secondary center of ossification. (B) Most fracture lines go between the condyles (Milch type II).

Harris type II (Fig. 22.2). By definition, because these fractures are intra-articular injuries, they should be considered type IV. However, the fracture line usually begins at the metaphysis (a characteristic of type II fractures), and the capitellar ossific nucleus usually is not split. In our opinion, most of these fractures act functionally like type II fractures. However, in the rare instance where the ossific nucleus is involved, they act more like type IV injuries.

Interestingly, Milch makes no reference to the relationship of the fracture line to the ossific nucleus except to where it crosses the cartilaginous epiphysis. Instead, he focuses on whether the fracture is associated with ulnar dislocation, showing that a dislocation is more likely with the fracture line lateral to the trochlear groove.[4]

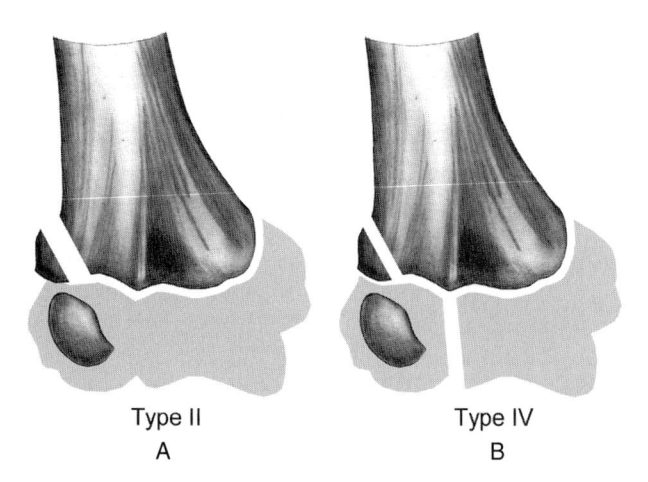

FIGURE 22.2. (A) A true Salter–Harris type II distal physeal separation and (B) a Salter–Harris type IV fracture. The radiographs are identical because the examiner only sees the detached metaphyseal chip. However, arthrography distinguishes between type II and IV. The shaded area depicts cartilage.

The amount of fracture displacement is more important than the location of the fracture. Rutherford described stages of displacement based on radiographs.[5] These stages are useful in determining treatment. Stage I fractures are nondisplaced with an articular hinge; the joint surface is intact. These fractures are considered stable. Stage II fractures are complete, with minimal to moderate displacement that usually occurs in rotation. These fractures are usually unstable. Stage III fractures are completely displaced and have significant rotation.

PHYSICAL EXAMINATION

A child who has a lateral condylar fracture often presents with only lateral swelling and tenderness accompanied by limited range of motion. Occasionally, these fractures are associated with elbow dislocation or an olecranon fracture. Sometimes only a posterior fat pad sign may be present. The diagnosis is made on the basis of plain radiographs in the anteroposterior, lateral, and oblique projections. Arthrography may be useful in distinguishing lateral condylar fractures from distal humeral physeal separations with a metaphyseal fragment (i.e., true Salter–Harris type II fractures).

Marzo et al. also showed that arthrography can be useful in characterizing the amount of displacement and rotation of the fracture, especially when plain films do not show these things. They caution that arthrography can only be interpreted successfully when the examination is performed within 24 hours of the injury.[6]

TREATMENT

Obviously, nondisplaced and severely displaced fractures are readily recognized on radiographs. However, fractures that are displaced from 2 to 4 mm are the most difficult to recognize, so the examining physician must carefully consider the appropriate treatment. Traditionally, the worst results occur with fractures displaced from 2 to 4 mm, because these fractures can displace later and because healing can be significantly delayed even with a very small amount of displacement.

Although guidelines are good to follow, the physician frequently treats patients whose injuries do not completely fit the typical fracture pattern described in the guidelines. For example, the fragment may be hinged so that it is displaced only 1 mm at the apex and 3 mm at the mouth of the hinge. Presentation of atypical fracture patterns can pose a problem to a surgeon who does not regularly treat these fractures. If the surgeon has concerns about or difficulty recognizing the fracture pattern, he or she should obtain a computed tomography scan or tomograms to better delineate the fracture pattern, especially at the articular surface.

Nonoperative Treatment

Treatment of lateral condylar fractures is based on stability of the fracture pattern. In fractures that are displaced 2 mm or less, long-arm cast immobilization and close initial follow-up is the treatment of choice. The senior author (ME) obtains serial tomography of the patient's fracture every 5 to 7 days until evidence of healing is seen on radiographs and elects to operate if displacement is evident. However, the other author obtains radiographs with the patient's arm out of the cast every 3 to 5 days until radiographs show evidence of healing or until the fracture displaces. Casting is continued for at least 6 weeks after injury. These fractures often can take longer to heal, and casting should be continued as long as necessary for bony union.[5,7,8] Traction is not an acceptable method of treatment.

The surgeon must recognize that the patient's elbow will be stiff when the cast is removed. We usually allow the child to regain motion on his or her own and examine the child 3 to 4 weeks after cast removal. If full motion is not exhibited at that time, we may refer the patient to a physical therapist for instruction in active range-of-motion exercises. We never recommend manipulation of the elbow to regain motion, because we may cause other problems, such as heterotopic ossification. We also do not let the child resume full activity until he or she has regained full motion and has been out of the cast usually for 2 months. The child's elbow becomes osteopenic with casting, and it is at a significant risk for fracture shortly after cast removal. We often have children lift light weights to strengthen the muscles and put stress on the bone to encourage remineralization.

Operative Treatment

Acute

For fractures initially displaced more than 2 mm or for fractures that displace within 2 weeks after injury, we generally perform an open reduction and fixation with lateral Kirschner wires (K-wires) (Figs. 22.3 and 22.4). We use a lateral approach, placing the incision over the palpable lateral condyle. Do not strip too much muscle off the fracture fragment, especially posteriorly, because this action disrupts the blood supply and may lead to avascular necrosis of the capitellum and to cubitus valgus (Fig. 22.5). Expose the joint surface anteriorly and reduce the fracture anatomically. In a classic Salter–Harris type IV fracture, the reason for fixing the fragments anatomically is to avoid bony bridge formation between the two portions of the ossific nucleus, leading to a growth arrest in that area.[2] In our experience, this is rare.

Next, drive two smooth K-wires across the fracture and check alignment with fluoroscopy. Often, some lateral comminution is present, and assessing the reduction can be difficult if the surgeon looks only at the metaphyseal portion. Therefore, the surgeon needs to adequately expose the articular surface anteriorly to assess reduction. The senior author prefers to bury the K-wires and to remove them in the operating room because of

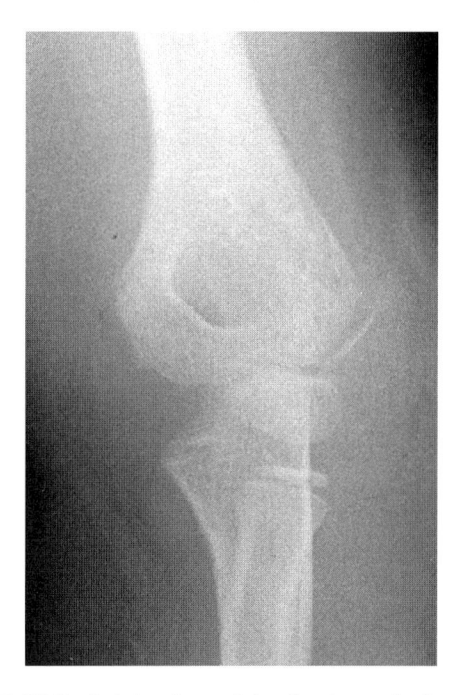

FIGURE 22.3. A lateral condylar fracture displaced 2 to 3 mm. Surgical treatment is usually indicated for a fracture displaced this much, because it can displace more and lead to a late nonunion.

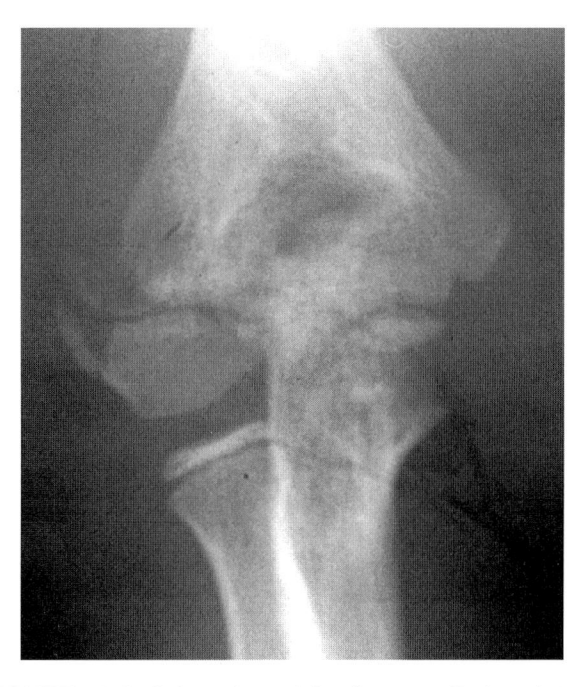

FIGURE 22.4. A lateral condylar fracture displaced 2 to 3 mm. This fracture was treated in a cast and went on to nonunion with all the complications.

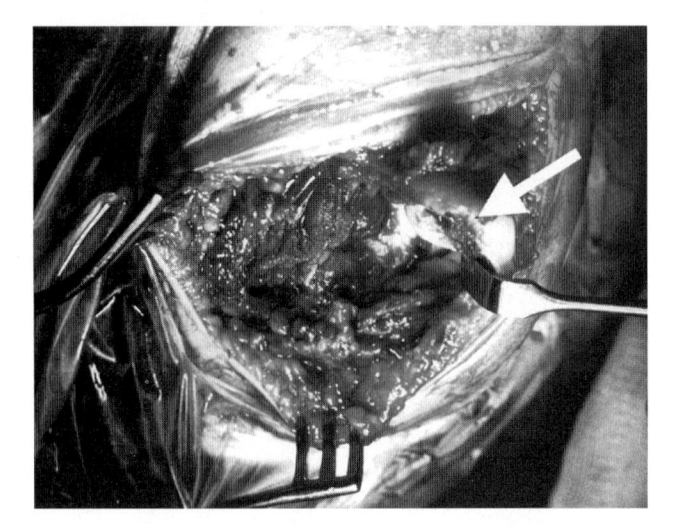

FIGURE 22.5. Intraoperative photograph of a displaced lateral condylar fracture. Most of the fragment represents the cartilaginous epiphysis. If the surgeon strips too much of the attached muscle to increase visualization, avascular necrosis results.

concerns with introducing infection into the fracture. The junior author leaves the wires out of the skin, applies a bulky dressing, and places the elbow in a long-arm cast. The wires generally are removed at 4 weeks, and splinting is continued for an additional 2 weeks. Closed reduction is almost never successful for the fractures displaced more than 1 cm, because the articular surface can be rotated up to 180° so that it faces the fracture line (Fig. 22.6A–C).

Makela et al. have described using self-reinforced polyglycolic acid (SR-PGA) pins for fixing these fractures.[9] Although we have no experience with SR-PGA pins, we believe that they may be an acceptable alternative to K-wires, with the potential benefit of not having to remove hardware. The main concern with biodegradable pins is the possibility of an inflammatory soft-tissue response from the degradation products. This response has been reported more with biodegradable screws, but there is insufficient literature on SR-PGA pins to determine if this response is also a possible sequela.

In some parts of the United States, surgeons are recommending closed reduction and percutaneous pin fixation. We agree with Hardacre et al.'s statement: "Anatomical reduction cannot be achieved by a closed manipulation."[7] However, in certain cases, fixing a nondisplaced or minimally displaced fracture may be advisable. This fixation should be done with an arthrogram to confirm that no articular step-off or significant gap is present. Because of technical problems, we would only recommend using this technique for fractures occurring less than 24 hours earlier.

Semi-acute

Fractures that displace 2 weeks after injury often are not detected in a timely fashion because they are in a cast. The surgeon should treat these fractures with open reduction and internal fixation, but he or she must recognize that reduction of the articular surface is vital to satisfactory outcome. The approach and fixation for semi-acute fractures is the same as for acute fractures.

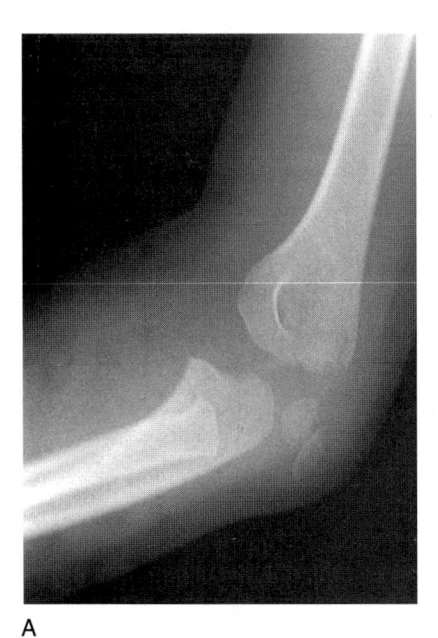

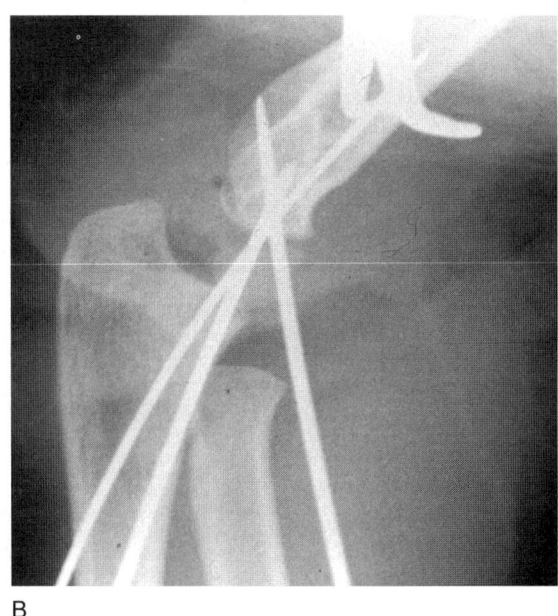

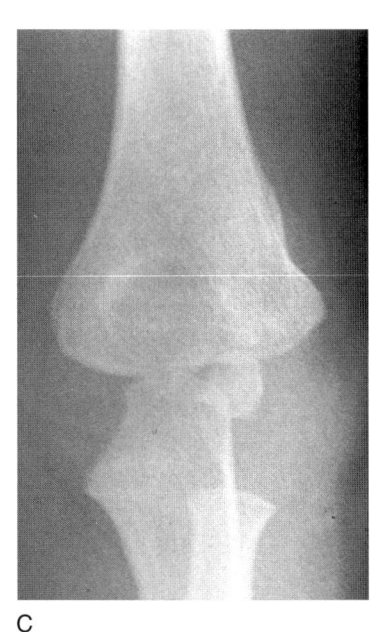

FIGURE 22.6. (A) Radiograph depicts a widely displaced lateral condylar fracture with the articular surface facing the fracture line. (B) Implanted Kirschner wires shown at the time of surgery. (C) Late result shows open growth plate with anatomic reduction.

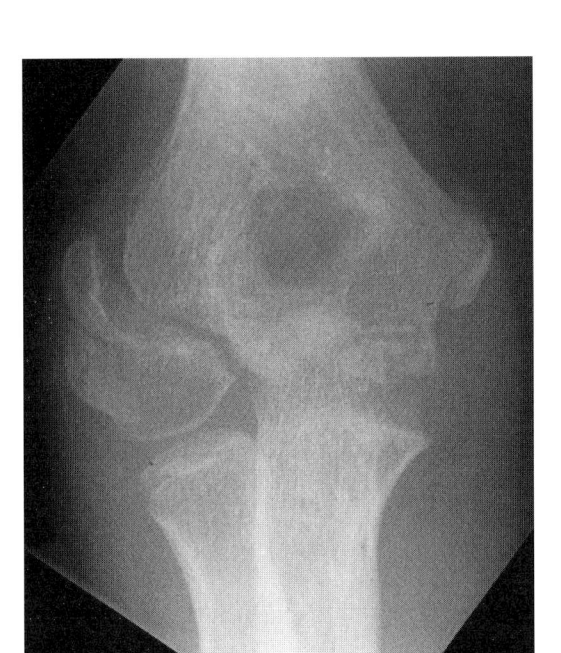

FIGURE 22.7. Late nonunion of a lateral condylar fracture.

Anatomic metaphyseal reduction is extremely difficult to achieve because of bone resorption and early callus formation. Intraoperative arthrography may be useful in assessing adequacy of reduction.

Chronic

Researchers debate the appropriate management of fractures that are displaced and ununited several months after injury (Fig. 22.7).[10–13] Recently, some researchers presented a new approach to the management of these fractures.[10–13] Good results have been reported with the new approach, but a number of pitfalls are involved. As indicated in Figure 22.7, many of these nonunions are seen months after injury. Traditionally, the approach has been to avoid taking down the nonunion and trying to anatomically repair it.[14–16] The argument for this approach is based on the belief that the blood supply to the fragment is tenuous at best and that putting screws across this fragment (which has to be stripped of soft tissues for manipulation into the appropriate alignment) further jeopardizes the blood flow and leaves the patient with avascular necrosis and, most likely, a stiff elbow.

Patients with nonunions usually report cosmetic deformity and, occasionally, pain or symptoms involving the ulnar nerve. Usually, these patients have a nearly full range of motion (they may lack 20° to 30° of extension). To treat these patients, we usually combine an anterior ulnar nerve transposition with a supracondylar varus osteotomy. We use a posterior approach through a V incision in the triceps tendon, extending it laterally and medially through the aponeurosis. We carefully expose the ulnar nerve, preserving its highest branches. Next, we remove a wedge of bone to correct the valgus deformity and, if we choose, address the flexion contracture. We fix

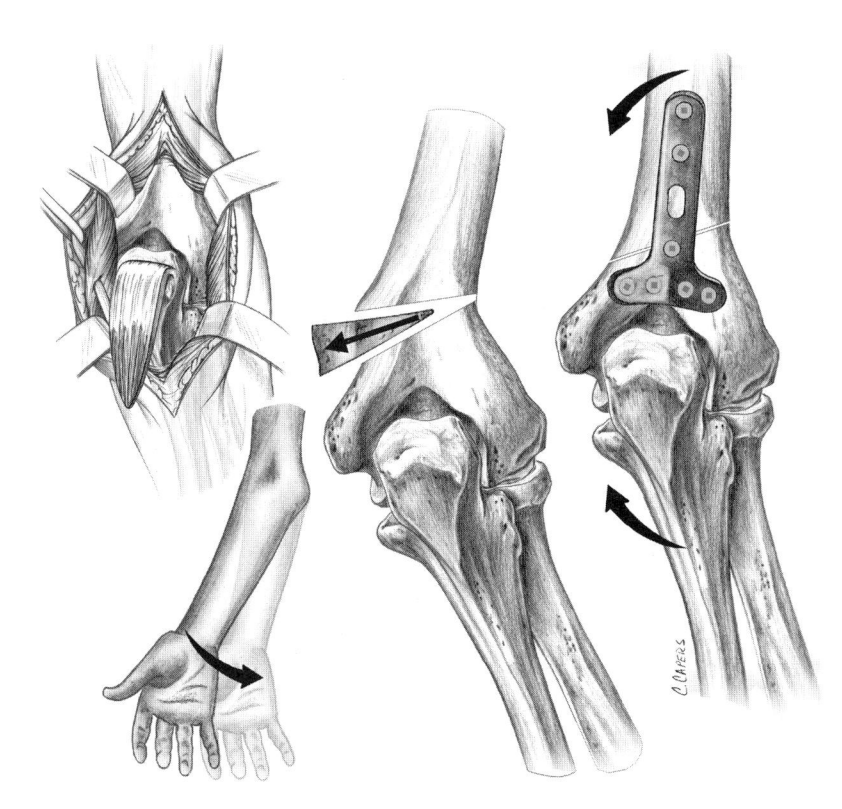

FIGURE 22.8. Wedge resection to correct cubitus valgus and placement of T-plate for fixation.

this osteotomy with a T-plate, using the transverse portion of the plate on the distal segment of the bone (Fig. 22.8). The ulnar nerve is transposed subcutaneously and sewn beneath some fat. The patient's arm is kept in a cast for 4 to 6 weeks.

Recently, some authors have reported using compression screws and bone graft to fix established nonunion in symptomatic patients.[10–13] They are careful not to disrupt the soft-tissue envelope of the epiphysis and have reported good healing in general, obtaining functional range of motion. However, this does not preclude the need for corrective osteotomy or ulnar nerve transposition. Although we have not yet changed our treatment regimen to include this option, a word of caution is in order. These authors often cite the need for soft-tissue or joint-capsule release to maintain range of motion of the elbow.[13] In fact, when we have viewed the elbow with fluoroscopy in a number of these patients before determining a surgical plan, the loose capitellar fragment has moved with the forearm, rather than with the humerus. Thus, if the forearm has significant decrease in flexion or extension with regard to the capitellum, fixing the capitellum to the humerus would decrease elbow motion. In accomplishing a "capsular release," the surgeon may destabilize the elbow joint. Therefore, we recommend careful examination before reconstruction.

In a few patients reporting pain, we have removed the capitellar fragment if it was small. We have only a few years of follow-up, but the adolescent patients do not appear to report pain or instability (Figs. 22.9 through 22.13).

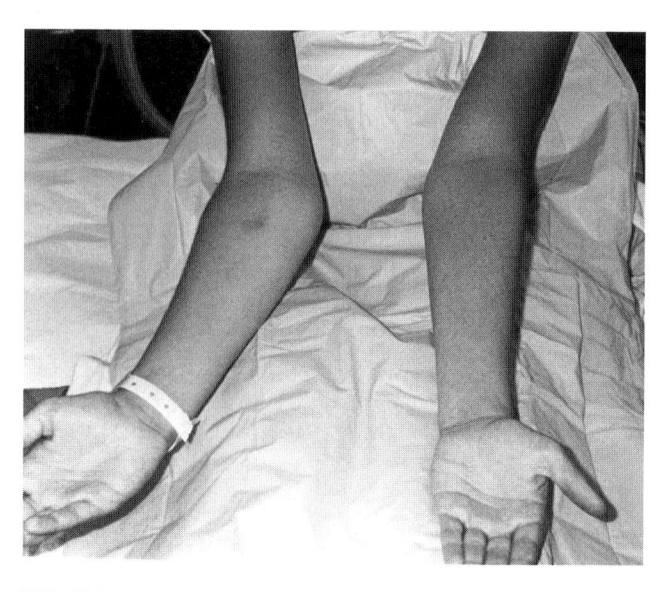

FIGURE 22.10. Clinical picture showing cubitus valgus in right arm of a 14-year-old patient.

COMPLICATIONS

Obtaining and maintaining reduction of an acute lateral condylar fracture and following the patient through to healing results in a uniformly good outcome. Complications arise when the fracture is unrecognized or when it displaces several months after injury.

Delayed union is not an infrequent occurrence with lateral condylar fractures. This problem is probably a combination of poor circulation to the metaphyseal fragment and bathing of the fracture by synovial fluid, which inhibits callus formation. Tension from the extensor muscles on the fragment also may contribute to this problem. This tension is seen most often in fractures treated nonoperatively. In this situation, we continue casting for up

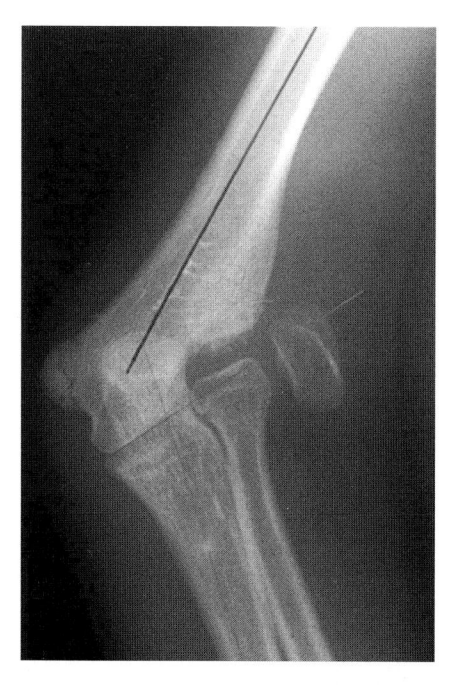

FIGURE 22.9. Late cubitus valgus with completely displaced condylar fragment in a 12-year-old girl (at least 10 years after the fracture).

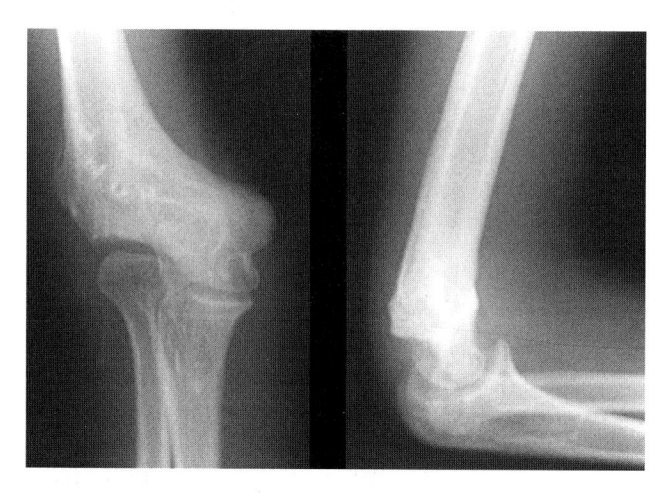

FIGURE 22.11. Radiograph of right arm 2 years after osteotomy and plate removal. Capitellar fragment has been removed.

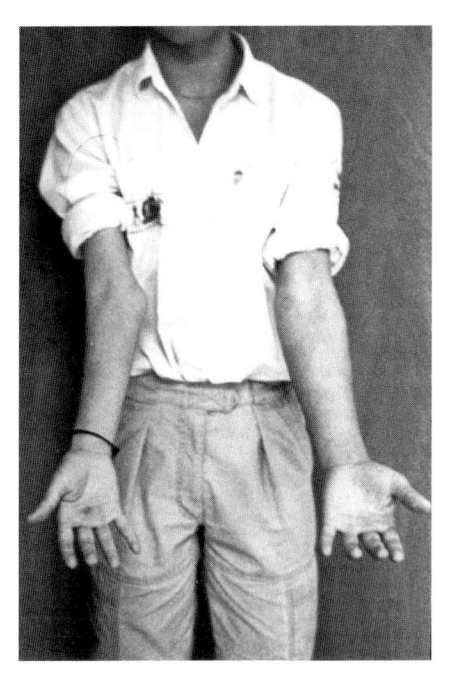

FIGURE 22.12. Note the cosmetic appearance of the right arm with the elbows in extension.

to 6 weeks after injury. At that time, the surgeon should consider bone grafting in addition to open reduction and internal fixation if the fracture is not healed.

Nonunion usually occurs with inadequate fixation of the fracture or failure to recognize a displaced fracture. The fracture is unstable and progressively displaces. It may or may not be symptomatic and may or may not be associated with angular deformity.

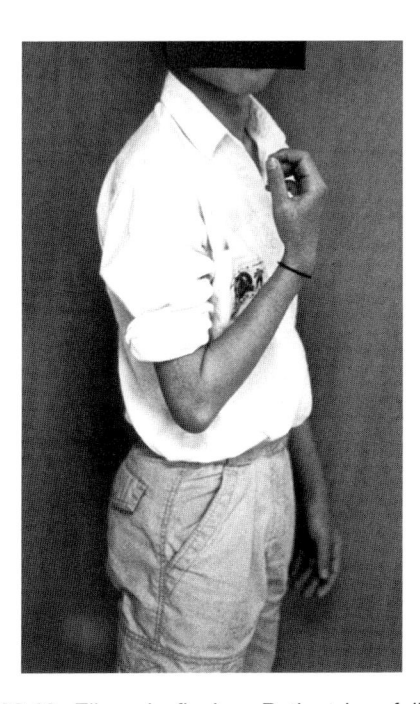

FIGURE 22.13. Elbow in flexion. Patient has full range of motion.

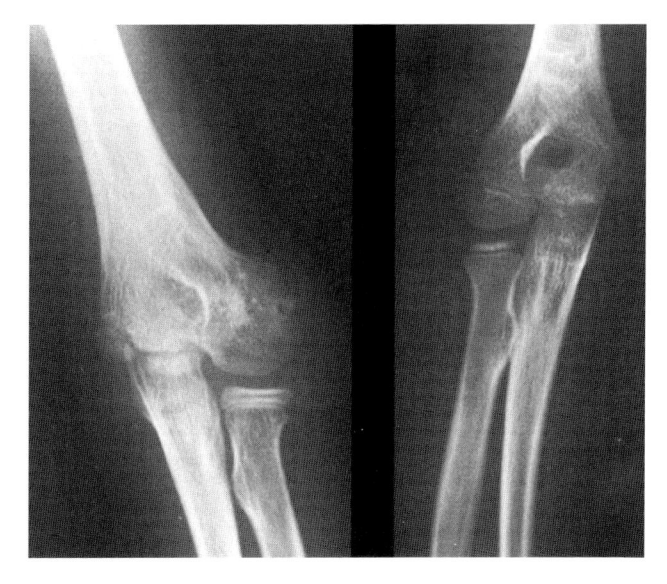

FIGURE 22.14. Radiographs show a rare case of cubitus varus secondary to overgrowth of lateral condyle after fracture. (A) Abnormal, (B) normal elbow.

Cubitus varus is an infrequent complication caused by overstimulation of the lateral condylar physis from the fracture. This deformity requires corrective osteotomy as well (Fig. 22.14).

CONCLUSION

It is important for the orthopedic surgeon to watch these pediatric lateral condylar fractures very carefully and to be alert to the many problems that can occur with them.

REFERENCES

1. Wilkins KE. Fractures and dislocation of the elbow region. In: Rockwood CA Jr, Wilkins KE, King RE, eds. *Fractures in children*. Philadelphia: JB Lippincott; 1984:447–457.
2. Tachdjian MO. *Pediatric orthopaedics*, 2nd ed. Philadelphia: WB Saunders, 1990.
3. Jakob R, Fowles JV, Rang M, et al. Observations concerning fractures of the lateral humeral condyle in children. *J Bone Joint Surg* 1975;57B:430–436.
4. Milch H. Fracture of the external humeral condyle. *JAMA* 1956;160:641–646.
5. Rutherford A. Fractures of the lateral humeral condyle in children. *J Bone Joint Surg* 1985;67A:851–856.
6. Marzo JM, d'Amato C, Strong M, et al. Usefulness and accuracy of arthrography in management of lateral humeral condyle fractures in children. *J Pediatr Orthop* 1990;10:317–321.
7. Hardacre JA, Nahigian SH, Froimson AI, et al. Fractures of the lateral condyle of the humerus in children. *J Bone Joint Surg* 1971;53A:1083–1095.
8. Foster DE, Sullivan JA, Gross RH. Lateral humeral condylar fractures in children. *J Pediatr Orthop* 1985;5:16–22.
9. Makela EA, Bostman O, Kekomaki M, et al. Biodegradable

fixation of distal humeral physeal fractures. *Clin Orthop* 1992; 283:237–243.
10. De Boeck H. Surgery for nonunion of the lateral humeral condyle in children. 6 cases followed for 1–9 years. *Acta Orthop Scand* 1995;66:401–402.
11. Inoue G, Tamura Y. Osteosynthesis for longstanding nonunion of the lateral humeral condyle. *Arch Orthop Trauma Surg* 1993;112:236–238.
12. Roye DP Jr, Bini SA, Infosino A. Late surgical treatment of lateral condylar fractures in children. *J Pediatr Orthop* 1991; 11:195–199.
13. Masada K, Kawai H, Kawabata H, et al. Osteosynthesis for old, established nonunion of the lateral condyle of the humerus. *J Bone Joint Surg* 1990;72A:32–40.
14. Flynn JC, Richards JF Jr. Non-union of minimally displaced fractures of the lateral condyle of the humerus in children. *J Bone Joint Surg* 1971;53A:1096–1101.
15. Flynn JC, Richards JF Jr, Saltzman RI. Prevention and treatment of non-union of slightly displaced fractures of the lateral humeral condyle in children. An end-result study. *J Bone Joint Surg* 1975;57A:1087–1092.
16. Flynn JC. Nonunion of slightly displaced fractures of the lateral humeral condyle in children: An update. *J Pediatr Orthop* 1989;9:691–696.

CHAPTER 23

Elbow Dislocation

Stuart H. Kuschner and Frances Sharpe

INTRODUCTION

Dislocations of the elbow are not uncommon, despite the fact that the elbow is a highly constrained, relatively stable joint.[1] They occur primarily in the young, with the peak incidence occurring in people from 10 to 20 years of age.[2] Among children, the elbow is the most commonly dislocated joint;[3] in adults, only the shoulder is dislocated more often.[4] Simple dislocations of the elbow (dislocations without elbow fracture) account for 18% to 28% of all injuries to the elbow.[5] The diagnosis is easily made on the basis of routine radiographs. The initial treatment involves closed reduction with careful assessment of the neurovascular status of the involved limb both before and after reduction.[6]

CLASSIFICATION

Elbow dislocations are classified by the direction of the forearm bones at the time of injury: posterior, anterior, divergent, medial, or lateral. Posterior dislocations are by far the most common type of injury. They frequently are subdivided into true posterior, posteromedial, or posterolateral. Some believe that whether the posterior dislocation is medial or lateral is irrelevant; that is, this subdivision does not influence ultimate treatment.[3] Anterior dislocations are rare and occur primarily in children. Linscheid and Wheeler[7] reported on 110 elbow dislocations in 105 patients; 108 dislocations were varieties of posterior dislocations, and two were anterior dislocations. Authors of other large series[5,8] have not reported on anterior dislocations. Divergent dislocations[9,10] (dislocations with concomitant separation of the proximal radius from the ulna) and pure medial and lateral dislocations are rare.

MECHANISM OF INJURY

Posterior dislocations typically occur following a fall on the outstretched upper extremity. Mehlhoff et al.[5] reported a fall as the mechanism of injury in 75% of patients. In young people, the injury frequently occurs during sports participation.[2] From 10% to 15% of elbow dislocations occur during automobile accidents.[2,5,7] Linscheid and Wheeler attributed posterior dislocation to hyperextension of the elbow.[7] With hyperextension, the olecranon acts as a fulcrum in the olecranon fossa, levering the semilunar notch of the ulna from the trochlea. The joint capsule is torn, and the collateral ligaments are torn at their attachment to the epicondyles. Additional valgus or varus forces result in lateral or medial displacement of the posterior dislocation.

Based on their study involving cadavers, O'Driscoll et al. proposed an alternative mechanism of injury.[11] They proposed that hyperextension of the elbow is not necessary to cause a posterior or posterolateral dislocation of the elbow. Instead, in their mechanism, falling on the outstretched hand is followed by elbow flexion and by internal rotation of the body and external rotation of the forearm. A valgus force also is applied, because the hand is lateral to the body's center of gravity. The result is soft-tissue disruption beginning laterally and extending medially, ultimately allowing dislocation of the elbow. Their work with cadavers also confirmed that the anterior medial collateral ligament is the major constraint to valgus instability of the elbow and that the elbow can dislocate without disrupting this ligament.

Anterior dislocations have been attributed to direct trauma on the olecranon when the elbow is flexed.[7] As discussed earlier, medial and lateral dislocations are thought by some to be a variation of posterior dislocations. (Linscheid and Wheeler describe only two anterior dislocations and 108 "*varieties* of posterior dislocations"[7]). Although not clearly described in the literature, medial and lateral dislocations result from a fall on an outstretched arm slightly flexed at the elbow. The divergent type, with ulna posterior and radius anterior, is the result of disruption of the medial collateral ligament, followed by pronation of the forearm and extension with a tear of the interosseous ligament.[6]

PHYSICAL EXAMINATION

The physical examination of a patient who has an elbow dislocation must focus on uncovering any neurovascular injury. Thomas and Noellert[12] stated that the incidence of neurovascular injury after closed posterior elbow dislocation was extremely rare. Others report that the rates of neurovascular injury range from 8% to 21%.[13] Injury to nerves and vessels can occur as a result of the trauma of dislocation and also as a consequence of reduction of the elbow. Therefore, the clinician needs to examine the involved limb both before and after reduction.

Injury to the brachial artery has long been recognized as a potential complication of elbow dislocation. In 1913, Sherrill[14] described brachial artery transection following elbow dislocation and successfully treated it with primary repair. Since then, the history of treatment has included observation (i.e., no repair), ligation of the brachial artery, interpositional vein graft with or without transarticular pin fixation, and direct suture repair.[15–24]

Linscheid and Wheeler[7] reported six brachial artery injuries occurring in 110 dislocations (105 patients). Three patients had a lacerated brachial artery, and three patients had stretching injuries of the brachial artery. Arterial repair was attempted in only one patient, but this repair was unsuccessful due to subsequent redislocation of the elbow. Ligations of the brachial artery were accomplished in two patients with lacerations. One patient, who had a stretch injury of the brachial artery, developed what appeared, by description, to be a Volkmann contracture of the forearm and hand.

Authors who promote the use of a nonoperative approach to brachial artery injury attribute successful outcome to the good collateral blood flow about the elbow, but clearly, this approach carries significant risk, such as late claudication, cold intolerance, and need for amputation.[12] Many authors recommend primary brachial artery repair with or without the use of a vein graft.[6,12,22,24]

Because of collateral blood flow around the elbow, radial and ulnar artery pulses may be present at the wrists even when the brachial artery has been disrupted. Therefore, the examiner should carefully evaluate each patient for this injury. Pain and swelling of the forearm should alert him or her to this possibility, which can be confirmed by arteriogram. The treating physician also needs to examine the patient for a compartment syndrome that accompanies vascular injury. If clinical symptoms warrant, fasciotomies of the forearm and hand should be performed.

Both the median nerve and, more commonly, the ulnar nerve can be injured as a result of an elbow dislocation.[25–35] Typically, the injury is a stretch injury that improves over time. For example, Mehlhoff et al.[5] reported nerve injury in 9 of 52 patients with elbow dislocations, which he treated nonoperatively. Five patients had ulnar nerve injury alone, three had median and ulnar nerve injury, and one had median nerve injury alone. One patient had mild ulnar dysesthesia 14 months after medial dislocation. Otherwise, all paresthesias resolved without sequelae.

Linscheid and Wheeler[7] reported a somewhat different experience after surgically treating several of their patients for ulnar nerve symptoms. Among the 110 patients with elbow dislocations who they treated, 24 patients had neurologic symptoms. Of these 24, 16 had ulnar nerve symptoms only, 3 had median nerve hypesthesia only, 4 had median and ulnar nerve symptoms, and 1 had brachial plexus stretch injury. Seven patients had surgery on the ulnar nerve; 6 had a translocation, and 1 had an exploration. Valgus stress to the elbow at the time of dislocation has been labeled as a cause of ulnar nerve injury, but cubital tunnel syndrome can develop as a late complication secondary to swelling, soft-tissue scarring, and heterotopic bone.

Ulnar nerve entrapment has not been reported; however intra-articular median nerve entrapment, typically in children, has been described.[31] This problem probably occurs during reduction; therefore, the examiner needs to assess neurological status before and after elbow reduction. Matev[33] described a radiologic sign of intra-articular median nerve entrapment as a depression, or "notch," in the cortex on the distal humeral metaphysis. To him, this depression looked as if the nerve were trying to "ulcerate its way back through bone into its proper position."[36] However, this radiologic sign is not obvious until 2 to 3 months after injury, before which time careful clinical evaluation should have alerted the examiner to the possibility of median nerve entrapment. Neurologic assessment should be performed immediately before and after elbow reduction. If nerve deficit is not worse following reduction, the patient should be followed closely. If the patient does not improve within 3 months, surgical exploration is appropriate. Serial electrodiagnostic studies may be helpful, but should not be a substitute for careful clinical evaluation. These studies can detect improvement before clinical recovery. In these circumstances, it may be reasonable to delay surgical intervention. Median nerve function that worsens after reduction, particularly in a child, is a strong indication for surgical exploration.

RADIAL HEAD FRACTURES

Radial head and radial neck fractures are not uncommon following elbow dislocations. Ten percent of the elbow dislocations have an associated radial head fracture.[37] Treatment of these injuries depends on the extent of displacement. Nondisplaced or minimally displaced fractures do not need specific intervention and do not preclude a program of early elbow motion. Displaced fractures should be treated by open reduction and internal fixation where feasible (Fig. 23.1). If the radial head is comminuted, excision can be performed. However, because valgus instability can follow, the surgeon should consider prosthetic radial head replacement and medial collateral ligament repair.[38] Chapter 20 presents a thorough discussion of radial head fractures and their treatment.

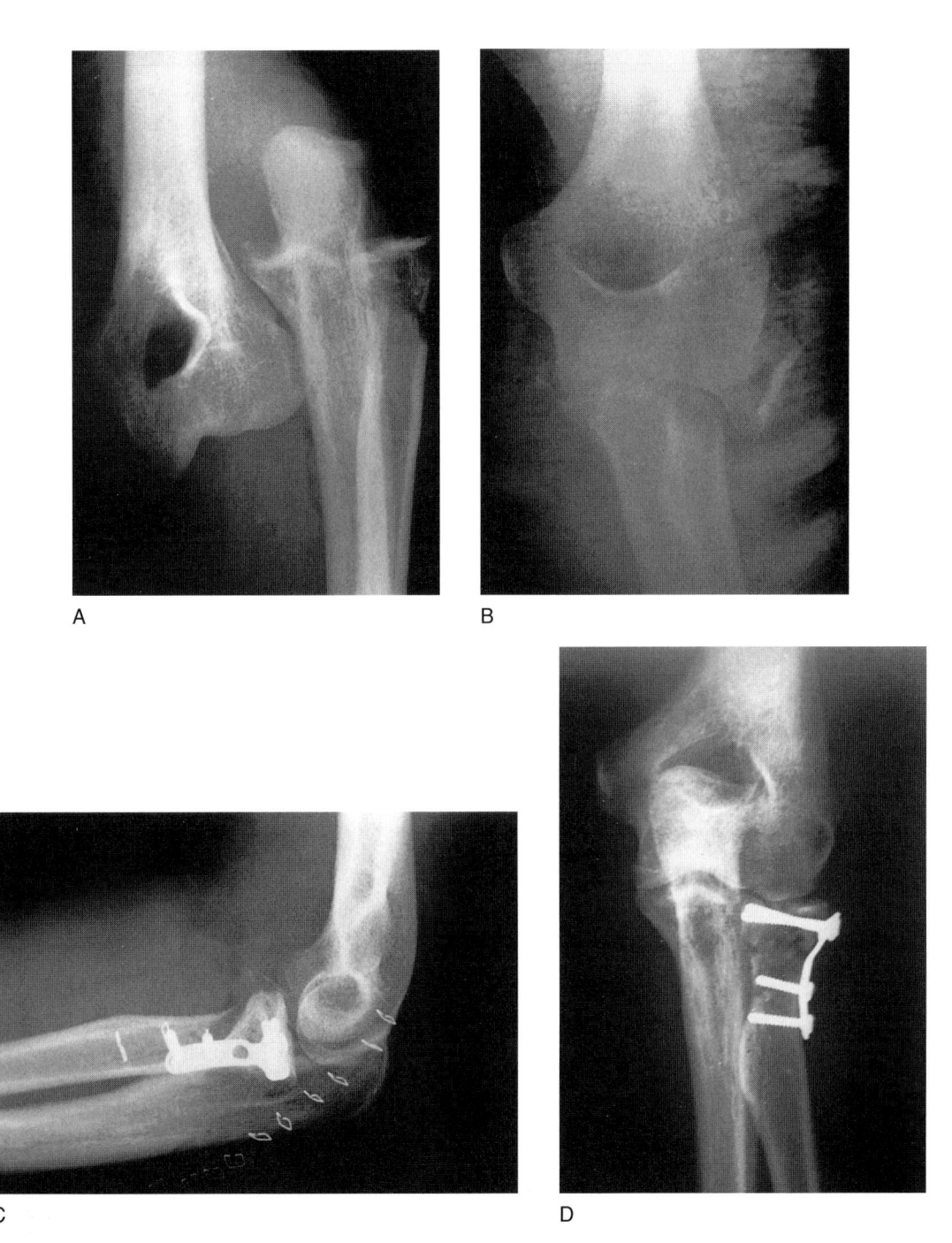

FIGURE 23.1. A 30-year-old woman fell approximately 25 feet out of a tree and sustained a posterior elbow dislocation and radial head fracture. (A) and (B) Closed reduction caused displacement of the radial head fracture. (C) and (D) The radial head fracture was treated by open reduction internal fixation.

TREATMENT

Closed reduction of posterior elbow dislocation is performed with gentle longitudinal traction on the forearm with the elbow in slight flexion. The examiner can feel the humerus slide into the olecranon notch (Fig. 23.2). Protzman[8] described performing most of his reductions without providing analgesics to the patient, but providing the patient with muscle relaxants and appropriate pain medication before reduction is more humane. Linscheid and Wheeler[7] stated that unlocking the coronoid by preliminary extension of the elbow was "occasionally necessary." Authors have condemned hyperextension as potentially injurious[39] and as the possible cause of median nerve entrapment.[31]

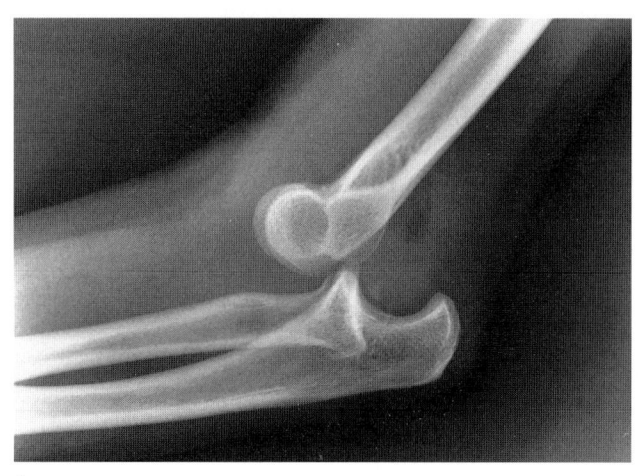

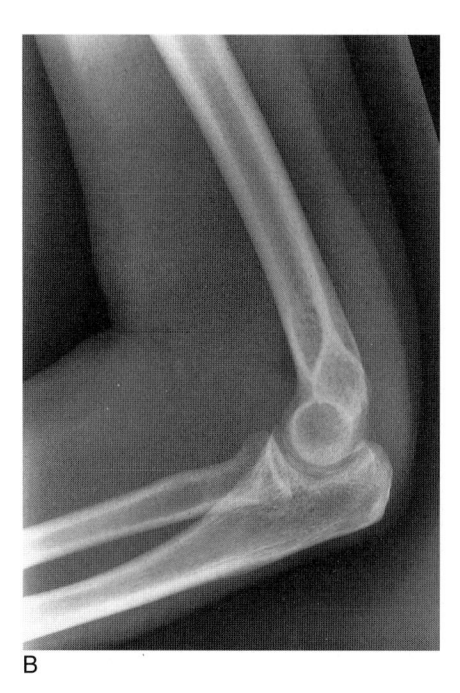

Following closed reduction, the physician addresses two important issues: whether to perform primary ligament repair and, if treating nonoperatively, the length of immobilization. Primary repair of elbow ligaments after dislocation has its advocates. Durig et al.[40] believed that surgery was necessary when there was "gross instability" of the elbow, loose bodies within the joint, or persistent subluxation after reduction. Rodgers et al.[41] repaired injured soft tissues in "severe, complicated elbow dislocations," most of which had associated fractures. However, most authors report good results with nonoperative treatment.[42,43] Studies comparing operative and nonoperative treatment show no difference in results between these two groups.[44,45] In a prospective study comparing operative and nonoperative treatment, Josefsson et al.[44] found no difference between the two methods regardless of the degree of ligamentous and muscular damage to the elbow.

With nonoperative treatment, the treating physician generally immobilizes the elbow with a posterior splint for up to 6 weeks after injury.[13] Mehlhoff[5] showed a significant correlation ($p < 0.001$) between increased degree of flexion contracture and increased duration of immobilization after reduction. In his study, six of seven patients who had elbow flexion contracture exceeding 30° had been immobilized for 4 or more weeks. Prevalence and severity of pain also increased with increased duration of immobilization.

Protzman[8] also noted a direct correlation between duration of immobilization and loss of extension. In his series, patients who had an elbow immobilized for less than 5 days had an average loss of 3° of elbow extension. Patients who had an elbow immobilized for more than 20 days had an average loss of 21° of elbow extension.

AUTHORS' PREFERRED METHOD

After neurovascular assessment and appropriate provision of analgesia, the patient is placed supine on the examining table. To reduce a posterior elbow dislocation, the surgeon applies longitudinal traction by grasping the patient's wrist and distal forearm, and an assistant provides countertraction on the upper arm. Medial or lateral displacement is corrected first. The surgeon continues longitudinal traction while flexing the patient's elbow and pushing downward on the anterior proximal forearm to help to bring the coronoid around the distal end of the humerus. Meanwhile, the assistant also can apply posteriorly directed pressure on the upper arm. Stability of the patient's elbow after reduction is assessed by passively flexing and extending it. Most elbows are stable beyond 30° of flexion. Radiographs are taken to confirm reduction. Neurovascular status is evaluated again.

FIGURE 23.2. (A) A 46-year-old woman slipped on level ground and sustained a posterior elbow dislocation. (B) The dislocation was reduced in the emergency room several hours after the injury.

To reduce an elbow dislocation with the patient positioned prone, the patient lies prone with the injured extremity (forearm and arm) hanging from the side of the bed. The surgeon pulls gently downward on the wrist and maintains the pressure. When the olecranon begins to move distally, upward force on the arm will reduce the elbow joint.

After reduction, the surgeon immobilizes the elbow in about 90° of flexion using a long-arm posterior splint. The patient is reexamined from 1 to 3 days after injury. At this time, the plaster splint is removed and a slightly bulky, soft dressing is applied around the elbow to help to limit the extremes of elbow motion. The patient begins gentle, active range-of-motion exercises. For 1 to 2 weeks, the patient wears a sling when not performing range-of-motion exercises.

The senior author (SHK) believes that elbow dislocations that are satisfactorily reduced can and should be treated nonoperatively. Josefsson et al. found in their study of operative versus nonoperative treatment of ligament injuries in dislocated elbows that "data do not support the view that surgical ligament repair is beneficial."[44] The authors agree.

After reduction, if the elbow is unstable or if the elbow has redislocated, then I (SHK) use a hinged brace that can be adjusted to limit extension. Over the course of several weeks, the amount of extension can be increased gradually.

Patients often present at the emergency room with an acute dislocation. If one attempt at closed reduction is unsuccessful, the patient should be taken to the operating room where the examiner can try closed reduction after administering appropriate analgesia and muscle relaxers to the patient and with the aid of the image intensifier. If the second attempt at closed reduction is unsuccessful, the surgeon accomplishes an open reduction with a lateral Kocher approach.

The surgeon reduces anterior dislocations by traction and extension.[7] Traction is applied to the patient's forearm. While pushing downward and then posteriorly on the forearm, the surgeon extends the patient's elbow. The patient should begin range-of-motion exercises shortly after reduction. To reduce the rare pure medial and lateral dislocations, the surgeon applies longitudinal traction on the forearm and countertraction on the upper arm, as described earlier. (Note that Linscheid and O'Driscoll group medial and lateral dislocations under "posterior dislocations" and state that "whether the forearm is medially or laterally displaced is irrelevant to the pathology seen or the ultimate treatment."[3] Hotchkiss believes that "pure lateral and medial dislocations are distinct."[6]) Next, the surgeon applies straight lateral or medial pressure. With divergent dislocations, the ulna typically dislocates posteriorly and the radius dislocates anteriorly. The ulna is reduced by longitudinal traction on the forearm and countertraction on the humerus, as with posterior dislocations.

As the ulna is being reduced, the surgeon applies pressure over the medial head to reduce the radius.[6]

Reduction of anterior dislocations, as described earlier, is different from posterior, medial, and lateral reductions. Postreduction treatment is similar for all types. Early motion reduces the chance of stiffness, which is manifested primarily by loss of terminal extension.

Complications of closed reduction are rare and may be due to overexuberant attempts at reduction. Traction-type nerve injury can occur. Matev has reported entrapment of the median nerve in the elbow joint after closed reduction of a posterior dislocation.[33] A careful neurovascular examination before and after reduction is appropriate. We know of no reports of complications directly related to early postreduction mobilization.

REFERENCES

1. Geissler WB, Freeland AE. Radial head fracture associated with elbow dislocation. *Orthopedics* 1992;15:874–877.
2. Josefsson PO, Nilsson BE. Incidence of elbow dislocation. *Acta Orthop Scand* 1986;57:537–538.
3. Linscheid RL, O'Driscoll SW. Elbow dislocations. In: Morrey BF, ed. *The elbow and its disorders*, 2nd ed. Philadelphia: WB Saunders; 1993:441–452.
4. Goldstock LE, Jupiter JB, Lins RE. Elbow trauma. In: Levine AM, ed. *Orthopaedic knowledge update: Trauma*. Rosemont, IL: American Academy of Orthopaedic Surgeons; 1996:47–55.
5. Mehlhoff TL, Noble PC, Bennett JB, et al. Simple dislocation of the elbow in the adult. Results after closed treatment. *J Bone Joint Surg* 1988;70A:244–249.
6. Hotchkiss RN. Fractures and dislocations of the elbow. In Rockwood CA, Bucholz RW, Green DP, Heckman JD, ed. *Fractures in adults*, 4th ed. Philadelphia: Lippincott–Raven; 1996:929–1024.
7. Linscheid RL, Wheeler DK. Elbow dislocations. *JAMA* 1965;194:1171–1176.
8. Protzman RR. Dislocation of the elbow joint. *J Bone Joint Surg* 1978;60A:539–541.
9. DeLee JC. Transverse divergent dislocation of the elbow in a child. Case report. *J Bone Joint Surg* 1981;63A:322–323.
10. Andersen K, Mortensen AC, Grøn P. Transverse divergent dislocation of the elbow. A report of two cases. *Acta Orthop Scand* 1985;56:442–443.
11. O'Driscoll SW, Morrey BF, Korinek S, et al. Elbow subluxation and dislocation. A spectrum of instability. *Clin Orthop* 1992;280:186–197.
12. Thomas PJ, Noellert RC. Brachial artery disruption after closed posterior dislocation of the elbow. *Am J Orthop* 1995;24:558–560.
13. Royle SG. Posterior dislocation of the elbow. *Clin Orthop* 1991;269:201–204.
14. Sherrill JG. Direct suture of the brachial artery following rupture. Result of traumatism. *Ann Surg* 1913;58:534–536.
15. Amsallem JL, Blankstein A, Bass A, et al. Brachial artery injury. A complication of posterior elbow dislocation. *Orthop Rev* 1986;15:379–382.

16. Aufranc OE, Jones WN, Turner RH. Dislocation of the elbow with brachial artery injury. *JAMA* 1966;197:719–721.
17. Friedmann E. Simple rupture of the brachial artery sustained in elbow dislocation. *JAMA* 1961;177:208–209.
18. Grimer RJ, Brooks S. Brachial artery damage accompanying closed posterior dislocation of the elbow. *J Bone Joint Surg* 1985;67B:378–381.
19. Henderson RS, Robertson IM. Open dislocation of the elbow with rupture of the brachial artery. *J Bone Joint Surg* 1952;34B:636–637.
20. Hofammann KE III, Moneim MS, Omer GE, et al. Brachial artery disruption following closed posterior elbow dislocation in a child: Assessment with intravenous digital angiography. A case report with review of the literature. *Clin Orthop* 1984;184:145–149.
21. Kilburn P, Sweeney JG, Silk FF. Three cases of compound posterior dislocation of the elbow with rupture of brachial artery. *J Bone Joint Surg* 1962;44B:119–121.
22. Louis DS, Ricciardi JE, Spengler DM. Arterial injury: A complication of posterior elbow dislocation. A clinical and anatomical study. *J Bone Joint Surg* 1974;56A:1631–1636.
23. Sturm JT, Rothenberger DA, Strate RG. Brachial artery disruption following closed elbow dislocation. *J Trauma* 1978;18:364–366.
24. Sullivan MF. Rupture of the brachial artery from posterior dislocation of the elbow treated by vein-graft. A case report. *Br J Surg* 1971;58:470–471.
25. Ayala H, De Pablos J, Gonzales J, et al. Entrapment of the median nerve after posterior dislocation of the elbow. *Microsurgery* 1983;4:215–220.
26. Beverly MC, Fearn CB. Anterior interosseous nerve palsy and dislocation of the elbow. *Injury* 1984;6:126–128.
27. Boe S, Holst-Nielsen F. Intra-articular entrapment of the median nerve after dislocation of the elbow. *J Hand Surg* 1987;12B:356–358.
28. Cotton FJ. Elbow dislocation and ulnar nerve injury. *J Bone Joint Surg* 1929;11:348–352.
29. Danielsson LG. Median nerve entrapment in elbow dislocation: A case report. *Acta Orthop Scand* 1986;57:450–452.
30. Malkawi H. Recurrent dislocation of the elbow accompanied by ulnar neuropathy: A case report and review of the literature. *Clin Orthop* 1981;161:270–274.
31. Hallett J. Entrapment of the median nerve after dislocation of the elbow. A case report. *J Bone Joint Surg* 1981;63B:408–412.
32. Mannerfelt L. Median nerve entrapment after dislocation of the elbow. Report of a case. *J Bone Joint Surg* 1968;50B:152–155.
33. Matev I. A radiological sign of entrapment of the median nerve in the elbow joint after posterior dislocation. A report of two cases. *J Bone Joint Surg* 1976;58B:353–355.
34. Pritchard DJ, Linscheid RL, Svien HJ. Intra-articular median nerve entrapment with dislocation of the elbow. *Clin Orthop* 1973;90:100–103.
35. Rana NA, Kenwright J, Taylor RG, et al. Complete lesion of the median nerve associated with dislocation of the elbow joint. *Acta Orthop Scand* 1974;45:365–369.
36. Strange FGSC: Entrapment of the median nerve after dislocation of the elbow. *J Bone Joint Surg* 1982;64B:224–225.
37. Ebraheim NA, Skie MC, Zeiss J, et al. Internal fixation of radial neck fracture in a fracture dislocation of the elbow. A case report. *Clin Orthop* 1992;276:187–191.
38. Broberg MA, Morrey BF. Results of treatment of fracture–dislocations of the elbow. *Clin Orthop* 1987;216:109–119.
39. Loomis LK. Reduction and after-treatment of posterior dislocation of the elbow, with special attention to brachialis muscle and myositis ossificans. *Am J Surg* 1944;63:56–60.
40. Durig M, Muller W, Ruedi TP, et al. The operative treatment of elbow dislocation in the adult. *J Bone Joint Surg* 1979;61A:239–244.
41. Rodgers WB, Kharrazi FD, Waters PM, et al. The use of osseous suture anchors in the treatment of severe, complicated elbow dislocations. *Am J Orthop* 1996;25:794–798.
42. Josefsson PO, Johnell O, Gentz CF. Long-term sequelae of simple dislocation of the elbow. *J Bone Joint Surg* 1984;66A:927–930.
43. Neviaser JS, Wickstrom JK. Dislocation of the elbow: A retrospective study of 115 patients. *South Med J* 1977;70:172–173.
44. Josefsson PO, Gentz CF, Johnell O, et al. Surgical versus nonsurgical treatment of ligamentous injuries following dislocation of the elbow joint. *Clin Orthop* 1987;214:165–169.
45. Lansinger O, Karlsson J, Körner L, et al. Dislocation of the elbow joint. *Arch Orthop Trauma Surg* 1984;102:183–186.

CHAPTER 24

Treatment of Olecranon, Coronoid, and Proximal Ulnar Fracture–Dislocation

James B. Bennett and Thomas L. Mehlhoff

INTRODUCTION

Elbow fractures and dislocations are common because of the longitudinal axial forces that are transmitted to the joint through the forearm during falls. The olecranon, trochlea, radial head, capitellum, and proximal radioulnar joint are susceptible to intra-articular and extra-articular fractures.

The humerus, ulna, and radial head meet in a tightly congruent joint at the elbow. The medial and lateral ligaments provide secondary soft-tissue support to the bony anatomy of the elbow. This support is further enhanced by the medial flexor–pronator muscle mass and the lateral extensor muscle mass. The triceps tendon attachment posteriorly and the brachialis and biceps tendon attachments anteriorly form anterior–posterior stabilizers that join with the joint capsule to support the bony architecture.

Few fractures about the elbow are isolated injuries. Most involve some soft tissue and joint injury in addition to the identified fracture. The evaluation of elbow fractures requires examination not only of the bony and cartilaginous lesions, but also of the ligamentous and muscular structures. Failure to address injury to all these structures can result in elbow instability.

OLECRANON FRACTURES

Olecranon fractures can result from a direct blow to the olecranon due to a fall on the flexed elbow or from a sudden contraction of the triceps due to a fall on the outstretched arm. Nondisplaced olecranon fractures can be treated by immobilizing the elbow in 30° of flexion for 3 weeks, followed by protected range of motion exercises until the fracture has healed. Displaced olecranon fractures, however, present two problems: (1) disrupted triceps tendon function and (2) a displaced intra-articular joint fracture. These fractures must be treated with surgery.

The surgical repair of displaced olecranon fractures must restore congruent, stable ulnohumeral joint motion, as well as triceps continuity to the ulna. Articular surface incongruity of more than 2 mm leads to posttraumatic arthritis, but a gap in the intra-articular surface of the ulnar semilunar notch may produce no ill effects.[1] Internal fixation must be stable to permit early range of motion and to minimize posttraumatic stiffness.[2] Symptoms, such as tenderness or bursal reaction, due to metal prominence are particularly common after AO tension-band wiring (as frequent as 80% in one series), but the hardware can be removed after the fracture heals.[1,3]

Olecranon fracture patterns can vary and include small avulsion, transverse or oblique olecranon, and comminuted olecranon fractures. They also can be combined with coronoid process or proximal ulnar fractures. Colton presented the original classification of these patterns.[4] Modifications to Colton's work have resulted in other classifications emphasizing displacement, comminution, and stability,[5] although no one classification has been universally accepted.

A small extra-articular avulsion of the olecranon process, in essence, represents a rupture of the triceps tendon insertion. This injury is best treated with excision of the bony fragment and reattachment of the triceps tendon to the olecranon with heavy nonabsorbable sutures through drill holes in bone[6] or with bone anchor sutures. Most of these fractured elbows are immobilized at 30° of flexion for 4 weeks. A night extension splint is used for 4 additional weeks. After this treatment, the patient begins graduated range-of-motion exercises and a strengthening program.[7]

Treatment of displaced transverse olecranon fractures includes internal fixation with tension-band wiring using parallel Kirschner wires (K-wires) or an intramedullary 6.5-mm cancellous screw (Fig. 24.1). Intramedullary screw fixation without tension banding is not a reliable treatment for these fractures. However, long oblique fractures of the proximal olecranon can be fixed internally and stabilized with bicortical screw fixation.

In an older patient (> than 60 years old) with a severely comminuted fracture, the surgeon can excise up to 50% of the proximal olecranon.[8] The triceps tendon must be repaired to the subarticular surface of the olecranon to minimize the anteroposterior instability of the elbow that can occur after excision of the proximal olecranon (Fig. 24.2).

Segmental fractures of the proximal ulnar shaft with a proximal olecranon process or a coronoid process fracture must be treated by open reduction and internal fixation with plate stabilization. The semilunar notch of the ulnohumeral joint should not be overly compressed. Bone grafting might be required to maintain the anatomic length and contour of the semilunar notch. The surgeon must obtain lag-screw fixation of the coronoid process to the proximal ulna in order to restore stability to the ulnohumeral joint. The coronoid process is a bony constraint for anteroposterior stability and the insertion for the medial collateral ligament for valgus stability.

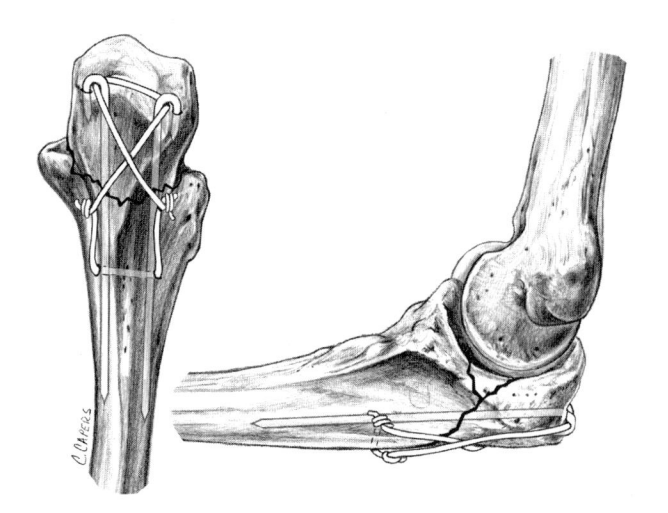

FIGURE 24.1. Tension-band wiring and pins.

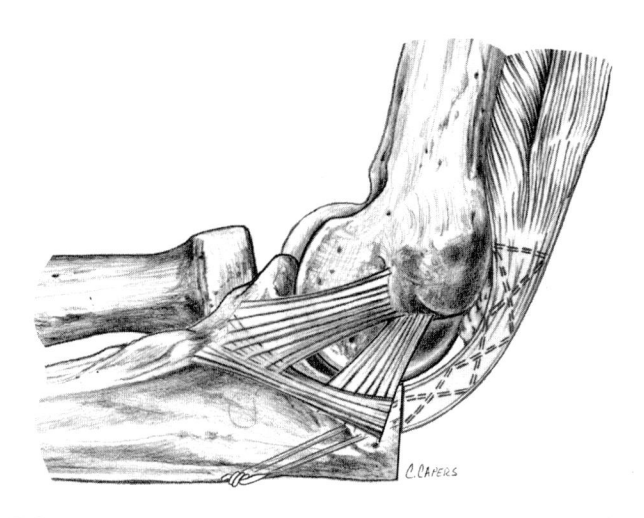

FIGURE 24.2. Excision of the olecranon and reattachment of the triceps tendon.

Surgical Technique

For surgery, the patient is placed in the supine or lateral decubitus position after general anesthesia. The supine position affords excellent access to the posterior aspect of the elbow and allows the surgeon to flex and extend the patient's elbow as needed. A previously calibrated pneumatic tourniquet is applied as proximal as possible on the upper extremity. The upper extremity is wrapped in a stockinette, placed across the chest, and attached to a 2-pound counterweight through a sterile Kerlex roll from the wrist (Fig. 24.3).

Tension-band Technique with Parallel K-wires

The tension-band technique with parallel K-wires is used most commonly for fixation of displaced proximal olecranon fractures. The surgeon makes a longitudinal incision over the posterior aspect of the elbow. If the surgeon desires, he or she can gently curve the incision around the tip of the olecranon. Full-thickness subcutaneous flaps are elevated. The superficial fascia of the ulna is incised in the midline to expose the fracture. After internal fixation, the surgeon can repair any accompanying partial tears of the extensor retinaculum from the triceps.

The fracture hematoma is irrigated and removed. The proximal fragment is reflected with a towel clip. Comminution of the fracture and the joint surface can be visualized (Fig. 24.4). Often, a central fracture fragment of the articular surface is present. This fragment should not be removed; rather, it should be elevated to restore articular congruity to the semilunar notch. If necessary, additional cancellous bone graft from the intramedullary canal, proximal olecranon, or distal radius can be packed into the deficit to support the articular surface fragment.

The surgeon further exposes the extra-articular frac-

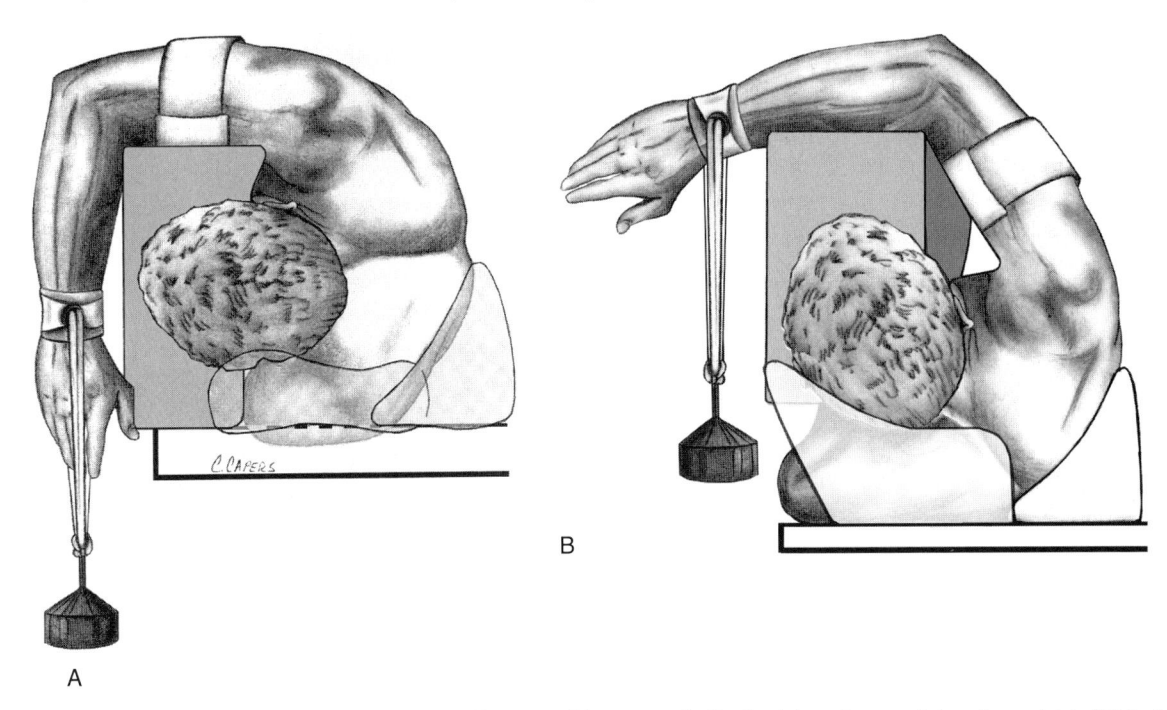

FIGURE 24.3. Patient's upper extremity is wrapped in a stockinette and attached to a 2-pound counterweight. (A) Lateral decubitus position. (B) Supine position.

ture line by elevating a 2-mm flap of periosteum on the medial, dorsal, and lateral aspects of the fracture. If the surgeon desires, he or she can identify the ulnar nerve. However, the ulnar nerve is not routinely released or transposed from the cubital tunnel during treatment of this fracture.

The extra-articular fracture alignment dictates the method of intra-articular reduction used. Temporary reduction of the proximal fragment is accomplished with a ratchet towel clip and is stabilized with the towel clip or temporary K-wire. The surgeon should use an intraoperative lateral radiograph to verify whether the articular joint surface reduction is stable and aligned.

Parallel Steinmann pins are passed through the proximal fragment, across the fracture, and into the intramedullary canal of the ulna. Two parallel Steinmann pins provide rotational control. Usually, pins of $\frac{5}{64}$-in. diameter are satisfactory. One pin is positioned, then the other pin is placed (Fig. 24.5).

Tension-band wiring in a figure-of-eight fashion is performed next. An 18-gauge malleable wire is preferred for most of these fractures in adults. A 2-mm drill bit is used to make a bicortical hole in the distal fragment approximately 4 cm distal from the fracture (Fig. 24.6). The surgeon passes the wire through this hole and over the fracture on the posterior aspect of the olecranon.

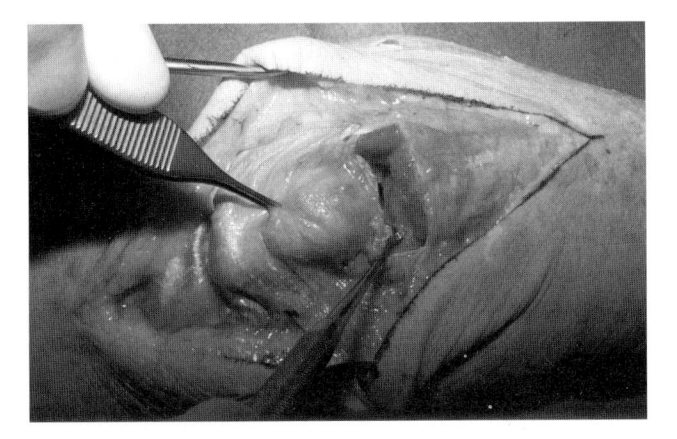

FIGURE 24.4. Incision over the posterior aspect of the elbow and elevation of the central fracture fragment.

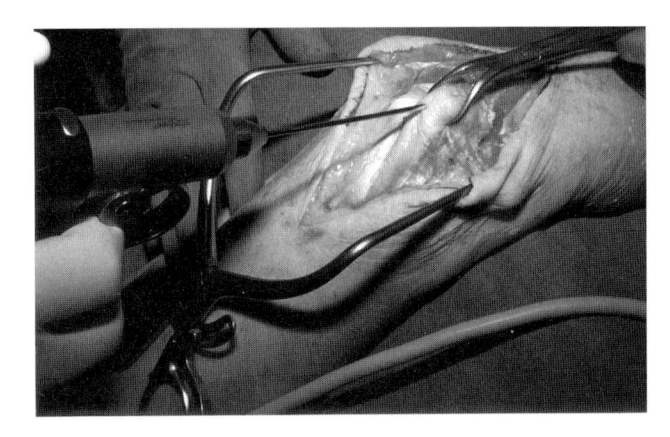

FIGURE 24.5. Steinmann pin placed into the proximal fracture fragment.

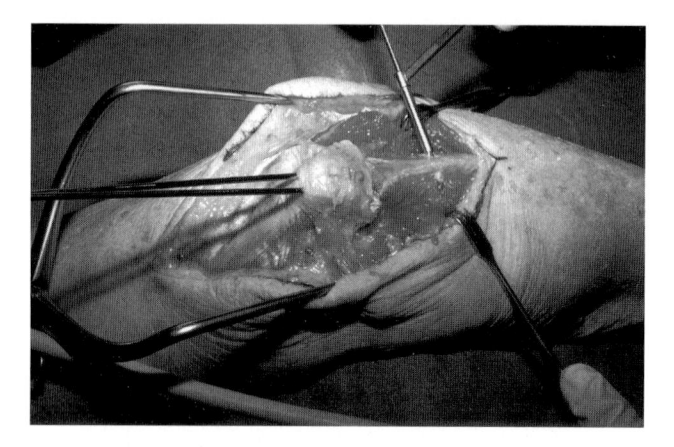

FIGURE 24.6. Drill hole for tension-band wire.

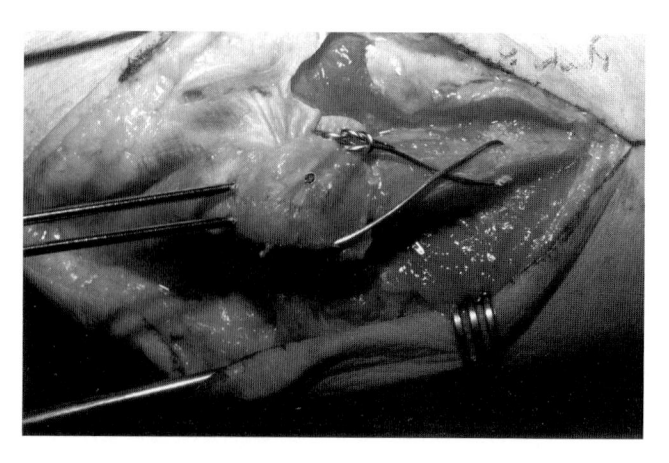

FIGURE 24.8. Completed figure-of-eight wiring.

A 14-gauge angiocatheter is used to assist passage of the wire under the triceps tendon. The metal needle is passed under the triceps tendon next to the bone, but anterior to the parallel Steinmann pins (Fig. 24.7). Next, the 18-gauge wire is passed through the catheter and safely and efficiently under the triceps tendon. The cather is removed. This step completes the figure-of-eight wiring. A Kirschner traction bow is used to tighten the tension band. Excellent compression is obtained when the wire is tightened after the first loop. The surgeon completes a square knot to secure the tension band and carefully positions the tails of the wire against the bone (Fig. 24.8). The hardware should not cause problems for the patient, such as a knot or prominence under the skin. The Kirschner traction bow provides more efficient tightening of the tension band than single or double loops provide.

The surgeon bends the Steinmann pins to 150° with a suction tip and longitudinally incises the triceps tendon for each pin (Fig. 24.9). The wires are rotated and advanced to the bone under the triceps tendon with a light mallet (Fig. 24.10). The triceps tendon is repaired over the pins with nonabsorbable sutures, minimizing the risk for proximal migration of the pins that later can become symptomatic tenderness or a prominence under the skin. The partial tears in the retinaculum of the extensor mechanism should be repaired as well.

An intraoperative lateral radiograph is recommended to confirm the position of the hardware and the anatomic reduction of the fracture. The semilunar notch must be congruent, and the pins should be in an intramedullary location. The proximal loop of the figure-of-eight wiring must be anterior to the parallel pins (Fig. 24.11).

The passive range of motion and stability of the elbow are tested. A well-padded sterile dressing and an extension splint are applied. The surgeon can decide whether to use a hemovac drain.

Tension-band Technique with Intramedullary Compression Screws

The tension-band technique with intramedullary compression screws is a well-suited treatment for transverse noncomminuted fractures of the proximal olecranon. It also is useful for repairing a proximal olecranon os-

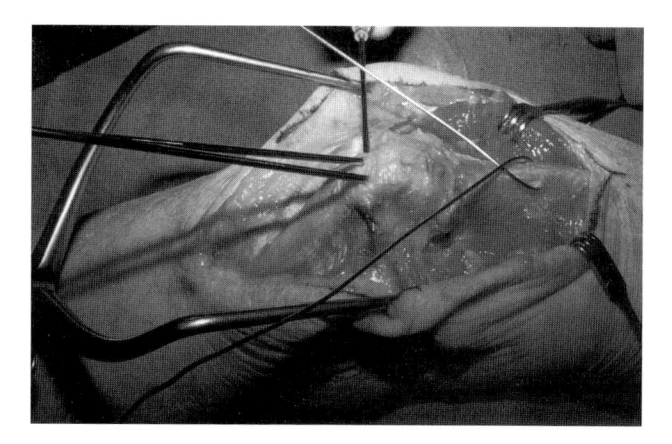

FIGURE 24.7. An angiocatheter placed under the triceps tendon.

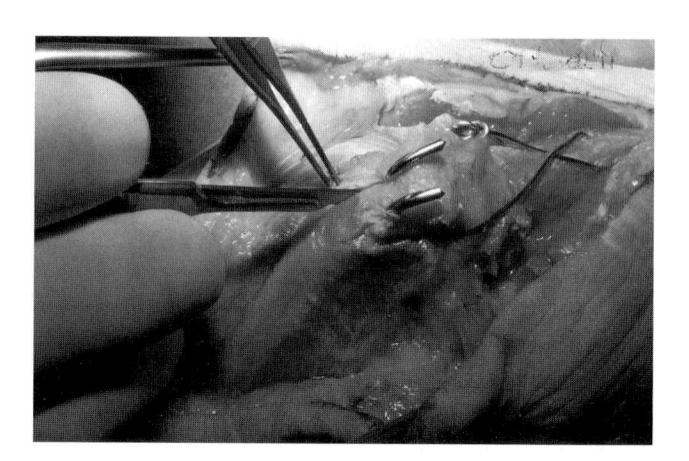

FIGURE 24.9. After bending the Steinmann pins, the surgeon longitudinally incises the triceps tendon to bury the pins.

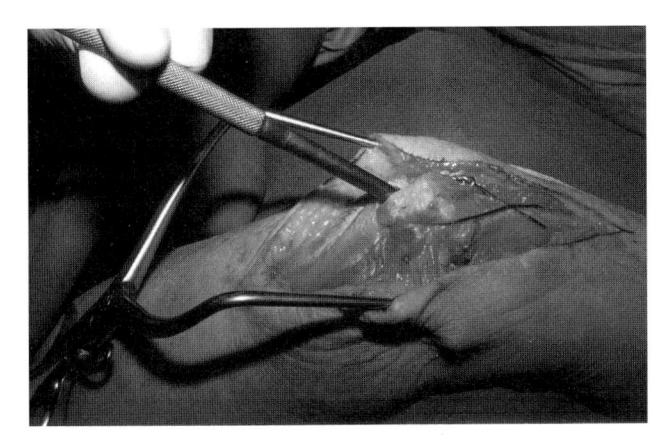

FIGURE 24.10. The surgeon uses a mallet to tap the Steinmann pins under the triceps tendon.

teotomy after exposure of a T-intercondylar fracture of the distal humerus.

The surgeon uses a 1.5-cm longitudinal incision through the triceps to expose the proximal olecranon tip. He or she uses a 3.2-mm drill bit to make a hole through the proximal fragment, across the fracture, and into the intramedullary canal (Fig. 24.12). Overdrilling with a 4.5-mm drill bit creates the proximal gliding hole. A 6.5-mm tap is passed through the proximal fragment and into the intramedullary canal. The tap should purchase the endosteal canal of the intramedullary canal and may require a cancellous screw that is 100 mm long. A 6.5-mm cancellous screw that is 65 to 100 mm long is positioned into the proximal fragment over a washer and then advanced and tightened to compress the fracture. To prevent rotation of the fracture, the surgeon should control the proximal fragment until the screw is tightened (Fig. 24.13). He or she must take care not to overcompress and shorten the normal anatomic contour of the semilunar notch. Finally, the surgeon may use an 18-gauge wire to accomplish tension-band wiring in the figure-of-eight fashion as previously described.

Bicortical Screw Fixation

Proximal olecranon fractures in adolescents commonly occur in an oblique, noncomminuted fracture pattern. Bicortical screw fixation is a treatment technique that is well suited to this fracture pattern.

The surgeon exposes the fracture through a posterior longitudinal incision. Full-thickness subcutaneous flaps are elevated. Fixation is obtained with a 4.5-mm interfragmentary bicortical screw that is oriented perpendicularly to the fracture and that achieves purchase on the anterior cortex distal to the coronoid (Fig. 24.14). If excellent purchase cannot be achieved with this screw, an alternative technique should be selected. Cannulated screw systems also are efficient in achieving good screw position for this technique, because the preliminary wire position can be checked on fluoroscan before the screw is inserted. Tension-band wiring is not necessary when the fracture is reduced anatomically and has rigid internal fixation. If the fracture is associated with a segmental fracture of the proximal ulna, the surgeon should address it with a plating technique, rather than bicortical screw fixation alone.

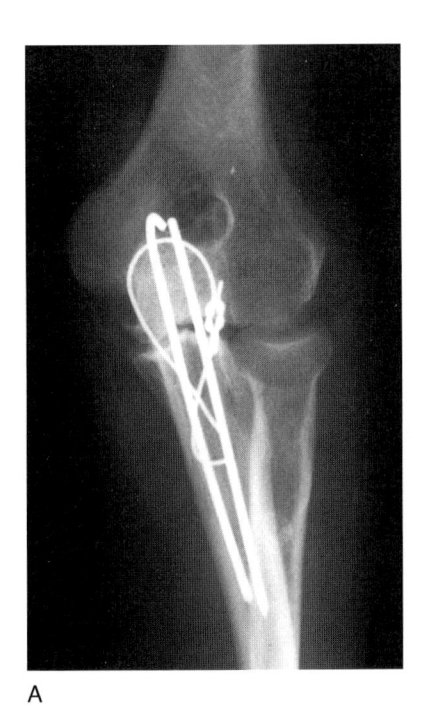

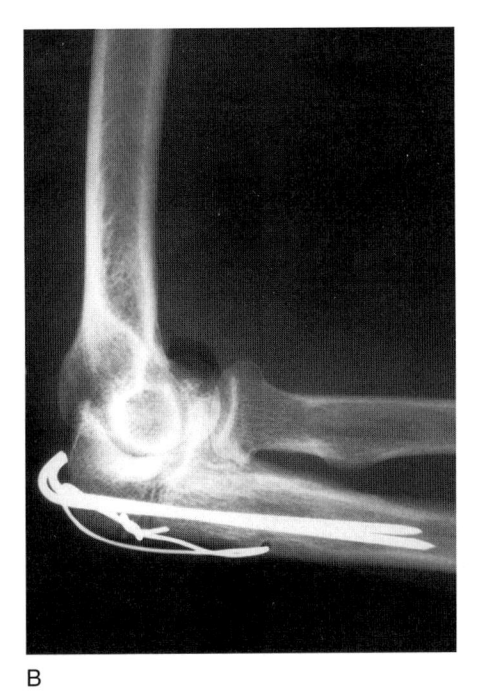

FIGURE 24.11. (A) Anteroposterior and (B) lateral radiographs of the tension-band wire and Steinmann pins.

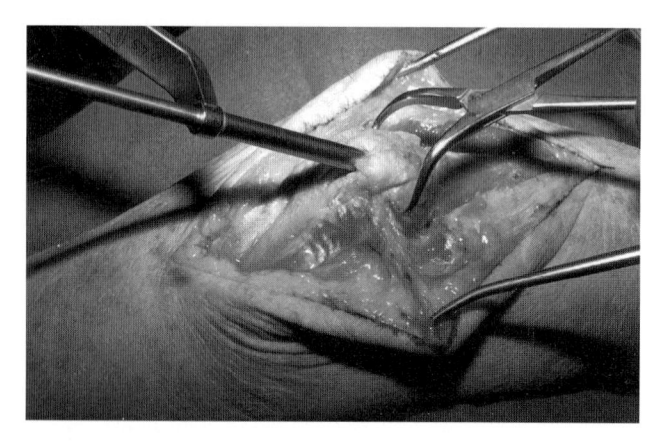

FIGURE 24.12. The surgeon drills a hole for the compression screw with a 3.2-mm drill bit.

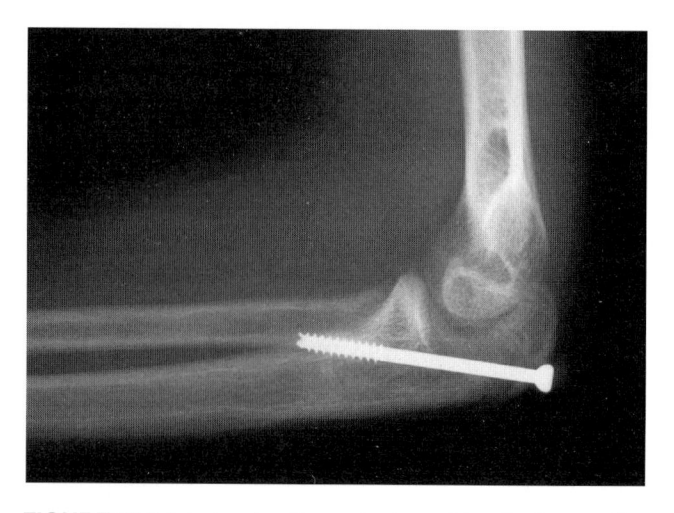

FIGURE 24.14. Lateral radiograph shows bicortical screw fixation of a proximal olecranon fracture.

Excision of Olecranon and Repair of Triceps Tendon

Excision of the proximal olecranon is a good technique for treating avulsion fractures or comminuted fractures involving less than 50% of the joint surface, particularly in older patients who have osteoporotic bone or who require salvage surgery to treat a failed nonunion. McKeever and Buck suggested excising up to 80% of the joint surface;[8] however, when excising more than 50% of the joint surface, the surgeon must carefully evaluate the joint for anteroposterior instability. The results of olecranon excision and repair of the triceps tendon are comparable to internal fixation, achieving similar strength and motion and fewer hardware complications.[9]

The proximal avulsion fragment, as well as other comminuted fragments, is excised (Fig. 24.15). Joint stability is tested with passive range of motion. Anteroposterior stability should be satisfactory, and subluxation should not be present. The medial collateral ligament must be intact to provide valgus stability (Fig. 24.16).

The triceps tendon is repaired to the articular joint surface with large nonabsorbable sutures placed through drill holes or bone tunnels in the proximal olecranon. These sutures can be passed into the triceps tendon with a modified Kessler or Bunnell technique, providing secure reattachment of the triceps tendon to the proximal ulna.

Contoured Plating Technique

Segmental fractures of the proximal ulna often are associated with olecranon and coronoid fractures. Neutralization plating of these fractures is necessary. Tension-band wiring techniques are not adequate alone. A 3.5-mm acetabular reconstruction plate can be contoured to wrap around the posterior aspect of the olecranon tip and ulnar shaft. Alternatively, a 3.5-mm dynamic compression plate can be placed on the lateral or medial cortex, providing transverse bicortical screw fixation (Fig. 24.17). Interfragmentary fixation of the coronoid process fracture through the proximal ulna is necessary for restoring stability to the ulnohumeral joint.

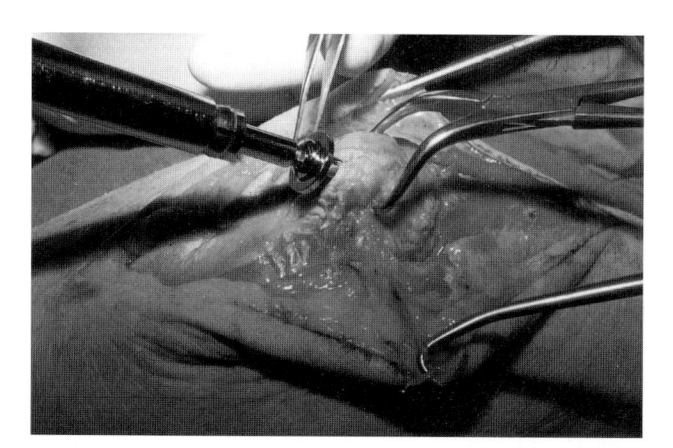

FIGURE 24.13. The surgeon holds the fragment with the tenaculum and positions a 6.5-mm cancellous screw and a washer.

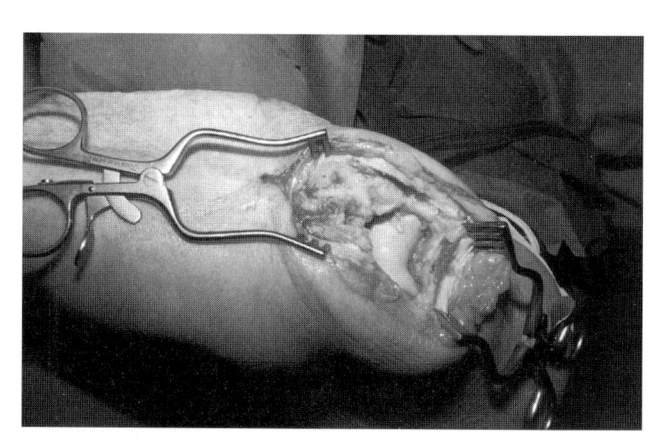

FIGURE 24.15. Excision of comminuted olecranon fracture fragment.

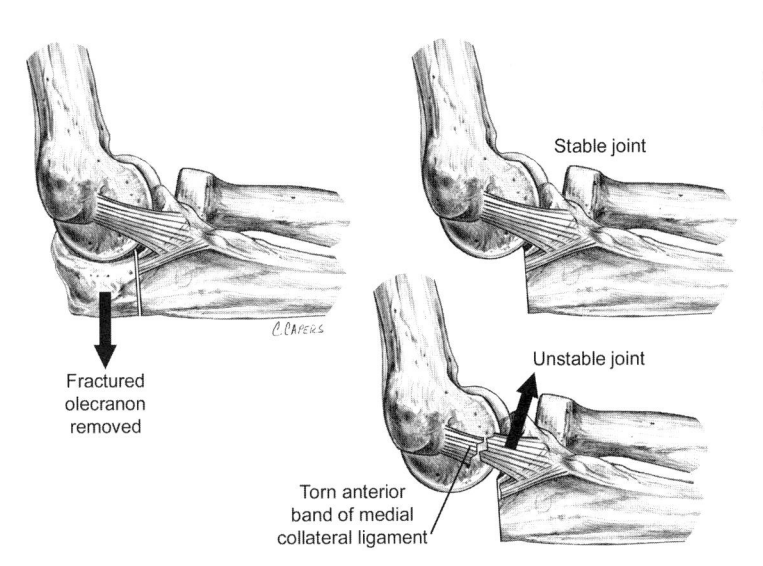

FIGURE 24.16. Stability of the joint depends on status of medial collateral ligament after excision of the fractured olecranon.

CORONOID PROCESS FRACTURES

A hyperextension injury to the elbow with high-force trauma can result in a coronoid process fracture of the elbow. Regan and Morrey[10] classified coronoid process fractures as types I, II, and III. Type I is an avulsion of the tip of the coronoid process, type II is a fragment involving less than 50% of the coronoid process, and type III is a fragment involving more than 50% of the coronoid process. Type I and type II coronoid process fractures do not need to be treated surgically; however, the surgeon should assume that they accompany a medial collateral ligament injury of the elbow and should treat them as a dislocated elbow. When these fractures are associated with dislocation of the elbow, they should be treated with closed reduction and early range of motion of the elbow and, if necessary, with a hinged brace.

Type III coronoid process fractures are highly unstable and are associated with a high rate of redislocation. These fractures must be treated with open reduction and internal fixation to restore anteroposterior stability, as well as valgus stability, because the medial collateral ligament inserts onto the fracture fragment.

One method for fixation of type III fractures is the compression-screw technique. The surgeon exposes the fracture through a longitudinal incision on the posterior aspect of the elbows as previously described. The superficial fascia is incised longitudinally along the shaft of the ulna. The subperiosteum is dissected on the medial aspect of the ulnar shaft, exposing the fracture at the base of the coronoid process (Fig. 24.18). The insertion of the medial collateral ligament can be seen on the large fragment of the coronoid process. Dissecting along the lateral aspect of the ulnar shaft through the same posterior

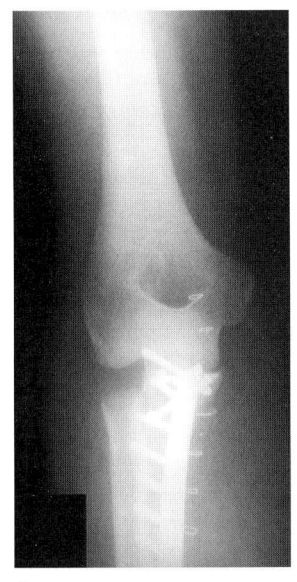

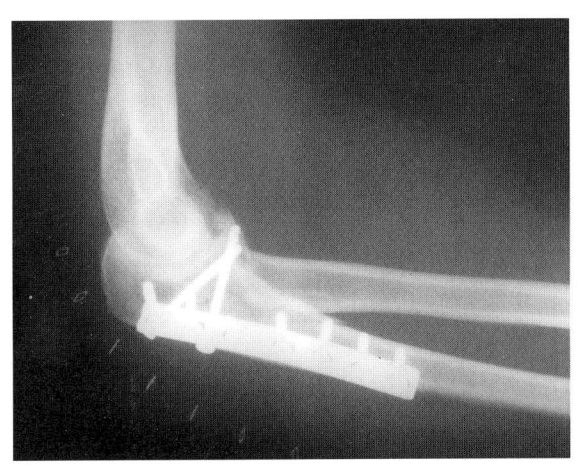

FIGURE 24.17. (A) Anteroposterior and (B) lateral radiograph of open reduction and internal fixation of the proximal ulna and coronoid and excision of the radial head.

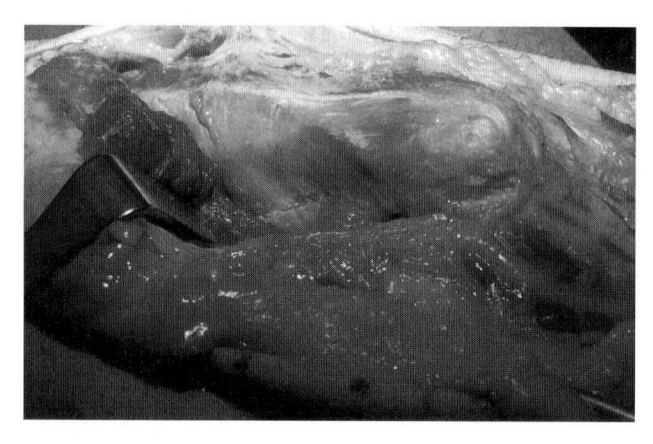

FIGURE 24.18. Exposure of a type III coronoid process fracture.

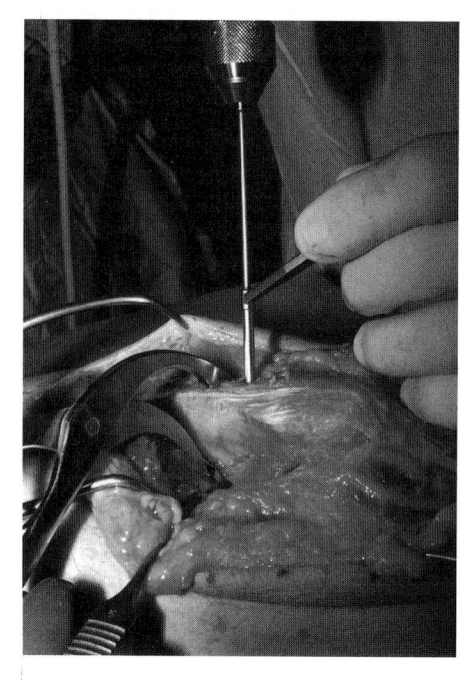

FIGURE 24.20. Interfragmentary screw fixation.

incision exposes the radial head for open reduction and internal fixation or for resection of the radial head, if needed. Alternatively, the coronoid process fracture fragment can also be exposed through an anterior approach by splitting the brachialis muscle in the midline over the antecubital fossa.

Temporary reduction of the coronoid process to the shaft is accomplished with a self-retaining tenaculum or Verbrugge clamp (Fig. 24.19). Interfragmentary fixation of the type III coronoid process fracture is accomplished with 3.5-mm bicortical screws. Using a 2.7-mm drill, the surgeon creates holes from the posterior cortex, through the coronoid process, and to the anterior cortex (Fig. 24.20). Overdrilling with a 3.5-mm drill bit creates the proximal gliding hole. The distal cortex is tapped, and a 3.5-mm bicortical screw is inserted by the interfragmentary technique. If possible, two screws should be placed for better fixation across the base of the coronoid process. Cannulated screw systems also provide another option for internal fixation of the coronoid fragment.

The passive range of motion and stability of the elbow are tested. Following fixation of the coronoid process, the medial collateral ligament should be competent. The humerus should not translate anteriorly on the ulnar shaft. An intraoperative radiograph should confirm a congruent ulnohumeral joint.

If a type III coronoid process fracture is associated with a segmental fracture of the proximal ulna, internal fixation of the ulnar shaft fracture with a contoured plate technique, as previously described, is necessary.

COMPLEX FRACTURE–DISLOCATION OF THE PROXIMAL ULNA

Direct trauma or a fall on the extended elbow and wrist can result in a complex fracture–dislocation of the elbow. These fracture–dislocations of the proximal ulna can range in complexity from a pure ligamentous and capsular injury, with an apparent avulsion fracture of the coronoid process, to a complex intra-articular fracture of the entire proximal ulna, including the coronoid process, olecranon process, and radial head.

In previous classifications of olecranon process, coronoid process, radial head, and proximal ulnar fractures, the authors do not consider fracture–dislocations.[4,10,11] In addition, Monteggia's classification of fracture–dislocations does not include the ulnohumeral articulation.[12,13] The Mayo Clinic's classification of olecranon fractures (i.e., type III unstable A and B) demonstrates the complexity of the lesion, including frank dislocation and associated radial head fracture.[5] The AO group's classification that recognizes both the proximal ulnar and proximal radial fractures includes the more complex in-

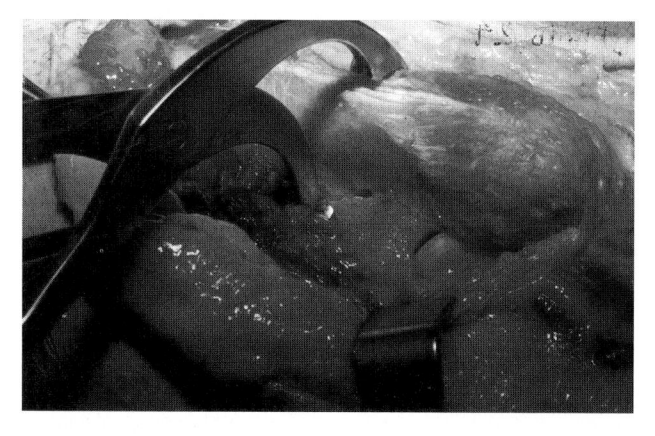

FIGURE 24.19. Reduction of a type III coronoid process fracture using a Verbrugge clamp.

tra- and extra-articular components of fracture–dislocation; however, it does not address instability and dislocation as a component of their fracture classification.

Fracture–dislocation about the elbow can include instability that requires diagnosis and treatment. Before treating this injury, the surgeon must assess the triad of ligaments consisting of the medial collateral ligament complex, the lateral collateral ligament complex, and the annular ligament. Likewise, the bony triad consisting of the olecranon process, coronoid process, and radial head are assessed and repaired for ligamentous and bony stability.

The extent to which the surgeon can reconstitute the articular surface of the elbow and the appropriate anatomic relationship with the distal humerus determines whether the surgeon uses fixation or excision of fracture components. Stability and fracture configuration dictate the type of fixation that the surgeon uses.

Deciding how to treat the fracture properly is difficult because of the complex issues of anterior elbow instability after olecranon fracture excision, forearm instability of the Essex–Lopresti lesion following radial head excision,[11] posterior dislocation of the elbow after resection, and untreated coronoid fractures. Critical assessment of the sigmoid notch in its relationship to the distal humerus, the proximal radioulnar joint, and the radiocapitellar joint are important in the treatment protocol.

When a fracture–dislocation is present, two of the three components of the bony triad must be stabilized, especially if comminution of the remaining component precludes fixation. If excision of the fractured bone is a component of operative intervention, ligament support and stability must be obtained and, if disrupted, must be repaired. In this complex situation, joint congruency must be maintained, and early range of motion must be initiated regardless of what type of fracture fixation or ligament reconstruction is performed.

In their study, Mehlhoff et al. demonstrated good and excellent results after simple dislocations when motion was initiated within the first 2 weeks after injury.[2] However, poor results were predominant when the elbow was immobilized for at least 4 weeks before motion was initiated. We believe these findings can be applied to patients who have complex fractures, as well. Therefore, to obtain good results, the surgeon should avoid cast immobilization in patients who have complex fractures. Instead, external hinge distraction systems, such as the dynamic joint distractor (Howmedica, Inc., Allendale, NJ) or the compass universal hinge device (Smith-Nephew, Memphis, TN), can be used to allow early motion.

Proximal ulnar fractures that include the olecranon and coronoid process fractures are treated by open reduction and internal fixation using a 3.5 distal compression plate that can be supplemented with interfragmentary screws as needed, as described earlier. The olecranon and coronoid processes are secured with the fixation. If comminution precludes the attachment of the olecranon process, the triceps is brought into the proximal fracture surface in alignment with the articular semilunar notch. If the coronoid process is comminuted and irreparable, it is reattached through comminuted fracture fragments and the brachialis insertion, or, in rare instances, it is reconstructed using a bone block. If reparable, the comminuted radial head is reconstructed with either screws or a plate. If comminution precludes reconstruction, the surgeon excises the radial head, considers a radial head implant, and then tests and repairs the medial collateral and lateral collateral ligaments as indicated. The longitudinal axial stress test that Davidson et al.[14] described is used to determine the status of the interosseous ligament and to indicate whether the treatment should include radial head replacement and pinning or repair of the distal radioulnar joint for an Essex–Lopresti lesion.

Proximal ulnar fractures that include coronoid process and radial head fractures result in an unstable configuration about the elbow. To stabilize the fractures and to enable the early range of motion required to produce functional elbow motion, the surgeon must use a combination of both internal and external fixation systems.

Hinged External Fixators

Distraction joint devices are external fixation systems that can be applied to a fracture–dislocation to provide stability, allow early motion, and maintain elbow congruency. Ligament and fracture healing occur while motion is maintained.[15]

Currently at our institution, we frequently use the dynamic joint distractor (Howmedica, Inc., Allentown, NJ) developed at the Mayo Clinic (Fig. 24.21) and the compass universal hinge (Smith-Nephew, Memphis, TN) developed at the Hospital for Special Surgery. Proper open reduction and internal fixation of the fracture instability pattern, application of the external fixation, and early motion have provided the most reliable and predictable results for these most difficult of elbow fractures.

The use of the dynamic joint distractor in the treatment of complex unstable fracture–dislocations is indicated if fracture fixation of the distal humerus or the proximal ulna does not interfere with pin placement. If it does, the compass elbow hinge, which technically bypasses the elbow joint and secures fixation proximal and distal to the joint, can be used with equal success in stabilization and early joint mobility.

Technique for Applying the Dynamic Joint Distractor

The surgical technique for applying the dynamic joint distractor requires the surgeon to accurately place the distal humeral transfixing pin through the rotational center. The surgeon uses a 3.2-mm drill bit to create a hole in the

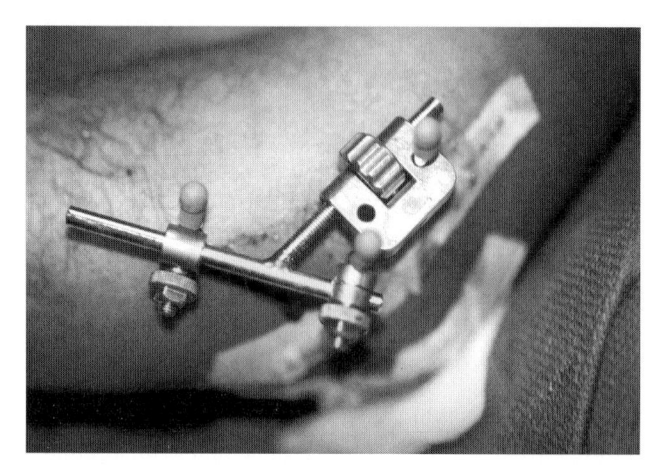

FIGURE 24.21. Dynamic joint distractor (Howmedica, Allentown, NJ).

anatomic axis of rotation at the projected rotational center of the capitellum. Drilling laterally to medially, the drill bit exits at the anterior–inferior aspect of the medial epicondyle. Before inserting the transfixing pin, the surgeon decompresses the ulnar nerve. The humeral guide is used during distal humeral pin placement.

The ulnar guide is used during the placement of the 3-mm smooth transfixing pins in the olecranon process and the proximal ulna. The surgeon places ulnar pins parallel to humeral transfixing pins (Fig. 24.22). The Y-body assembly is inserted medially and laterally and is secured in place with appropriate coupling devices. Distraction is applied to maintain joint separation of 3 to 5 mm. Either

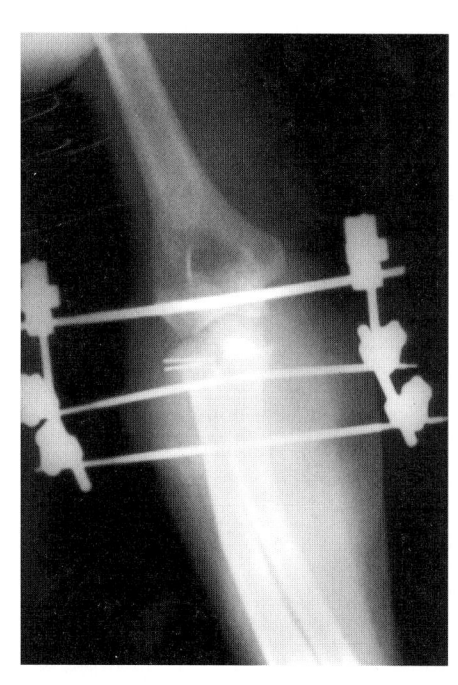

FIGURE 24.22. AP radiographic view of the patient with a dynamic joint distractor device (Howmedica) shows placement of ulnar pins.

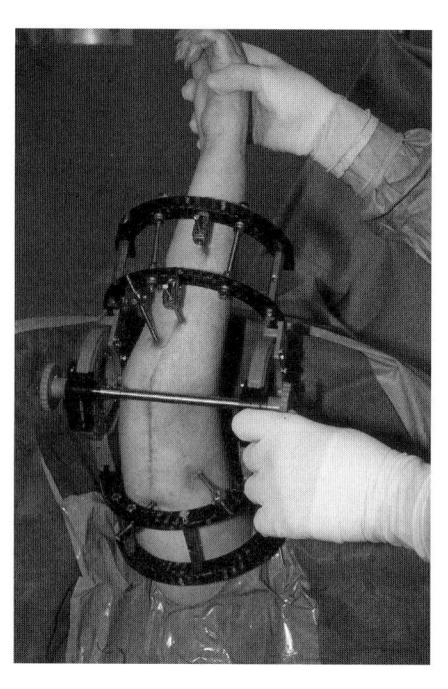

FIGURE 24.23. Compass elbow (universal) hinge (posterior view) (Smith-Nephew, Memphis, TN).

under direct observation or fluoroscopy, the upper extremity is moved through an arc of motion to evaluate the concentric range of motion of the elbow joint through the distraction device. The collateral ligaments and the brachialis or triceps muscles are reattached as the injury and the fracture fixation indicate.

The patient should participate in a physical therapy program for the first 4 to 6 weeks after surgery; after this

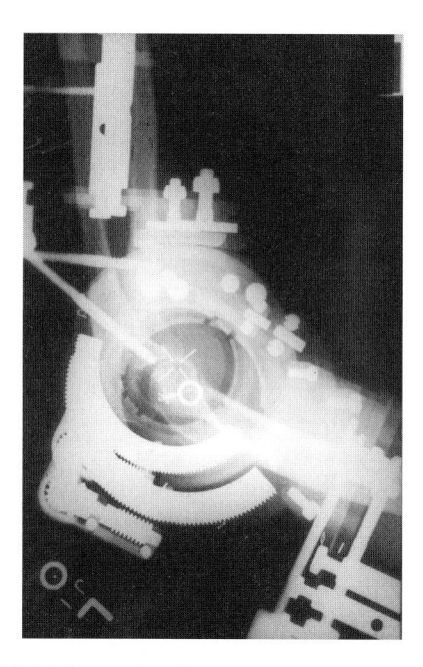

FIGURE 24.24. Lateral radiograph of patient with the compass elbow hinge device in place.

time, distraction device removal is recommended. An appropriate flexion–extension splint, dynamic brace, or hinged brace device may be used when the external fixation is terminated. The complete surgical techniques of the dynamic joint distractor are provided in the Howmedica surgical techniques manual.[16]

Technique for Applying the Compass Elbow Hinge

Application of the compass elbow hinge device involves the placement of half-pins proximal and distal to the elbow after the rotational axis is determined and verified by radiograph. After accomplishing secure humeral and ulnar pin placement, the surgeon applies the humeral and ulnar rings (Fig. 24.23), removes the axis of rotation pin, applies distraction, and verifies the arc of motion through C-arm imaging (Fig. 24.24). Postoperative dressings are applied, and the mobilization program is initiated. The complete surgical techniques for the application of the compass universal hinge are provided in the Smith-Nephew manual.[17]

COMPLICATIONS

Complications associated with elbow injuries, whether for an isolated fracture, a ligament injury, or a complex fracture–dislocation, consist of decreased range of motion, soft-tissue and heterotopic bone contractures, and traumatic arthritis. Vascular insult can occur acutely, resulting in compartment syndrome, and chronically, resulting in Volkmann's ischemic contracture; fortunately it is rare. Compression neuropathy of the ulnar, radial, and median nerve can occur. Unaddressed ligament disruptions may result in chronic instability patterns. Failure of bone healing resulting in nonunion, or malunion can occur. The hardware can cause symptoms, such as pain, infection, or bursal reaction and therefore might necessitate removal.

CONCLUSION

Stabilizing these complex injuries about the elbow adequately to initiate early range-of-motion exercises and providing careful follow-up will maximize the functional recovery of the elbow and minimize complications. The use of internal and external fixation devices, cast braces, hinged braces, and continuous passive motion machines may be indicated in specific cases. The recent trend of more aggressive treatment for these complex injuries has provided improved function and more predictable outcomes than prolonged cast treatment or neglect.

REFERENCES

1. Murphy DF, Greene WB, Dameron TB Jr. Displaced olecranon fractures in adults. Clinical evaluation. *Clin Orthop* 1987; 224:215–223.
2. Mehlhoff TL, Noble PC, Bennett JB, et al. Simple dislocation of the elbow in the adult. Results after closed treatment. *J Bone Joint Surg* 1988;70A:244–249.
3. Wolfgang G, Burke F, Bush D, et al. Surgical treatment of displaced olecranon fractures by tension band wiring technique. *Clin Orthop* 1987;224:192–204.
4. Colton CL. Fractures of the olecranon in adults: Classification and management. *Injury* 1973;5:121–129.
5. Morrey BF. Current concepts in the treatment of fractures of the radial head, the olecranon, and the coronoid. *Instr Course Lect* 1995;44:175–185.
6. Farrar EL III, Lippert FG III. Avulsion of the triceps tendon. *Clin Orthop* 1981;161:242–246.
7. Bach BR, Warren RF, Wickiewicz TL. Triceps rupture. A case report and literature review. *Am J Sports Med* 1987;15:285–289.
8. McKeever FM, Buck RN. Fractures of the olecranon process of the ulna. Treatment by excision of fragment and repair of triceps. *JAMA* 1947;135:1.
9. Gartsman GM, Sculco TP, Otis JC. Operative treatment of olecranon fractures. Excision or open reduction with internal fixation. *J Bone Joint Surg* 1981;63A:718–721.
10. Regan W, Morrey B. Fractures of the coronoid process of the ulna. *J Bone Joint Surg* 1989;71A:1348–1354.
11. Mason ML. Some observations on fractures of the head of the radius with a review of one hundred cases. *Br J Surg* 1954; 42:123–132.
12. Bado JL. The Monteggia lesion. *Clin Orthop* 1967;50:71–86.
13. Reckling FW. Unstable fracture–dislocations of the forearm. (Monteggia and Galeazzi lesions). *J Bone Joint Surg* 1982; 64A:857–863.
14. Davidson PA, Moseley JB, Tullos HS. Radial head fracture; a potentially complex injury. *Clin Orthop* 1993;297:224–230.
15. Cobb TK, Morrey BF. Use of distraction arthroplasty in unstable fracture dislocations of the elbow. *Clin Orthop* 1995; 312:201–210.
16. Morrey BF. *Howmedica surgical techniques. Dynamic joint distractor surgical technique.* Howmedica, Allentown, NJ; 1994.
17. Hotchkiss RN. *Compass universal hinge.* Smith-Nephew Catalog, Memphis, TN; 1998.

CHAPTER 25

Nonunions of the Elbow

David Ring and Jesse B. Jupiter

INTRODUCTION

To a large degree, optimal function of the elbow depends on maintenance of the dimensions, contour, and integrity of its osseous and articular elements. Failure of an elbow fracture to unite can diminish function as a result of pain, loss of motion, instability, or arthrosis. Although pain relief alone may be an appropriate goal for patients who have limited functional demands, usually it is necessary to address the need for stability and motion.

Nonunion about the elbow is seen most often as a result of inadequate immobilization, particularly instability following operative fixation.[1–5] The appeal of operative fixation is substantial for fractures about the elbow when immobilization of fracture fragments to gain healing must be balanced with the propensity of this articulation to develop capsular contracture with even brief periods of inactivity. In the development of internal fixation, fractures about the elbow commonly were secured with a limited number of screws, wires, or suture. This approach led to poor results, because the stabilization of the fracture was insufficient to allow functional aftercare, while the operative devitalization of the fracture fragments and their surrounding soft tissues compromised healing. Recent years have witnessed substantial improvements in the techniques and implants for fixation of small articular fracture fragments.[6–12] When an experienced surgeon applies them appropriately, current techniques do not often result in nonunion. The occurrence of nonunion is often related to technical errors, extensive soft-tissue injury, infection, or bone loss.[13–16] As a result, ununited fractures about the elbow represent complex reconstructive problems.

A number of general principles should be considered in the operative treatment of nonunions about the elbow.

1. Before resection of fracture fragments (e.g., of the radial head or olecranon) can be considered, the stability of the elbow must be assured.

2. Fixation should be of sufficient rigidity to allow active mobilization.

3. Contracture release for stiff elbows is important not only to optimize function, but also to reduce the stresses encountered by the implants.

4. In general, restoration of the contour and dimensions of the articulating surfaces takes precedence over congruity of articular surfaces; residual defects should be filled with autogenous bone graft.

5. Malalignment of the fracture fragments is commonplace, and restoration of anatomic alignment is as important as obtaining healing to the ultimate functional result.

6. In situations with real or potential instability, restoration of the osseous and articular anatomy should take precedence over maintenance of motion, because the results of later capsular release are more predictable than those for reconstruction of chronic posttraumatic instability.[17]

HISTORY

Although nonunions about the elbow may be painful due to instability of fracture fragments or articular incongruity, the proximity of the ulnar nerve to the cubital articulation should be kept in mind, because it is susceptible to fibrosis and painful neuritis following elbow trauma. Pain hinders active mobilization and contributes to stiffness. Malalignment of fracture fragments, particularly articular fragments, also may contribute to stiff-

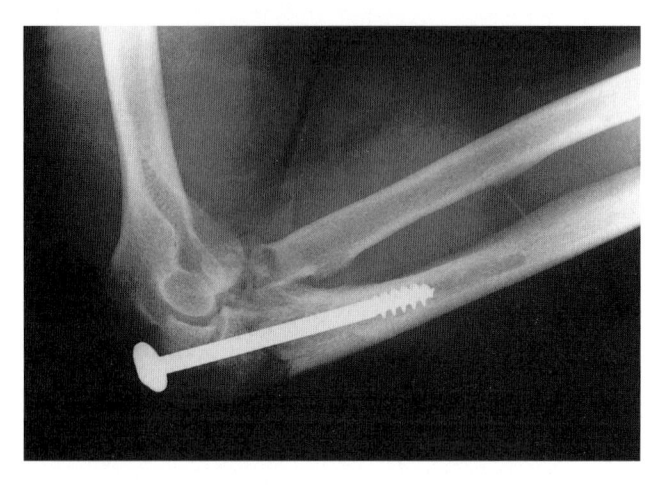

FIGURE 25.1. A complex high-energy injury to the elbow in a 47-year-old mechanic resulted in an ununited olecranon with deformity and elbow instability.

ness. Malalignment (e.g., narrowing of the trochlear notch or residual angulation of the ulna) also may cause articular instability, particularly in the setting of capsuloligamentous injury.

Nonunion of the Proximal Ulna

Failure of olecranon fractures to unite is uncommon when current techniques of operative fixation are applied correctly. Coonrad noted nonunion of simple olecranon fractures in 1.67% (1 of 60) of patients[18] treated at his institution; Papagelopoulos and Morrey, in 1% (2 of 196) of patients.[19] In the past, nonunion was far more common when closed reduction and cast immobilization were used. Many of these nonunions resulted in pain and weakness of elbow extension, but some authors contended that a large percentage represented relatively asymptomatic fibrous unions.[18]

Nonunion of the proximal ulna now is encountered most often following complex, comminuted fractures of the proximal ulna, many of which are fracture–dislocations (Figs. 25.1 and 25.2). Recounting the Mayo Clinic experience between 1976 and 1991, Papagelopoulos and Morrey noted that, among 24 consecutive patients treated for an ununited fracture of the proximal ulna, 18 (75%) had either comminution (11 patients, 46%) or associated fracture–dislocation (12 patients, 50%).[19] The most common patterns of proximal ulnar fracture–dislocation, which include the anterior or transolecranon fracture–dislocation of the elbow[20,21] and the posterior Monteggia fracture–dislocation of the forearm[22–24] (Fig. 25.3), often involve the ulnar metaphysis distal to the trochlear notch, frequently with a large coronoid fracture fragment and occasionally with extension into the diaphysis. Nonunion following these more complex injuries, not unexpectedly, is much more problematic than fibrous nonunion of a simple olecranon fragment. In the Mayo Clinic series, 16 of 24 patients (67%) had pain, 8 (33%) had stiffness, and 7 (29%) had instability.[19] Twenty of 24 patients (83%) requested operative treatment on the basis of one or more of these problems.[19]

Nonunion of the Proximal Radius

Failure of a fracture of the proximal radius to unite may be more common than has been reported.[25–30] The proximal radial epiphysis is analogous to the proximal femoral epiphysis because it is contained entirely within the joint capsule. As a result, its blood supply is derived from a limited number of vessels entering through the proximal radial metaphysis, as well as from an interosseous supply. This tenuous vascularity is likely disrupted in many

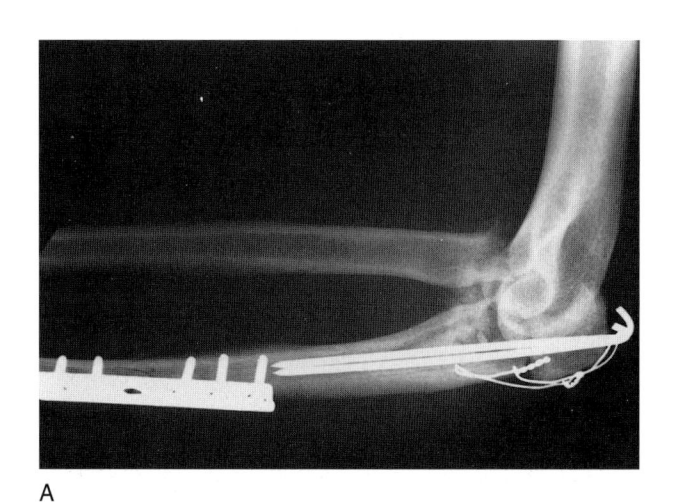

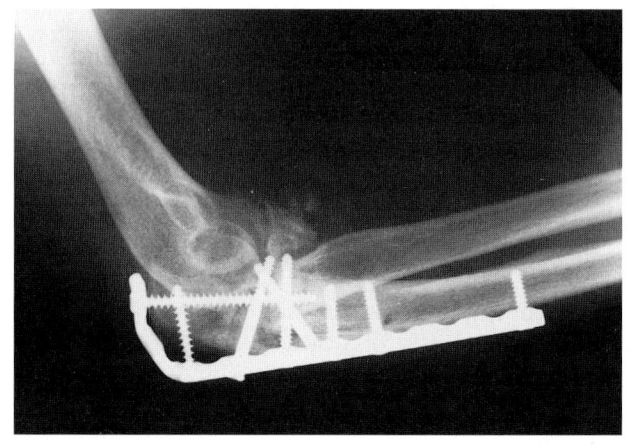

FIGURE 25.2. A complex nonunion of the proximal ulna following failed internal fixation. (A) Lateral radiograph of the displaced ununited ulna. (B) Lateral radiograph taken postoperatively.

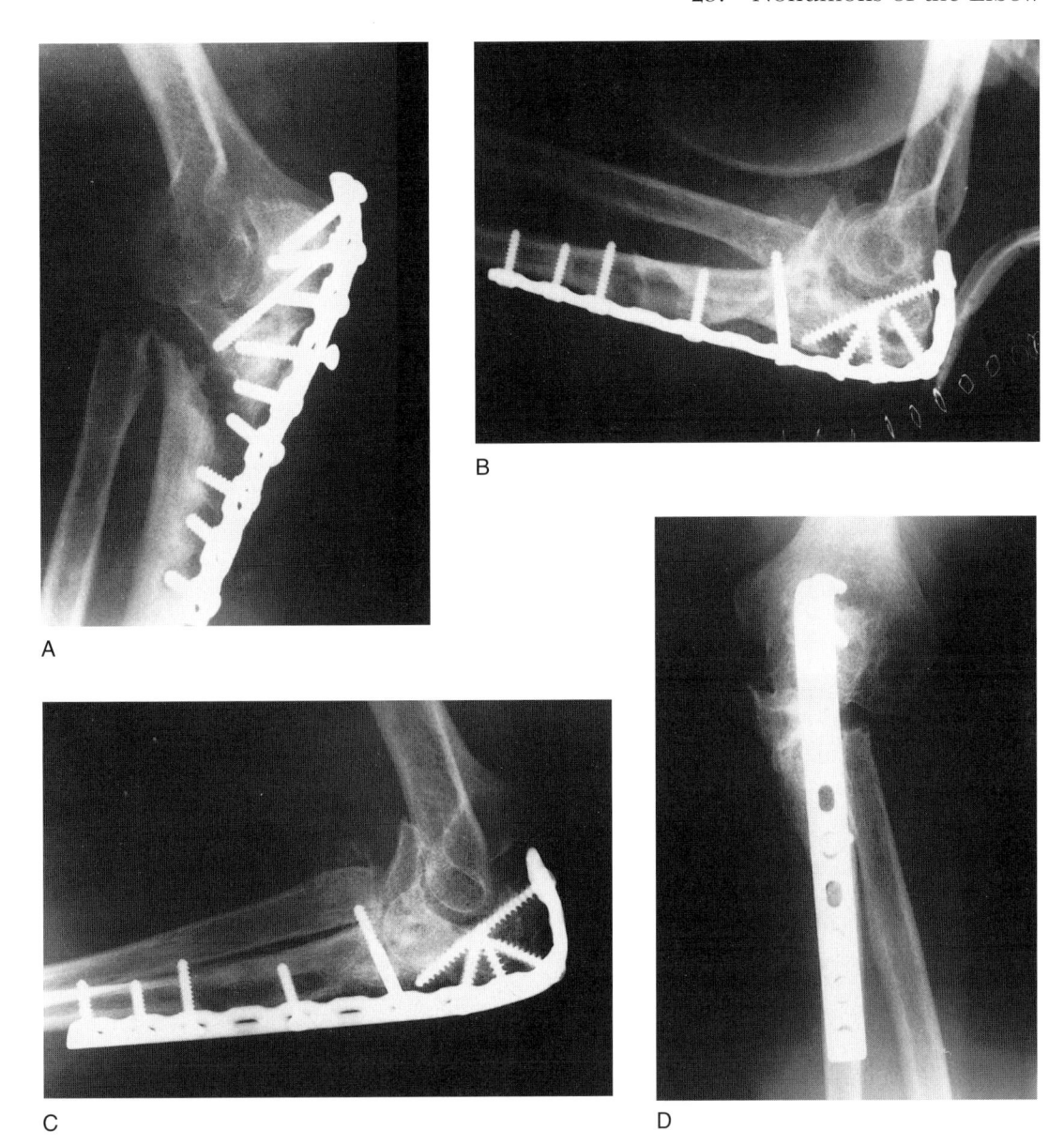

FIGURE 25.3. A posterior Monteggia fracture–dislocation involving the dominant limb of a 72-year-old woman was treated with a plate and screws, leading to nonunion and deformity as well as elbow stiffness. (A) Radiograph of the nonunion with loose internal fixation and deformity. (B) Operative fixation included realignment of the nonunion, stable internal fixation, autogenous bone graft, and elbow capsulectomy. (C) Lateral and (D) anteroposterior radiographs taken at 2-year followup.

high-energy injuries and may be further jeopardized by operative dissection. As a result of the increased emphasis on the importance of preserving the radial head in the presence of capsuloligamentous injury and the improvements in techniques and implants for internal fixation, attempts to salvage the radial head are now common, even in the face of comminution.[31–35] We have encountered nonunion of the radial head and neck following operative fixation of high-energy radial head fractures on a sufficient number of occasions to suspect an increased risk for nonunion in this setting (Fig. 25.4). Nonunion of the proximal radius may contribute to pain, restriction of motion (particularly forearm rotation), and arthrosis.

Nonunion of the Distal Humerus

Nonunion of the distal humerus is often the result of inadequate fixation (Figs. 25.5 and 25.6), but it also can be related to the severity of the initial injury (Fig. 25.7) and the presence of infection.[13–16] Nonunion most frequently involves the junction between the articular and columnar

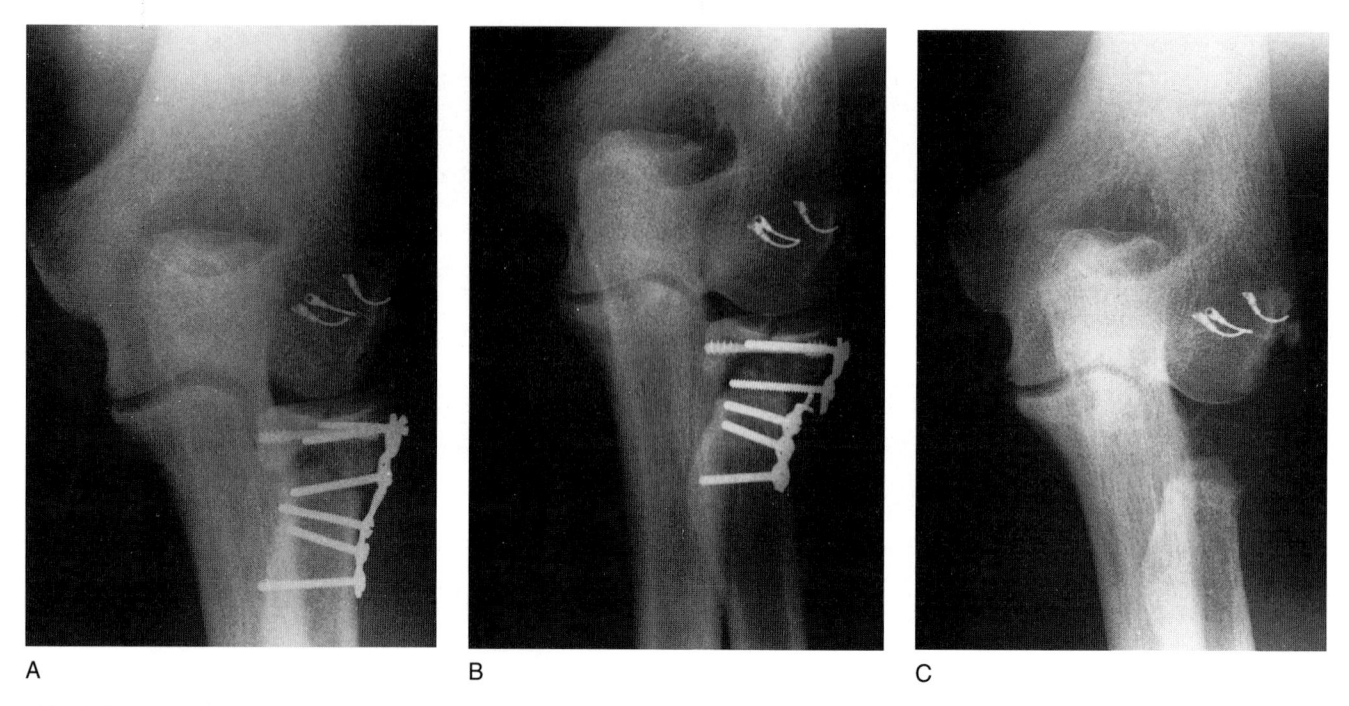

FIGURE 25.4. A nonunion of a radial head and neck fracture associated with internal fixation of a complex fracture–dislocation of the elbow. (A) Open reduction and internal fixation permitted functional motion after surgery. (B) Failure to unite was noted at 4 months. (C) The nonunion was treated by radial head resection 6 months after surgery.

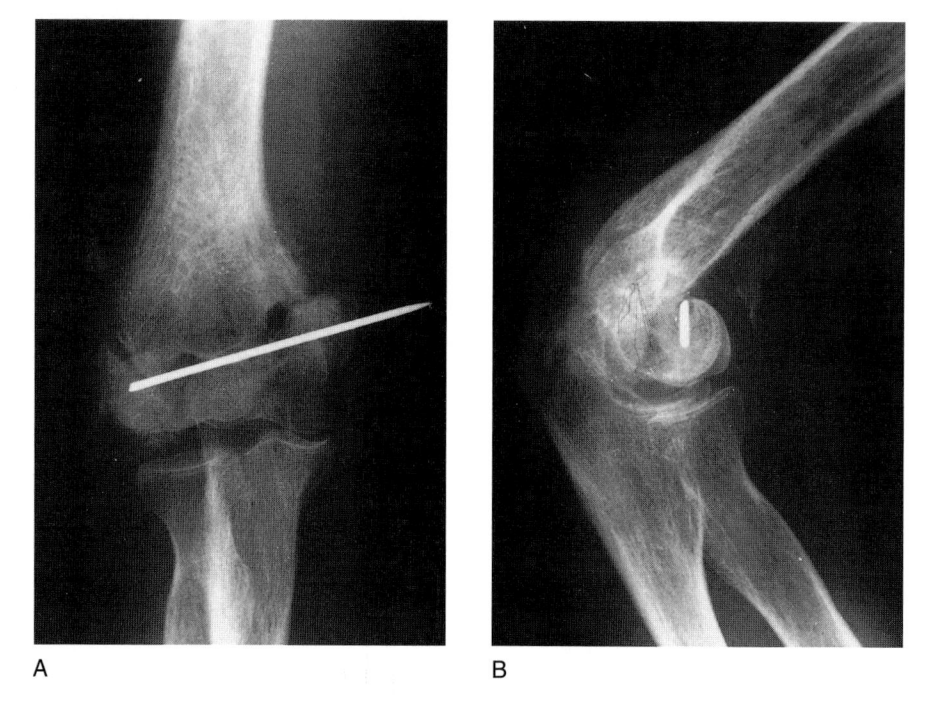

FIGURE 25.5. A distal humeral intra-articular fracture in a 68-year-old retired nurse was treated with Kirschner wire fixation, resulting in instability and nonunion. (A) Anteroposterior and (B) lateral radiographs show that unstable fixation resulted in failure to unite both the intra-articular and extra-articular components of the fracture.

A   B   C

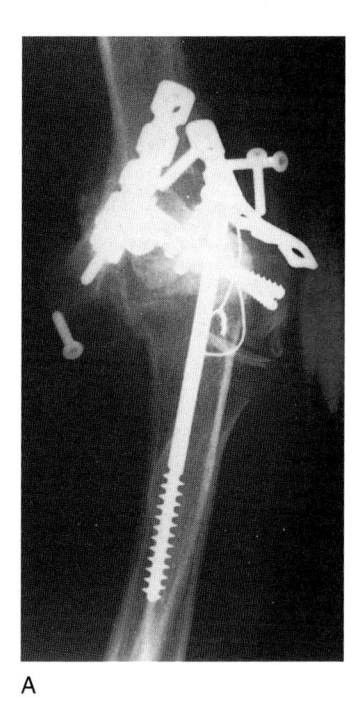

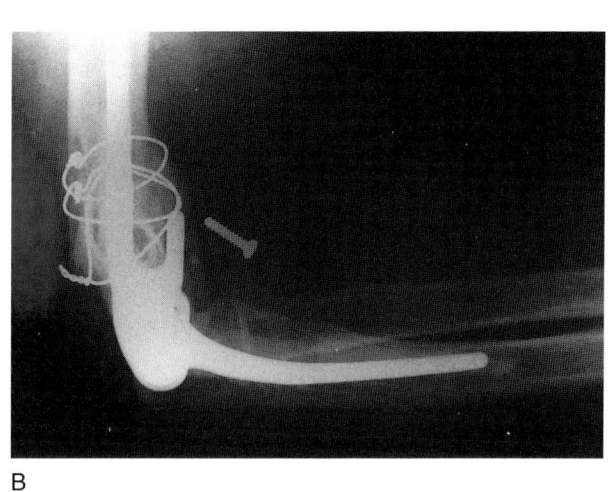

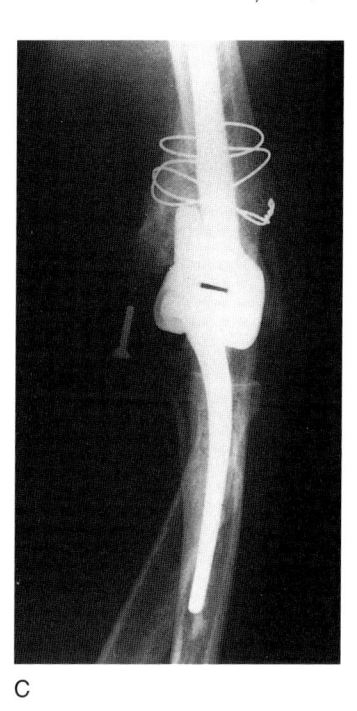

FIGURE 25.6. Nonunion of an intra-articular fracture of the distal humerus in a 63-year-old man was treated with total elbow arthroplasty. (A) Unstable internal fixation led to failure of union and severe elbow instability, along with a profound ulnar nerve neuropathy. (B) Lateral and (C) anteroposterior radiographs show the total elbow arthroplasty.

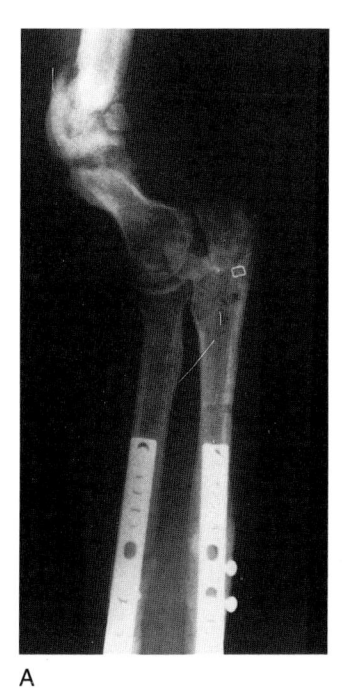

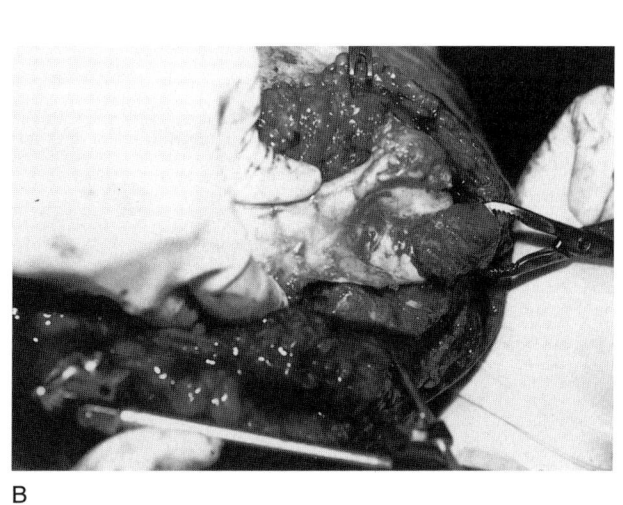

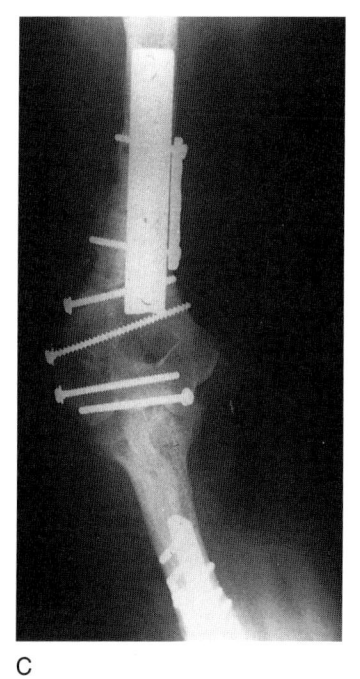

A   B   C

FIGURE 25.7. A high-energy road accident led to severe dysfunction, nonunion, and bone loss in the elbow of a 26-year-old truck driver. (A) A radiograph reveals extensive bone loss of the distal humerus. (B) An allograft distal humerus was contoured to replace the missing component of the distal humerus. (C) Anteroposterior radiograph shows the allograft internally fixed to the remaining distal humerus.

fragments, but it also may involve the articular surfaces. Pain, loss of motion, and instability are frequent symptoms. Symptoms related to ulnar nerve dysfunction are also common.

PHYSICAL EXAMINATION

To assure appropriate coverage of implants and nourishment of autogenous bone grafts, the examiner should evaluate the status of the soft tissues, particularly with respect to the location of previous incisions, the presence or absence of a draining sinus indicating chronic infection, and the viability of the overlying skin and muscle. Active and passive ulnohumeral and forearm motion are recorded, and a complete neurologic examination is performed. The examiner should attempt to document the stability of the elbow and the integrity of the capsuloligamentous structures; however, he or she may have difficulty isolating the ligaments if the ununited fracture is grossly unstable.

NONOPERATIVE TREATMENT

Nonoperative treatment is appropriate for some asymptomatic nonunions and for nonpainful nonunions in patients who have very low functional demands. This treatment consists of support or immobilization in a brace or splint.

OPERATIVE TREATMENT

Indications

Failure of a fracture about the elbow to unite nearly always requires operative treatment to relieve pain, to restore stability, or to improve motion and strength. The time at which a nonhealing fracture of metaphyseal bone can be deemed a nonunion has been arbitrarily set at 3 to 4 months, but it may be clear at a much earlier stage that healing is unlikely or, at best, will be delayed for a prolonged period. In these situations, earlier intervention may be warranted to limit stiffness and to restore functional use of the upper extremity. Electrical stimulation or other modalities usually are not used, because they require immobilization and cannot address deformity, instability, or stiffness.

In general, we make every effort to restore the osseous and articular anatomy of the elbow. In certain circumstances, alternative treatment approaches are warranted. Total elbow arthroplasty appears to represent a viable treatment option for some distal humeral and olecranon nonunions, especially for older patients who have limited functional demands. In a recent review of the Mayo Clinic experience treating distal humeral nonunion with total elbow arthroplasty, 86% of the patients (31 of 36) had satisfactory results.[36] The average arc of ulnohumeral motion was 111°, all elbows were stable, and only 9% of patients had more than mild pain. Papagelopoulos and Morrey also had good results when treating three olecranon nonunions with total elbow arthroplasty.[19] However, arthroplasty remains a poor option for the younger, active individual.

Patients who have low functional demands and ununited fractures of the olecranon process also may do well after excision of the olecranon and advancement of the triceps. Avulsion-type fractures of the olecranon tip are particularly amenable to this technique (see Chapter 24).

Allograft replacement of the distal humerus has generated some enthusiasm among surgeons, but problems with infection, nonunion, and instability have restricted the use of this technique.[37,38]

Contraindications

Before definitive skeletal fixation, the surgeon should ensure stable soft-tissue coverage and eradication of infection. Serial debridement, temporary external fixation, and local tissue flaps or free microvascular tissue transfer may be needed. In some cases, stable fixation allowing functional mobilization and eradication of infection or colonization at the fracture site can be addressed simultaneously using an Ilizarov construct.

After fracture–dislocations, the radial head and olecranon should not be excised until complete healing of the capsuloligamentous structures with physiologic tension has occurred. If the ligaments are attenuated, ligamentous reconstruction or temporary hinged elbow distraction may be required.[39–41]

In some patients, particularly those who have rheumatoid arthritis, the small size and extreme osteopenia of articular fracture fragments can preclude operative fixation. The surgeon should be prepared to use total elbow arthroplasty or, if necessary, allograft replacement in these situations.

Techniques

Positioning the patient in the lateral decubitus position with the involved extremity superior and draped over a bolster facilitates posterior exposure of the ulna or distal humerus. The iliac crest should be sterilized and draped into the operative field in case the surgeon encounters bony defects requiring autogenous bone graft. A sterile pneumatic tourniquet is used to improve visualization.

Exposure of nearly the entire elbow can be achieved through a single posterior midline skin incision (incorporating old incisions when possible) with the elevation of broad, full-thickness medial and lateral skin flaps (Fig. 25.8).[42,43] Access to various anatomic structures is es-

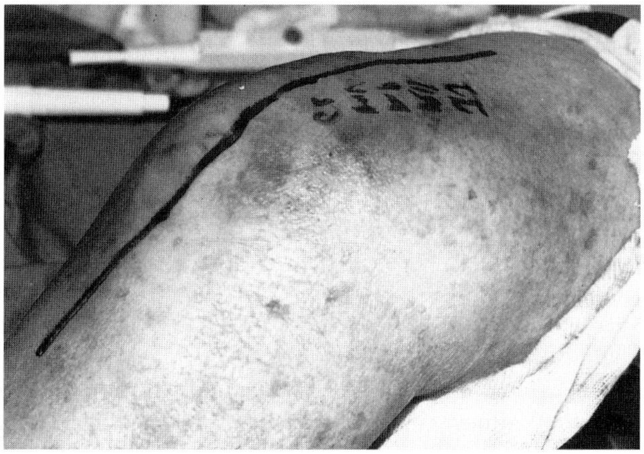

FIGURE 25.8. Nonunions about the elbow are preferentially approached through a straight posterior incision with the patient in the lateral decubitus position.

tablished through separate muscular intervals. For isolated radial head excision, a lateral skin incision is used.

When required, elbow release can be performed from the lateral aspect of the elbow by elevating the brachialis off the anterior capsule and the triceps off the posterior capsule.[17,44–47] Complete capsulectomy is also possible directly through a nonunion of the distal humerus.[48,49]

Open Reduction and Internal Fixation of the Proximal Ulna

The ulna is exposed along its dorsal subcutaneous border. This border represents the interval between the flexor carpi ulnaris and the extensor carpi ulnaris (the anconeus muscle proximally); however, elevation of these muscles is limited to preserve the blood supply to the bones. The periosteum is elevated only at the site of the nonunion so that devitalized tissue can be resected and deformity can be corrected.

All dysvascular bone and soft tissue should be removed from the nonunion site. This removal can result in a substantial bony defect, because most proximal ulnar nonunions represent complex problems involving bone loss. The bone loss results either from resorption of initial comminution or from debridement of previous infection and disruption of the vascular supply to the bone and surrounding soft tissues, due to the initial trauma and subsequent operative attempts to gain union. Failure of previous internal fixation is also problematic, because it causes further bony resorption and contributes to an inflammatory response that can lead to a dysvascular, noncompliant, soft-tissue envelope.

By using a small distractor, the surgeon can more easily realign the ulna with less soft-tissue dissection and without the use of devascularizing circumferential clamps.[50] The proximal ulnar (olecranon) fragment is first placed in anatomic position with the elbow flexed to 90° and is pinned to the distal humerus with a 0.062-in.

smooth Kirschner wire. Distraction is applied between this pin and a 2.5- or 4.0-mm Schanz screw placed in the ulnar diaphysis distal to the anticipated margin of the plate. The trochlea of the distal humerus is used as a template for restoring the contour and dimensions of the trochlear notch. This restoration is verified under image intensification. The distractor serves to maintain the reduction while the plate is applied.

Stable anatomic fixation of the proximal ulna is achieved most predictably using a 3.5-mm plate placed on the dorsal (tension) surface. The plate is contoured and then applied to the dorsal surface of the ulna with the proximal 0.062-in. Kirschner wire placed through one of the plate holes before definitive distraction. The olecranon fragment is often small and osteopenic. To achieve stable fixation, the surgeon must contour the proximal extent of the plate so that it extends to the tip of the olecranon. This contouring provides for an increased number of screws in the proximal fragment. The most proximal screws are oriented at 90° to more distal screws, thereby creating an interlocking construct. In most cases, inserting a long screw through the most proximal hole is possible.

We prefer 3.5-mm, limited-contact dynamic compression plates (Synthes, Paoli, PA) for their balance of strength and rigidity, with uniform stiffness, ability to be contoured, and variability in screw direction.[51] We advise against using semitubular and one-third tubular plates, because these plates are more susceptible to fatigue failure when exposed to cyclic loading at the elbow. The contoured proximal portion of the plate is applied to the tip of the olecranon through a longitudinal incision in the triceps insertion. After provisional fixation of the fragments, the distractor is removed and plain radiographs are obtained to document the quality of the reduction.

A large ununited coronoid fragment can contribute to instability, pain, and stiffness. Occasionally, this fragment is seen in isolation, but more often the fracture of the coronoid is part of a more complex fracture–dislocation of the elbow or forearm. Following mobilization and subcutaneous anterior transposition of the ulnar nerve, the coronoid process can be exposed either by osteotomizing the medial epicondyle and reflecting the origin of the flexor–pronator mass distally or, alternatively, by elevating the ulnar origin of the flexor carpi ulnaris anteriorly off the medial aspect of the ulna. Devascularized bone can be excised and replaced with autogenous cancellous bone graft. Stable fixation in anatomic alignment can be achieved either with interfragmentary compression screws placed through the dorsal aspect of the ulna or with a wire or stout suture placed through drill holes.

Nonunion of the Radial Head or Neck

Although union of an ununited radial head or neck fracture can be achieved in unique situations, we usually prefer resection. A number of operative techniques can be used to expose the radial head. Recent emphasis has been placed on the need to minimize the risk of operative disruption of the lateral collateral ligament complex.[52–54] If the surgeon uses Kocher's[55] exposure through the interval between the extensor carpi ulnaris and the anconeus, he or she should ensure that the capsular incision remains anterior to the anterior margin of the anconeus and parallel to the fascial limit of the extensor carpi ulnaris.[52] Hotchkiss described an alternative exposure in which the elbow joint is entered initially by elevating the capsule off the anterior aspect of the lateral humerus in a safe area anterior to the origin of the lateral collateral ligament complex.[56] This exposure allows visualization of the articular surface of the radial head. More distal exposure is accomplished by incising the capsule longitudinally along a line that bisects the anteroposterior diameter of the radial head. The lateral collateral ligament complex and annular ligament can be elevated anterior, but not posterior, to this line. More distal exposure of the neck requires entrance into the common extensor muscle compartment, mobilization of the muscle fibers anteriorly, and incision of the facial floor of the compartment.[56] This exposure uncovers the supinator muscle that is incised at its posterior margin and swept anteriorly with the forearm in full pronation to protect the posterior interosseous nerve.[57,58] Long right-angled retractors, rather than Bennett or Hohmann retractors, should be used to avoid injury to the posterior interosseous nerve. If the surgeon uses a long plate, he or she should expose and protect the posterior interosseous nerve.[56] Another option for exposure is osteotomy of the origin of the lateral collateral ligament from the lateral condyle of the distal humerus, with later repair using a 3.5-mm screw.[31,43,59]

After exposing the radial head, the surgeon removes all hardware and ununited fracture fragments. Resection to the distal margin of the annular ligament is sufficient. Bone wax can be placed over the cut end of the radial neck to prevent bone reformation and to limit the risk of proximal radioulnar synostosis. With the patient's forearm placed in pronation to ensure optimal tension, the surgeon carefully repairs the lateral collateral ligament complex with interrupted nonabsorbable sutures.[52,54]

Open Reduction and Internal Fixation of the Distal Humerus

Operative reconstruction of an ununited fracture of the distal humerus is a demanding procedure that involves mobilization and neurolysis of the ulnar nerve, resection of the nonunion site if it is atrophic or synovial, anterior and posterior capsulectomy, and realignment and stabilization of the distal fragments, which are almost always small and osteoporotic.[48,49] The ulnar nerve is isolated and mobilized over a sufficient distance of at least 6 cm proximal and distal to the cubital tunnel to permit the nerve to rest in the subcutaneous tissues anteromedially to the cubital tunnel. Neurolysis is performed on the basis of preoperative evaluation or presence of extensive scarring.

The operative repair of complex extra- or intra-articular nonunions, particularly those involving articular components sheared off in the coronal plane or in the presence of underlying osteopenia, requires extensile exposure of the joint surface, preferably through an osteotomy of the olecranon. We usually perform olecranon osteotomy; however, if total elbow arthroplasty is necessary, we use a medial triceps elevating exposure.

Careful attention to the details of creating and fixing the olecranon osteotomy reduces the incidence of complications associated with osteotomy healing. A chevron-shaped osteotomy with the apex pointing distally facilitates anatomic repositioning, enhances stability, and provides a broader interface of cancellous bone. The osteotomy should be located at the depth of the semilunar notch where the least amount of articular cartilage is present. This location is identified precisely under direct visualization following partial elevation of the anconeus from its insertion on the olecranon. The osteotomy is initiated with a thin oscillating saw. The articular surface and subchondral bone are cracked with a thin-bladed osteotome, resulting in a rough interdigitating surface that further facilitates anatomic repositioning of the fragment. Next, the triceps is elevated from the posterior humeral surface.

Complete anterior and posterior elbow capsulectomy can be performed through the operative exposure to reduce the stresses on the implants and improve the ultimate motion and functional status of the patient (Fig. 25.9). The nonunion site is inspected, and avascular and synovial tissues are excised.

The surgeon also should carefully inspect the articular surface. Ununited articular fragments (e.g., coronal shear fractures) can be fixed with self-compressing screws inserted deep to the articular surface (e.g., Herbert screws); small, threaded Kirschner wires; or bioabsorbable pins. Malalignment of articular fragments, such as narrowing of the trochlear spool, should be corrected with an osteotomy, if necessary. Resulting gaps can be filled with autogenous cancellous or corticocancellous bone, and the realigned trochlea can be held through its center with a screw. This screw is fully threaded so that it engages the medial and lateral fragments and holds them in proper alignment.

Fixation of the articular fragments onto the osseous columns represents the potential weak point of the internal fixation of distal humeral nonunions. The challenge is to ensure a secure hold on the distal fragments while avoiding both the articular surfaces and the central fossae and preserving the attachments of the collateral ligaments. Nonunion is associated with disuse osteopenia and resorption, so the distal fragments are small, are nearly

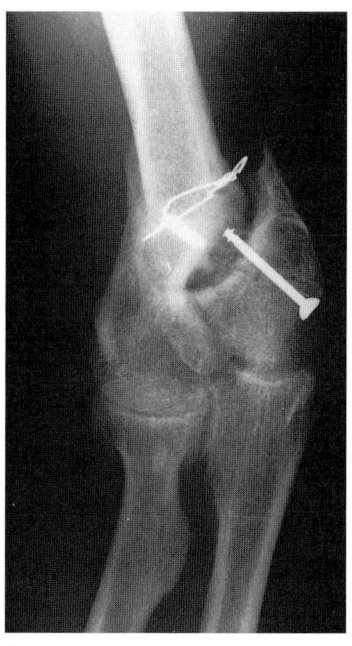

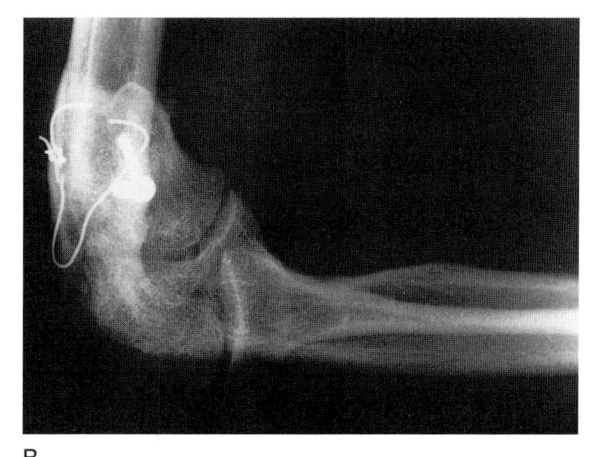

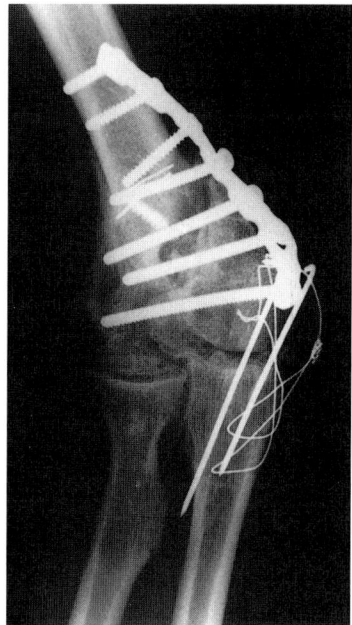

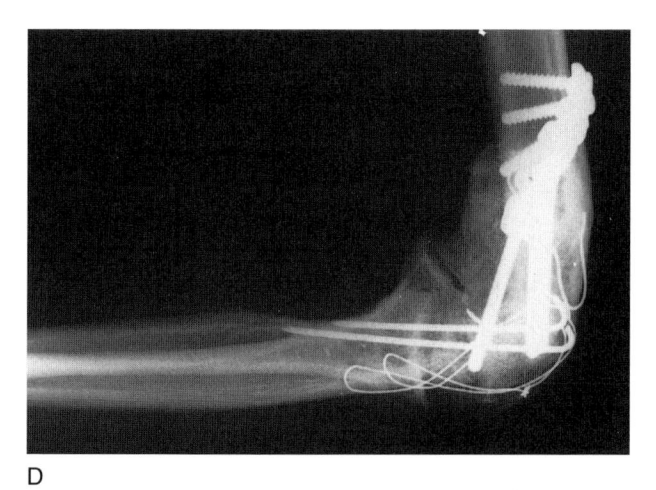

FIGURE 25.9. A complex intra-articular fracture of the distal humerus in a 37-year-old man was treated with autogenous bone graft, internal fixation, and capsular release. (A) Anteroposterior and (B) lateral radiographs of the nonunion. (C) Anteroposterior and (D) lateral radiographs of the healed nonunion.

entirely articular, and have very poor bone quality. The keys to success include the use of well-contoured plates, fixation with plates oriented as closely as possible to 90° to one another,[60–63] and adequate purchase in the articular fragments (Fig. 25.10).

We prefer 3.5-mm reconstruction plates because they are stout enough to resist the deforming forces in this region, and yet they are contoured easily in three dimensions. This is particularly important in the distal humerus, because the complex bony surfaces require equally complex and exacting contour of the plates.

Certain operative tactics can facilitate the stable fixation of small, articular fracture fragments. Given the fact that the medial column is entirely nonarticular, the inferior surface of the medial column at the level of the medial epicondyle can accommodate an internal fixation device. Following elevation of the ulnar nerve, a 3.5-mm reconstruction plate can be contoured into a semicircle at its distal end so that it can cradle the medial epicondyle. A screw placed through the most distal hole of the plate is oriented superiorly and can be directed either at a 90° angle to the more proximal screws, which creates an interlocking construct, or obliquely to obtain purchase into the lateral bony column.[64]

On the lateral column, the anterior capitellar articular surface imposes limitations. Nonetheless, a plate that extends to the posterior limit of the capitellar articular surface provides for screws directed anterosuperiorly, above the superior limit of the capitellum and nearly orthogonal to more proximal screws.[64] Being mindful of the triangular shape of these columns, which taper in anteroposterior width toward the olecranon and coronoid fossae,

FIGURE 25.10. A complex nonunion of a distal humerus fracture in a 64-year-old school teacher. (A) Anteroposterior and (B) lateral radiographs show the nonunion that occurred following unstable internal fixation. (C) Anteroposterior and (D) lateral radiographs show that stable fixation was provided using three strategically contoured plates.

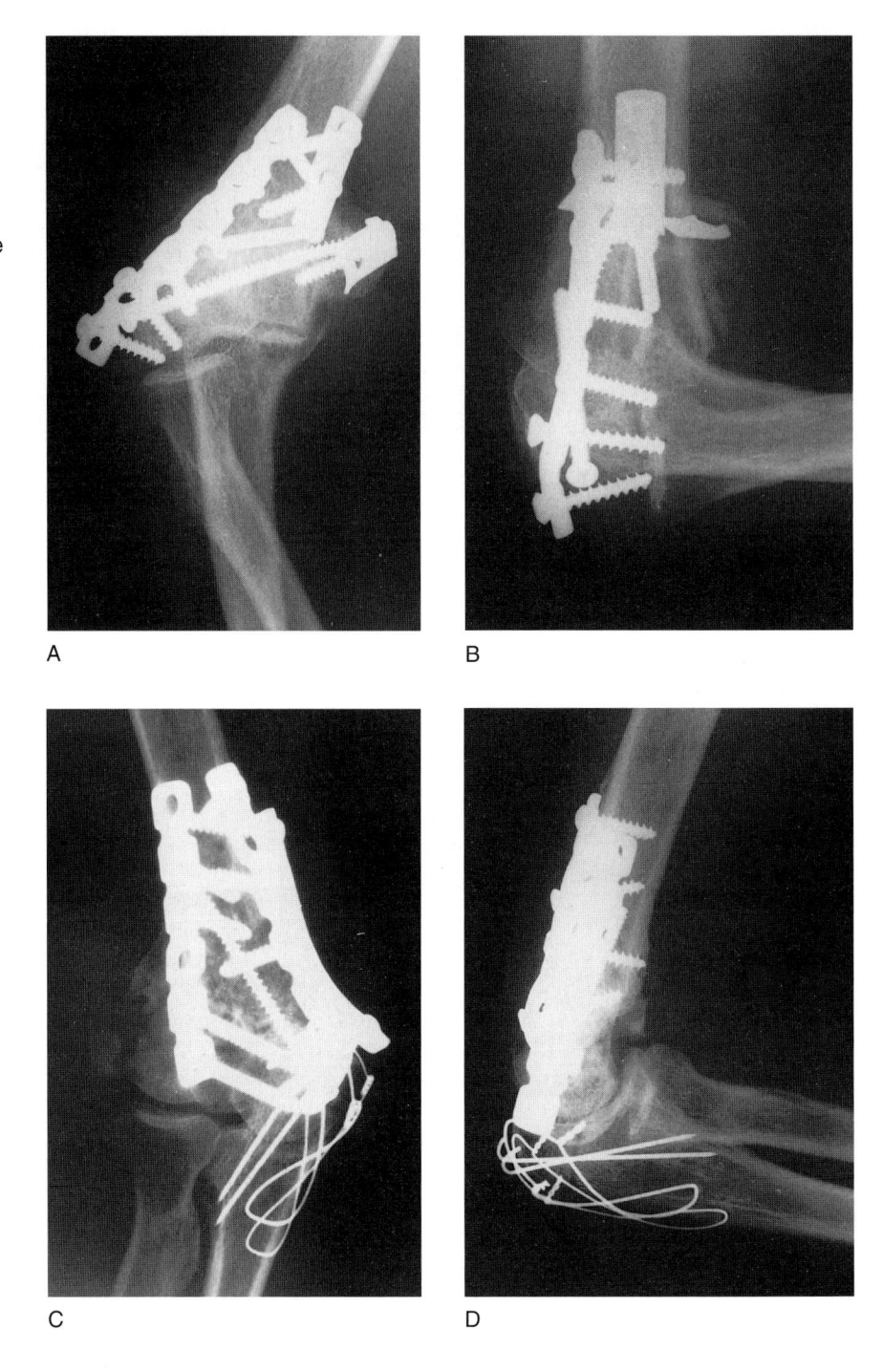

screws obtain better purchase when directed away from the fossae and into the cortical bone of the thickest portion of the columns.

The stability of the internal fixation is evaluated intraoperatively by placing the elbow through a complete range of motion and looking for movement between the fragments. A few options should be considered if inadequate stability exists following operative fixation. One alternative is to add a third plate (see Fig. 25.10).[48] The most distal screw is located distal to the lateral epicondyle and obtains purchase in the firm cancellous bone of the trochlea. This third plate achieves multiple foci of fixation oriented in numerous directions.

A second consideration is to reinforce poor screw fixation with polymethyl methacrylate.[59,65] The cement must be injected into the screw holes in a relatively liquid phase through a syringe. Next, the screw is placed into the cement, and a final turn is applied to the screw when the cement becomes firm.[59] Extrusion of cement into the fracture site should be avoided.

Despite these efforts, if stability is deemed insufficient for the initiation of early motion, the treatment options include (1) placement of a total elbow arthroplasty either as a primary procedure (if the surgeon is well versed in the technique) or as a reconstructive elective procedure and (2) supplementation with iliac crest cancellous autograft bone followed by immobilizing the limb in an above-elbow cast. A later elbow capsulectomy[17,44–47,65] may be required to help the patient to regain functional motion if healing is successful.

We prefer to fix the olecranon osteotomy with a tension-band wire construct. Two parallel Kirschner wires are inserted through the olecranon and are aimed into the anterior ulnar cortex just beyond the limit of the coronoid process. Fixation in the anterior cortex may limit the risk for pin migration. After the pins are placed satisfactorily, they are backed out slightly in anticipation of subsequent impaction of the bent tips into the olecranon. An 18- or 20-gauge wire is passed through a hole drilled in the dorsal ulnar cortex at a site that is at least as distal to the fracture as the entrance of the Kirschner wires is proximal to the fracture. Using a 14-gauge angiocatheter to facilitate wire passage, the surgeon passes this wire deep to the triceps insertion just proximal to the insertion point of the Kirschner wires. Alternatively, two separate tension-band wires can be applied with narrower (e.g., 20- or 22-gauge) wire. The tips of the Kirschner wires are bent twice at 90° so that the tip is parallel with the remainder of the wire. Using a tamp, the surgeon drives these tips into bone under small incisions in the triceps insertion.

Infected or Contaminated Fractures of the Distal Humerus

In an unpublished series of four such cases, we used an Ilizarov construct to stabilize infected or contaminated fractures of the distal humerus; two fractures were nonunions. This construct provided sufficient stability to allow functional aftercare. The Ilizarov construct consists of two posterior five-eighths rings attached by four bars. The distal ring is attached to the distal fragment with two thin olive wires; one olive is on the lateral and one olive is on the medial aspect of the distal humerus. We used olive wires so that the wires would provide some compression of articular fragments and so that the wires could be crossed at a relatively acute angle (approximately 30°) to avoid impaling muscle-tendon units, while still providing stable attachment to the distal ring. The proximal fragment is secured to the proximal ring with a second set of olive wires or, on occasion, with Schanz screws. When possible, fashioning the distal fracture surface so that it interlocks with the proximal fracture surface in a tongue-and-groove fashion improves fracture stability and enhances bony healing by means of the greater apposition of the fracture surfaces. Compression is applied across the fracture through the frame. This construct provides sufficient stability to allow functional elbow motion.

RESULTS

Very few published data document the prognosis following surgical treatment of nonunions of the proximal ulna. Our experience is similar to that of others documenting good function when skeletal continuity and alignment are restored. Among sixteen patients who had proximal ulnar nonunion treated by osteosynthesis at the Mayo Clinic, seven patients had an excellent result; three patients, a good result; four patients, a fair result; and two patients, a poor result.[19] The arc of ulnohumeral motion averaged 89°. The poor results were related to persistent nonunion and stiffness in one patient and stiffness and residual instability in the other patient.[19]

According to the Mayo Clinic experience, more than 75% of patients undergoing late resection of the radial head will have decreased pain and increased motion.[66] The results are less predictable if the radial head is resected after arthrosis has become established.[66]

Improvements in the operative approach to distal humeral nonunions have led to improved results. An early report on the treatment of ununited fractures of the distal humerus at Massachusetts General Hospital over a 16-year period was published in 1988.[67] Of the 20 patients included in this series, most patients had an extra-articular nonunion, and only 13 patients had their nonunion treated with dual-plate fixation and autogenous iliac crest bone graft. This review suggested the need for routine elbow capsulectomy because, although union was achieved frequently (94% of elbows), elbow stiffness was a common residual problem (76° average arc of ulnohumeral motion), and most patients continued to have a major long-term disability. This was particularly the case in patients who had an intra-articular fracture, because residual stiffness, instability, and residual deformity were commonplace.

A subsequent series based on the practice of the senior author (JBJ) and others have demonstrated substantial improvement in the results of operative treatment with the addition of routine elbow capsulectomy and ulnar nerve transposition and neurolysis.[48,49] One series of six patients demonstrated the benefits of operative treatment even when the patient was elderly and the fracture presented small, osteopenic distal fragments.[48] Complete anterior and posterior elbow capsulectomy restored motion and limited the stress on the fracture fixation. The addition of a third plate was used to provide sufficient stability to allow early mobilization of the elbow. All six fractures healed following the index operation, and an average of 102° of ulnohumeral motion was obtained.[48]

The reconstruction of intra-articular nonunions and malunions of the distal humerus was addressed in a series of 13 patients. The authors used osteotomy for malunion or debridement for nonunion, realignment with stable fixation and autogenous bone grafts, anterior and posterior elbow capsulectomy, ulnar nerve transposition, and neurolysis.[49] Healing occurred in all patients, and ulnohumeral motion averaged 97°. Ten of 13 patients had a good or excellent overall rating according to the scale of Broberg and Morrey.[66] The authors' experience with this technique now extends to more than 20 patients. The improved results in this series, compared with the results in the older series, were ascribed to the improved motion following capsulectomy. The presence of intra-articular malunion or nonunion did not prevent a good result owing to the restoration of normal elbow mechanics and stability following stable realignment of the articular surface. Progressive arthrosis was not demonstrated in any patient after a mean follow-up of 25 months.

The results of fixation for infected fractures of the distal humerus with an Ilizarov construct have been encouraging.[68] This technique allows early elbow motion, resulting in an average of 80° of ulnohumeral motion at an average follow-up of 2 years. Two of five patients had a fibrous union of the lateral condyle that healed following plate and screw or cannulated screw fixation. Of the five patients, one who had a vascularized fibular graft needed another operation for delayed union at the distal host graft junction. The infection was eradicated in each patient. Improvements in hand and nerve function also were achieved.

COMPLICATIONS

When elbow fracture nonunions are treated with surgery, the elbow is no more prone to infection, hematoma, and other wound problems and seems less prone to developing heterotopic ossification than when these nonunions are treated with primary fracture surgery. If the fracture fails to heal, the fixation eventually loosens, and pain, stiffness, and instability return. If the fracture heals, the most common complications are related to persistent stiffness, ulnar neuropathy, and symptomatic hardware.

Stiffness

Persistent stiffness may occur if healing is delayed, pain is slow to resolve, or postoperative immobilization is used. Passive splinting (turnbuckle) may help to restore motion in the early postinjury period after the fractures have healed.[69] Elbow capsular release has proved to be a very predictable method of restoring elbow motion, provided that no intrinsic contributions (i.e., articular incongruity or adhesions) to the contracture exist.[17,44–47]

Ulnar Neuropathy

Ulnar nerve dysfunction is one of the most common complications of operative treatment for distal humeral fractures. Our experience with reconstruction of nonunions and malunions of the distal humerus has revealed that the nerve tends to become fibrosed and adherent in the medial epicondylar region as a result of scar formation and the fracture healing response. This problem can be minimized by adequate mobilization and anterior subcutaneous transposition at the initial operation.

Mobilization of the ulnar nerve during a reconstructive operation requires careful dissection, because the nerve is typically bound up in scar and even bone. The nerve can be freed from the bone with careful application of a small osteotome. The ulnar nerve has proved remarkably responsive to neurolysis and mobilization at the time of reconstruction. Experience with reconstruction of ununited fractures of the distal humerus has proved that improvements in ulnar nerve function contribute invaluably to both pain relief and improved upper extremity function following reconstruction.

Recently, researchers reviewed the treatment results of posttraumatic ulnar neuropathy after periarticular elbow injury in the senior author's (JBJ) practice.[70] This review documented how gratifying the results of ulnar neurolysis and transposition can be in this setting for both patient and surgeon. In the 22 patients studied, the Gabel and Amadio[71] score improved from an average of 3.2 preoperatively to an average of 6.5 postoperatively, reflecting improvements in grip strength (67% of uninvolved side), lateral pinch strength (71%), and tip pinch strength (73%). On the NERVEPACE® Nerve Conduction Monitor (NeuMed®, West Trenton, NJ), motor nerve conduction velocity measured an average of 31.8 m/s of the affected side and 39.9 m/s on the unaffected side. The results were good or excellent in 20 of 22 patients, and satisfaction was high, averaging 8.0 on a 10-point visual analog scale.

Symptomatic Hardware

Distal humeral fixation devices are rarely symptomatic, but patients frequently request removal of prominent ulnar plates. Plate removal should be delayed at least 12 months (preferably 18 months) to reduce the risk of refracture.

Some authors have documented problems with tension-band wire fixation of the olecranon.[8] If fixation is performed correctly with the smooth Kirschner wires driven through the anterior ulnar cortex and bent and driven into the olecranon below the triceps insertion, proximal migration and symptomatic prominence should be uncommon.

SUMMARY

Ununited fractures about the elbow represent uncommon, but complex, reconstructive problems. Skeletal union in anatomic alignment represents the best opportunity for younger, active individuals to regain function and maintain it long term. Stable fixation is difficult to achieve, but the techniques described herein have been used with good results. Capsulectomy and ulnar nerve neurolysis may be essential to a good result, particularly in the treatment of distal humeral nonunions.

REFERENCES

1. Bickel WH, Perry RE. Comminuted fractures of the distal humerus. *JAMA* 1963;184:553–557.
2. Bryan RS, Bickel WH. "T" condylar fractures of distal humerus. *J Trauma* 1971;11:830–835.
3. Cassebaum WH. Operative treatment of T and Y fracture of the lower end of the humerus. *Am J Surg* 1952;83:265–270.
4. Evans EM. Supracondylar-Y fractures of the humerus. *J Bone Joint Surg* 1953;35B:381–385.
5. Johansson H, Olerud S. Operative treatment of intercondylar fractures of the humerus. *J Trauma* 1971;11:836–843.
6. Aitken GK, Rorabeck CH. Distal humeral fractures in the adult. *Clin Orthop* 1986;207:191–197.
7. Gabel GT, Hanson G, Bennett JB, et al. Intraarticular fractures of the distal humerus in the adult. *Clin Orthop* 1987;216:99–108.
8. Henley MB, Bone LB, Parker B. Operative management of intra-articular fractures of the distal humerus. *J Orthop Trauma* 1987;1:24–30.
9. Holdsworth BJ, Mossad MM. Fractures of the adult distal humerus. Elbow function after internal fixation. *J Bone Joint Surg* 1990;72B:362–365.
10. Jupiter JB, Neff U, Holzach P, et al. Intercondylar fractures of the humerus. An operative approach. *J Bone Joint Surg* 1985;67A:226–239.
11. Sanders RA, Sackett JR. Open reduction and internal fixation of delayed union and nonunion of the distal humerus. *J Orthop Trauma* 1990;4:254–259.
12. Waddell JP, Hatch J, Richards R. Supracondylar fractures of the humerus—results of surgical treatment. *J Trauma* 1988;28:1615–1621.
13. Mitsunaga MM, Bryan RS, Linscheid LR. Condylar nonunions of the elbow. *J Trauma* 1982;22:787–791.
14. Södergård J, Sandelin J, Böstman O. Mechanical failures of internal fixation in T and Y fractures of the distal humerus. *J Trauma* 1992;33:687–690.
15. Södergård J, Sandelin J, Böstman O. Postoperative complications of distal humeral fractures: 27/96 adults followed up for 6 (2–10) years. *Acta Orthop Scand* 1992;63:85–89.
16. Wang KC, Shih HN, Hsu KY, et al. Intercondylar fractures of the distal humerus: Routine anterior subcutaneous transposition of the ulnar nerve in a posterior operative approach. *J Trauma* 1994;36:770–773.
17. Modabber MR, Jupiter JB. Reconstruction for post-traumatic conditions of the elbow joint. *J Bone Joint Surg* 1995;77A:1431–1446.
18. Coonrad RW. Nonunion of the olecranon and proximal ulna. In: Morrey BF, ed. *The elbow and its disorders*. Philadelphia: WB Saunders; 1995:429–440.
19. Papagelopoulos PJ, Morrey BF. Treatment of nonunion of olecranon fractures. *J Bone Joint Surg* 1994;76B:627–635.
20. Biga N, Thomine JM. La luxation trans-olecranienne du coude. *Rev Chir Orthop Reparatrice Appar Mot* 1974;60:557–567.
21. Ring D, Jupiter JB, Sanders RW, et al. Transolecranon fracture–dislocation of the elbow. *J Orthop Trauma* 1997;11:545–550.
22. Jupiter JB, Leibovic SJ, Ribbans W, et al. The posterior Monteggia lesion. *J Orthop Trauma* 1991;5:395–402.
23. Pavel A, Pitman JM, Lance EM, et al. The posterior Monteggia fracture: A clinical study. *J Trauma* 1965;5:185–199.
24. Penrose JH. The Monteggia fracture with posterior dislocation of the radial head. *J Bone Joint Surg* 1951;33B:65–73.
25. Horne G, Sim P. Nonunion of the radial head. *J Trauma* 1985;25:452–453.
26. Karpinski MR. Ununited radial neck fracture. *Injury* 1982;13:447–448.
27. Middleton RW, Miles NM. A report of a case of non-union following fracture of the neck of the radius. *Injury* 1976;8:31–34.
28. Reidy JA, Van Gorder GW. Treatment of displacement of the proximal radial epiphysis. *J Bone Joint Surg* 1963;45A:1355–1372.
29. Scudder CL. *Treatment of fractures*. Philadelphia: WB Saunders, 1922:297.
30. Thomas T. Fracture of the head of the radius. *U Pa Med Bull* 1915;18:184.
31. Geel CW, Palmer AK, Rüedi T, et al. Internal fixation of proximal radial head fractures. *J Orthop Trauma* 1990;4:270–274.
32. McArthur RA. Herbert screw fixation of the head of the radius. *Clin Orthop* 1987;224:79–87.
33. Odenheimer K, Harvery JP Jr. Internal fixation of fracture of the head of the radius. Two case reports. *J Bone Joint Surg* 1979;61A:785–787.
34. Sanders RA, French HG. Open reduction and internal fixation of comminuted radial head fractures. *Am J Sports Med* 1986;14:130–135.
35. Shmueli G, Herold HZ. Compression screwing of displaced fractures of the head of the radius. *J Bone Joint Surg* 1981;63B:535–538.
36. Morrey BF, Adams RA. Semiconstrained elbow replacement for distal humeral nonunion. *J Bone Joint Surg* 1995;77B:67–72.
37. Breen T, Gelberman RH, Leffert R, et al. Massive allograft replacement of hemiarticular traumatic defects of the elbow. *J Hand Surg* 1988;13A:900–907.
38. Urbaniak JR, Black KE Jr. Cadaveric elbow allografts. A six year experience. *Clin Orthop* 1985;197:131–140.
39. Cobb TK, Morrey BF. Use of distraction arthroplasty in unstable fracture dislocations of the elbow. *Clin Orthop* 1995;312:201–210.
40. McKee MD, Richards RR, King GJW, Patterson SD, Jupiter JB. The compass elbow hinge for complex, acute elbow instability (abstract). *J Bone Joint Surg* 1997;79B(Suppl I):75.
41. McKee MD, Bowden SH, King GJ, Patterson SD, Jupiter JB, Bamberger HB, Paksima N. Management of recurrent complex instability of the elbow with a hinged external fixator. *J Bone Joint Surg Br* 1998;80:1031–1036.

42. Dowdy PA, Bain GI, King GJ, et al. The midline posterior elbow incision. An anatomical appraisal. *J Bone Joint Surg* 1995; 77B:696–699.
43. Patterson SD, King GJ, Bain GI. A posterior global approach to the elbow (abstract). *J Bone Joint Surg* 1995;77B(Suppl III): 316.
44. Gates HS III, Sullivan FL, Urbaniak JR. Anterior capsulotomy and continuous passive motion in the treatment of post-traumatic flexion contracture of the elbow. A prospective study. *J Bone Joint Surg* 1992;74A:1229–1234.
45. Husband JB, Hastings H II. The lateral approach for operative release of posttraumatic contracture of the elbow. *J Bone Joint Surg* 1990;72A:1353–1358.
46. Morrey BF. Post-traumatic contracture of the elbow. Operative treatment, including distraction arthroplasty. *J Bone Joint Surg* 1990;72A:601–618.
47. Urbaniak JR, Hansen PE, Beissinger SF, et al. Correction of post-traumatic flexion contracture of the elbow by anterior capsulotomy. *J Bone Joint Surg* 1985;67A:1160–1164.
48. Jupiter JB, Goodman LJ. The management of complex distal humerus nonunion in the elderly by elbow capsulectomy, triple plating, and ulnar nerve neurolysis. *J Shoulder Elbow Surg* 1992;1:37–46.
49. McKee MD, Jupiter JB, Toh CL, et al. Reconstruction after malunion and nonunion of intra-articular fractures of the distal humerus. Methods and results in 13 adults. *J Bone Joint Surg* 1994;76B:614–621.
50. Mast J, Jakob RP, Ganz R. *Planning and reduction techniques in fracture surgery.* Heidelberg: Springer-Verlag; 1979.
51. Simpson NS, Goodman LA, Jupiter JB. Contoured LCDC plating of the proximal ulna. *Injury* 1996;27:411–417.
52. Cohen MS, Hastings H II. Rotatory instability of the elbow: The anatomy and role of the lateral stabilizers. *J Bone Joint Surg* 1997;79A:225–233.
53. Nestor BJ, O'Driscoll SW, Morrey BF. Ligamentous reconstruction for posterolateral rotatory instability of the elbow. *J Bone Joint Surg* 1992;74A:1235–1241.
54. O'Driscoll SW, Bell DF, Morrey BF. Posterolateral rotatory instability of the elbow. *J Bone Joint Surg* 1991;73A:440–446.
55. Kocher T. *Text book of operative surgery.* London: Adam and Charles Black; 1911.
56. Hotchkiss RN. Displaced fractures of the radial head: Internal fixation or excision. *J Am Acad Orthop Surg* 1997;5:1–10.
57. Strachan JC, Ellis BW. Vulnerability of the posterior interosseous nerve during radial head resection. *J Bone Joint Surg* 1971;53B:320–323.
58. Sunderland S. Metrical and nonmetrical features of the muscular branches of the radial nerve. *J Comp Neurol* 1946;85: 93–97.
59. Müller ME, Allgöwer M, Schneider R, Willenegger H, eds. *Manual of internal fixation: Techniques recommended by the AO-ASIF group,* 3rd ed. Berlin: Springer-Verlag; 1991.
60. Helfet DL, Hotchkiss RN. Internal fixation of the distal humerus: A biomechanical comparison of methods. *J Orthop Trauma* 1990;4:260–264.
61. Kirk P, Goulet JA, Freiberg A, et al. A biomechanical evaluation of fixation methods for fractures of the distal humerus. *Orthop Trans* 1990;14:674.
62. Schemitsch EH, Tencer AF, Henley MB. Biomechanical evaluation of methods of internal fixation of the distal humerus. *J Orthop Trauma* 1994;8:468–475.
63. Self J, Viegas SF, Buford WL Jr, et al. A comparison of double-plate fixation methods for complex distal humerus fractures. *J Shoulder Elbow Surg* 1995;4:10–16.
64. Jupiter JB, Mehne DK. Fractures of the distal humerus. *Orthopedics* 1992;15:825–833.
65. Jupiter JB. Complex fractures of the distal part of the humerus and associated complications. *J Bone Joint Surg* 1994;76A: 1252–1264.
66. Broberg MA, Morrey BF. Results of delayed excision of the radial head after fracture. *J Bone Joint Surg* 1986;68A:669–674.
67. Ackerman G, Jupiter JB. Non-union of fractures of the distal end of the humerus. *J Bone Joint Surg* 1988;70A:75–83.
68. Ring D, Jupiter JB, Toh S. Salvage of contaminated fractures of the distal humerus with thin wire external fixation. *Clin Orthop* 1999;359:203–208.
69. Green DP, McCoy H. Turnbuckle orthotic correction of elbow-flexion contractures after acute injuries. *J Bone Joint Surg* 1979;61A:1092–1095.
70. McKee MD, Jupiter JB, Bosse G, Goodman L. Outcome of ulnar neurolysis during post-traumatic reconstruction of the elbow. *J Bone Joint Surg Br* 1998;80:100–105.
71. Gabel GT, Amadio PC. Reoperation for failed decompression of the ulnar nerve in the region of the elbow. *J Bone Joint Surg* 1990;72A:213–219.

SUMMARY

Ununited fractures about the elbow represent uncommon, but complex, reconstructive problems. Skeletal union in anatomic alignment represents the best opportunity for younger, active individuals to regain function and maintain it long term. Stable fixation is difficult to achieve, but the techniques described herein have been used with good results. Capsulectomy and ulnar nerve neurolysis may be essential to a good result, particularly in the treatment of distal humeral nonunions.

REFERENCES

1. Bickel WH, Perry RE. Comminuted fractures of the distal humerus. *JAMA* 1963;184:553–557.
2. Bryan RS, Bickel WH. "T" condylar fractures of distal humerus. *J Trauma* 1971;11:830–835.
3. Cassebaum WH. Operative treatment of T and Y fracture of the lower end of the humerus. *Am J Surg* 1952;83:265–270.
4. Evans EM. Supracondylar-Y fractures of the humerus. *J Bone Joint Surg* 1953;35B:381–385.
5. Johansson H, Olerud S. Operative treatment of intercondylar fractures of the humerus. *J Trauma* 1971;11:836–843.
6. Aitken GK, Rorabeck CH. Distal humeral fractures in the adult. *Clin Orthop* 1986;207:191–197.
7. Gabel GT, Hanson G, Bennett JB, et al. Intraarticular fractures of the distal humerus in the adult. *Clin Orthop* 1987;216:99–108.
8. Henley MB, Bone LB, Parker B. Operative management of intra-articular fractures of the distal humerus. *J Orthop Trauma* 1987;1:24–30.
9. Holdsworth BJ, Mossad MM. Fractures of the adult distal humerus. Elbow function after internal fixation. *J Bone Joint Surg* 1990;72B:362–365.
10. Jupiter JB, Neff U, Holzach P, et al. Intercondylar fractures of the humerus. An operative approach. *J Bone Joint Surg* 1985;67A:226–239.
11. Sanders RA, Sackett JR. Open reduction and internal fixation of delayed union and nonunion of the distal humerus. *J Orthop Trauma* 1990;4:254–259.
12. Waddell JP, Hatch J, Richards R. Supracondylar fractures of the humerus—results of surgical treatment. *J Trauma* 1988;28:1615–1621.
13. Mitsunaga MM, Bryan RS, Linscheid LR. Condylar nonunions of the elbow. *J Trauma* 1982;22:787–791.
14. Södergård J, Sandelin J, Böstman O. Mechanical failures of internal fixation in T and Y fractures of the distal humerus. *J Trauma* 1992;33:687–690.
15. Södergård J, Sandelin J, Böstman O. Postoperative complications of distal humeral fractures: 27/96 adults followed up for 6 (2–10) years. *Acta Orthop Scand* 1992;63:85–89.
16. Wang KC, Shih HN, Hsu KY, et al. Intercondylar fractures of the distal humerus: Routine anterior subcutaneous transposition of the ulnar nerve in a posterior operative approach. *J Trauma* 1994;36:770–773.
17. Modabber MR, Jupiter JB. Reconstruction for post-traumatic conditions of the elbow joint. *J Bone Joint Surg* 1995;77A:1431–1446.
18. Coonrad RW. Nonunion of the olecranon and proximal ulna. In: Morrey BF, ed. *The elbow and its disorders*. Philadelphia: WB Saunders; 1995:429–440.
19. Papagelopoulos PJ, Morrey BF. Treatment of nonunion of olecranon fractures. *J Bone Joint Surg* 1994;76B:627–635.
20. Biga N, Thomine JM. La luxation trans-olecranienne du coude. *Rev Chir Orthop Reparatrice Appar Mot* 1974;60:557–567.
21. Ring D, Jupiter JB, Sanders RW, et al. Transolecranon fracture–dislocation of the elbow. *J Orthop Trauma* 1997;11:545–550.
22. Jupiter JB, Leibovic SJ, Ribbans W, et al. The posterior Monteggia lesion. *J Orthop Trauma* 1991;5:395–402.
23. Pavel A, Pitman JM, Lance EM, et al. The posterior Monteggia fracture: A clinical study. *J Trauma* 1965;5:185–199.
24. Penrose JH. The Monteggia fracture with posterior dislocation of the radial head. *J Bone Joint Surg* 1951;33B:65–73.
25. Horne G, Sim P. Nonunion of the radial head. *J Trauma* 1985;25:452–453.
26. Karpinski MR. Ununited radial neck fracture. *Injury* 1982;13:447–448.
27. Middleton RW, Miles NM. A report of a case of non-union following fracture of the neck of the radius. *Injury* 1976;8:31–34.
28. Reidy JA, Van Gorder GW. Treatment of displacement of the proximal radial epiphysis. *J Bone Joint Surg* 1963;45A:1355–1372.
29. Scudder CL. *Treatment of fractures*. Philadelphia: WB Saunders, 1922:297.
30. Thomas T. Fracture of the head of the radius. *U Pa Med Bull* 1915;18:184.
31. Geel CW, Palmer AK, Rüedi T, et al. Internal fixation of proximal radial head fractures. *J Orthop Trauma* 1990;4:270–274.
32. McArthur RA. Herbert screw fixation of the head of the radius. *Clin Orthop* 1987;224:79–87.
33. Odenheimer K, Harvery JP Jr. Internal fixation of fracture of the head of the radius. Two case reports. *J Bone Joint Surg* 1979;61A:785–787.
34. Sanders RA, French HG. Open reduction and internal fixation of comminuted radial head fractures. *Am J Sports Med* 1986;14:130–135.
35. Shmueli G, Herold HZ. Compression screwing of displaced fractures of the head of the radius. *J Bone Joint Surg* 1981;63B:535–538.
36. Morrey BF, Adams RA. Semiconstrained elbow replacement for distal humeral nonunion. *J Bone Joint Surg* 1995;77B:67–72.
37. Breen T, Gelberman RH, Leffert R, et al. Massive allograft replacement of hemiarticular traumatic defects of the elbow. *J Hand Surg* 1988;13A:900–907.
38. Urbaniak JR, Black KE Jr. Cadaveric elbow allografts. A six year experience. *Clin Orthop* 1985;197:131–140.
39. Cobb TK, Morrey BF. Use of distraction arthroplasty in unstable fracture dislocations of the elbow. *Clin Orthop* 1995;312:201–210.
40. McKee MD, Richards RR, King GJW, Patterson SD, Jupiter JB. The compass elbow hinge for complex, acute elbow instability (abstract). *J Bone Joint Surg* 1997;79B(Suppl I):75.
41. McKee MD, Bowden SH, King GJ, Patterson SD, Jupiter JB, Bamberger HB, Paksima N. Management of recurrent complex instability of the elbow with a hinged external fixator. *J Bone Joint Surg Br* 1998;80:1031–1036.

42. Dowdy PA, Bain GI, King GJ, et al. The midline posterior elbow incision. An anatomical appraisal. *J Bone Joint Surg* 1995; 77B:696–699.
43. Patterson SD, King GJ, Bain GI. A posterior global approach to the elbow (abstract). *J Bone Joint Surg* 1995;77B(Suppl III): 316.
44. Gates HS III, Sullivan FL, Urbaniak JR. Anterior capsulotomy and continuous passive motion in the treatment of post-traumatic flexion contracture of the elbow. A prospective study. *J Bone Joint Surg* 1992;74A:1229–1234.
45. Husband JB, Hastings H II. The lateral approach for operative release of posttraumatic contracture of the elbow. *J Bone Joint Surg* 1990;72A:1353–1358.
46. Morrey BF. Post-traumatic contracture of the elbow. Operative treatment, including distraction arthroplasty. *J Bone Joint Surg* 1990;72A:601–618.
47. Urbaniak JR, Hansen PE, Beissinger SF, et al. Correction of post-traumatic flexion contracture of the elbow by anterior capsulotomy. *J Bone Joint Surg* 1985;67A:1160–1164.
48. Jupiter JB, Goodman LJ. The management of complex distal humerus nonunion in the elderly by elbow capsulectomy, triple plating, and ulnar nerve neurolysis. *J Shoulder Elbow Surg* 1992;1:37–46.
49. McKee MD, Jupiter JB, Toh CL, et al. Reconstruction after malunion and nonunion of intra-articular fractures of the distal humerus. Methods and results in 13 adults. *J Bone Joint Surg* 1994;76B:614–621.
50. Mast J, Jakob RP, Ganz R. *Planning and reduction techniques in fracture surgery*. Heidelberg: Springer-Verlag; 1979.
51. Simpson NS, Goodman LA, Jupiter JB. Contoured LCDC plating of the proximal ulna. *Injury* 1996;27:411–417.
52. Cohen MS, Hastings H II. Rotatory instability of the elbow: The anatomy and role of the lateral stabilizers. *J Bone Joint Surg* 1997;79A:225–233.
53. Nestor BJ, O'Driscoll SW, Morrey BF. Ligamentous reconstruction for posterolateral rotatory instability of the elbow. *J Bone Joint Surg* 1992;74A:1235–1241.
54. O'Driscoll SW, Bell DF, Morrey BF. Posterolateral rotatory instability of the elbow. *J Bone Joint Surg* 1991;73A:440–446.
55. Kocher T. *Text book of operative surgery*. London: Adam and Charles Black; 1911.
56. Hotchkiss RN. Displaced fractures of the radial head: Internal fixation or excision. *J Am Acad Orthop Surg* 1997;5:1–10.
57. Strachan JC, Ellis BW. Vulnerability of the posterior interosseous nerve during radial head resection. *J Bone Joint Surg* 1971;53B:320–323.
58. Sunderland S. Metrical and nonmetrical features of the muscular branches of the radial nerve. *J Comp Neurol* 1946;85: 93–97.
59. Müller ME, Allgöwer M, Schneider R, Willenegger H, eds. *Manual of internal fixation: Techniques recommended by the AO-ASIF group*, 3rd ed. Berlin: Springer-Verlag; 1991.
60. Helfet DL, Hotchkiss RN. Internal fixation of the distal humerus: A biomechanical comparison of methods. *J Orthop Trauma* 1990;4:260–264.
61. Kirk P, Goulet JA, Freiberg A, et al. A biomechanical evaluation of fixation methods for fractures of the distal humerus. *Orthop Trans* 1990;14:674.
62. Schemitsch EH, Tencer AF, Henley MB. Biomechanical evaluation of methods of internal fixation of the distal humerus. *J Orthop Trauma* 1994;8:468–475.
63. Self J, Viegas SF, Buford WL Jr, et al. A comparison of double-plate fixation methods for complex distal humerus fractures. *J Shoulder Elbow Surg* 1995;4:10–16.
64. Jupiter JB, Mehne DK. Fractures of the distal humerus. *Orthopedics* 1992;15:825–833.
65. Jupiter JB. Complex fractures of the distal part of the humerus and associated complications. *J Bone Joint Surg* 1994;76A: 1252–1264.
66. Broberg MA, Morrey BF. Results of delayed excision of the radial head after fracture. *J Bone Joint Surg* 1986;68A:669–674.
67. Ackerman G, Jupiter JB. Non-union of fractures of the distal end of the humerus. *J Bone Joint Surg* 1988;70A:75–83.
68. Ring D, Jupiter JB, Toh S. Salvage of contaminated fractures of the distal humerus with thin wire external fixation. *Clin Orthop* 1999;359:203–208.
69. Green DP, McCoy H. Turnbuckle orthotic correction of elbow-flexion contractures after acute injuries. *J Bone Joint Surg* 1979;61A:1092–1095.
70. McKee MD, Jupiter JB, Bosse G, Goodman L. Outcome of ulnar neurolysis during post-traumatic reconstruction of the elbow. *J Bone Joint Surg Br* 1998;80:100–105.
71. Gabel GT, Amadio PC. Reoperation for failed decompression of the ulnar nerve in the region of the elbow. *J Bone Joint Surg* 1990;72A:213–219.

CHAPTER 26

Elbow Contracture Release: Open Operative Strategies

Kenneth J. Faber and Graham J.W. King

INTRODUCTION

Elbow stiffness is an uncommon problem that can interfere with a patient's ability to perform activities of daily living. The elbow's primary function is to position and stabilize the hand in space. Unfortunately, patients do not tolerate elbow stiffness well because adjacent joints cannot provide adequate compensatory motion. Morrey et al. showed that a functional arc of motion from 30° to 130° of elbow flexion is required to perform most activities of daily living.[1] Patients who have elbow stiffness have varying degrees of impairment in functional abilities, depending on the location in the arc of motion and the magnitude of the contracture. A recent study of volunteers with healthy elbows revealed an ability to adapt to an arc of 70° to 120° for 12 activities of daily living.[2] In spite of the marked stiffness that can be tolerated when adjacent joints have full motion, most patients report functional disability and request treatment when flexion contractures approach 40°. Patients who have an arc of motion from 40° to 120° rarely require surgery unless their employment or athletic activity specifically requires terminal elbow flexion or extension.

In this chapter, we focus on operative treatment of elbow contracture. We discuss open capsular release and distraction interposition arthroplasty.

ETIOLOGY

Contractures of the elbow are encountered most frequently following elbow trauma.[3-10] In Mohan's report on 200 patients who had elbow ankylosis, 38% of the patients had a previous fracture–dislocation, 30% had isolated fractures, and 20% had a previous dislocation.[11] Elbow contractures also are seen in patients who have inflammatory, degenerative, or septic arthritis.[12,13] The presence of an underlying head injury is associated with the formation of an elbow contracture.[4,14-16] Congenital contractures of the elbow are rare; arthrogryposis is the most frequent cause. Paralytic contractures are seen most frequently in older patients following a cerebral vascular accident and in younger patients who have cerebral palsy. In the past, upper limb burns were a frequent cause of elbow contractures; however, now, they cause contractures less frequently due to rapid joint mobilization in these patients.[17-19]

The severity of elbow contractures following elbow dislocations has been correlated with a greater duration of immobilization following reduction.[20] In the series of simple elbow dislocations by Mehlhoff et al., 15% of the patients treated with closed reduction had a residual flexion contracture of more than 30°.[21] In recent years, one goal of operative treatment of displaced elbow fractures in adults has been to minimize stiffness by providing internal fixation that is sufficiently stable to allow early postoperative mobilization.

CLASSIFICATION

Elbow stiffness can be classified by etiology, pathoanatomy, and location of stiffness within the arc of motion. Contracture pathoanatomy can be extrinsic to the joint, intrinsic to the joint, or mixed.[9] Extrinsic contractures do not involve the joint; they are the most common type and arise in the soft tissue, bone, or both. Extrinsic causes include heterotopic ossification following closed head injuries, burns, or elbow fracture–dislocations. Intrinsic contractures involve intra-articular adhesions with articular cartilage destruction. Regardless of cause, almost all stiff elbows have a thickened anterior and posterior elbow capsule. With the development of elbow stiffness, secondary contractures of the collateral ligaments and muscles around the elbow can occur. Hastings and Graham proposed a classification for heterotopic ossification of the elbow. Type I heterotopic ossification involves no functional deficits, type II results in some functional deficits, and type III results in elbow ankylosis.[22] Only ankylosis or a functional loss of flexion–extension or pro-supination must be treated surgically.

EVALUATION

When evaluating a patient who has elbow stiffness, the physician should take an appropriate history, physical examination, and imaging before proceeding with treatment. The duration, as well as any possible progression, of symptoms should be determined. The cause of the contracture is usually clear from the history. The physician should determine the impact of the contracture on the patient's elbow function, as well as any limitation of activities of daily living. Any previous treatment of the contracture, including duration and appropriateness of physical therapy or surgery, should be noted. The presence of residual internal fixation devices and the history of any remote infection should be considered when planning treatment.

The physical examination should include a general physical evaluation and a focused evaluation of the involved joint and adjacent joints in the upper extremity. The skin should be examined, and any previous incisions, skin grafts, or areas of wound breakdown should be noted. Before considering surgical release of an elbow contracture, the surgeon must ensure that the patient has an adequate soft-tissue envelope. Elbow motion should be measured with a goniometer, and joint stability should be evaluated. Where appropriate, active and passive motion should be compared. The surgeon carefully evaluates motor strength of the upper limb muscles. A joint without adequate strength is unlikely to maintain motion following an elbow release; in fact, the patient may become more disabled as a result of weakness induced by the surgical procedure. A neurologic examination should be performed, because many patients who have traumatic and inflammatory elbow contractures have associated involvement of the ulnar nerve, which often requires treatment at the time of surgery.

Imaging studies of the elbow should be performed before proceeding with operative treatment. Anteroposterior, lateral, and oblique radiographs of the elbow provide most of the information about the cause and appropriate management of the contracture. Spiral tomography or computed tomography scanning should be employed in selected cases to evaluate the extent of articular congruity and in other cases to evaluate the extent and location of heterotopic ossification around the elbow. Magnetic resonance imaging may be useful in identifying soft-tissue problems that have caused the contracture and in identifying any associated loose bodies. Nerve conduction studies and electromyography should be considered if associated neurologic involvement of the upper limb is present. Technetium bone scans have not been useful in predicting the chances of heterotopic ossification recurring after excision.[22] Before making a decision to procede with surgery, we consider the length of time elapsed since injury and the radiographic maturity of the heterotopic bone. The persistence of a functional brain injury has been correlated with the risk of heterotopic ossification.[4,14–16] The surgeon must assess the patient's understanding of his or her disability and must assess the potential for patient compliance if treatment is initiated.

NONOPERATIVE MANAGEMENT

Nonoperative management of elbow stiffness can be successful if it is initiated during the first year after onset of the contracture; however, most improvement is achieved if treatment is initiated within the first 6 months. The best outcome for nonoperative treatment of a contracture occurs if the contracture is of recent onset and if the endpoint of the range of motion is springy.[23] In contrast, if the range-of-motion endpoint is firm and painless, nonoperative treatment likely will be unsuccessful.

In the nonoperative treatment of elbow contractures, researchers have proposed various strategies, including physical therapy with active-assisted range of motion, manipulation under anesthesia, serial casting, static-progressive splinting, and dynamic splinting.[23–28] Static-progressive splinting involves the application of a molded thermoplastic splint at a fixed flexion or extension angle (Fig. 26.1). The angle of the splint is adjusted periodi-

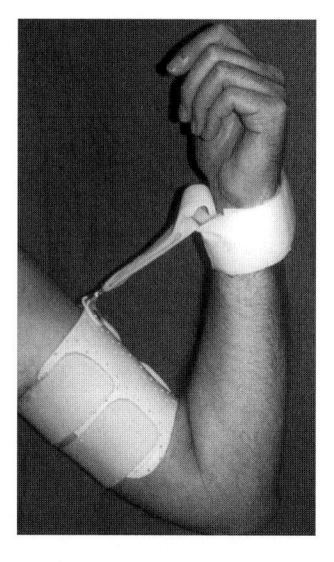

FIGURE 26.1. Static-progressive flexion splint made in our rehabilitation department. The patient adjusts the Velcro strap on the two-part flexion splint to provide a gentle passive stretch to the elbow.

cally as elbow motion improves. Dynamic splinting involves the use of a splint with a spring mechanism that the patient can adjust throughout the day to regain motion. Both splinting techniques have been demonstrated to be efficacious, and one technique is not superior to the other.[23,24]

Some authors warn that passive range-of-motion exercises that are too aggressive can result in increased stiffness, swelling, and pain and possibly in the development of heterotopic ossification.[14,29] Other authors have reported success with manipulation of stiff elbows.[25] However, most authors recommend against passive stretching due to the risk of heterotopic ossification and periarticular fractures.[13] If signs of elbow inflammation develop, the physical therapy program should be tapered, passive manipulation should be avoided, and efforts should be directed toward minimizing edema. The use of ice and nonsteroidal anti-inflammatory drugs can be helpful. Use of mild, nonnarcotic analgesics often enables a patient to wear the splint through the night.

Our preferred nonoperative treatment consists of active-assisted range of motion under the supervision of an experienced physical therapist and the use of splinting. Static-progressive splinting in the flexed and extended positions should be used between therapy periods. Although the duration of splinting required for management of the contracture is not known, we recommend a 20-hour cycle alternating flexion with extension splinting and four 1-hour periods involving active motion exercises without the splint. Through the night, the patient wears the splint in the direction where motion is most lacking.

A modification to static-progressive splinting is the addition of a turnbuckle to the orthosis (Fig. 26.2).[23] The patient controls the force in the turnbuckle to allow gradual, progressive stretching of the elbow joint. Note that as patients gain motion in one direction they often lose motion in the opposite direction. Therefore, treatment of any elbow contracture must focus on range of motion in both directions to achieve an optimal result.

OPERATIVE MANAGEMENT

Arthroscopic Capsular Release

Nowicki and Shall first reported on arthroscopic release of the stiff elbow in 1992.[30] Subsequently, other authors have reported their experience with larger series.[31,32] The indications, technique, and outcome of arthroscopic capsular release are discussed in detail in Chapter 17.

Open Capsular Release

The key to a successful outcome for an open capsular release involves adequate surgical exposure and the systematic evaluation of all potential structures and underlying abnormalities that may be impeding motion. Various approaches for joint exposure have been described and include anterior, lateral, and medial approaches.[6,7,10,33]

Urbaniak et al. popularized an anterior capsulotomy using an anterior (Henry) approach for release of elbow flexion contractures.[10] If necessary, release of the anterior portions of the lateral and medial collateral ligaments can be performed to improve extension. Lengthening of the biceps and release of the brachialis can be performed through this approach in selected cases of more severe contractures. Although this procedure may be useful in patients who have an isolated flexion contracture due to scarring of the anterior capsule, it does not allow for exposure of the ulnar nerve or for treatment of abnormalities in the posterior capsule without a second incision. In addition, Urbaniak et al. reported reduced postoperative

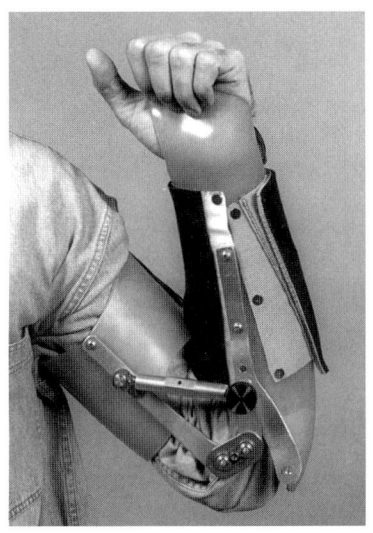

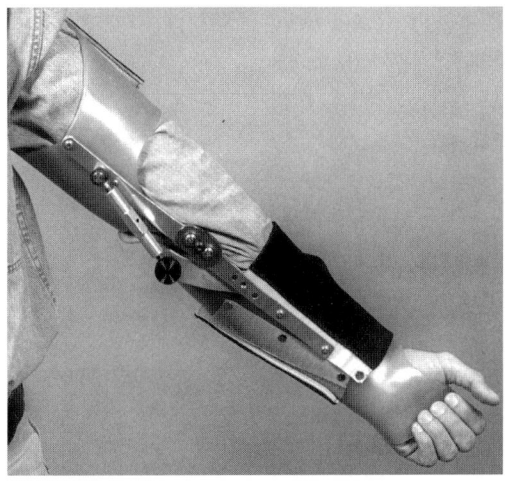

FIGURE 26.2. Turnbuckle splint. The custom turnbuckle orthosis has an adjustable bolt to provide patient-controlled, passive stretching of the elbow. The device is used both for elbow flexion (A) and extension (B) by changing the attachment site of the bolt.

elbow flexion with this approach; therefore, the approach has limited clinical usefulness.[10]

The lateral surgical approach has become increasingly popular for the management of elbow contractures (Fig. 26.3).[6,7] For milder contractures, surgery can be done through a limited approach, elevating the brachialis, brachioradialis, and extensor carpi radialis longus off the lateral supracondylar ridge to expose and excise the anterior capsule. The lateral approach enables the surgeon to expose the posterior aspect of the elbow between the anconeus and extensor carpi ulnaris without a supplemental incision. If olecranon osteophytes or loose bodies in the olecranon fossa are restricting extension, they can be excised. If the posterior capsule is restricting flexion, it can be excised.

Hotchkiss et al. popularized the use of a medial approach for the treatment of patients who have established elbow contracture (Fig. 26.4).[33] After isolation of the ulnar nerve, excellent exposure of the anterior aspect of the elbow can be achieved between the flexor carpi ulnaris and the pronator teres. After displacing the ulnar nerve anteriorly, the surgeon can view the posterior aspect of the elbow by elevating the triceps, and he or she can remove the posterior capsular tissues under direct visualization.

No authors have compared surgical techniques used for open capsular release of the elbow. To treat uncomplicated extrinsic contractures, we prefer to use a lateral ligament-sparing approach that Hastings and Cohen recently reported.[6] If the underlying abnormality is more extensive, the surgeon should choose an approach that allows all the relevant abnormality to be treated. The isolated use of one approach may not be the best choice in all patients. We advocate the use of a midline posterior skin incision in patients who have elbow contractures.[34] The skin flaps can be elevated on the deep fascial plane to protect adjacent cutaneous nerves while allowing wide exposure of both the medial and lateral aspects of the elbow joint, as needed. This incision avoids the need for both a medial and lateral incision.

In each case, the procedure must be individualized and may require more than one type of surgical intervention to ensure an optimal outcome. For example, if the elbow will not fully flex following a posterior capsular release, the surgeon should consider the anterior structures, such as an impinging coronoid osteophyte or loose body within the coronoid fossa. After each surgical intervention, elbow motion is reevaluated, and additional interventions are accomplished until a satisfactory arc of motion is achieved. An important principle to remember is that the postoperative range of motion is never greater, and is usually less, than that achieved at the time of surgery.

In general, the anterior or posterior elbow capsule needs to be excised. The triceps and brachialis often are scarred down to the distal humerus, and subperiosteal el-

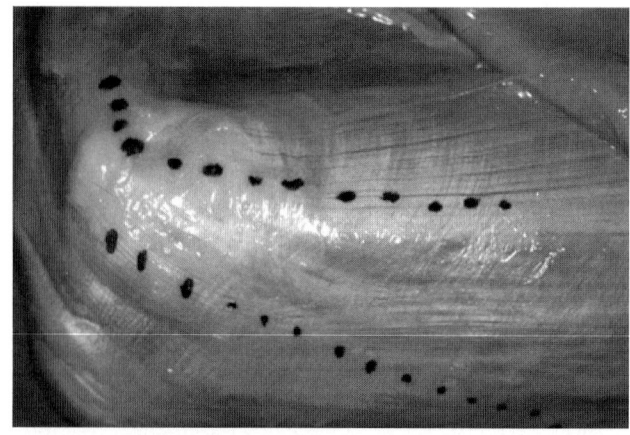

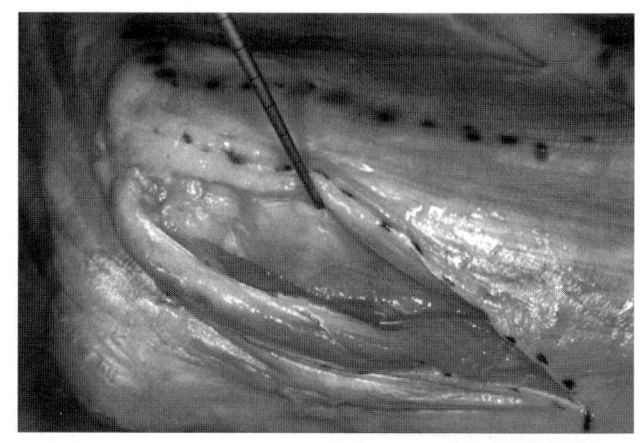

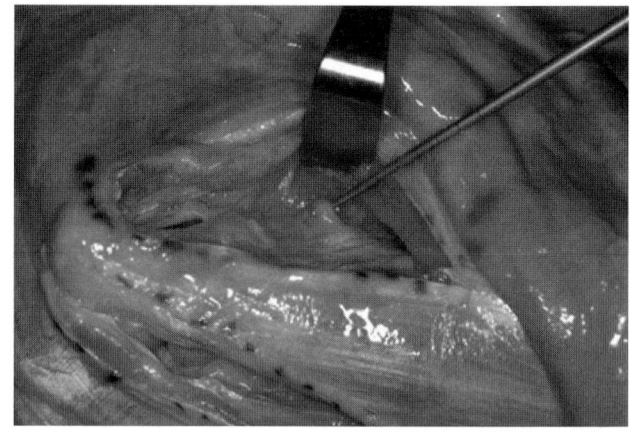

FIGURE 26.3. Lateral approach. (A) A posterior incision is made, and a full-thickness fasciocutaneous flap is elevated to expose the lateral musculature. (B) The interval between the anconeus and extensor carpi ulnaris muscles is developed to expose the radiocapitellar joint and the posterior capsule. (C) The interval between the extensor carpi radialis longus and extensor digitorum communis is developed to expose the anterior capsule. Note the proximity of the posterior interosseous nerve. The lateral ulnar collateral ligament is protected between the posterior and anterior exposures.

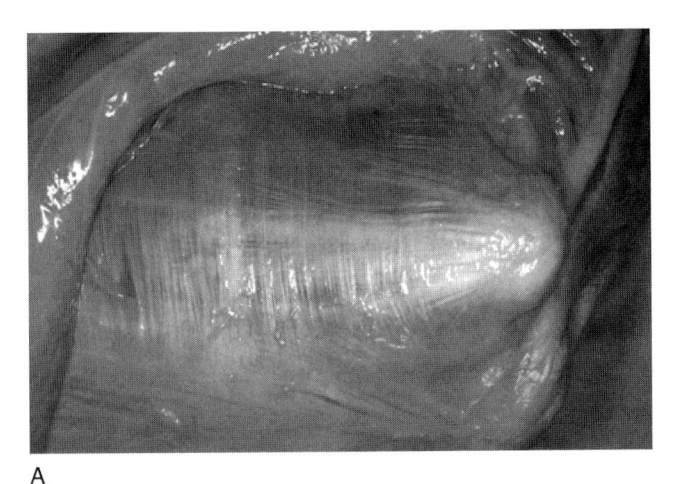

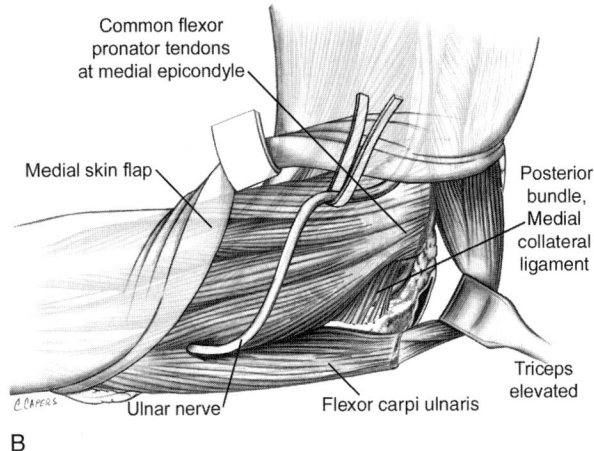

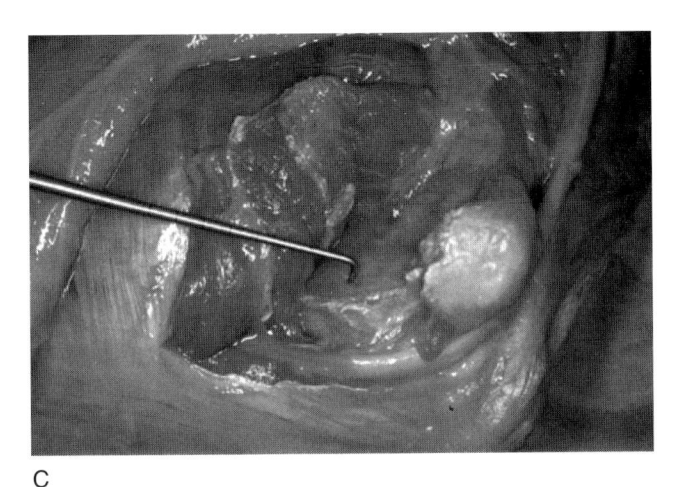

FIGURE 26.4. Medial approach. (A) The posterior incision allows for elevation of a medial skin flap and exposure of medial structures. (B) The ulnar nerve is mobilized and protected. (C) The anterior aspect of the elbow is exposed by developing the interval between the flexor carpi ulnaris and pronator teres. The biceps and brachialis are retracted anteriorly. The posterior aspect of the elbow is exposed by elevating the triceps posteriorly.

evation of these muscles may be necessary to achieve improved joint motion. Only rarely is fractional or step-cut lengthening of the elbow musculature required to achieve motion in elbows with a posttraumatic contracture. All heterotopic bone should be excised through an appropriate surgical approach. Commonly, the tip of the olecranon or coronoid needs to be removed to allow full extension or flexion, respectively. Bone wax is applied to bleeding cancellous surfaces to minimize postoperative hematoma formation.

Portions of the collateral ligaments are released when necessary to achieve elbow motion, particularly in patients who have more severe contractures. The posterior bundle of the medial collateral ligament is not isometric, and it often needs to be released in patients who have persistent limitation of elbow flexion in spite of capsular release.[13] Controlled partial surgical release of the collateral ligaments is preferable to intraoperative disruption by manipulation. The surgeon must intraoperatively evaluate elbow stability following partial division of collateral ligaments, and, if instability is identified, he or she should consider applying an articulated external fixator or postoperative protection in a hinged orthosis.

The Mayo distraction device (Howmedica, East Rutherford, NJ) is an articulated external fixator that is useful for treating the unstable elbow (Fig. 26.5).[13] After the surgeon isolates and protects the ulnar nerve, he or she places a threaded transfixion pin through the axis of rotation of the elbow joint under fluoroscopic control. The elbow is reduced, and an alignment guide is used for placement of the ulnar transfixion pins. The pin clusters are linked with medial and lateral bars that rotate about the humeral pin.

The compass universal hinge (Smith and Nephew, Memphis, TN) is a newer device that relies on the placement of a temporary transfixion pin through the axis of rotation in the distal humerus (Fig. 26.6). Definitive fixation is achieved with half-pins placed remote to the joint. Fluoroscopy is used to ensure appropriate application of the hinge. The surgeon places three pins in the humerus and two to three pins in the ulna. Following application of the hinge, the distal humeral transfixion pin is removed.

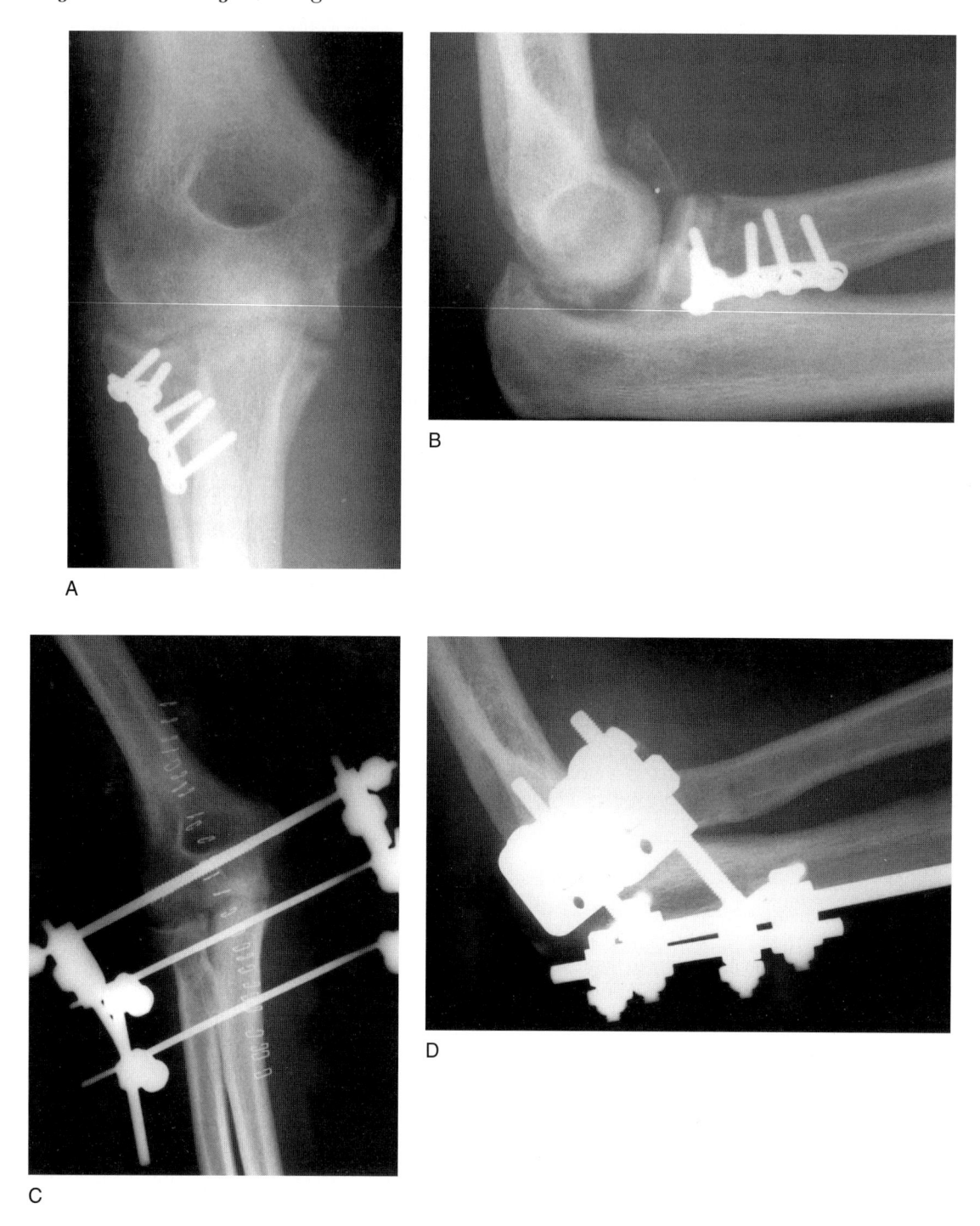

FIGURE 26.5. Mayo distraction device. **(A)** Anteroposterior (AP) radiograph of a 21-year-old man 1 year after open reduction and internal fixation of a radial neck fracture in association with an elbow dislocation. The patient has a flexion–extension arc from 60° to 90°, pronation of 50°, and no supination of the elbow and forearm. **(B)** Lateral radiograph demonstrating extensive heterotopic ossification. **(C)** Postoperative AP radiograph following excision of heterotopic bone and application of Mayo distraction device to control posterolateral rotatory instability induced by the surgical release. **(D)** Lateral radiograph following excision of heterotopic bone and debridement of the radial head. (*Continues*)

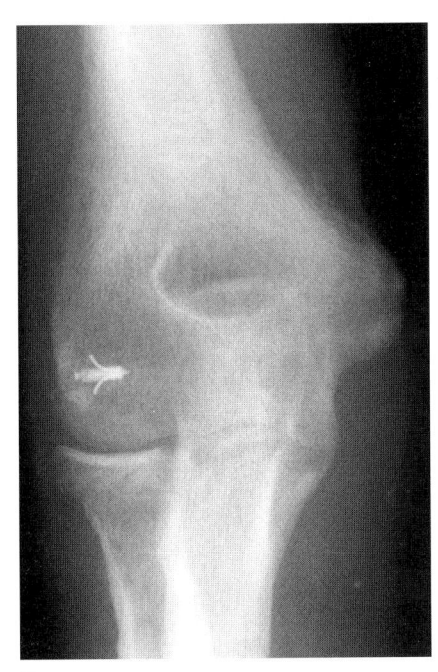

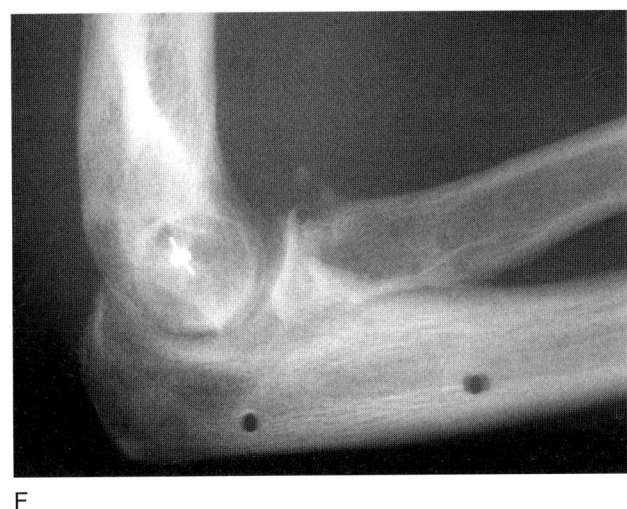

FIGURE 26.5. (*Continued*) Mayo distraction device. (E) AP radiograph following removal of the external fixation device 6 weeks after surgery. (F) Lateral radiograph after removal of the external fixation device.

Removal of internal fixation at the time of elbow contracture release is controversial. Some authors have suggested that hardware removal leads to a higher risk of stiffness and recurrent heterotopic ossification; however, we have not experienced this problem. If the internal fixation is removed, it should be accomplished after the contracture release has been completed. Removal at this point minimizes the risk of iatrogenic fracture through stress risers that empty screw holes create.

Distraction Interposition Arthroplasty

If the surgeon identifies the presence of significant articular abnormalities and underlying elbow contractures when making the preoperative clinical and radiographic assessment, he or she should consider performing an interposition arthroplasty at the time of contracture release. Interposition arthroplasty is an established procedure for the treatment of joints that posttraumatic arthritis has damaged. Morrey et al. suggested that, if half of the articular surface of the joint is not covered with hyaline cartilage, interposition arthroplasty should be considered.[12,19] Patients who need their articular surface reshaped due to an intra-articular malunion also are candidates for interposition arthroplasty. The current interposition materials of choice are fascia lata and dermis. The efficacy of collagen scaffolds as an interposition material is currently under investigation.

As with any surgical procedure, adequate exposure of the elbow joint is required for interposition arthroplasty. Division of the humeral origin of the lateral collateral ligament complex allows the elbow to be hinged open on the intact medial collateral ligament. The articular surfaces can then be debrided and reshaped as necessary. Radial head excision should be avoided due to the increased instability that can occur following this procedure. A 4 cm by 15 cm fascia lata graft is harvested, folded into a three-ply graft, and sutured to the distal humerus through drill holes to prevent graft dislodgement. At the end of the operative procedure, the lateral ligament complex is repaired back to bone through drill holes.

In addition to providing elbow stability, the previously mentioned articulated elbow fixators also can distract the joint space and protect the interposition material. The joint is distracted approximately 3 to 5 mm by the device and then the wound is closed in layers.

The Mayo device is simple to apply, available for repeated use, and amenable to use with a continuous passive motion machine. Unfortunately, the distal humeral transfixion pin can loosen, especially in patients who have disuse osteoporosis. If the transfixion pin loosens, the patient is at increased risk for infection that can lead to septic arthritis. In contrast, the compass hinge elbow brace is bulky, is recommended only for single use, and is more difficult to apply. This brace has the significant advantage of leaving no axis pin in the distal humerus, so the

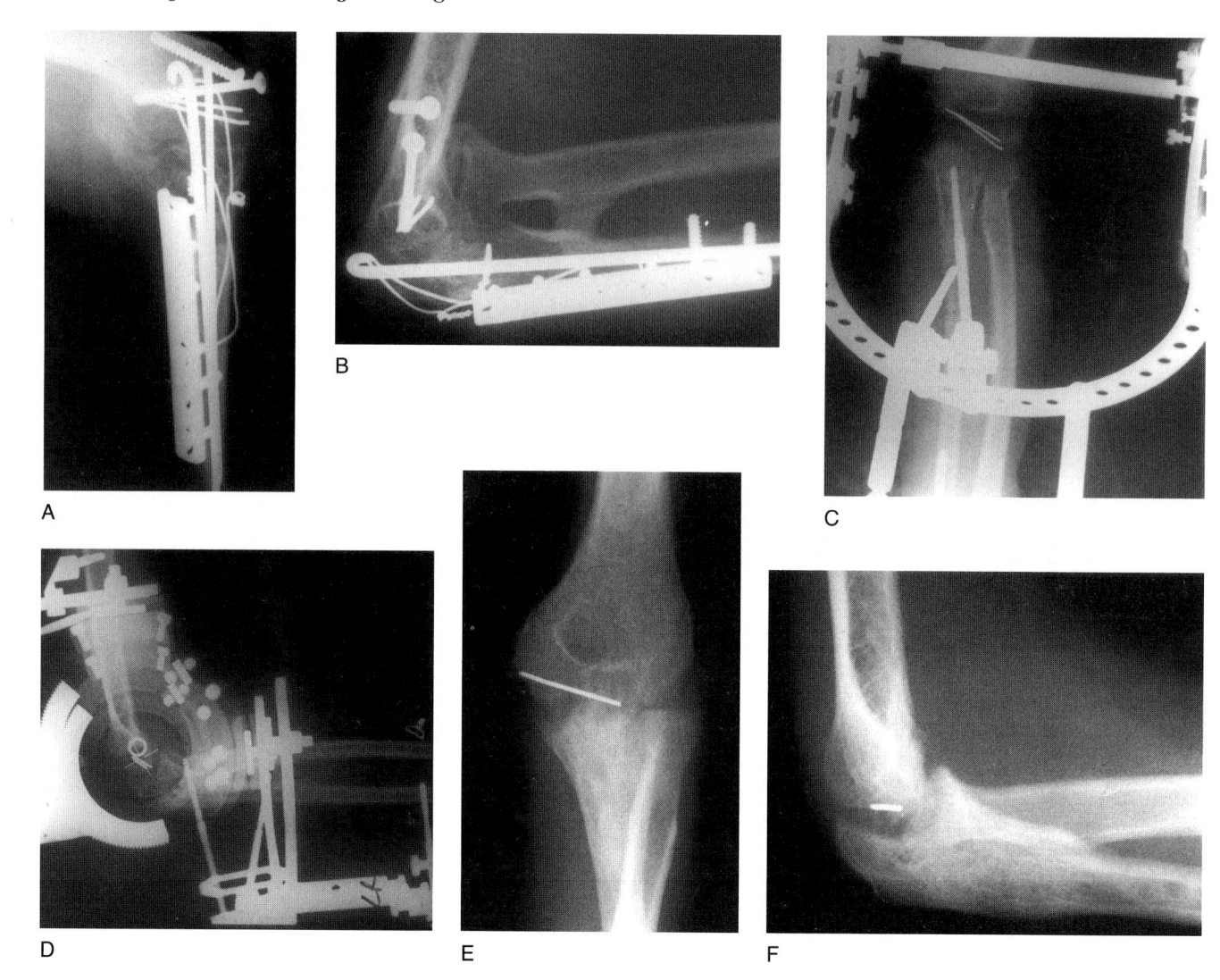

FIGURE 26.6. Compass hinge distraction device. (A) Anteroposterior (AP) radiograph of a 26-year-old woman 1 year after a supracondylar humeral fracture. The patient has significant elbow pain and a flexion–extension arc from 90° to 130°. (B) Lateral radiograph demonstrating posttraumatic arthritis and heterotopic ossification. (C) Postoperative AP radiograph after elbow contracture release, hardware removal, and interposition arthroplasty with application of compass elbow hinge. (D) Postoperative lateral radiograph illustrating cross hairs on device that ensure proper replication of axis of rotation. (E) AP radiograph 20 months after surgery. Patient has a flexion extension arc from 22° to 138° and minimal activity-related elbow pain. (F) Lateral radiograph 20 months after removal of distraction device.

risk of pin loosening and possible joint infection are reduced. The compass hinge brace, in addition, allows for gradual, progressive, patient-controlled stretching of the joint because of its worm-gear mechanism; this mechanism also can be disengaged for active range-of-motion exercises. Further experience and development of such devices will clarify their ultimate place in the management of elbow contractures.

At the conclusion of the procedure, the surgeon deflates the tourniquet, obtains hemostasis, and places suction drains within the joint and the subcutaneous tissue. Wound closure is followed by application of a compressive dressing to minimize postoperative swelling.

POSTOPERATIVE CARE

The goals of postoperative care include minimization of swelling, control of pain, and maintenance of elbow motion. Use of ice and nonsteroidal anti-inflammatory medications helps to control postoperative swelling. Some anti-inflammatory medications possess analgesic properties and also may help to prevent heterotopic ossification.[35,36] For additional pain control, continuous brachial plexus blockade may be helpful in the early postoperative period (from 24 to 48 hours) and may facilitate early mobilization of the elbow.[37] Some evidence exists that continuous passive motion may be helpful in obtaining and maintaining elbow motion in the postoperative period.[5,37] Alternatively, early active motion combined with a flexion and extension splinting program can be considered. The flexion and extension splints are alternated during the day, and the extension splint usually is worn at night because extension tends to be the hardest motion to maintain postoperatively. We do not permit the patient to have passive stretching by a physical therapist for the first 6 weeks after surgery. The role of turnbuckle splinting following open contracture release is not yet determined. We advocate the use of this device after the elbow pain and swelling have subsided and if the patient is not progressing following a 6-week trial of conventional physical therapy. If the patient has an interposition arthroplasty, he or she should use a continuous passive motion device for 20 hours each day; during the remaining 4 hours, the patient should participate in active range-of-motion exercises.

The risk of recurrent heterotopic ossification is low. Nevertheless, we recommend prophylaxis for recurrence with a nonsteroidal anti-inflammatory medication, such as 25-mg indomethacin three times each day for 6 weeks, in combination with a gastric cytoprotective agent.[38] For patients who are intolerant of the anti-inflammatory medication and are at a higher risk of recurrence (e.g., short duration from the development of the heterotopic bone to its excision, the need for repeated surgery, and poor preoperative cognitive function), the surgeon can consider using postoperative radiation.[35,39,40] Significant evidence in the literature supports the efficacy of postoperative radiation in patients who have acetabular fractures and hip replacement arthroplasty, but its use in heterotopic ossification of the elbow has not been defined.[38]

COMPLICATIONS

Numerous complications have been reported following elbow contracture release.[9,29,41] Local skin complications occasionally are seen in patients whose elbow stiffness was caused by previous trauma. Whenever possible, the surgeon should use a previous incision to avoid skin flap necrosis. Pressure over the posterior incision should be avoided by careful splinting in the postoperative period (from 24 hours up to 6 weeks). Deep infections occasionally are seen due to extensive operative exposures and long operating times in patients who have a more severe elbow contracture. Prophylactic antibiotics should be used routinely to reduce the risk of this complication. Pin tract infections are common with the use of elbow distraction devices and usually can be treated with pin site care and oral antibiotics. Neurologic injuries are uncommon if the surgeon uses careful technique. Neuropraxias, especially of the ulnar nerve, due to nerve dissection and retraction can be encountered. Fortunately, they usually resolve with time. Vessel injury due to direct trauma is rare but can occur in older patients who have long-standing, severe flexion contractures due to intimal tears. Periarticular fractures can occur through the previous site of hardware as a consequence of aggressive manipulation both intraoperatively and postoperatively.

Recurrence of the contracture is uncommon with careful patient selection. Employing an experienced physical therapist to assist with splinting and active motion in the postoperative period is essential. Heterotopic ossification occasionally can recur, particularly if the previous elbow injury that caused the contracture is recent and the initial heterotopic ossification is radiographically immature. Reflex sympathetic dystrophy usually occurs in association with an intraoperative nerve injury and should be treated by aggressive sympathetic blocks and supervised physical therapy. Ligament instability is uncommon following routine elbow contracture release, but it can occur following an interposition arthroplasty. Appropriate splinting and activity modification usually allow the ligaments to heal adequately; however, ligament reconstructions occasionally are required. Extensive soft-tissue stripping and denervation of the elbow joint can result in a neurotrophic joint. Weakness of the elbow may be more apparent following contracture release, particularly if the patient had weakness before surgery.

RESULTS

Elbow contracture release, regardless of the surgical approach, has been highly successful, with an overall improvement in motion ranging from 29° to 65°.[3,6,7,9,10,42] Most patients achieve a functional arc of motion, and patient satisfaction is high. Patients who have greater restriction of elbow motion before surgery have a greater improvement in the arc of motion after surgery. Pain usually subsides following the release of an intrinsic elbow contracture with interposition arthroplasty.[9] About half of the patients report some residual, mild elbow discomfort; however, more significant pain is uncommon.[6] Elbow stability usually is maintained, given appropriate intraoperative ligament preservation or postoperative protection with an articulated external fixator or orthosis.[43]

REFERENCES

1. Morrey BF, Askew LJ, Chao EY. A biomechanical study of normal functional elbow motion. *J Bone Joint Surg* 1981;63A: 872–877.
2. Vasen AP, Lacey SH, Keith MW, et al. Functional range of motion of the elbow. *J Hand Surg* 1995;20A:288–292.
3. Boerboom AL, de Meyier HE, Verburg AD, et al. Arthrolysis for post-traumatic stiffness of the elbow. *Int Orthop* 1993;17: 346–349.
4. Garland DE, Hanscom DA, Keenan MA, et al. Resection of heterotopic ossification in the adult with head trauma. *J Bone Joint Surg* 1985;67A:1261–1269.

5. Gates HS III, Sullivan FL, Urbaniak JR. Anterior capsulotomy and continuous passive motion in the treatment of post-traumatic flexion contracture of the elbow. A prospective study. *J Bone Joint Surg* 1992;74A:1229–1234.
6. Hastings H, Cohen MS. Post-traumatic contracture of the elbow: Operative release using a lateral collateral sparing approach. *J Bone Joint Surg* 1998;80B:805–812.
7. Husband JB, Hastings H. The lateral approach for operative release of post-traumatic contracture of the elbow. *J Bone Joint Surg* 1990;72A:1353–1358.
8. Lamine A, Fikry T, Essadki B, et al. L'artholyse du coude— a propos de 70 cas, *Acta Orthop Belgica* 1993;59:352–356.
9. Morrey BF. Post-traumatic contracture of the elbow. Operative treatment, including distraction arthroplasty. *J Bone and Joint Surg* 1990;72A:601–618.
10. Urbaniak JR, Hansen PE, Beissinger SF, et al. Correction of post-traumatic flexion contracture of the elbow by anterior capsulotomy. *J Bone and Joint Surg* 1985;67A:1160–1164.
11. Mohan K. Myositis ossificans traumatica of the elbow. *Int Surg* 1972;57:475–478.
12. Ljung P, Jonsson K, Larsson K, et al. Interposition arthroplasty of the elbow with rheumatoid arthritis. *J Shoulder Elbow Surg* 1996;5:81–85.
13. Morrey BF. *The elbow and its disorders*, 2nd ed. Philadelphia: WB Saunders; 1993.
14. Garland DE, O'Hollaren RM. Fractures and dislocations about the elbow in the head-injured adult. *Clin Orthop* 1982;168:38–41.
15. Moore TJ. Functional outcome following surgical excision of heterotopic ossification in patients with traumatic brain injury. *J Orthop Trauma* 1993;7:11–14.
16. Roberts JB, Pankratz DG: The surgical treatment of heterotopic ossification following long-term coma. *J Bone and Joint Surg* 1979;61A:760–763.
17. Engber WD, Reynen P. Post-burn heterotopic ossification at the elbow. *Iowa Orthop J* 1994;14:38–41.
18. Evans EB. Orthopaedic measures in the treatment of severe burns. *J Bone Joint Surg* 1966;48A:643–669.
19. Seth MK, Khurana JK. Bony ankylosis of the elbow after burns. *J Bone and Joint Surg* 1985;67B:747–749.
20. Josefsson PO, Johnell O, Gentz CF. Long-term sequelae of simple dislocation of the elbow. *J Bone Joint Surg* 1984;66A:927–930.
21. Mehlhoff TL, Noble PC, Bennett JB, et al. Simple dislocation of the elbow in the adult. Results after closed treatment. *J Bone Joint Surg* 1988;70A:244–249.
22. Hastings H II, Graham TJ. The classification and treatment of heterotopic ossification about the elbow and forearm. *Hand Clin* 1994;10:417–437.
23. Green DP, McCoy H. Turnbuckle orthotic correction of elbow-flexion contractures after acute injuries. *J Bone Joint Surg* 1979;61A:1092–1095.
24. Bonutti PM, Windau JE, Ables, BA, et al. Static progressive stretch to reestablish elbow range of motion. *Clin Orthop* 1994;303:128–134.
25. Duke JB, Tessler RH, Dell PC. Manipulation of the stiff elbow with patient under anesthesia. *J Hand Surg* 1991;16A:19–24.
26. Karachalios T, Maxwell-Armstrong C, Atkins RM. Treatment of post-traumatic fixed flexion deformity of the elbow using an intermittent compression garment. *Injury* 1994;25:313–315.
27. O'Driscoll SW, Shankland SW, Beaton D. Patient-adjusted static elbow splints for elbow contractures [Abstract]. *J Shoulder Elbow Surg* 1996;5:S73.
28. Zander CL, Healy NL. Elbow flexion contractures treated with serial casts and conservative therapy. *J Hand Surg* 1992;17A:694–697.
29. Jupiter JB. Heterotopic ossification about the elbow. *Instr Course Lect* 1991;40:41–44.
30. Nowicki KD, Shall LM. Arthroscopic release of a posttraumatic flexion contracture in the elbow: A case report and review of the literature. *Arthroscopy* 1992;8:544–547.
31. Jones GS, Savoie FH III. Arthroscopic capsular release of flexion contractures (arthrofibrosis) of the elbow. *Arthroscopy* 1993;9:277–283.
32. Timmerman LA, Andrews JR. Arthroscopic treatment of post-traumatic elbow pain and stiffness. *Am J Sports Med* 1994;22:230–235.
33. Hotchkiss RN, An K-N, Weiland AJ, et al. *Treatment of severe elbow contractures using the concepts of Ilizarov*. Presented at the 61st annual meeting of the American Academy of Orthopaedic Surgeons, New Orleans, Louisiana, February 1994.
34. Dowdy PA, Bain GI, King GJ, et al. The midline posterior elbow incision. An anatomical appraisal. *J Bone Joint Surg* 1995;77B:696–699.
35. Hedley AK, Mead LP, Hendren DH. The prevention of heterotopic bone formation following total hip arthroplasty using 600 rad in a single dose. *J Arthroplasty* 1989;4:319–325.
36. Segstro R, Morley-Forster PK, Lu G. Indomethacin as a postoperative analgesic for total hip arthroplasty. *Can J Anaesth* 1991;38:578–581.
37. Rymaszewski L, Glass K, Parikh R. Post-traumatic elbow contracture treated by arthrolysis and continual passive motion under brachial plexus anaesthesia [Abstract]. *J Bone Joint Surg* 1996;76B:S30.
38. McLaren AC. Prophylaxis with indomethacin for heterotopic bone after open reduction of fractures of the acetabulum. *J Bone Joint Surg* 1990;72A:245–247.
39. Cullen JP, Pellegrini VD Jr., Miller RJ, et al. Treatment of traumatic radioulnar synostosis by excision and postoperative low-dose irradiation. *J Hand Surg* 1994;19A:394–401.
40. McAuliffe JA, Wolfson AH. Early excision of heterotopic ossification about the elbow followed by radiation therapy. *J Bone Joint Surg* 1997;79A:749–755.
41. Modabber MR, Jupiter JB. Reconstruction for post-traumatic conditions of the elbow joint. *J Bone Joint Surg* 1995;77A:1431–1446.
42. Mih AD, Wolf FG. Surgical release of elbow-capsular contracture in pediatric patients. *J Pediatr Orthop* 1994;14:458–461.
43. Faber KJ, Patterson SD, King GJW. Post-traumatic elbow contracture release through a posterior midline longitudinal incision. *J Bone Joint Surg* 1998;80B:S6.

CHAPTER 27

Tumors of the Elbow

Dempsey S. Springfield and Stephanie Sweet

INTRODUCTION

Although bone and soft-tissue tumors about the elbow and forearm are rare, the general orthopedist must be aware that these tumors can occur and must be prepared to manage them appropriately. These tumors present challenging oncologic and reconstructive issues even for the tumor surgeon, and early recognition and evaluation make management easier. The purpose of this chapter is to review the general principles in managing bone and soft-tissue tumors, to suggest an appropriate approach to diagnosis and biopsy, and to review specific tumors that afflict the upper extremity.

The differential diagnosis of a patient who has a bone or soft-tissue mass includes infection, neoplasia, trauma, and inflammatory processes; pain is the most common, but a nondiscriminatory, presenting symptom. Usually, with physical examination, medical history, and review of systems, the differential diagnostic list can be shortened, and, with good-quality plain radiographs (at least two views taken at 90° to each other), the diagnosis often can be made or at least the possibilities can be limited to three or four specific conditions.

Plain radiographs are invaluable diagnostic tools, particularly for bone lesions. According to Enneking,[1] four questions must be answered when looking at a plain radiograph of a tumor:

1. Where is the tumor, that is, long or flat bone; epiphysis, metaphysis, or diaphysis; or cortex, medullary cavity, or surface?

2. What is the tumor doing to the bone?

3. What is the bone doing to the tumor, that is, endosteal or periosteal reaction?

4. Does the tumor have intrinsic characteristics, such as, bone formation or calcification, that indicate its histology?

Answering these four fundamental questions is critical to the orthopedic surgeon in terms of making the correct diagnosis and managing the tumor. For example, in Figure 27.1, the lesion is clearly in the metaphysis of a long bone. The cortex has been destroyed. The periosteal reaction is well developed, but endosteal reaction is minimal. Various septations within the tumor, which actually are corrugations in the irregular wall, are present. No intralesional ossifications or calcifications exist. The lesion has all the hallmarks of a typical aneurysmal bone cyst. It could be a giant cell tumor of bone, but giant cell tumor rarely occurs in a patient who has open growth plates. Telangiectatic osteosarcoma also can present with these radiographic findings; however, without an accompanying soft-tissue mass, telangiectatic osteosarcoma is unlikely. Thus, a differential diagnosis has been formulated in this patient simply by addressing Enneking's four questions.[1]

EVALUATION

Most diagnoses can be made on the basis of the patient's history, physical examination, and plain radiographs. Additional studies are obtained either when the diagnosis cannot be made this way or when surgical resection is planned. Serum values are usually normal in patients who have a musculoskeletal neoplasia. Despite this fact, as a rule the surgeon needs to obtain at least a serum calcium, erythrocyte sedimentation rate, alkaline phosphatase, lactic dehydrogenase, immunoelectrophoresis, and complete blood count (CBC). The erythrocyte sedimentation rate may be elevated, but this is nonspecific. Myeloma may be recognized by the protein spike on immunoelectrophoresis.

A technetium bone scan is an excellent method for evaluating the primary lesion and for surveying the en-

FIGURE 27.1. (A) Anteroposterior and (B) lateral radiographs of a six-year-old child with elbow pain show an aneurysmal bone cyst.

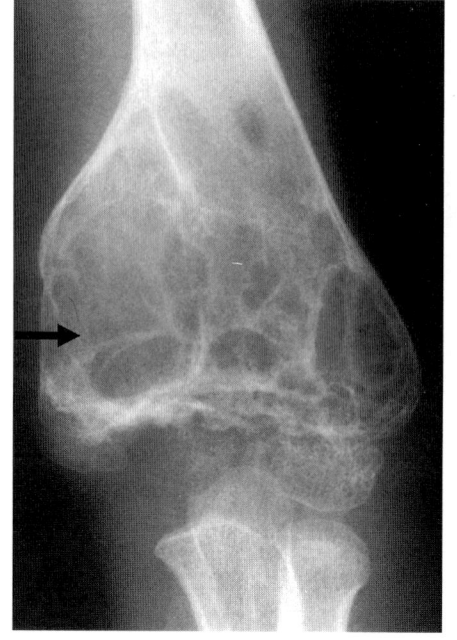

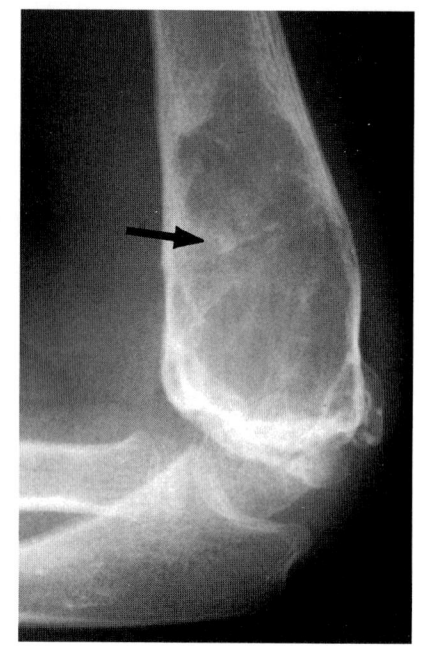

tire skeleton. Some active small round cell lesions (eosinophilic granuloma, metastatic neuroblastomas, and myeloma) may not produce hot spots on bone scan, but, otherwise, a lesion without increased uptake of technetium is unlikely to be active.

Magnetic resonance imaging (MRI) or computed tomography (CT) scans, rarely both, are often necessary for complete evaluation of a musculoskeletal tumor. Pettersson et al.[2] compared radiographs, bone scan, MRI, CT, and angiography in the evaluation of 92 patients who had soft-tissue tumors and found MRI to be superior in the assessment of extent, detection of hemorrhage and necrosis, and evaluation of the relationship of the tumor to adjacent vascular structures. Bloem et al.[3] also prospectively studied MRI in 56 patients who had primary bone sarcomas and, based on findings at surgery, reported MRT to be superior to bone scan, angiography, and CT. Specifically, MRI was superior in the assessment of intraosseous extent of the tumor and comparable with CT in the assessment of cortical destruction. MRI is the modality of choice in defining extraosseous extent, skip lesions, epiphyseal extension, and joint involvement. CT still remains superior for assessing calcification and ossification.

Figure 27.2A shows a lucent lesion in the metaphysis of the proximal ulna, largely within the medullary cavity. This lesion is difficult to see on plain radiographs, but the endosteal surface is scalloped. An MRI scan was obtained to further delineate the lesion (Figs. 27.2 B and C). The exact extent of the tumor can be seen clearly on the MRI scan. No significant extraosseous component exists. The bright signal seen on the gradient echo image suggests a cartilage tumor. A biopsy was performed, and the lesion proved to be a chondromyxoid fibroma.

STAGING

Enneking[1] and his associates developed a useful surgical staging system (Table 27.1). Malignant tumors are separated into two histologic stages (I, low; II, high) and two anatomic locations (A, intracompartmental; B, extracompartmental). Metastatic disease is considered stage III. Surgical margins are defined as intralesional, marginal, wide, or radical. An intralesional excision involves violating the tumor's pseudocapsule and removing the specimen from within (i.e., incisional biopsy, curettage). A marginal excision is obtained by dissecting in the plane between normal tissue and the tumor's pseudocapsule. A wide surgical margin is achieved when the tumor is removed with a surrounding cuff of normal tissue (en bloc). A radical excision removes the tumor and the entire compartment or compartments.

Enneking[1] also recommended a staging system for benign bone tumors. This system is based on the radiographic appearance of a lesion and usually suggests the appropriate treatment (Fig. 27.3). Stage 1 (benign, latent) lesions occur within the bone and are surrounded by a well-developed reactive rim of bone. They are usually inactive, spontaneously resolving lesions that do not require surgery. Stage 2 (benign, active) lesions continue to grow slowly and are also well encapsulated, although the reactive zone around the capsule is thicker and less mature than in stage 1 lesions. Stage 3 (benign, aggressive) le-

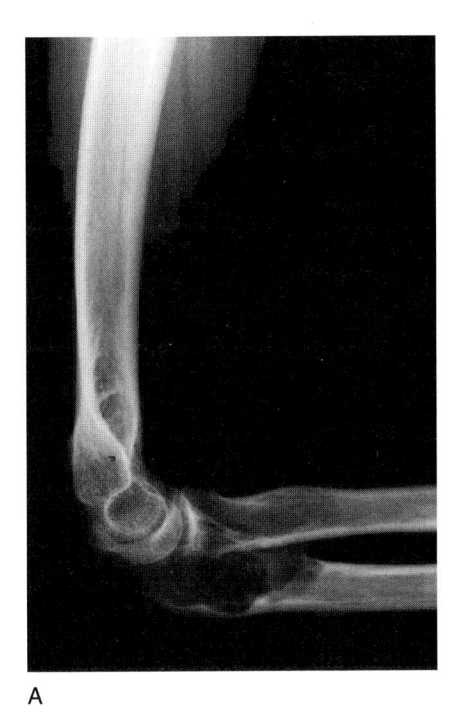

FIGURE 27.2. (A) Lateral radiograph; (B) sagittal T1 image, and (C) gradient echo image of a 25-year-old woman with pain in her left elbow.

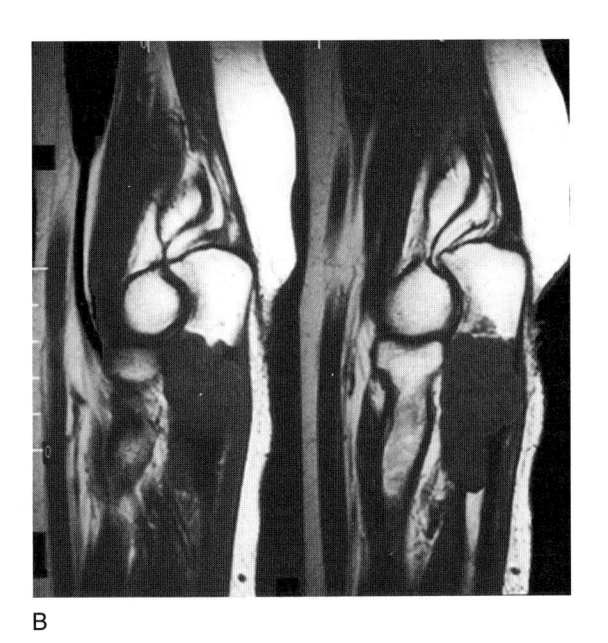

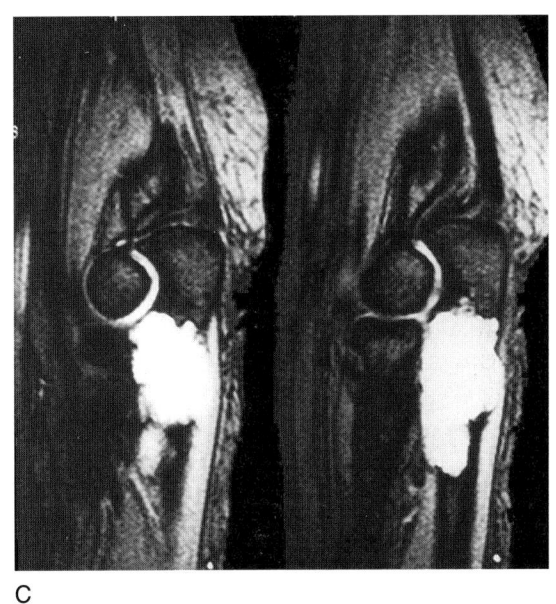

sions pursue a much more aggressive local course. The reactive zone around the tumor is much more biologically active, is thicker, and may be penetrated by neoplastic cells. Stage 3 tumors demonstrate local growth behavior similar to that of a malignant tumor and often need to be treated surgically, with resection obtaining a wide margin.

TABLE 27.1. *Staging of musculoskeletal tumors[1]*

Stage	Description
I-A	Low grade, intracompartmental, no metastases
I-B	Low grade, extracompartmental, no metastases
II-A	High grade, intracompartmental, no metastases
II-B	High grade, extracompartmental, no metastases
III-A	Any grade, intracompartmental, with metastases
III-B	Any grade, extracompartmental, with metastases

PRINCIPLES OF BIOPSY

A biopsy of the lesion should be the last step in the evaluation of the tumor and should be used to confirm the prebiopsy diagnosis. Many tumors are heterogeneous, and the specific site of the biopsy is important. Complications related to biopsy occur when it is performed with-

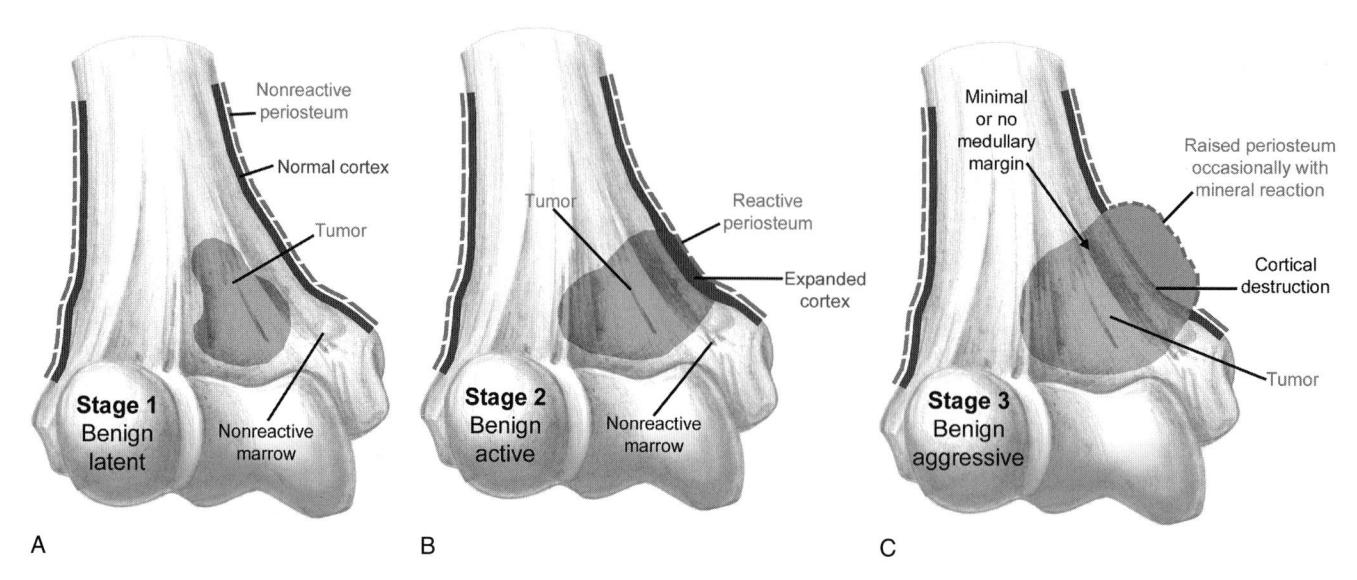

FIGURE 27.3. The three stages of benign tumors as they appear in the distal humerus. (A) Stage 1, benign latent; (B) stage 2, benign active; (C) stage 3, benign aggressive.

out exact knowledge of the anatomic extent of the tumor. In 1982, Mankin et al.[4] reviewed the results of 329 biopsies of bone and soft-tissue neoplasms. They found an 18% incidence of major error in diagnosis and a 10% incidence of nondiagnostic specimens. In 8.5% of the entire group, improper biopsy adversely affected outcome, and 4.5% of the group had unnecessary amputation because of biopsy-related problems. The results were essentially unchanged when this study was repeated in 1996.[5]

Needle biopsies can be done. They require the same preoperative planning as an open biopsy. The tissue obtained is limited, and histologic grading usually cannot be done. Skrzynski et al.[6] reported that, in selected instances, needle biopsy accomplished on an outpatient basis could save $6000 per patient when compared with open biopsy. The diagnostic accuracy of closed needle biopsy in their study was 84% compared with 96% for open biopsy. Of the 62 lesions on which closed needle biopsy was performed, 10 were incorrectly diagnosed. All 10 were soft-tissue sarcomas, and 8 of the 10 did not have diagnostic tissue obtained with the needle biopsy.

If the closed needle biopsy method is chosen and if resection of the tumor is necessary, the site of needle aspiration and the contaminated tissue must be excised during definitive resection. If the radiologist performs a biopsy under CT guidance, the surgeon must plan the biopsy with the radiologist and direct the path of the needle. Three cores of tumor-containing tissue are recommended: one core for frozen section, immunohistochemical analysis, and molecular genetic studies; one core for electron microscopy; and one core for routine paraffin studies.

Open biopsy must be planned even more carefully than needle biopsy, especially if limb salvage is an option; when the tumor is malignant, the tissue exposed during an open biopsy must be resected with the definitive resection of the tumor. Usually, the biopsy incision should be longitudinal, because this incision is easier to incorporate into a limb salvage resection (Fig. 27.4).

Dissection during the biopsy should be as limited as possible, taking care not to raise skin flaps or to expose neurovascular bundles. The dissection should be through muscle, not between two muscles. Sharp incision of a specimen with a piece of pseudocapsule is recommended. A frozen section should be performed to assure that diagnostic tissue has been obtained. The use of a tourniquet is acceptable if the limb is not exsanguinated with

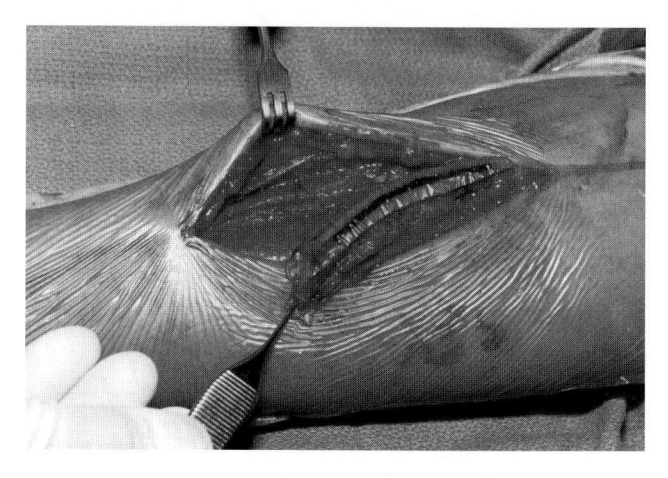

FIGURE 27.4. Biopsy incision being excised during definitive resection of a subcutaneous sarcoma. Fortunately, this biopsy was performed through a longitudinal incision, which made definitive resection relatively easy.

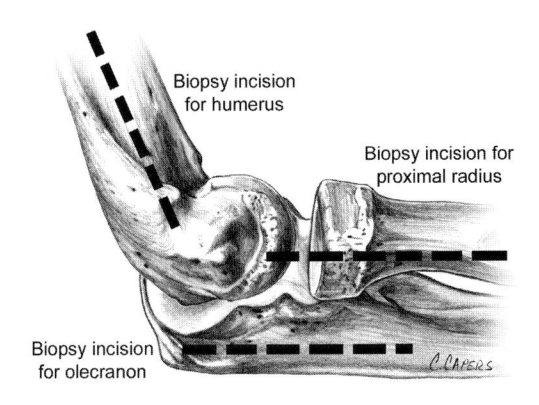

FIGURE 27.5. Location of bone lesion biopsies about the elbow.

an Esmarch bandage. The tourniquet is released before wound closure, and meticulous hemostasis is critical; wound hematoma contains tumor cells and increases the extent of contamination. Placement of the drain site should be close to and in line with the skin incision.

Biopsies of bone lesions about the elbow should be done through a lateral longitudinal incision for the distal humerus and proximal radius or through the subcutaneous tissue over the proximal lateral olecranon (Fig. 27.5). The obvious caveat is that the biopsy site should be adjusted to fit the definitive resection. If the definitive surgery calls for a medial approach to the elbow, then a medial biopsy should be done. Conversely, even if the tumor is largely medial, but the resection will be done through a lateral approach, then a lateral biopsy should be accomplished. Knowledge of the anatomy and the common surgical approaches about the elbow is important.[7] Sometimes the surgeon must make the biopsy more difficult to make the resection easier.

Excisional biopsies are indicated only when the lesion is small and easily removable. The decision whether to perform incisional or excisional biopsy should be individualized and must take the patient's wishes into account, realizing that excisional biopsy may occasionally lead to overtreatment.

Finally, when doing a biopsy some material should be sent for culture, and when doing an incision and drainage for a suspected infection, tissue should be sent for pathologic examination.

OPERATIVE TREATMENT

Benign bone tumors are treated most often with a curettage with or without bone graft. The exposure for these procedures is usually the same as for an open biopsy. Malignant bone tumors and some aggressive benign tumors (benign stage 3) should be treated with a resection (wide surgical margin). These resections are done most commonly through a posterior or posterolateral approach. The biopsy incision is ellipsed, and all tissue exposed at the time of biopsy is resected with the tumor.

BENIGN AND MALIGNANT TUMORS

No benign or malignant tumors have a predilection for the elbow, and no benign lesions have a predilection for the forearm. Benign lesions include ganglion cyst, lipoma, fibromatosis, hemangioma, arteriovenous malformation, lipofibromatous hamartoma of nerve, neurilemmoma, neurofibroma, enchondroma, osteochondroma, chondroblastoma, chondromyxoid fibroma, eosinophilic granuloma, osteoid osteoma, unicameral bone cyst, osteoblastoma, giant cell tumor of bone, and aneurysmal bone cyst.

All malignant lesions can occur in the upper extremity and include synovial sarcoma, epithelial sarcoma, clear cell sarcoma, fibrosarcoma, malignant fibrohistiocytic tumors (malignant fibrous histiocytoma, dermatofibrosarcoma protuberans), liposarcoma, angiosarcoma, Kaposi's sarcoma, malignant schwannoma, chondrosarcoma, osteosarcoma, rhabdomyosarcoma, small round cell tumors (lymphoma, myeloma, and Ewing's sarcoma), and metastatic tumor. Epithelial sarcoma is the only one of these lesions that has a predilection for the upper extremity, especially the forearm. Synovial cell sarcoma occurs in the hand more often than other soft-tissue sarcomas.

Benign Tumors

Fibromatosis is a fibroblastic tumor that occurs primarily in adults and is firm, nonencapsulated, and locally invasive. It does not metastasize. When superficial, it arises from fascia, may be familial, and grows slowly. When deep, it is referred to as aggressive fibromatosis or an extra-abdominal desmoid tumor. Extra-abdominal fibromatosis primarily occurs in young adults and is more common in women.[8] In the upper extremity, it occurs most commonly around the brachium and shoulder. Its margins are difficult to define. Patients may present with pain or a mass, or both. Occasionally, the soft-tissue mass causes cortical pressure and bony erosion. The tumor consists of fibroblasts and collagen. Treatment is difficult. Although wide resection is the treatment of choice, recurrence within the first 2 years after surgery ranges from 20% to 100%. Posner et al.[9] reported a 5-year survival rate of 92%, but suggested that surgeons should treat aggressive fibromatosis as if it were a low-grade sarcoma because of this frequent local recurrence. McCollough et al.[10] reported that 70% to 90% of aggressive lesions can be controlled by administering 50 γ of radiation in fractional doses; they recommended adjunctive postoperative radiation if wide surgical excision with adequate margins was not achieved. We recommend treating the initial tumor with a wide resection and reserving irradiation for those patients who develop a local recurrence.

Lipomas usually present as an asymptomatic, slowly enlarging mass. They often are subcutaneous, but may be deep. A tissue-specific diagnosis usually can be made with CT or MRI. Removal is not required and is recommended only for cosmesis or if the mass is an irritant.

Congenital arteriovenous (AV) malformations may occur in deep or superficial locations. Rarely, the deep lesion will result in significant shunting and, when this occurs, the lesion should be treated to eliminate the effects of the blood flow. Large shunts result in a bruit over the mass and reflex bradycardia when the feeding vessel is compressed (Branham's sign). Most AV malformations do not have significant blood flow and are only important because they may be mistaken for a sarcoma. Only those causing symptoms need excision. Rarely is the AV malformation so extensive that the only acceptable treatment is an amputation.

Neurilemmoma is a common benign nerve tumor that arises from the Schwann cell. It is encapsulated, usually arises from the peripheral aspect of the nerve, grows slowly, and presents as a mass that is sensitive to touch. These tumors usually are associated with a lacerating pain or electric shock sensation when tapped (a positive Tinel sign). Treatment consists of surgical enucleation when they arise from a major motor nerve; a surgical microscope may be necessary. However, most neurilemmomas are associated with a terminal sensory branch and can be excised simply. Recurrence is rare, and these tumors have an extremely low incidence of malignant degeneration.

Neurofibroma arises from nerve sheath, as does the neurilemmoma, but is not encapsulated. It can be localized, diffuse, or plexiform. Neurofibroma, unlike neurilemmoma, is intimately associated with the nerve fascicles, and resection can easily result in sacrifice of some fascicular bundles. When a major peripheral nerve is involved, the neurofibroma should be resolved only if symptomatic. Usually, by carefully dissecting between the nerve fascicles, the surgeon can remove the mass. An alternative approach is to completely resect the lesion and perform primary nerve repair or nerve grafting; however, we do not recommend this treatment.

Giant cell tumor of the bone occurs in the epiphysis and metaphysis of the bone and almost always extends to the articular surface. Patients are usually more than 20 years of age. The tumors may be indolent, active, or aggressive. Radiographically, giant cell tumor presents as a well-defined lucent defect that is eccentrically located in the epiphysis and metaphysis. The endosteal margin rarely has a reactive rim, and often periosteal reaction is minimal even when the cortex is eroded. Grossly, the lesion is homogeneous, tan in color, and firm in consistency; microscopically, the tumor contains a background of proliferating, homogeneous, mononuclear cells with multinucleated giant cells dispersed throughout the lesion.[11] Standard treatment is curettage. Cryosurgery can be used, but is controversial. Polymethyl methacrylate packing can be used to provide immediate stability but bone graft is acceptable. The tumor may recur locally after currettage in up to 25% of cases.[12] Resection may be necessary in more advanced or recurrent cases.

On plain radiographs, aneurysmal bone cyst is a tumor that sometimes is confused with giant cell tumor. The patients are usually less than 20 years of age and present with an aching pain. On plain radiographs, the tumor is a solitary, expansile, eccentric lesion. The periphery of the lesion often is indistinct. Fluid–fluid levels are seen on CT and MRI. Grossly, the wall of the tumor is soft and fibrous, and friable brownish blood clot often is found inside the cyst. Aneurysmal bone cyst comprises giant cells, blood-filled spaces, fibrous tissue, and osteoid. It may arise de novo or in preexisting lesions. In the Mayo Clinic experience, 78% of the patients were less than 20 years of age, and only 8 of 134 lesions arose in the elbow region.[12] Telangiectatic osteosarcoma must be considered in the differential diagnosis. Treatment of an aneurysmal bone cyst consists of curettage and bone grafting.

Eosinophilic granuloma, now more properly called Langerhan's cell histiocytosis, is a lesion of unknown cause that can present a unifocal lesion, multifocal osseous lesions, or systemic soft-tissue involvement (Fig. 27.6). About 80% of patients have a solitary lesion.[11] Classically, the lesion presents in men less than 20 years of age. Patients often report pain. Radiographically, the lesion is a circumscribed lytic defect without a reactive rim. In the long bones, the tumor is often diaphyseal, and the cortex is often eroded. The histology is characterized by eosinophils, plasma cells, and Langerhan's histiocytes. Unifocal lesions may spontaneously regress, and treatment is not always necessary.

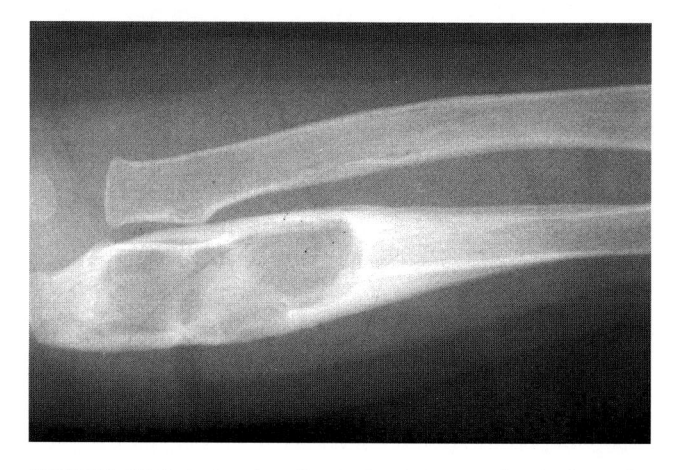

FIGURE 27.6. Lateral radiograph of the proximal ulna of a 3-year-old child who had pain and swelling in the upper forearm for 1 month. This lesion is a solitary Langerhan's cell histiocytosis.

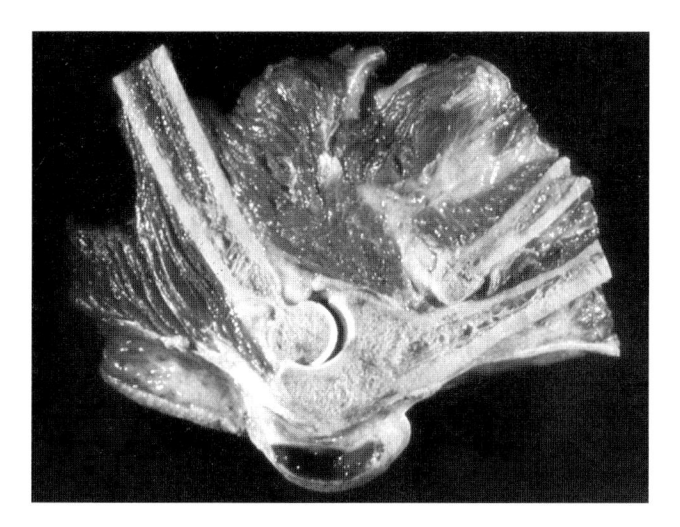

FIGURE 27.7. Specimen from an above-elbow resection of a malignant fibrous histiocytoma around the elbow of a 55-year-old man.

Malignant Tumors

Epithelial sarcoma is a highly malignant lesion often found in the upper extremity. It is the most common soft-tissue sarcoma of the hand.[13] This sarcoma is not infrequently confused with granuloma or squamous cell carcinoma because it is often subcutaneous and ulcerated. Microscopically, the tumor consists of nodules of epithelioid tumor cells and central necrosis associated with an inflammatory cellular response.[14] Adequate treatment is a wide surgical resection. Irradiation seems not to be as effective as it is in other sarcomas. Metastasis to lymph nodes is not uncommon and heralds a poor prognosis.[15]

Synovial sarcoma occurs in periarticular locations, but almost never within the joint cavity. It is most prevalent in persons from age 15 to 40 years and shows a slight predilection for men. Patients present with a deep, palpable mass that sometimes is painful. Growth is slow, and the tumor may be mistaken as bursitis or arthritis. These tumors occur principally in the extremities, with 23% arising in the upper extremity.[16] Bone erosion may be seen in poorly differentiated, long-standing lesions, but usually the bone is uninvolved. Multiple stippled areas of calcification often are visible on plain radiographs. Microscopic evaluation shows epithelial cells and spindle cells that can mimic fibrosarcoma, metastatic carcinoma, melanoma, and epithelial sarcoma. Synovial sarcomas are high-grade malignancies that require a wide surgical resection. A more limited excision combined with adjuvant irradiation can be used to salvage a limb that otherwise would be amputated. Metastasis occurs in more than 50% of patients. The lung is the most common site of a distant site of metastasis, but synovial cell sarcoma has a more frequent (approximately 25%) incidence of metastasis to lymph nodes than have other sarcomas.

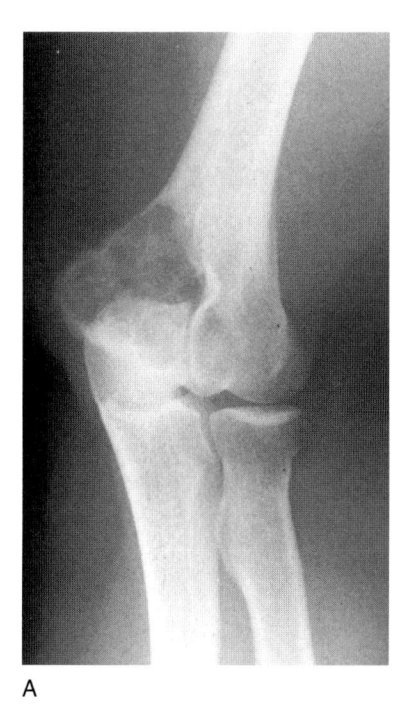

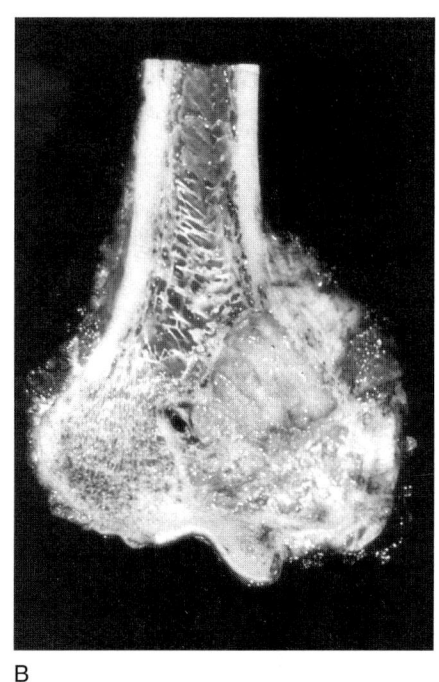

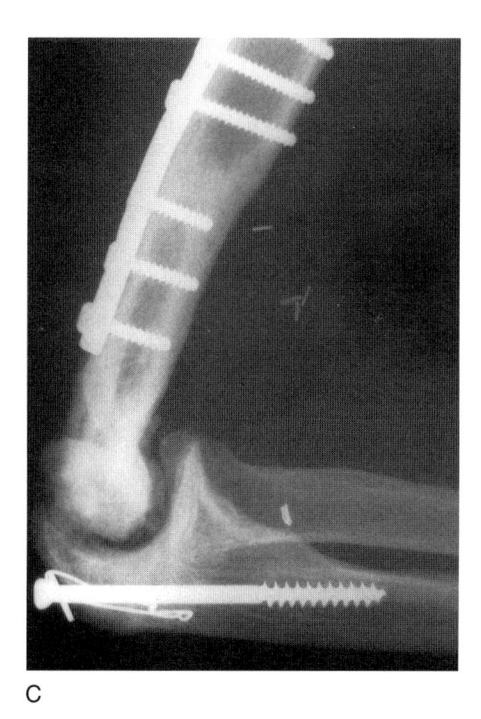

FIGURE 27.8. (A) Anteroposterior radiograph of the elbow of a 40-year-old man who had pain in his elbow. The radiograph shows an eccentric metaphyseal–epiphyseal lesion in the humerus. Giant cell tumor was suspected. Subsequent biopsy proved this to be a chondrosarcoma. (B) The patient underwent nonamputative resection with allograft reconstruction. (C) Reconstruction shown 4 years after surgery. There was no recurrence.

Approximately 9% of liposarcomas occur in the arm or forearm.[17] The mass usually is painless and slow growing. The myxoid liposarcoma is more common in patients younger than 50 years of age. Round cell liposarcoma and pleomorphic liposarcoma are more aggressive subtypes. Treatment includes wide surgical resection or a marginal resection combined with adjuvant irradiation.

Malignant fibrous histiocytoma is the most common soft-tissue sarcoma in adults. It usually affects persons from age 50 to 70 years. The location is variable; it can arise in subcutaneous tissue, within deep muscle and fascia, or within bone. The tumor is multinodular and may contain small satellite lesions surrounding the mass. Histologically, both histocytes and fibrocytes are present, and the cells are arranged in a storiform pattern. Immunohistochemical stains help to distinguish these tumors from poorly differentiated liposarcomas and malignant muscle tumors.[11] To treat these tumors, use wide surgical resection (Fig. 27.7). As with most other soft-tissue sarcomas, adjuvant irradiation can be used to reduce the need for amputation.

Central chondrosarcoma is the fourth most common primary malignancy of the skeleton. Approximately 27% of chondrosarcomas affect the upper extremity.[18] This slow-growing intraosseous tumor sometimes has intralesional calcifications that can be seen on plain radiographs. The endosteal surface of the bone may be scalloped. A soft-tissue mass may be present. Treatment involves surgical resection (Fig. 27.8).

CONCLUSION

Bone and soft-tissue tumors of the elbow are rare. The first principle in treatment is to recognize the lesion. After recognizing it, the surgeon must carefully evaluate the tumor. This evaluation may require a plain radiograph and follow-up, or it may require a more thorough evaluation (plain radiograph, bone scan, laboratory values, MRI, and biopsy). Biopsy should be the last evaluation performed and should be accomplished only after specific planning. Patients who have tumors suggestive of an aggressive benign or a malignant tumor probably should be treated at a regional medical center with expertise in musculoskeletal oncology. Following this recommendation, the most important principles of management are as follows: (1) do not biopsy and always refer any patient who has a lesion that the surgeon is not comfortable treating definitively, (2) take the biopsy very seriously, and (3) avoid compromising definitive treatment by inappropriate or poorly performed biopsy.

REFERENCES

1. Enneking WF. *Musculoskeletal tumor surgery*. New York: Churchill Livingstone; 1983.
2. Pettersson H, Gillespy T III, Hamlin DJ, et al. Primary musculoskeletal tumors: Examination with MR imaging compared with conventional modalities. *Radiology* 1987;164:237–241.
3. Bloem JL, Bluemm RG, Taminiau AH, et al. Magnetic resonance imaging of primary malignant bone tumors. *Radiographics* 1987;7:425–445.
4. Mankin HJ, Lange TA, Spanier SS. The hazards of biopsy in patients with malignant primary bone and soft-tissue tumors. *J Bone Joint Surg* 1982;64A:1121–1127.
5. Mankin HJ, Mankin CJ, Simon MA. The hazards of biopsy, revisited. Members of the Musculoskeletal Tumor Society. *J Bone Joint Surg* 1996;78A:656–663.
6. Skrzynski MC, Biermann JS, Montag A, et al. Diagnostic accuracy and charge-savings of outpatient core needle biopsy compared with open biopsy of musculoskeletal tumors. *J Bone Joint Surg* 1996;78A:644–649.
7. Bass RL, Stern PJ. Elbow and forearm anatomy and surgical approaches. *Hand Clin* 1994;10:343–356.
8. Rock MG, Pritchard DJ, Reiman HM, et al. Extra-abdominal desmoid tumors. *J Bone Joint Surg* 1984;66A:1369–1371.
9. Posner MC, Shiu MH, Newsome JL, et al. The desmoid tumor. Not a benign disease. *Arch Surg* 1989;124:191–196.
10. McCollough WM, Parsons JT, van der Griend R, et al. Radiation therapy for aggressive fibromatosis. The experience at the University of Florida. *J Bone Joint Surg* 1991;73A:717–725.
11. Bullough PJ. *Orthopaedic pathology*. London: Mosby-Wolfe; 1997.
12. Morrey BF. *The elbow and its disorders*, 2nd ed. Philadelphia: WB Saunders; 1993.
13. Bryan RS, Soule EH, Dobyns JH, et al. Primary epithelioid sarcoma of the hand and forearm. A review of thirteen cases. *J Bone Joint Surg* 1974;56A:458–465.
14. Enzinger FM. Epithelioid sarcoma. A sarcoma simulating a granuloma or carcinoma. *Cancer* 1970;26:1029–1041.
15. Dell PC, Stern PJ. Benign and malignant neoplasms of the upper extremity. In: Peimer CA, ed. *Surgery of the hand and upper extremity*. New York: McGraw-Hill, 1996:2231–2263.
16. Enzinger FM, Weiss SW. *Soft tissue tumors*, 2nd ed. St. Louis, MO: CV Mosby; 1988.
17. Orson GG, Sim FH, Reiman HM, et al. Liposarcoma of the musculoskeletal system. *Cancer* 1987;60:1362–1370.
18. Campanacci M. *Bone and soft tissue tumors*. New York: Springer-Verlag; 1990.

CHAPTER 28

Olecranon Bursitis

Champ L. Baker Jr. and Peter W. Hester

INTRODUCTION

The function of the olecranon bursa, an underappreciated structure, is to limit friction in the elbow during the performance of everyday activities. The olecranon is the most common site of superficial bursitis.[1] Because there has been scant coverage of the condition in the literature, especially in recent work, we believe its pathologic state and treatment options should be addressed in this text.

CLINICAL ANATOMY

In an anatomic study, Chen and associates found no olecranon bursae in 47 cadavers of less than 7 years old.[2] A minute unilateral bursa was appreciated in 4 of 6 cadavers that were 7 to 10 years old. All specimens older than 10 years had a bursa present.

Buck et al. differentiated between adventitious bursae, such as the olecranon bursa, that lacked an endothelial lining and synovial bursae.[3] They noted that adventitious bursae, which are not present before birth, develop by "myxomatous degeneration in the fibrous tissue between skin and underlying bone." The bursal walls consist of fibroblasts surrounded by collagen fibrils, with lymphocytes, macrophages, and plasma cells.

The olecranon bursa is a subcutaneous synovial sac overlying the olecranon process (see Fig. 1.6B). When distended, it measures approximately 6 to 7 cm in length and 2.5 cm in width. The upper half usually lies proximal to the olecranon on the triceps tendon.[4] Bursae about the elbow are labeled deep or superficial. Deep bursae lie between muscles or between muscle and bone. Superficial bursae are those that lie over the epicondyles and the olecranon.

Deep bursae, which are difficult to define anatomically, are rarely pathologic. The bicipital radial bursa, a deep bursa located at the radial tuberosity between the tuberosity and biceps tendon, can be a confounding structure. Inflammation of the bursa can occur with pronation and supination, causing it to be misdiagnosed as distal biceps tendinitis. Among the superficial bursae, the medial epicondylar bursa may become inflamed in association with chronic subluxation of the ulnar nerve.[5]

ETIOLOGY

Traumatic Etiology

Repetitive valgus stressing of the elbow in the throwing athlete produces a shear force in the olecranon fossa that can lead to degenerative processes and the formation of osteophytes and loose bodies.[6] Extensor valgus overload syndrome, experienced primarily in the deceleration and follow-through phases of throwing, results in impingement of the olecranon on the posteromedial aspect of the olecranon fossa.[7] A direct blow can cause a fracture or can be the instigating event of olecranon bursitis.

Several conditions should be considered in a differential diagnosis for olecranon bursitis. An acute, forceful hyperextension locking of the elbow, as in football line blocking, can cause an avulsion fracture of the olecranon tip. Chronic overuse with repetitive extension can result in triceps tendinitis. Spontaneous rupture of the triceps tendon and disruption of the biceps at its insertion often mimic bursitis.

Infectious Etiology

Bacterial organisms that can cause olecranon bursitis are brucellosis, fusobacterium, mycobacterium, staphylococcus (*S. aureus*, which is the most common, occurring in 75% to 90% of cases, and *S. epidermidis*), streptococcus (group A β-hemolytic), and syphilis.[8]

Among the fungal organisms that have been found in patients with olecranon bursitis are blastomyces, *Candida*, *Sporothrix*, and tuberculosis.[8]

Inflammatory Etiology

Viggiano et al. reported three cases of septic arthritis in patients with rheumatoid arthritis that presented initially as olecranon bursitis.[9] Acute exacerbation of rheumatoid arthritis with pain, erythema, and swelling can be difficult to distinguish from septic arthritis. It is often difficult for the physician to differentiate between rheumatoid arthritis exacerbation and septic arthritis on the basis of radiographs and in the presence of fever, elevated erythrocyte sedimentation rate, and systemic leukocytosis.[6] Petrie and Wigley described proximal dissection of the bursal contents after rupture that presented as triceps swelling in patients with rheumatoid arthritis.[10]

Gerster and coworkers presented a case of nonseptic bursitis thought to be an extra-articular manifestation of calcium pyrophosphate dihydrate crystal deposition disease (chondrocalcinosis).[11] They believed that crystalline material had migrated from the triceps tendon toward a more superficial site, the bursa.

HISTORY AND PHYSICAL EXAMINATION

A distended olecranon bursa is usually painless and develops slowly. Traumatic bursitis is normally painless after the initiating event. When it is associated with a septic or crystalline inflammatory process, olecranon bursitis presents with pain and tenderness. Pien et al. reported associated local cellulitis and lymphadenitis in 41% of patients with septic bursitis.[1] The percentage of these patients who have fever ranges from 15%[1] to 86%.[12] In a series of 12 patients who had septic bursitis, Thompson and associates found the following concomitant conditions: diabetes (2), cirrhosis (2), end-stage renal disease (1), superficial burn to the elbow (1), lung cancer (1), alcoholism (1), and C-6 quadriplegia (1).[6]

Penetrating trauma or infections in proximity to the bursa are not prerequisites to septic bursitis.[8] Superficial bursae are usually more susceptible to infection because they are more vulnerable to trauma, such as the repeated or persistent pressure and friction caused by writing.[2]

Because posterior elbow pain associated with olecranon bursitis may be the result of traumatic, inflammatory, infectious, or noninfectious etiologic factors, the physician should examine the patient's history for a plausible mechanism and associated risk factors. Is the patient a baseball pitcher, a football lineman, a horticulturist, an end-stage renal patient on dialysis, or a middle-aged patient with a history of gout?

Understanding the nature of the patient's occupation and daily activities, such as those of a gardener, carpet layer, carpenter, housemaid, tailor, or truck driver, that makes them most vulnerable assists the physician in making the diagnosis and in preventing future episodes. A patient's medical history can alert the examiner to who is at greatest risk for operative complications, such as recurrence and infection. Dialysis elbow has been found in 7% of patients with an ipsilateral shunt.[13] Rheumatoid arthritis and gout are the two conditions most frequently associated with olecranon bursitis.[14]

Olecranon bursitis is signaled by the appearance of soft-tissue swelling (Fig. 28.1); however, differentiation between nonseptic and septic bursitis by appearance is not as straightforward. When a patient with septic bursitis is symptomatic, flexing the elbow to greater than 90° causes the most pronounced discomfort. Loss of motion, however, is an inconsistent finding.[5]

Before providing antibiotics to a patient, the bursa should be aspirated and the aspirate should be evaluated for gram stain, cell count with differential, culture and sensitivity, crystals (polarized light microscopy), and fungus (acid fast preparation). Glucose testing is of little value and is not necessary.[11] A low leukocyte count is to be expected with posttraumatic bursitis and helps to differentiate it from septic bursitis.

Blood studies include routine complete blood count with differential, electrolytes, erythrocyte sedimentation rate, serum uric acid level, and rheumatoid factor. Pathologic evaluation of acute bursitis shows a watery mucoid fluid. In the chronic condition, the fluid is darkened and marked by granular calcific densities. The bursal wall becomes thick and fibrous as the condition progresses.[15]

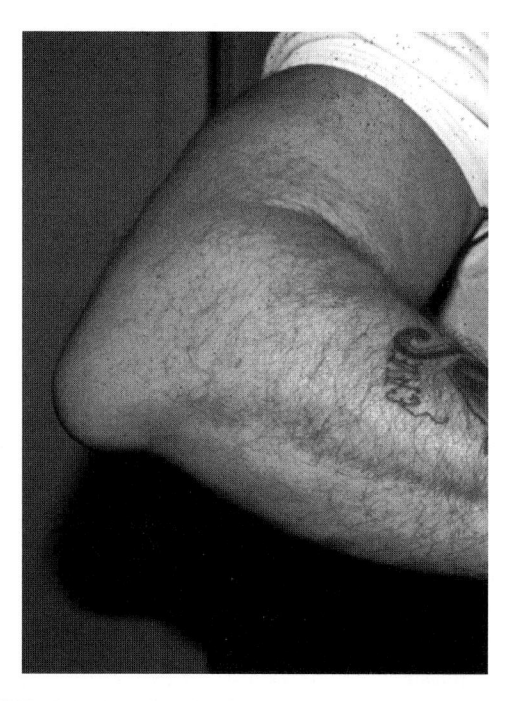

FIGURE 28.1. Localized soft-tissue swelling in a patient with olecranon bursitis.

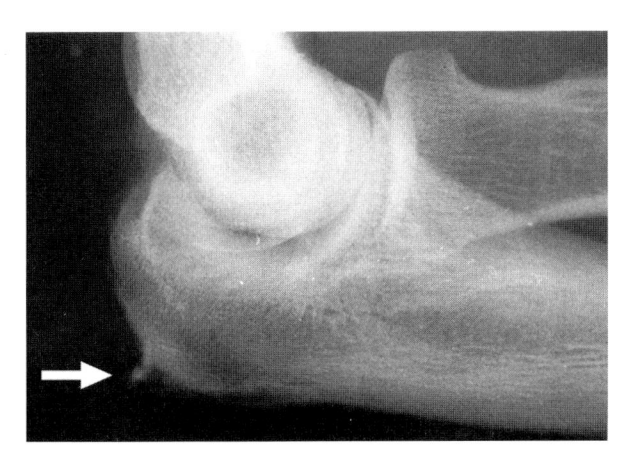

FIGURE 28.2. Olecranon spurring is seen frequently in the patient with olecranon bursitis.

Osteophytes, in particular olecranon spurs, can be seen on anteroposterior or lateral radiographic views (Fig. 28.2). The repetitive irritation caused by the spur is associated with traumatic bursitis.

To determine the best treatment course, the physician must consider the variables of overall patient condition, time course, response to previous treatments, and cause of the bursitis. Questions to be answered include the following:

1. Who is best treated with an oral antibiotic versus a parenteral antibiotic?
2. Who is best treated by aspiration versus surgical debridement?
3. Who is best treated with open debridement versus endoscopic excision?
4. Is bony excision necessary?

On reviewing the literature, we found authors who espoused very different treatment preferences for very similar conditions. The limited number of affected patients affords the practitioner few subjects on which to base treatment decisions.

NONOPERATIVE TREATMENT

Most patients with aseptic olecranon bursitis respond well to nonoperative treatment. Initially, the patient should be treated with any combination of immobilization, padding from pressure, limiting trauma, compression dressing, splinting, anti-inflammatory medication, aspiration, and corticosteroid injection.

Pien and coworkers reported successful treatment with oral antibiotics alone in 51% of 34 patients with septic olecranon bursitis.[1] The authors used dicloxacillin sodium, 4g, and probenecid, 2g, daily for at least 4 weeks. The patients in their study, however, had no fever, leukocytosis, or extensive cellulitis before treatment.

Fisher suggested placing a size 16 angiocath into the bursa and leaving it in place for 3 days.[16] His experience was that the recurrence rate was diminished compared with that of a single aspiration. Others use aspiration and corticosteroid injections to treat the disorder. Jaffe and Fetto treated four of twelve patients with aspiration and an injection of 40 mg methylprednisolone acetate.[17] One patient had resolution of pain, and two had recurrent painless swelling. In a second group of five patients treated with aspiration, oral indomethacin, 25 mg, 3 times a day; and compression dressings, they reported that three patients had resolution and no recurrence. No patient in either of these two groups was thought to have an infection. For bursitis without infection in this small population, oral anti-inflammatory medication was as effective as intrabursal injection. Weinstein and associates found that, although the injection of corticosteroids reduced the frequency of recurrence in their patients, there was an increased complication rate.[18] Infections and subdermal atrophy were most notable. Quayle and Robinson aspirated 4 of 11 elbows in their patients with olecranon bursitis.[4] All were without resolution and required surgery. Kerr recommends application of a compressive wrap to be maintained for several weeks.[19]

Complications

Triceps tendon ruptures have been linked to nonoperative treatment of olecranon bursitis. In 1993, Stannard and Bucknell reported a case of triceps rupture in a patient treated with local steroid injections.[20] The fact that he was a weight lifter with a history of anabolic steroid use increased this patient's vulnerability to this injury. Treating strength athletes with local injections for pain relief can place injured or compromised tissues at risk.

Clayton and Thirupathi proposed proliferation of the bursal synovial lining membrane extending to and then posterior to the triceps tendon, creating a "collar stud-shaped bursa," as the precursor for triceps tendon rupture in an elderly man.[21] They suggested that patients with chronic olecranon bursa problems should be carefully examined for triceps function.

OPERATIVE TREATMENT

When aspiration and corticosteroid injection do not eradicate olecranon bursitis, surgical excision of the bursa is the remaining option. Some authors recommend a second or third aspiration before deciding on surgery,[19] whereas others proceed with surgery after one unsuccessful aspiration.[1] If the condition does not respond quickly to aspiration with or without steroid injection and the discomfort and pain persist, the physician should assume that the condition is septic bursitis and, as such, requires greater intervention.

Open Technique

In their patients with septic bursitis, Pien et al. reported that 6 of 34 patients required surgical drainage.[1] Knight and coworkers used a suction-drainage antibiotic (1% kanamycin and 0.1% polymyxin) irrigation system through 3-mm percutaneous tubes.[22] In 10 patients treated by this method, there were no recurrences or chronic sinus tract formation.

Quayle and Robinson recommended excision of a prominent olecranon process or spur for their patients with chronic bursitis.[4] They also leave the bursal substance intact to avoid skin compromise. A curved lateral incision is made 3 cm proximal and 5 cm distal to the olecranon. The triceps tendon and its periosteal attachment are divided longitudinally in the midline and elevated from the olecranon and proximal end of the ulna. Nine of 11 patients had normal function after prominence excision. They reported no recurrences.

Stewart et al. recommend a lateral incision and complete excision of the bursa as a single structure to ensure complete removal of the bursal lining.[23] Osteophytes were removed when present. They reviewed the cases of 21 patients with chronic olecranon bursitis who had had no aspirations or steroid injections. Five of these patients had a history of rheumatoid arthritis. Only 2 of the 5 had long-lasting relief, compared with 94% of the remaining patients who had no systemic conditions.

Postoperatively, the elbow is maintained in flexion from 45° to 90° for 1 to 2 weeks.

Endoscopic Technique

The most commonly reported complications of an open olecranon bursectomy are problems related to the surgical wound.[4] Because of the morbidity associated with open surgical excision of the bursa, other authors have proposed endoscopic excision.[19,24–26]

Ogilvie-Harris and Gilbart recently reported the results of their endoscopic technique for bursal resection in 31 patients.[25] With their technique, the patient was positioned supine and given either a general or regional anesthetic. Before inserting the 5.0-mm arthroscope, the bursa is expanded with saline through a small needle. The authors recommend not inserting the scope directly into the skin over the bursa, which could collapse the bursa, but rather placing the portals 1 cm away from the bursal sac. By doing so, the arthroscope passes subcutaneously through a tunnel into the sac. A sharp, rather than blunt, obturator is used to avoid bursal rupture. To optimize visualization of the bursa, the elbow is flexed to 45° and a pressure irrigation system is used.

A 4.5-mm curved shaver is introduced medially. The subcutaneous portion of the bursa is resected first, followed by the deep portion. Resection is complete when triceps tendon fibers can be seen. After the scope is removed, any remaining bursa quickly collapses.

Twenty-five of the 31 patients had no postoperative pain. One recurrence was reported in a patient with rheumatoid arthritis. The bursa was found to communicate with the elbow joint in this patient. The authors recommend caution when considering bursal excision in patients with rheumatologic conditions.

Kerr used a similar arthroscopic bursectomy technique, but recommends the prone position.[19] He felt it was most important to remove the anterior and posterior walls of the bursa and to avoid removing too much subcutaneous fat. He mentions increasing transillumination of the skin as a guide to determining the amount of wall removed.

In 1993, Kerr reported the results of his four patients treated with endoscopic excision.[19] Three of the four had satisfactory results with no recurrence, no pain, no loss of motion, and no complication after endoscopic excision. The one unsatisfactory result was in a patient who had gout as an underlying condition and developed an infection postoperatively that required open incision and drainage and intravenous antibiotics.

Authors' Preferred Technique

We also recommend prone positioning of the patient for arthroscopic olecranon bursectomy.[24] The three portals used are the lateral, proximal central, and distal central. Medial portals are not used because of the risk of injury to the ulnar nerve. The portals are created using a no. 11 surgical blade, and a hemostat is used to spread the soft tissues. Initial examination of the bursal sac usually reveals chronic granulomatous inflammatory tissue. Rheumatoid tophi or gouty crystals may be present. A total

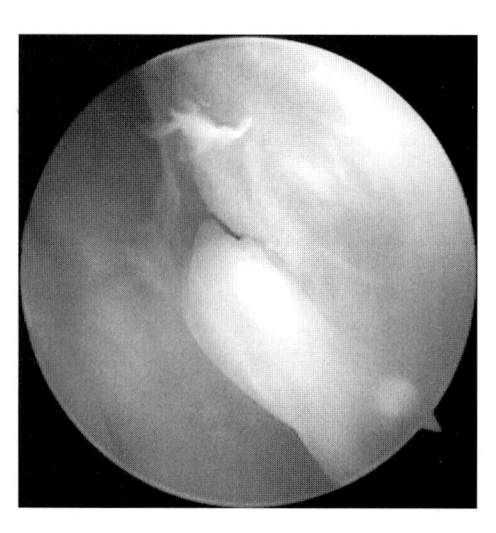

FIGURE 28.3. Osteophyte formation on the olecranon tip.

bursectomy is performed, with the surgeon exchanging operative and visualization portals as necessary. After the bursal tissue has been removed, an increase in light can be appreciated through the skin and the triceps tendon can be seen. Any spurs on the olecranon tip should be removed with an arthroscopic burr (Fig. 28.3).

The portals are closed with 3-0 nylon sutures. The portals are not injected with anesthetic because of the need for a postoperative neurological evaluation. A compression dressing is worn for 7 to 10 days. Mobilization of the extremity is started immediately.

COMPLICATIONS

From the few data available detailing treatment results of this condition, we can see that complications occur frequently. Quayle and Robinson reported adherence of scars to tendon and bone in 2 of 11 patients treated with open excision.[4] Thompson and coworkers found that open surgical drainage produced a chronic synovial-cutaneous fistula in 2 of their 5 patients.[6]

When treating olecranon bursitis by the endoscopic method, the surgeon should be aware that patients with a rheumatologic condition are more susceptible to recurrence and infection and rarely do well.[19,24]

CONCLUSIONS

Olecranon bursitis remains a condition that is infrequently encountered, and treatment options are less than dogmatic. We encourage nonoperative management of this condition initially. However, operative treatment for recalcitrant cases can be successful and produce long-lasting results. We believe that arthroscopic resection of the bursa lessens the frequency of complications of skin incisions and infections and loss of joint mobility.

To be effective in treating olecranon bursitis, the physician needs to recognize the patient at risk for complications. The physician should be familiar with basic bursal histopathology, elbow anatomy, and treatment options for acute, aseptic bursitis. He or she should be able to recognize septic bursitis, which is potentially fatal, and take the appropriate steps to make the diagnosis and treat the patient.

REFERENCES

1. Pien FD, Ching D, Kim E. Septic bursitis: experience in a community practice. *Orthopedics* 1991;14:981–984.
2. Chen J, Alk D, Eventov I, Weintroub S. Development of the olecranon bursa: an anatomic cadaver study. *Acta Orthop Scand* 1987;58:408–409.
3. Buck RM, McDonald JR, Ghormley RK. Adventitious bursae. *Arch Surg* 1943;47:344.
4. Quayle JB, Robinson MP. A useful procedure in the treatment of chronic olecranon bursitis. *Injury* 1978;9:299–302.
5. Morrey BF. Bursitis. In: Morrey, BF, ed. *The elbow and its disorders*, 3rd ed. Philadelphia: WB Saunders; 2000:901–908.
6. Thompson GR, Manshady BM, Weiss JJ. Septic bursitis. *JAMA* 1978;240:2280–2281.
7. Andrews JR, Schemmel SP, Whiteside JA. Evaluation, treatment, and prevention of elbow injuries in throwing athletes. In: Nicholas JA, Hershman EB, eds. *The upper extremity in sports medicine*. St. Louis, MO: CV Mosby; 1990:793.
8. Ho G Jr, Tice AD, Kaplan SR. Septic bursitis in the prepatellar and olecranon bursae. An analysis of 25 cases. *Ann Internal Med* 1978;89:21–27.
9. Viggiano DA, Garrett JC, Clayton ML. Septic arthritis presenting as olecranon bursitis in patients with rheumatoid arthritis. A report of three cases. *J Bone Joint Surg* 1980;62A:1011–1012.
10. Petrie JP, Wigley RD. Proximal dissection of the olecranon bursa in rheumatoid arthritis. *Rheumatol Int* 1984;4:139–140.
11. Gerster JC, Lagier R, Boivin G. Olecranon bursitis related to calcium pyrophosphate dihydrate crystal deposition disease. *Arthritis Rheum* 1982;25:989–996.
12. Soderquist B, Hedstrom SA. Predisposing factors, bacteriology and antibiotic therapy in thirty-five cases of septic bursitis. *Scand J Infect Dis* 1986;18:305–311.
13. Jain VK, Cestero RV, Baum J. Septic and aseptic olecranon bursitis in patients on maintenance hemodialysis. *Clin Exp Dial Apheresis* 1981;5:405–414.
14. Bensen WG, Laskin CA, Little HA, Fam AG. Hemochromatotic arthropathy mimicking rheumatoid arthritis. A case with subcutaneous nodules, tenosynovitis, and bursitis. *Arthritis Rheum* 1978;21:844–848.
15. Robbins SL. *Pathologic basis of disease*. Philadelphia:WB Saunders; 1974:1474–1475.
16. Fisher, RH. Conservative treatment of distended patellar and olecranon bursae. *Clin Orthop* 1977;123:98.
17. Jaffe L, Fetto JF. Olecranon bursitis. *Contempor Ortho* 1984;8: 51–54.
18. Weinstein PS, Canoso JJ, Wohlgethan JR. Long-term follow-up of corticosteroid injection for traumatic olecranon bursitis. *Ann Rheum Dis* 1984;43:44–46.
19. Kerr DR. Prepatellar and olecranon arthroscopic bursectomy. *Clin Sports Med* 1993;12:137–142.
20. Stannard JP, Bucknell AL. Rupture of the triceps tendon associated with steroid injections. *Am J Sports Med* 1993;21: 482–485.
21. Clayton ML, Thirupathi RG. Rupture of the triceps tendon with olecranon bursitis. A case report with a new method of repair. *Clin Orthop* 1984;184:183–185.
22. Knight JM, Thomas JC, Maurer RC. Treatment of septic olecranon and prepatellar bursitis with percutaneous placement of a suction-irrigation system: a report of 12 cases. *Clin Orthop* 1986;206:90–93.
23. Stewart NJ, Manzanares JB, Morrey BF. Surgical treatment of aseptic olecranon bursitis. *J Shoulder Elbow Surg* 1997;6:49–54.
24. Baker CL Jr, Cummings PD. Arthroscopic management of miscellaneous elbow disorders. *Oper Tech Sports Med* 1998;6: 16–21.
25. Ogilvie-Harris DJ, Gilbart M. Endoscopic bursal resection: the olecranon bursa and prepatellar bursa. *Arthroscopy* 2000;16: 249–253.
26. Savoie FH. Miscellaneous disorders. In: Savoie FH, Field LD, eds. *Elbow arthroscopy*. New York: Churchill-Livingstone; 1996:145–149.

CHAPTER 29

Rehabilitation of Elbow Injuries in Overhead-throwing Athletes

Kevin E. Wilk and Terese Chmielewski

INTRODUCTION

Rehabilitation plays a significant role in restoring complete, unrestricted, and pain-free elbow function following elbow injury or surgery. The elbow is susceptible to a variety of injuries because of the excessive forces that are generated and transferred to this joint during sports. The athlete who participates in sports involving overhead throwing motions is susceptible to both macrotraumatic and microtraumatic injuries of the elbow. Baseball pitchers are particularly susceptible to elbow injuries because of the significantly high forces generated at the elbow joint complex. According to biomechanical studies, each time the pitcher throws a fast ball, the force that occurs on the medial side of the elbow joint is sufficient to rupture the ulnar collateral ligament. Tennis players are most susceptible to overuse injuries, such as tendinitis.[1] Javelin throwers also are susceptible to specific elbow injuries, such as ligament ruptures and osseous spurring.[2]

Some elbow injuries can be treated nonoperatively, but others require surgical intervention to restore full, pain-free function. The rehabilitation process often is challenging to clinicians due to the unique anatomic orientation of the elbow joint complex, particularly the high degree of joint congruency and the role of the dynamic stabilizers. The purpose of this chapter is to discuss the rehabilitation programs for various elbow injuries in the overhead athlete.

REHABILITATION OVERVIEW

Before focusing on each rehabilitation program, several basic principles of elbow rehabilitation should be recognized. Two of these principles include the following: the effects of immobilization should be minimized, and healing tissue should never be overstressed.

Next, the rehabilitation specialist should follow a rehabilitation program that is progressive, has multiple phases, and is based on specific criteria. In this approach, the clinician outlines objective goals that the patient must meet before advancing to the next phase of rehabilitation. This approach decreases the likelihood that healing tissue will be exposed to stresses for which it is not ready. In addition, the rehabilitation program should be based on current clinical and basic science research. The program also should be adaptable to the individual and the individual's goals. For example, with an athlete, the program must progress to a sport-specific program. Finally, a team approach should be used. The team comprises the athlete, physician, physical therapist, athletic trainer, coach, and any ancillary staff, including a biomechanist or strength and conditioning coach. By following this type of approach, the goal of returning the athlete to his or her sport can be achieved in the safest and most expeditious manner possible.

Often, deciding when an athlete is ready to progress to sport-specific rehabilitation can be difficult. This decision becomes more objective when specific criteria are outlined. At our center, the athlete must exhibit full, nonpainful range of motion (ROM); a satisfactory clinical examination; and isokinetic assessment results within a specific range (Table 29.1). Additionally, the athlete must have progressed through the necessary phases of rehabilitation, particularly the advanced phase. An interval sport program can be initiated when the athlete exhibits all the outlined criteria and when adequate healing has occurred.

The rehabilitation programs that we discuss next are based on the rehabilitation principles and guidelines. We briefly discuss the nonoperative rehabilitation of elbow injuries frequently applied in sports medicine.

TABLE 29.1. *Isokinetic assessment*

	180°/s	300°/s
Bilateral comparison		
Elbow flexor	110%–120%	105%–115%
Elbow extensor	105%–115%	100%–110%
Flexor–extensor ratio	70%–80%	63%–69%

Medial Pathology

Structures on the medial aspect of the elbow are subject to tensile overload forces. Of great concern is the large valgus torque applied to the elbow during the overhead throwing motion.[3] Morrey and An[4] reported that the ulnar collateral ligament (UCL) accounted for 54% of the restraint to a valgus stress. Thus, the UCL is one of the medial elbow structures commonly injured during the overhead throwing motion. During each pitch, the tensile forces generated on the medial aspect of the elbow are significant enough to rupture the ulnar collateral ligament.[3] However, the medial forearm musculature and osseus structures help to dissipate these forces and prevent ulnar collateral ligament failure.

UCL Sprain or Tear

Nonoperative treatment is employed for suspected UCL sprains and occasionally for partial tears. Controversy exists regarding whether immobilization is required or whether immediate motion can be used in the treatment of this injury. Table 29.2 provides the complete rehabil-

TABLE 29.2. *Conservative rehabilitation for ulnar collateral ligament sprains*

Phase	Goals	ROM[1]	Exercises and modalities
I: Immediate motion (weeks 0–2)	Increase ROM[1] Promote UCL[2] healing Retard muscular atrophy Decrease pain, inflammation	Brace (optional) and nonpainful ROM (20°–90°) AAROM,[3] PROM[4] for elbow and wrist (nonpainful ROM)	Isometrics for wrist and elbow musculature Shoulder strengthening (no ER) Ice and compression
II: Intermediate (weeks 3–6)	Increase ROM Improve strength, endurance Decrease pain, inflammation	Gradually increase motion 0°–90° (10°/week)	Initiate isotonic exercises Wrist curls Wrist extensions Pronation, supination Biceps, triceps Dumbbells: ER, IR, deltoid, supraspinatus, rhomboids Rhythmic stabilization drills Ice and compression
III: Advanced (weeks 6/7–12/14)	Increase strength, power, endurance Improve neuromuscular control Initiate high-speed exercise drills To progress to: Full ROM No pain or tenderness No increased laxity Strength 4/5[1] of elbow flexors, extensors	Initiate tubing, shoulder program Thrower's Ten Biceps, triceps Supination, pronation Wrist flexion, extension Plyometric throwing drills	
IV: Return to activity (week 12/14)	To return to throwing: Full, nonpainful ROM No increased laxity Isokinetic test fulfills criteria Satisfactory clinical examination	Initiate interval throwing Continue Thrower's Ten Continue plyometrics	

ROM, range of motion; UCL, ulnar collateral ligament; AAROM, active assisted range of motion; PROM, passive range of motion; ER, external rotation; IR, internal rotation.
[1]Manual muscle testing grade of good/normal.

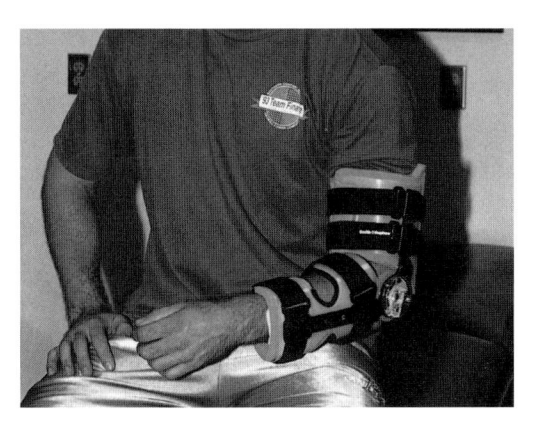

FIGURE 29.1. Elbow range of motion brace (Smith and Nephew, Carlsbad, CA).

proprioceptive and dynamic stabilization abilities of the elbow joint complex before a throwing program is started.

The third phase is initiated approximately 6 to 7 weeks after injury. In this phase, the goals are to increase muscular strength and endurance and to improve neuromuscular control. The athlete follows the Thrower's Ten program (Table 29.3), which is an isotonic strengthening program focusing on muscle groups specific to the throwing athlete. This program may be modified based on the individual's deficiencies. Exercises that are initiated during this phase include exercise-tubing drills for the wrist, elbow, shoulder, and plyometrics (any exercise in which the muscle is contracted eccentricly then, immediately concentrically). Specific plyometrics that can be performed include two-hand overhead soccer throw, two-hand chest pass, two-hand side-to-side throw, one-hand

itation program. During the first phase, which usually lasts 2 to 3 weeks, we use a program that limits motion in a range from 20° to 90° immediately following injury. This program may allow the inflamed tissue to calm and may promote collagen formation along the medial capsule and UCL without generating excessive stress on the UCL. This approach is used for acute UCL injury only. A ROM brace is most often used to assist in controlling the ROM and the valgus stress applied to the elbow joint (Fig. 29.1); the athlete can perform active assisted or passive ROM exercises while in the brace. Isometric strengthening exercises also are allowed during this phase. Isometrics are performed for the entire upper extremity. Modalities, especially cryotherapy, are used to control pain and inflammation.

The second phase usually begins during week 3 and progresses through week 6 of treatment. The athlete's ROM is gradually progressed with the goal of obtaining full ROM. Motion usually is progressed by 5° of extension and 10° of flexion per week. Thus, by the end of 6 weeks, the patient should exhibit full motion. Often a flexion contracture is present in the overhead pitcher before the injury. Therefore, full elbow extension is occasionally not possible. The clinician should ask the athlete if he or she was able to extend the arm fully before the injury. Isotonic strengthening is initiated for the entire upper extremity. Particular focus is placed on the flexor–pronator muscles, shoulder external rotators, and scapular muscles. We emphasize the flexor carpi ulnaris and flexor digitorum muscles because of their origin overlying the UCL and their role in improving medial elbow stability. To enhance proprioception, neuromuscular control, and dynamic stability of the medial aspect of the elbow, rhythmic stabilization drills and manual resistance drills also are included in this phase (Figs. 29.2 and 29.3). These drills use principles of proprioceptive neuromuscular facilitation.[5] Our goal is to enhance the athlete's

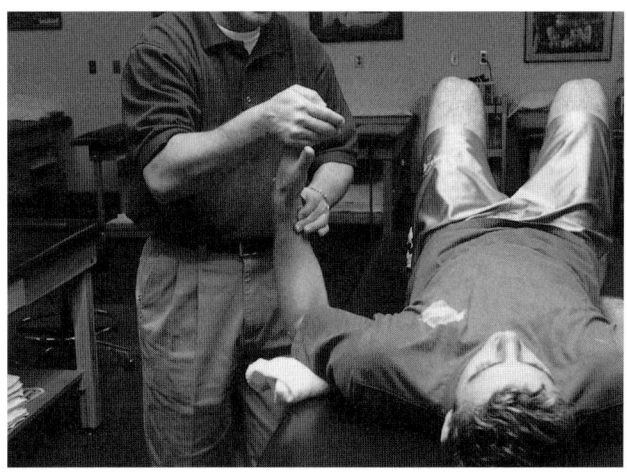

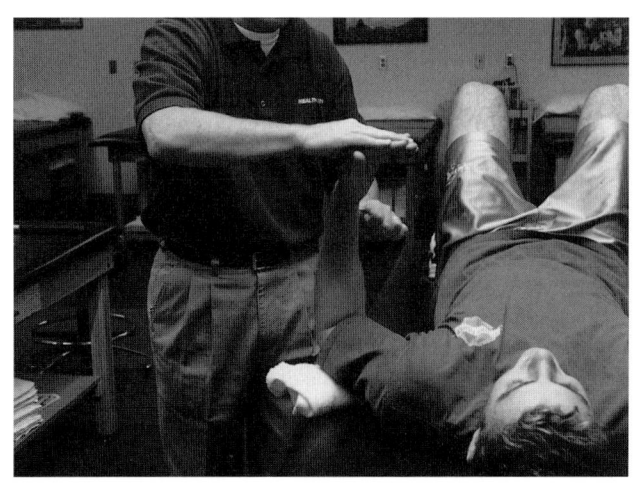

FIGURE 29.2. Rhythmic stabilization drill performed for the elbow musculature. The clinician gently applies force to elbow flexion (A) and extension (B). The patient attempts to control the force so that no movement occurs at the elbow.

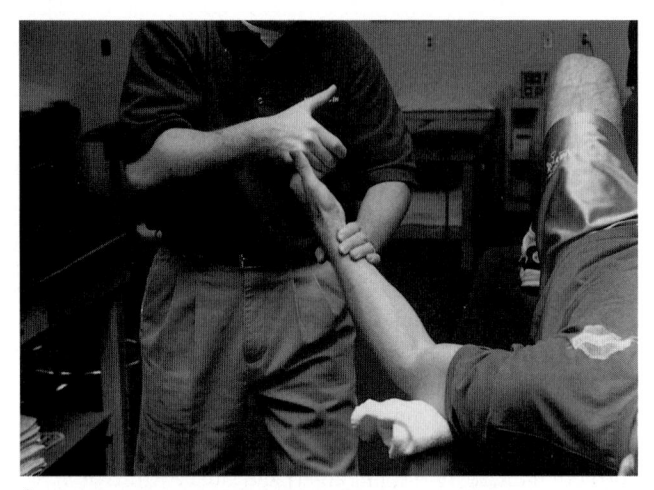

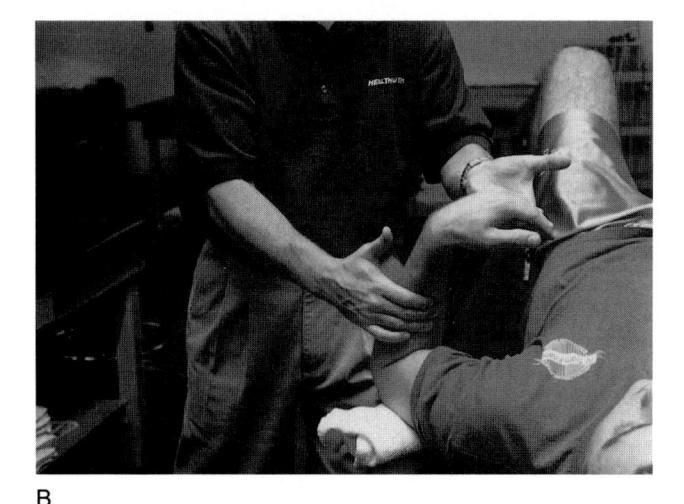

FIGURE 29.3. Manual resistance is applied during (A) elbow and (B) wrist flexion.

baseball throw, wrist flips, wall dribble, and side throw (Figs. 29.4 through 29.10). These exercises promote and enhance proprioception, neuromuscular control, and reactive neuromuscular control; they also prepare the athlete for the final phase of the rehabilitation program by gradually increasing the stresses applied to the elbow joint. The rehabilitation specialist should develop a sport-specific plyometric program.

Once the athlete exhibits the criteria to enter the fourth phase, an interval sport program is initiated. The overhead thrower initiates an interval throwing program, starting with phase I, the long-toss program (Table 29.4), and progressing to phase II, off-the-mound throwing (if the athlete is a pitcher) (Table 29.5). After the interval throwing program has been completed, the athlete can gradually return to competition. Often a pitcher is placed on a progressive pitch count program when he or she returns to competitive play. This program is designed to control the amount of stress applied to the elbow while gradually increasing the demands.

Ulnar Neuritis

Ulnar neuritis can be divided into three stages.[2] The acute onset of radicular symptoms characterizes the first stage. In the second stage, the athlete experiences a recurrence of symptoms when he or she attempts to return to throwing. A persistence of motor weakness and sensory changes characterize the third stage. If an athlete has progressed to the third stage, reversing symptoms through nonoperative methods is difficult.[6] Clinically, most throwers present either in stage 1 or, more frequently, in stage 2 of ulnar neuropathy.

Initially, the goal of the rehabilitation program for ulnar neuritis is to decrease inflammation of the ulnar nerve (Table 29.6). This goal is accomplished with modalities, such as cryotherapy, whirlpool, and high-voltage galvanic

TABLE 29.3. Thrower's Ten program

Exercise	Exercise
Diagonal pattern (D2) extension	Press-ups
Diagonal pattern (D2) flexion	Prone rowing
External rotation at 0° abduction	Push-ups
Internal rotation at 0° abduction	Elbow flexion
External rotation at 90° abduction (slow)	Elbow extension
External rotation at 90° abduction (fast)	Wrist extension
Internal rotation at 90° abduction (slow)	Wrist flexion
Internal rotation at 90° abduction (fast)	Supination
Shoulder abduction to 90°	Pronation
Scaption* ("full can")	
Prone horizontal abduction (neutral)	
Prone horizontal abduction (full ER, 100° ABD)	

*Elevation of the shoulder in the plane of the scapula.

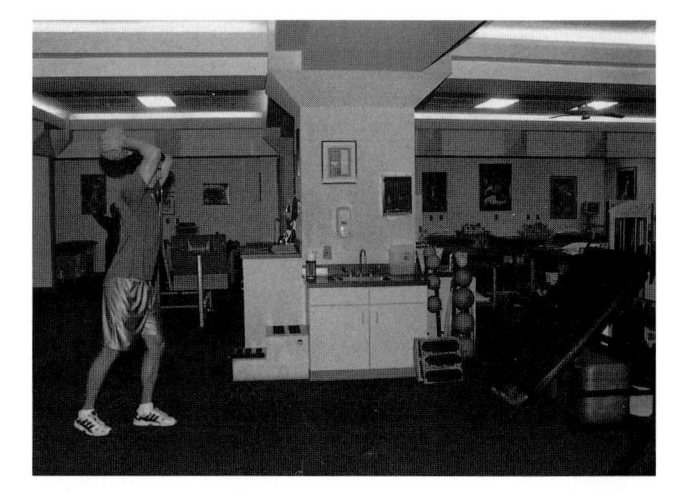

FIGURE 29.4. Two-hand overhead soccer throw plyometric exercise drill.

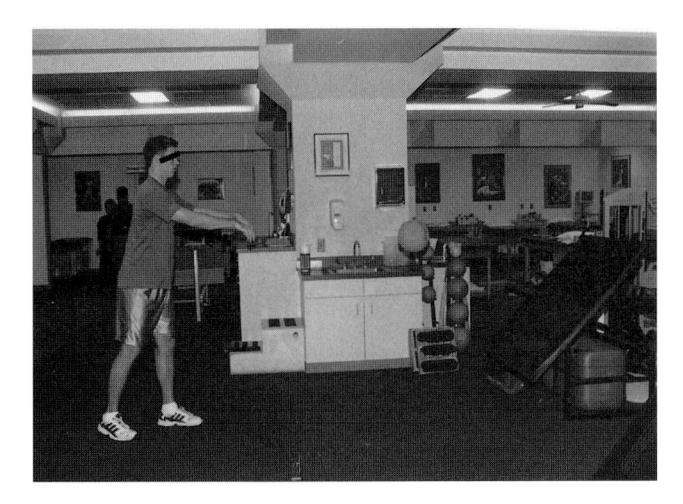

FIGURE 29.5. Two-hand chest pass plyometric exercise drill.

stimulation. Brace use is optional and may be used for patients who have more complicated cases or who exhibit pronounced irritability. Motion can be restricted if ulnar nerve instability is present. Often humeral rotation combined with elbow extension and flexion is restricted by the clinician. Isometric strengthening may be required if the elbow is extremely painful; otherwise, isotonics can be initiated. The musculature of the entire upper extremity should be included in the strengthening program. Exercises to improve gripping also should be included, particularly for the muscles of the hypothenar eminence: adductor pollicis, flexor pollicis brevis, and the interossei muscles. These muscles receive motor supply from the ulnar nerve. Strengthening exercises, such as elbow flexion–extension and shoulder internal–external rotation should be monitored carefully to ensure that ulnar nerve irritability or instability does not occur. Flexibility exercises should be performed to prevent muscular tightness and to restore full ROM. The acute phase usually lasts

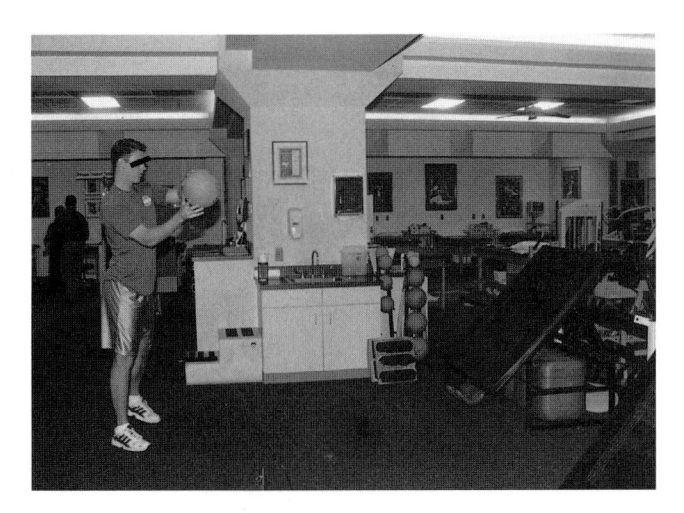

FIGURE 29.6. Two-hand side-to-side throw plyometric exercise drill.

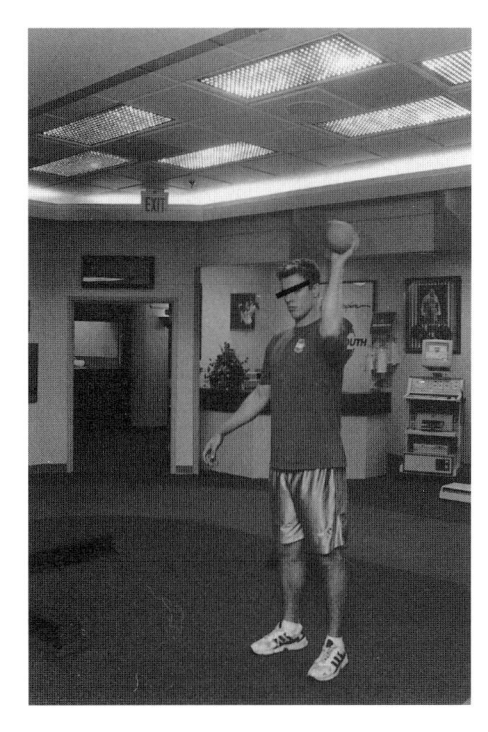

FIGURE 29.7. One-hand baseball throw (90° of shoulder abduction) plyometric exercise drill.

approximately 2 weeks or until the ulnar neuritis symptoms have subsided.

An important consideration in rehabilitation for ulnar neuritis is restoring dynamic stability to the medial elbow. This component, along with increasing muscular strength and endurance, is the focus of the advanced strengthening phase. Neuromuscular drills aid in restor-

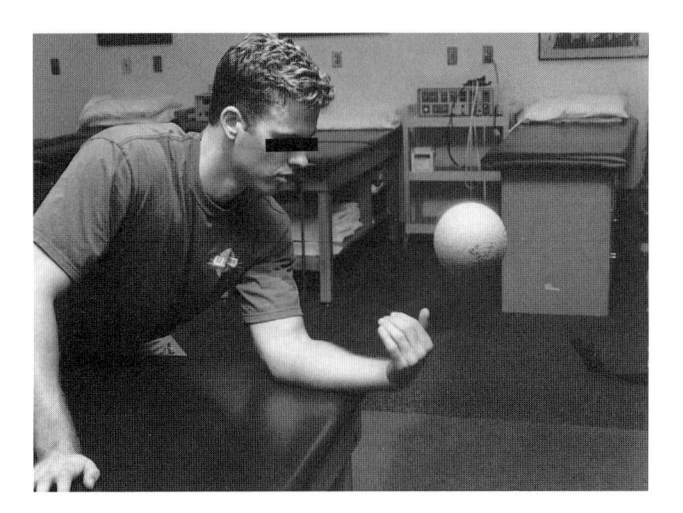

FIGURE 29.8. Wrist extension plyometric exercise drill. The patient lays his wrist across the edge of a table, tosses the ball into the air, and catches the ball. This drill also can be performed with the forearm supinated, working the wrist flexors.

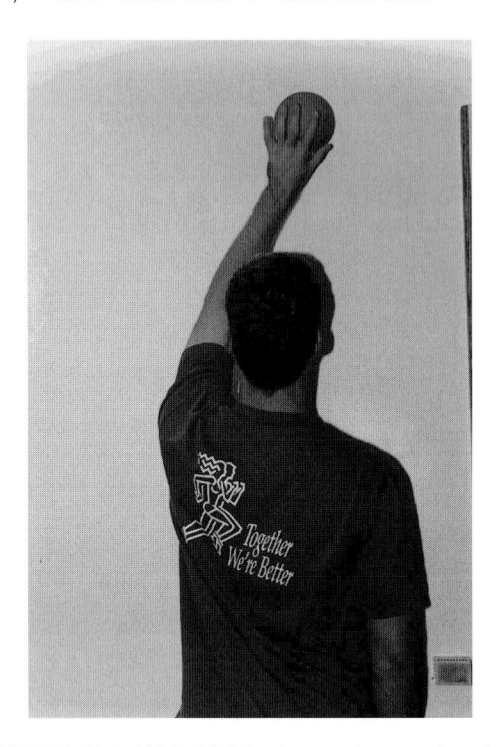

FIGURE 29.9. Wall dribble plyometric exercise drill.

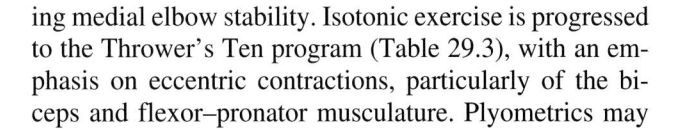

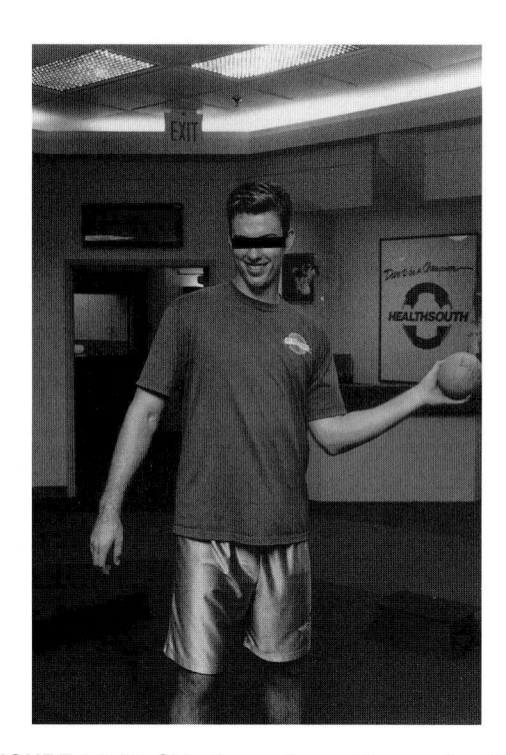

FIGURE 29.10. Side throw plyometric exercise drill.

ing medial elbow stability. Isotonic exercise is progressed to the Thrower's Ten program (Table 29.3), with an emphasis on eccentric contractions, particularly of the biceps and flexor–pronator musculature. Plyometrics may be initiated, provided that the athlete does not report pain or recurrent ulnar neuropathy symptoms.

The return-to-activity phase usually is initiated after 4 to 6 weeks of treatment. The athlete must exhibit all cri-

TABLE 29.4. *Interval throwing program, Phase I: Long-toss program*

Distance (ft)	Step	Program
45	1	Warm-up throwing
		25 throws at 45 ft
		Rest 15 minutes
		25 throws at 45 ft
	2	Warm-up throwing
		25 throws at 45 ft
		Rest 10 minutes
		Repeat
		Repeat
60	3	Same as step 1 but substitute 60 ft for 45 ft
	4	Same as step 2 but substitute 60 ft for 45 ft
90	5	Same as step 1 but substitute 90 ft for 45 ft
	6	Same as step 2 but substitute 90 ft for 45 ft
120	7	Same as step 1 but substitute 120 ft for 45 ft
	8	Same as step 2 but substitute 120 ft for 45 ft
150	9	Same as step 1 but substitute 150 ft for 45 ft
	10	Same as step 2 but substitute 150 ft for 45 ft
180	11	Same as step 1 but substitute 180 ft for 45 ft
	12	Same as step 2 but substitute 180 ft for 45 ft
	13	Same as step 12
	14	Begin throwing off the mound or return to respective position

Note: Throwing is performed every other day unless specified otherwise by physician, physical therapist, or athletic trainer.

TABLE 29.5. *Interval throwing program, Phase II: Off-the mound throwing*

Stage	Step	Program
1 Fastball only	1	Interval throwing[1] 15 throws off mound[2] at 50%
	2	Interval throwing 30 throws off mound at 50%
	3	Interval throwing 45 throws off mound at 50%
	4	Interval throwing 60 throws off mound at 50%
	5	Interval throwing 30 throws off mound at 75%
	6	30 throws off mound at 75% 45 throws off mound at 50%
	7	45 throws off mound at 75% 15 throws off mound at 50%
	8	60 throws off mound at 75%
2 Fastball only	9	45 throws off mound at 75% 15 throws in batting practice
	10	45 throws off mound at 75% 30 throws in batting practice
	11	45 throws off mound at 75% 45 throws in batting practice
3	12	30 throws off mound at 75% (warm-up) 15 throws off mound at 50% (breaking balls) 45–60 throws in batting practice (fastball only)
	13	30 throws off mound at 75% 30 breaking balls at 75% 30 throws in batting practice
	14	30 throws off mound at 75% 60–70 throws in batting practice, 25% breaking balls
	15	Simulated game: Progress by 15 throws per workout

[1] Use interval throwing to 120 feet as warm-up.

[2] All throwing off the mound should be done in the presence of the pitching coach to stress proper throwing mechanics. Use speed gun to aid in effort control.

teria necessary to enter this phase, including full, nonpainful ROM; satisfactory clinical examination; and satisfactory isokinetic performance (see Table 29.1). The athlete must complete both phases I and II of the interval throwing program before he or she can return to competition. If the athlete continues to report and exhibit symptoms of ulnar neuritis once a sport-specific program has been initiated, further diagnostic tests may be necessary to determine an underlying cause. Often, UCL insufficiency causes recurring ulnar neuritis symptoms. Occasionally, surgical intervention is required.

Medial Epicondylitis and Flexor–Pronator Tendinitis

Characteristics of flexor–pronator tendinitis include pain over the tendon insertion site as well as pain produced with resisted wrist flexion and pronation. It can exist in isolation (primary disorder) or in combination with another disorder (secondary disorder). Associated ulnar neuropathy is often found in patients with medial epicondylitis. Overhead throwers with this condition may have an underlying sprain or partial tear of the UCL, and the flexor–pronator tendinitis becomes a secondary condition. Thus, the differential diagnosis in medial elbow pain is not only difficult, but also vital to successful treatment.

The initial phase of treatment for these disorders focuses on decreasing inflammation, promoting tissue healing, retarding muscle atrophy, and allowing the patient to be involved in activities that are not irritating to the involved area. Modalities, such as cryotherapy, iontophoresis, phonophoresis, high-voltage galvanic stimulation, and warm whirlpool, can be used to control pain and inflammation. Isometrics may be used in this phase for muscular strengthening. Flexibility exercises are essential to ensure tendon healing and proper alignment of newly synthesized collagen tissue. Transverse, or friction, massage has been suggested as a treatment approach for

TABLE 29.6. *Nonoperative rehabilitation for ulnar neuritis*

Phase	Goals	Program

I: Acute (weeks 0–2)	Diminish ulnar nerve inflammation
	Restore normal motion
	Maintain, improve muscular strength
		Brace (optional): Only used if extreme inflammation
		Range of motion (ROM)
		  Restore full, nonpainful ROM as soon as possible
		  Initiate stretching exercises for wrist, forearm, elbow musculature
		Strengthening exercises: If extreme pain and inflammation, use isometrics for approximately one week; otherwise, initiate isotonic strengthening
		    Wrist flexion, extension
		    Forearm pronation, supination
		    Elbow flexion, extension
		    Shoulder program
		Pain and inflammation control
		  Warm whirlpool
		  Cryotherapy
		  High-voltage galvanic stimulation

II: Advanced strengthening (weeks 3–4)	Improve strength, power, endurance
	Enhance dynamic joint stability
	Initiate high-speed training
		Exercises: Thrower's Ten
		  Eccentrics for wrist, forearm muscles
		  Rhythmic stabilization drills for elbow joint
		  Plyometric exercise drills
		Continue stretching exercises

III: Return to activity (weeks 4–6)	Gradual return to functional activities
	Enhance muscular performance
	Criteria to begin throwing:
	  Full, nonpainful ROM
	  Satisfactory clinical examination
	  Satisfactory muscular performance
		Initiate interval sport program
		Continue Thrower's Ten
		Continue all stretching exercises

this condition;[7,8] however, the senior author (KEW) has noted clinically that transverse massage performed too aggressively can produce an increase in inflammation and symptoms. During this early phase, the patient is encouraged not to perform activities that require forceful gripping or gripping of a racquet or golf club. This avoidance is encouraged until symptoms are reduced and controlled.

In the subacute phase, muscular strength and endurance are increased. Isotonics are initiated for the entire upper extremity, with an emphasis on the flexor and pronator muscle groups. Concentric contractions are used initially and progressed to more eccentric contractions as the patient is able to tolerate. If medial elbow instability also is present, rhythmic stabilization and other neuromuscular drills are incorporated into treatment. As the patient's strength and endurance progress, plyometrics can be added to treatment.

Once the patient has reached the chronic phase, where he or she has full, nonpainful ROM and sufficient muscle strength, a gradual return to sport is permitted. The athlete begins an interval sport program. Successful completion of the interval sport program results in a return to competition. It is often beneficial to instruct the patient in proper gripping techniques of the golf club or tennis racquet. Frequently, patients who exhibit tendinitis grip the racquet or golf club with excessive force. This pathomechanical behavior pattern should be modified.

Lateral Pathology

Abnormality of the lateral aspect of the elbow primarily is found at the capitellum (e.g., osteochondritis dissecans) or at the extensor tendon (e.g., lateral epicondylitis). These injuries can occur in isolation or concomitantly with other lesions.

Osteochondritis Dissecans

Rehabilitation for osteochondritis dissecans (OCD) lesions usually involves an initial period of immobilization with the elbow flexed to 90° for approximately 3 to 6 weeks. Duration of immobilization is based on the severity of the lesion and the healing response. During this time, the patient is allowed to perform active assisted ROM exercises three to four times each day to prevent loss of motion and, in particular, flexion contracture (Table 29.7). Modalities can be used as indicated to decrease pain and inflammation and to promote motion restoration. Overhead activities or forceful weight-lifting activities are strongly discouraged until approved by the physician.

TABLE 29.7. *Nonoperative rehabilitation for elbow injuries*

Phase	Goals	Exercises

I: Acute (weeks 0–1)	Improve range of motion (ROM)
	Diminish pain and inflammation
	Retard muscular atrophy
		Week 1
		Stretching for wrist, elbow, shoulder
		Isometrics for wrist, elbow, shoulder musculature
		Modalities
		    Cryotherapy
		    High-voltage galvanic stimulation
		    Ultrasound
		    Whirlpool

II: Subacute (weeks 2–4)	Normalize motion Improve muscular strength, power, endurance	*Week 2* Initiate isotonic strengthening for wrist, elbow muscles Initiate exercise tubing for shoulder Continue use of modalities *Week 3* Initiate rhythmic stabilization drills for elbow, shoulder joints Progress isotonic strengthening for entire upper extremity Initiate isokinetic strengthening for elbow flexion, extension *Week 4* Initiate Thrower's Ten Emphasize eccentric biceps, concentric triceps, wrist flexor exercises Progress endurance training Initiate light plyometric drills Initiate swinging drills

III: Advanced strengthening (weeks 4–8)	Prepare to return to functional activities
	To progress to next phase:
	  Full, nonpainful ROM
	  No pain, tenderness
	  Satisfactory isokinetic test
	  Satisfactory clinical examination
		Weeks 4–5
		Continue strengthening, endurance, flexibility daily
		Thrower's Ten
		Progress plyometric drills
		Emphasize maintenance program based on pathology
		Progress swinging drills (i.e., hitting)
		Weeks 6–8
		Initiate interval sport program when physician determines

IV: Return to activity (weeks 6–9)	Physician determines return to play	Thrower's Ten Flexibility Progress functional drills to unrestricted play

Strengthening exercises are initiated only when symptoms resolve. Usually, isometrics for the elbow and wrist musculature are performed before isotonics are initiated. In this subacute phase, flexibility exercises also are performed at the elbow and wrist. If medial elbow instability was a contributing factor to lateral elbow compression and, subsequently, OCD, then neuromuscular exercises for dynamic stability should be initiated as well. Neuromuscular exercises may include light plyometrics, if the drills can be performed asymptomatically.

In the advanced strengthening phase, strength and endurance of the entire upper extremity are progressed. The plyometric program is advanced as the athlete prepares to begin sport-specific exercise. Near the end of this phase, an interval sport program can be initiated if the athlete does not exhibit symptoms with the plyometric program. The athlete gradually resumes play upon completion of the interval sport program.

Lateral Epicondylitis

The rehabilitation program for lateral epicondylitis is outlined in Table 29.8. Acutely, modalities, such as cryotherapy, high-voltage galvanic stimulation, phonophoresis, or iontophoresis, are used to help to control inflammation and pain. Additionally, the patient should avoid aggravating activities. A cock-up splint may be used to help to rest the wrist extensors.[9] More commonly, a counterforce brace, or tennis elbow strap, is used to alleviate the patient's symptoms.[10] According to Wadsworth,[11] this brace can effectively increase wrist extensor and grip strength, possibly by dispersing stress away from the lesion and thus reducing pain. Glazebrook et al.[12] reported no change in the electromyographic activity of the forearm musculature during the golf swing in individuals wearing a counterforce brace compared with individuals not wearing a brace. We judiciously use a counterforce

TABLE 29.8. *Epicondylitis rehabilitation protocol*

Phase	Goals	Program

I: Acute	Decrease inflammation, pain
	Promote tissue healing
	Retard muscle atrophy
		Cryotherapy
		Whirlpool
		Stretching to increase flexibility
		    Wrist flexion, extension
		    Elbow flexion, extension
		    Forearm pronation, supination
		Isometrics
		    Wrist flexion, extension
		    Elbow flexion, extension
		    Forearm pronation, supination
		High-voltage galvanic stimulation
		Phonophoresis
		Friction massage
		Iontophoresis (with anti-inflammatory, e.g., dexamethasone)

II: Subacute	Improve flexibility
	Increase muscular strength, endurance
	Increase functional activities, return to function
		Emphasize concentric, eccentric strengthening
		    Concentrate on involved muscle group
		    Wrist flexion, extension
		    Elbow flexion, extension
		    Forearm pronation, supination
		Initiate shoulder strengthening (if deficiencies noted)
		Continue flexibility exercises
		May use counterforce brace
		Continue use of cryotherapy after exercise, activity
		Gradually return to stressful activities
		Gradually reinitiate once-painful movements

III: Chronic	Improve muscular strength, endurance Maintain and enhance flexibility Gradual return to sport, high-level activities	Continue strengthening exercises (concentric, eccentric) Emphasize deficiencies in shoulder and elbow strength Continue flexibility exercises Gradually diminish use of counterforce brace Use cryotherapy as needed Gradually return to sport activity Modify equipment (grip size, string tension, playing surface) Conduct biomechanical analysis if needed Emphasize maintenance program

brace for patients with lateral epicondylitis. Isometrics are used for strengthening in the acute phase, and flexibility exercises are used to promote full ROM and to discourage tendon shortening during healing. Stretching exercises to improve wrist extensor muscle flexiblity are emphasized with the elbow in terminal extension and slightly flexed to 25°. Patients are encouraged to perform these stretches at least four to five times a day.

In the subacute phase, strength and endurance are increased. Isotonic exercises are initiated for the entire upper extremity. Strengthening exercises are progressed to incorporate eccentric and concentric muscular contractions at the elbow and wrist. Eccentric muscle training as advocated by Curwin and Stanish[13] is emphasized for the wrist extensors. This muscle training helps to improve musculotendinous strength and flexibility. As the patient's pain decreases and strength increases, sport-specific training may be initiated.

Once the athlete reaches the advanced stage where full, nonpainful ROM is present and appropriate strength is demonstrated, sport-specific exercise is initiated. Often, tennis players benefit from modifications that can help to control the force loads at the elbow. For instance, the athlete can benefit from using a racquet with a mid- to large-sized head or a large grip size, using a lighter-weight racquet, and reducing string tension by 3 to 5 lb.[2,14,15] In addition, an analysis of the swing technique may be necessary to ensure proper playing technique. Kelly et al.[16] noted altered mechanics in tennis players who had a history of lateral epicondylitis, including wrist extension at ball impact and exaggerated wrist pronation at ball impact in the lower portion of the string area; these mechanical faults could be a predisposing factor in lateral epicondylitis. Furthermore, Kelly et al.[16] reported that players who had lateral epicondylitis exhibited significantly greater electromyographic activity of the wrist extensors and pronator teres muscles during ball impact and early follow-through than did asymptomatic players. The clinician should remember that a large percentage of all patients presenting with this abnormality have symptoms due to activities other than tennis. Thus, an analysis of functional activities is often necessary to properly counsel the patients regarding aggravating activities. During functional activities, the use of a biofeedback unit can assist the patient in reducing extensor muscle activity especially during activities that require grasping an object or gripping a handle.

Posterior Pathology

Valgus Extension Overload

The rehabilitation program for valgus extension overload is outlined in Table 29.7. Similar to the previously discussed protocols, the acute phase focuses on decreasing pain and inflammation, normalizing ROM, and retarding muscle atrophy. Modalities previously mentioned in the acute phase of the other various protocols (cryotherapy, high-voltage galvanic stimulation, and phonophoresis) can be used for decreasing pain and inflammation. If the elbow is extremely painful, isometrics for the wrist, elbow, and shoulder may be necessary; otherwise, light isotonics can be initiated. Flexibility exercises can be prescribed as indicated. We strongly advise the patient against rigid elbow extension exercises, such as triceps pushdowns and triceps extensions. Often, the bench press or press-ups aggravate the elbow and should be restricted until the patient is pain free.

In the subacute phase, the concentration is placed on strengthening. Specifically, rehabilitation targets the wrist flexors and pronators and the elbow flexors. These muscle groups are important in controlling either the valgus stress or rapid elbow extension that occurs during throwing. Improved eccentric strength of the biceps, brachioradialis, and brachialis may help to reduce the compressive load posteriorly. Also, by training the elbow flexors eccentrically, the athlete may be able to learn to decelerate elbow extension more effectively. Tubing exercises can be used for eccentric strengthening. Rhythmic stabilization exercises also can be used to improve dynamic stability of the medial elbow. As the athlete progresses with the isotonic program, light plyometrics can be added to rehabilitation.

Advanced strengthening can be initiated when the athlete no longer exhibits pain and when he or she has full ROM and adequate strength. At this time, the patient can begin the full plyometric program and batting drills. Once the patient progresses through the advanced strengthening phase, a return to sport can begin with an interval sport program. At this point, a biomechanical analysis may be necessary to determine if faulty or undesirable mechanics are contributing to abnormalities at the elbow.

The analysis and subsequent correction of mechanics may be necessary for a successful return to sport. If nonoperative treatment fails, surgical excision of the posterior and posteromedial olecranon tip may be necessary. This treatment can be accomplished arthroscopically or through an open approach. Additionally, exercises that enhance the elbow's medial stability are essential. We believe there is an association between the valgus extension overload pathology and medial elbow instability.

SUMMARY

The athlete who uses the overhead motion can sustain numerous injuries to the elbow joint complex. The differential diagnosis of the specific disorder is vital to a successful outcome and to establish a proper nonoperative rehabilitation program. Thus, specific rehabilitation programs and time frames for the nonoperative treatment of various elbow injuries are available. In this chapter, we discussed nonoperative treatment for several common elbow injuries. The physician must communicate with the rehabilitation specialist regarding the differential diagnosis, rehabilitation program, and expected outcome. Many elbow maladies can be successfully managed nonoperatively. When nonoperative treatment fails, further clinical examination, diagnostic testing, and, possibly, surgical intervention are necessary.

REFERENCES

1. Nirschl RP. Prevention and treatment of elbow and shoulder injuries in the tennis player. *Clin Sports Med* 1988;7:289–308.
2. Alley RM, Pappas AM. Acute and performance-related injuries of the elbow. In: Pappas AM, ed. *Upper extremity injuries in the athlete*. New York: Churchill Livingstone; 1995: 339–364.
3. Fleisig G, Escamilla R. Biomechanics of the elbow in the throwing athlete. *Operative Tech Sports Med* 1996;4:62–68.
4. Morrey BF, An KN. Articular and ligamentous contributions to the stability of the elbow joint. *Am J Sports Med* 1983;11: 315–319.
5. Voss DE, Ionta MK, Myers BJ. Techniques for facilitation. In: *Proprioceptive neuromuscular facilitation*. Philadelphia: Harper & Row; 1985:289–314.
6. Azar FM, Wilk KE. Nonoperative treatment of the elbow in throwers. *Operative Tech Sports Med* 1996;4:91–99.
7. Cyriax JH. The pathology and treatment of tennis elbow. *J Bone Joint Surg* 1936;18:921–940.
8. Chamberlain GL. Cyriax's friction massage. A review. *J Orthop Sports Phys Ther* 1982;4:16–22.
9. Noteboom T, Cruver R, Keller J, et al. Tennis elbow: A review. *J Orthop Sports Phys Ther* 1994;19:357–366.
10. Froimson AI. Treatment of tennis elbow with forearm support band. *J Bone Joint Surg* 1971;53A:183–184.
11. Wadsworth CT, Nielson DH, Burns LT, et al. Effect of the counterforce armband on wrist extension and grip strength and

pain in subjects with tennis elbow. *J Orthop Sports Phys Ther* 1989;11:192–197.
12. Glazebrook MA, Curwin S, Islam MN, et al. Medial epicondylitis: An electromyographic analysis and an investigation of intervention strategies. *Am J Sports Med* 1994;22:674–679.
13. Curwin S, Stanish WD. *Tendinitis. Its etiology and treatment.* Lexington, MA: Collamore Press; 1984.
14. Nirschl RP, Pettrone FA. Tennis elbow. The surgical treatment of lateral epicondylitis. *J Bone Joint Surg* 1979;61A:832–839.
15. Lehman RC. Surface and equipment variables in tennis injuries. *Clin Sports Med* 1988;7:229–232.
16. Kelley JD, Lombardo SJ, Pink M, et al. Electromyographic and cinematographic analysis of elbow function in tennis players with lateral epicondylitis. *Am J Sports Med* 1994;22:359–363.

Index

Note: Page numbers followed by *f* or *t* denote figures or tables, respectively.

Abduction, force in, 31
Abductor pollicis longus muscle, posterior interosseous nerve compression syndrome and, 150
Acceleration, of arm, 29
　in baseball pitching, 31*f*–33*f*, 34–35, 70, 71*f*, 124, 124*f*
　　muscle activity in, 32*t*
　in football passing, 36
　pain with, characterization of, 42
　in underhand throw (softball pitching), 37
Accessory anterior oblique ligament, as landmark in medial epicondylitis surgery, 85, 86*f*
Accessory collateral ligament, 186*f*
Accessory lateral collateral ligament, 10, 10*f*
Achilles tendon
　strips of, for ulnar collateral ligament reconstruction, 95
　Vulpius lengthening technique for, 121
Acute injuries, 41
Adduction, force in, 31
Adipose tissue, of subcutaneous plane, 1–2, 3*f*
Adventitious bursae, 87, 303
Air bubbles, mimicking loose bodies, in magnetic resonance imaging, 61–62
Alkaline phosphatase, serum levels of, with tumors of elbow, 295
Alonso-Llames surgical approach, 13*t*, 15*f*, 15*t*
Anatomy, clinical, of elbow, 1–10
Anconeus epitrochlearis, 8
　replacement of cubital tunnel retinaculum by, 64–65, 66*f*
Anconeus muscle, 4, 7*f*
　action of, 4, 5*t*, 30, 34
　insertion of, 5*t*
　in lateral collateral ligament reconstruction, 105–107, 106*f*–107*f*
　nerve supply to, 5*t*, 149

Anconeus muscle (*continued*)
　origin of, 5*t*
Aneurysmal bone cyst, 295, 296*f*, 299–300
Angiofibroblastic tendinitis, 59, 80
Angiosarcoma, 299
Angular displacement, in throwing, 29
Angular velocity
　in baseball pitching, 34
　in javelin throw, 37
　in tennis, 36
Ankylosis of elbow. *See also* Contracture(s)
　arthroscopic treatment of, 177–184, 287
　　contraindications to, 178
　　indications for, 178
　　versus open surgical release, 183
　　patient positioning for, 178, 179*f*
　　precautions in, 182–183
　　results of, 183
　　technique for, 178–181, 179*f*–182*f*
　with collateral ligament injury, 178
　contracture release in, open operative strategies for, 285–294
　etiology of, 177
　frank, as contraindication to diagnostic arthroscopy, 163
　incidence of, 177
　nonoperative treatment of, 178
　with nonunion of fractures, 271–272, 282
　postoperative management of, 182
　posttraumatic, pathogenesis of, 177–178
Annular ligament, 9–10, 9*f*–10*f*, 186, 186*f*, 208
　arthroscopy of, 165*f*
　in joint stabilization, 101–102, 102*f*–103*f*
　in lateral collateral ligament reconstruction, 105
　reconstruction of, Boyd's approach in, 16
　step-cut (Z) incision of, in modification of Kocher's lateral approach, 21
　in trochlear shear fracture surgery, 203, 203*f*

Antecubital fossa, 109–110
　biceps tendon rupture and, 110–111
Anterior bundle, of ulnar collateral ligament, 9–10, 10*f*, 89, 186
　arthroscopy of, 89
　clinical anatomy of, 89–90, 90*f*–91*f*
　histology of, 89
　mean length of, 89
　mean width of, 89
　reciprocal tightening of anterior and posterior bands of, 90, 91*f*
　strength of, 30
　undersurface partial tears of, magnetic resonance imaging of, 56, 57*f*
Anterior capsular release, arthroscopic, for ankylosis, 179*f*–182*f*, 179–184
Anterior capsulitis, palpation of, 43
Anterior dislocation, 253
　mechanism of injury, 253
Anterior force, in baseball pitching, 33, 33*f*
Anterior humeral line, for radiography, of supracondylar fracture, 225, 225*f*
Anterior interosseous artery, relationship to medial and lateral intermuscular septa, 4*f*
Anterior interosseous nerve, 142
　compression/entrapment of, 47, 145, 146*f*
　injury, with supracondylar fractures, 226, 237
Anterior provocative tests, 50–51
Anterior surgical approaches, 11–12, 13*t*, 15*t*, 24–26
　in open capsular release, 287–288
　to radial nerve, 152–153, 152*f*–154*f*
Anterior symptoms, 41
Anterolateral approach to humerus, 15*t*
Anterolateral portal, for arthroscopy, 160–161, 161*f*, 165–166
　for capsular release, in ankylosis, 179–180, 179*f*–180*f*

Anterolateral portal (continued)
    for loose body removal, 173f, 173–174
    in radial head excision, 190–192, 191f
Anteromedial portal, for arthroscopy, 159–160
    in radial head excision, 190–192, 191f
Anteroposterior Jones view, in fluoroscopy, of supracondylar fracture, 235, 236f
Anteroposterior radiographic views, 51f, 51–52
Antibiotic therapy, for olecranon bursitis, 304–305
AO classification, of distal humerus fractures, 196f, 196–197
Apophyseal injury, in Little League elbow, 69
Arcade of Frohse, 6, 8
    radial nerve compression by, 65, 150, 150f, 152, 154
Arcade of Osborne, 8, 8f
Arcade of Struthers, 8f
    ulnar nerve compression at, 132, 132f
Arm acceleration, 29
    in baseball pitching, 31f–33f, 34–35, 70, 71f, 124, 124f
        muscle activity in, 32t
    in football passing, 36
    pain with, characterization of, for diagnosis, 42
    in underhand throw (softball pitching), 37
Arm cocking
    in baseball pitching, 31f–33f, 32–34, 35f, 70, 71f, 90
        muscle activity in, 32t
    in football passing, 36, 36f
    pain with, 42
Arm deceleration
    in baseball pitching, 31f–33f, 35
        muscle activity in, 32t
    in football passing, 36
Art of surgery, 1
Arteriography, in vascular injury, with supracondylar fracture, 238
Arteriovenous malformation, 299–300
Arthritis
    arthroscopic radial head excision for, 188–189, 193
    as contraindication to operative treatment of nonunions, 276
    magnetic resonance imaging of, 57
    olecranon bursitis with, 304, 306
    olecranon osteotomy and, 19
    radiocapitellar joint degeneration with, 185, 187–189, 193
Arthrofibrosis. *See also* Contracture(s)
    arthroscopic treatment of, 177–184
        contraindications to, 178
        indications for, 178
        versus open surgical release, 183
        patient positioning for, 178, 179f
        precautions in, 182–183
        results of, 183
        technique for, 178–181, 179f–182f
    nonoperative treatment of, 178
    postoperative management of, 182
    posttraumatic, pathogenesis of, 177–178
Arthrography, 51, 53, 61
    of lateral condylar fractures, 246, 249
    of medial collateral ligament injury, 56
    of osteochondritis dissecans of capitellum, 73
Arthroplasty
    for distal humerus fractures
        nonunited, 276, 278, 281
        semiconstrained implant, 204, 204f
    distraction interposition, for contractures, 291–292

Arthroplasty (continued)
    for olecranon fractures, nonunited, 276
    radial head, 19
    surgical approaches in, 15t
        Bryan and Morrey's extensive posterior, 15t, 16
        Campbell's posterolateral, 13, 15t
        Kocher's lateral, 15t, 19
        Wadsworth's posterolateral, 14, 15t
    ulnohumeral, 181, 189, 192
Arthroscopic removal
    of loose bodies, 171–176
        complications in, 175
        contraindications to, 172
        indications for, 172
        postoperative management of, 175
        in radial head excision, 191, 193–194
        results of, 175
        techniques for, 173–175, 173f–175f
    of osteophytes
        with capsular release, for ankylosis, 180–182, 181f–182f
        in olecranon bursitis, 306f, 307
        with radiocapitellar joint degeneration, 192–194
        in valgus extension overload syndrome, 126–128, 127f–128f, 175, 175f
Arthroscopy, 157–162
    advantages of, 126
    of anterior bundle of ulnar collateral ligament, 89
    diagnostic, 163–169
        complications of, 167–168
        contraindications to, 163
        indications for, 163
        neurologic complications of, 168
        nonneurologic complications of, 168
        results of, 167
        techniques for, 163–167, 165f–167f
        value of, 163
    equipment for, 157–158, 164–165, 165f
    fluid leakage in, 161–162
    operating room setup for, 157–158, 158f, 173, 173f
    patient positioning for, 158, 158f, 164, 164f, 173, 173f, 178, 179f, 190, 306
    portals for, 158–162, 164
        lateral, 160–161, 161f, 165–167
        for loose body removal, 173–175, 173f–175f
        medial, 159–160, 159f–160f, 164–165
        midlateral or direct lateral, 161f, 161–162
        in olecranon bursectomy, 306–307
        posterior, 161f, 162, 166–167, 166f–167f
        in radial head excision, 190–193, 191f
        soft spot, 166–167, 167f, 180, 191, 191f
    postoperative rehabilitation with, 127–128, 128t
    for radial head excision, 185–194
    surgical anatomy in, 158–162
    for treatment
        of ankylosis/contractures, 177–184, 179f–182f, 287
        of lateral epicondylitis, 83–85, 84f
        of olecranon bursitis, 306f, 306–307
        of osteochondritis dissecans of capitellum, 74, 171, 172f, 174
        of radial head fractures, 189, 215, 219
        of radiocapitellar/radioulnar degeneration, 185–194
        of ulnar collateral ligament injuries, 95–98
        of valgus extension overload syndrome, 123, 125–128, 127f–128f, 171–172, 175, 175f

Articular capsule, 9f
Articulations, 1, 2f
Aspiration
    needle, of tumors, 298
    for olecranon bursitis, 304–305
    in radial head fractures, 211, 216
Athletes. *See also* specific sports
    overhead-throwing, rehabilitation of injuries in, 309–320
Avascular necrosis
    baseball pitching and, 33
    of capitellum, lateral condylar fracture surgery and, 247, 248f
Avulsion
    medial epicondylar, 72–73, 73f
    triceps, palpation of, 44, 44f
Avulsion fractures
    of coronoid process, 265
    epicondylar, 72–73
        fluoroscopy of, 53
    of olecranon, 264–265f
    with posterolateral rotatory instability, 103, 103f
    with triceps tendon rupture, 119
Axial plane, magnetic resonance imaging in, 56
Axial radiographic view, 52–53, 53f
Axillary artery, 141

Bardinet's ligament, 9–10, 10f. *See also* Posterior bundle
Baseball pitching
    arm acceleration in, 31f–33f, 32t, 34–35, 70, 71f, 124, 124f
    arm cocking in, 31f–33f, 32t, 32–34, 35f, 70, 71f, 90
    arm deceleration in, 31f–33f, 32t, 35
    biomechanics of elbow during, 31f, 31–36, 70, 71f–72f, 124
    comparison of different pitches, 33–35, 34t, 70
    follow-through in, 31f–33f, 32t, 35–36
    versus football passing, 36
    muscle activity in, 32t
    overhand versus sidearm, 69
    poor technique of, and injury, 69
    stride in, 31, 31f–33f, 32t
    time-matched measurements during, 35f
    too much, too soon training phenomenon in, 69
    windup in, 31, 31f–33f, 32t
Baseball pitching injuries, 37, 51, 80
    lateral compression, 33, 73–75
    magnetic resonance imaging of, 56–58, 57f–58f
    medial tension, 71–73
    olecranon bursitis, 303
    pain with, 42
        localization and characterization of, for diagnosis, 42
    palpation in, 45
    posterior extension, 75–76
    rehabilitation of, 309–329
        basic principles of, 309
        interval throwing program in, 312, 314t–315t
        isokinetic assessment in, 309, 310f, 315
        in lateral pathology, 316–319
        long-toss program in, 312, 314t
        in medial pathology, 310–316
        off-the-mound throwing program in, 312, 315t
        overview of, 309
        plyometrics in, 311–312, 312f–314f, 314, 317, 319

Baseball pitching injuries *(continued)*
  in posterior pathology, 319
  sport-specific, determining readiness for, 309
  team approach in, 309
  Thrower's Ten program for, 311–312, 312t, 314
  of ulnar collateral ligament, 32–33, 42, 56–57, 57f, 73, 89–100, 186–187. *See also* Ulnar collateral ligament injuries
  rehabilitation of, 98–99, 310t, 310–312, 311f–312f, 312t, 314t–315t
  ulnar nerve compression with, 132–133
  valgus extension overload, 123–130. *See also* Valgus extension overload syndrome
  in young athletes (Little League elbow), 69–77. *See also* Little League elbow
Baseball throw, one-hand, in plyometric exercise drill, 311–312, 313f
Basilic vein, 1, 3f
Baumann's angle, for radiography
  modified, 224, 224f
  of supracondylar fracture, 224, 224f
Benign tumors, 299–300
  staging of, 296–297, 298f
Biceps brachii muscle, 109–110
  action of, 5t, 30
  in baseball pitching, 32t
  insertion of, 5t
  nerve supply to, 5t
  origin of, 5t
  palpation of, 43
  proximal migration of, with biceps tendon rupture, 110f, 110–112
  strength testing of, 46, 46f
Biceps reflex, assessment of, 47
Biceps tendinitis
  distal, versus olecranon bursitis, 303
  palpation in, 43
  provocative tests for, 50–51
Biceps tendon, 7f, 259
  bicipital aponeurosis and, 2, 4f
  clinical anatomy of, 109–110
  injury, magnetic resonance imaging of, 56, 62–63, 64f–65f
  palpation of, 43
  repair of, 111–118, 112f–117f
    anatomic, 109, 111–118, 112f–117f
    complications in, 112, 118
    delayed diagnosis as contraindication to, 111
    Henry's anterior approach in, 24
    nonanatomic, 111
    postoperative management of, 116–117, 117t
    results of, 117–118
  as surgical landmark, in Henry's anterior approach, 25–26
Biceps tendon rupture, 109–118
  distal, 109–118
  magnetic resonance imaging of, 56, 111
  mechanism of injury in, 109
  nonoperative treatment of, 111
  operative treatment of, 111–118, 112f–117f
    anatomic, 111–118, 112f–117f
    authors' preferred technique for, 112–117, 112f–117f
    complications in, 112, 118
    delayed diagnosis as contraindication to, 111
    indications for, 111
    nonanatomic, 111
    results of, 117–118

Biceps tendon rupture *(continued)*
    techniques for, 111–112
  pain with, 41, 110
  palpation of, 43, 110–111
  physical examination in, 110f, 110–111
  postoperative management of, 116–117, 117t
  proximal, 109
  radiographic findings in, 109, 111
Bicipital aponeurosis (lacertus fibrosus), 2, 4f, 7, 7f, 110
  biceps tendon secured to, in nonanatomic repair of rupture, 111
  magnetic resonance imaging of, 63, 65f
  median nerve compression by, 142f, 142–143, 145–146
  palpation of, 43
Bicipital radial bursa, 303
  enlargement of, magnetic resonance imaging of, 63, 64f–65f
  and radial nerve entrapment, 65
Bicortical screw fixation, of proximal olecranon fractures, 263–264, 264f
Bioabsorbable polyglycolide pins
  for lateral condylar fractures, 248
  for radial head fracture fixation, 212
Biomechanics, 29–31
  during baseball pitching, 31f, 31–36, 70, 71f–72f, 124
    comparison of different pitches, 33–35, 34t, 70
  during football passing, 36, 36f
  of javelin throw, 37
  of tennis, 36–37
  and throwing mechanism, 29–39
  and ulnar collateral ligament injury, 89–91
Biopsy
  complications related to, 297–298
  needle, 298
  open, 298–299, 298f–299f
  in tumor evaluation, principles of, 297–299, 302
Bipolar electrocautery, in radial nerve decompression, 152–154
Blade plate, in distal humerus fracture fixation, 203
Blastomyces infection, olecranon bursitis with, 304
Blunt-tipped trocars, for arthroscopy, 157, 164
Bone cement, for distal humerus fractures, 204, 204f, 280–281
Bone cyst
  aneurysmal, 295, 296f, 299–300
  unicameral, 299
Bone grafts
  for distal humerus fractures, 200–201, 202f, 204
  for lateral condylar fractures, 250–251
  for nonunions of elbow, 276–277
  for olecranon fractures, 260
  in tumor treatment, 299–300
Bone marrow, magnetic resonance imaging of, 55
Bone tumors, 295–302
Bony morphology, 11, 12f
Boyd-Anderson surgical approach, in biceps tendon repair, 112
Boyd's surgical approach, 13t, 16–18, 18f
  indications for, 15t, 16
  modifications in, 18
Brachial artery, 7, 7f–8f, 110
  injury
    with elbow dislocation, 254
    with supracondylar fractures, 225–226, 226f, 237, 238f

Brachial artery *(continued)*
    treatment of, 254
  pulse, palpation of, 43
  relationship to medial and lateral intermuscular septa, 4f
Brachialis muscle
  action of, 30
  in baseball pitching, 32t
  biceps tendon secured to, in nonanatomic repair of rupture, 111
  injury
    magnetic resonance imaging of, 60f
    with posterior dislocation injury, 60, 60f
    with supracondylar fractures, 225–226, 234–235, 237
  nerve supply to, 149
  potential contractile strength of, 30
  splitting of, in coronoid process reduction and fixation, 266
  work capacity of, 30
Brachialis tendinitis, provocative tests for, 50–51
Brachialis tendon, 259
Brachioradialis muscle, 8
  action of, 5t, 30
  in baseball pitching, 32t
  in border of cubital fossa, 7, 7f
  insertion of, 5t
  nerve supply to, 5t, 149
  origin of, 5t
  palpation of, 43
  splitting of, in radial nerve surgery, 154
Brachioradialis reflex, assessment of, 47
Brachioradialis-extensor carpi radialis longus interval approach, in radial nerve surgery, 155
Branham's sign, 300
Brucellosis infection, olecranon bursitis with, 303
Bryan and Morrey's extensive posterior surgical approach, 13t, 16, 17f, 198
  for distal humerus fractures, 16, 198, 205
  indications for, 15t, 16
  modifications in, 16
Bunnell sutures
  in biceps tendon repair, 113, 113f–114f
  in triceps tendon repair, 120
Burns, contractures with, 285
Bursae
  adventitious, 87, 303
  bicipital radial, 303
    enlargement of, magnetic resonance imaging of, 63, 64f–65f
    and radial nerve entrapment, 65
  deep, 303
  olecranon, 2, 6f, 44, 44f, 303
    collar shaped, 305
  superficial, 303–304
  synovial, 303
Bursitis
  cubital, magnetic resonance imaging of, 63, 64f–65f
  medial epicondylar, 303
  olecranon, 303–307
    arthroscopic/endoscopic treatment of, 306f, 306–307
    concomitant conditions with, 304
    versus distal biceps tendinitis, 303
    etiology of, 303–304
    history and physical examination in, 304–305, 304f–305f
    laboratory findings in, 304
    nonoperative treatment of, 305
    operative treatment of, 305–307

Bursitis *(continued)*
    osteophytes with, 305f–306f, 305–307
    palpation of, 44
    septic, 304–307
    swelling with, 42, 304, 304f
    throwing/pitching and, 303
    triceps tendon rupture with, 118, 305

Cadenat's surgical approach, 20–21
Calcium, serum levels of, with tumors of elbow, 295
Campbell's posterolateral surgical approach, 13t, 13–14, 15t, 16f
    indications for, 13, 15t
Cancellous bone graft, for distal humerus fractures, 200
Candida infection, olecranon bursitis with, 304
Cannula systems, for arthroscopy, 157, 164, 164f, 174, 179
Cannulated screw system
    for coronoid process fractures, 266
    for distal humerus fractures, 201
Capitellum, 11, 12f
    arthroscopy of, 160–162, 165–167, 167f
    in radial head excision, 191
    avascular necrosis of, lateral condylar fracture surgery and, 247, 248f
    in axis of rotation, 90
    injury, with radial head fractures, 209, 216, 218
    ossification of, 245
    osteochondritis dissecans of
        arthroscopic radial head excision for, 188
        arthroscopy of, 74, 171, 172f, 174
        complications of, 74
        loose bodies with, 171, 172f
        magnetic resonance imaging of, 57, 61, 73–74, 74f
        pain with, 41
        versus Panner's disease, 61
        physical findings of, 73
        radiographic findings of, 73, 74f
        rehabilitation of, 316–317, 317t
        staging of, 74
        treatment of, 74
        with ulnar collateral ligament injuries, 93f, 95
        in young athletes (Little League elbow), 42, 45, 73–74, 74f
    osteochondrosis of (Panner's disease)
        loose bodies with, 171–172
        versus osteochondritis dissecans, 61
        palpation in, 45
        radiographic findings in, 75, 75f
        in young athletes (Little League elbow), 74–75, 75f
Capitellum fractures, 197f, 259
    surgical approaches in
        alternative, 15t
        global, 15t, 23
        recommended, 15t
Capsular contracture, as contraindication to diagnostic arthroscopy, 163
Capsular release/capsulectomy
    arthroscopic
        for ankylosis/contractures, 179f–182f, 179–184, 287
        versus open surgical release, 183
        compass elbow hinge in, 289, 292f
        for lateral condylar fractures, 250
        Mayo distraction device in, 289, 290f–291f
        for nonunions of elbow, 277–278, 279f, 281
    open
        for contractures, 287–291, 288f–292f

Capsular release/capsulectomy *(continued)*
    surgical approaches in, 287–288, 288f–289f
Capsule(s), 9f, 9–10, 259
    arthrography of, 53
    arthroscopy of, 161–163, 166
    inflammation of, pain with, 41–42
    magnetic resonance imaging of, 56
    thickened, with contractures, 285
Capsulitis, anterior, palpation of, 43
Carrying angle, 11, 29
    decrease in (cubitus varus), 42
    increase in (cubitus valgus), 42
    inspection of, 42, 42f
    maintenance of, in distal humerus fracture fixation, 201
    with supracondylar fractures, 42, 224f–225f, 224–226, 233–234, 236, 236f, 238–240, 239f–241f
    ulnar nerve compression and, 134
Cartilage
    arthroscopy of, 163
    growth, injury to, in Little League elbow, 69
    hyaline articular, magnetic resonance imaging of, 56
    unossified, magnetic resonance imaging of, 55
Catching and locking, 41, 73, 171–172
Center of rotation, 90, 90f
Centrifugal force
    in baseball pitching, 34–35
    in underhand throw (softball pitching), 37
Cephalic vein, 1, 3f
    protection of, in surgery, in Henry's anterior approach, 25
Chair test, for lateral epicondylitis, 49, 49f
Change-up pitch, biomechanics of, 33–34, 34t
Chest pass, two-hand, in plyometric exercise drill, 311–312, 313f
Chevron olecranon osteotomy, 18–19, 19f
    complications of, 19
    for distal humerus fractures, 18–19, 19f, 198–199, 199f, 205, 278, 281–282
    indications for, 15t, 18
    modifications in, 19
Children
    lateral condylar fractures in, 245–252
    supracondylar fractures of humerus in, 15, 223–243
Chondroblastoma, 299
Chondromalacia
    baseball pitching and, 34–35
    radiocapitellar, with valgus extension overload syndrome surgery, 126
    of trochlea, with valgus extension overload syndrome, 127, 128f
Chondromyxoid fibroma, 296, 297f, 299
Chondrosarcoma, 299, 301f, 302
Chronic injuries, 41
Cinematography, of throwing, 29
Clear cell sarcoma, 299
Clinical anatomy, of elbow, 1–10
Closed reduction
    of coronoid process fractures, 265
    of dislocation, complications of, 257
    of dislocation injury, 253, 255f–256f, 256–257
    of lateral condylar fractures, 248
    of supracondylar fractures, 230–233
    technique for, 235–237, 235f–237f
Cloward drill, 181, 192
Cobra retractor, in biceps tendon repair, 113–114, 115f

Cocking, of arm
    in baseball pitching, 31f–33f, 32–34, 35f, 70, 71f, 90
        muscle activity in, 32t
    in football passing, 36, 36f
    pain with, 42
Coffee cup test, 80
Collagen, as interposition material, 291
Collar shaped bursa, 305
Combined medial and lateral surgical approaches, 11–12, 13t, 23–24
Comminution
    of distal humerus fractures, 195–196, 196f, 198, 200
        treatment of, 200–201, 201f–202f, 204
    of lateral condylar fractures, 247–248
    of olecranon fractures, 259–260, 264
    of radial head fractures, 209–210, 210f, 212, 216, 217f, 267, 273
Common extensor origin, in trochlear shear fracture surgery, 203, 203f
Common extensor tendon, 186f
Common flexor tendonitis, with medial epicondylitis, 57–58
Common interosseous artery, relationship to medial and lateral intermuscular septa, 4f
Compartment syndrome, with Henry's anterior approach, 26
Compass hinge device
    for complex fracture-dislocation of proximal ulna, technique for applying, 268f, 269
    for contractures
        in distraction interposition arthroplasty, 291–292
        in open capsular release, 289, 292f
Complete blood count (CBC)
    in olecranon bursitis, 304
    with tumors of elbow, 295
Complex fracture-dislocation of proximal ulna, 266–269
    classification of, 266–267
    compass elbow hinge for, technique for applying, 268f, 269
    complications of, 269
    dynamic joint distractor for, 267–269, 268f
        technique for applying, 267–269, 268f
    hinged external fixators for, 267–269, 268f
Composite epiphysis, 11
Compression injury, lateral
    baseball pitching and, 33, 73–75
    in young athletes (Little League elbow), 73–75
Compression screws
    for coronoid process fractures, 265–266, 266f
    with tension-band wiring, for olecranon fractures, 262–263, 264f
Compressive force, in baseball pitching, 33, 33f, 35
Compressive neuropathies, 131. *See also specific nerves*
Computed tomography (CT), 51, 53
    for biopsy guidance, 298
    of contractures, 286
    of distal humerus fractures, 197, 205
    of fractures, 61
    of lateral condylar fractures, 246
    of loose bodies, 172
    of medial collateral ligament injury, 56
    of medial epicondylar avulsion, 72
    of osteochondritis dissecans of capitellum, 73
    of radial head fractures, 209

Computed tomography *(continued)*
  of radial nerve compression, 152
  of tumors, 296, 300
Condyle(s), lateral, 11. *See also* Lateral
    condylar fractures
Congenital contractures, 285
Congenital medial supracondylar process,
    palpation of, 43
Continuous passive motion, 182, 205
Contoured plating technique
  for distal humerus fractures, nonunited,
      279–280, 280*f*
  for nonunion of proximal ulna, 277
  for olecranon fractures, 264, 265*f*
Contracture(s)
  capsular release for
    arthroscopic, 177–184, 179*f*–182*f*, 287
    open, 287–291, 288*f*–292*f*
  classification of, 285–286
  compass hinge device for in, 289, 291–292, 292*f*
  congenital, 285
  distraction interposition arthroplasty for, 291–292
  etiology of, 285
  evaluation of, 286
  extrinsic, 285
  flexion
    arthroscopic treatment of, 177–184, 179*f*–182*f*
    with collateral ligament injury, 178
    nonoperative treatment of, 178
    open capsular release for, 287–291
    with osteochondritis of capitellum, 74
    postoperative management of, 182
    posttraumatic, pathogenesis of, 177–178
    soft endpoints with, 46
    with valgus extension overload syndrome, 123–124
  history of, 286
  imaging studies of, 286
  intrinsic, 285
  Mayo distraction device for, 289, 290*f*–291*f*, 291
  nonoperative management of, 286–287, 286*f*–287*f*
  operative management of, 287–292
    complications in, 293
    results of, 293
  paralytic, 285
  physical examination in, 286
  postoperative care in, 292–293
  recurrence of, 293
  release of
    anterior, 24
    with nonunion of fractures, 271
    open operative strategies for, 285–294
  secondary, of ligaments and muscles, 285–286
  static-progressive splinting in, 286*f*, 286–287
  surgical approaches in, 287–288, 288*f*–289*f*
Coronal plane, magnetic resonance imaging in, 55–56
Coronoid fossa, 9*f*, 223
  fat pad within, 9*f*
Coronoid hypertrophy, palpation of, 43
Coronoid process, 9*f*, 11, 12*f*
  arthroscopy of, 160–161, 166, 166*f*, 173
  injury, flexion contracture with, 178
  osteophytes in
    arthroscopic inspection for, 166, 166*f*
    with radiocapitellar joint degeneration, 193
  with radial head fracture, 218*f*, 219, 265–266

Coronoid process *(continued)*
  radiography of, 51
Coronoid process fractures, 259, 265–266
  avulsion, 265
  classification of, 265
  closed reduction of, 265
  compression-screw technique for, 265–266, 266*f*
  medial collateral ligament injury with, 265–266
  nonunion of, operative treatment of, 277
  olecranon fractures with, 259
  open reduction and internal fixation of, 260, 265–266, 266*f*
  with proximal ulnar fracture-dislocation, 264, 265*f*, 266–267
  radiographically occult, magnetic resonance imaging of, 63*f*
  surgical approaches in
    alternative, 15*t*
    global, 15*t*, 23
    Henry's anterior, 15*t*, 24
    recommended, 15*t*
  type I, 265
  type II, 265
  type III, 265–266, 266*f*
Corticocancellous bone graft, for distal humerus fractures, 200
Corticosteroids
  for epicondylitis, 81
  hypopigmentation with, 81, 81*f*
  for olecranon bursitis, 305
Counterforce bracing, for epicondylitis, 81, 81*f*, 86, 317–318
Crepitation/crepitus, 41, 46, 91, 187
Crescent sign, in radiographic evaluation of supracondylar fracture, 225, 225*f*, 236
Cross section through elbow, for developing understanding of surgical approaches, 14*f*
Cross-pinning, of supracondylar fractures, 234, 234*f*, 236
Cryotherapy, 312–313, 315, 317, 319
Crystalline inflammatory process, olecranon bursitis with, 304
CT. *See* Computed tomography
Cubital bursa, inflammation of, magnetic resonance imaging of, 63, 64*f*–65*f*
Cubital fossa, 6–7, 7*f*
  palpation of, 43
  tumors in, excision of, 24
Cubital retinaculum, 8, 8*f*
  absence or redundancy of, 8
Cubital tunnel, 8, 8*f*
Cubital tunnel retinaculum
  replacement/absence of, 64–65, 66*f*
  and ulnar neuropathy, 64–65, 66*f*
Cubital tunnel syndrome, 131–139. *See also* Ulnar nerve compression/entrapment
  classic presentation of, 133
  clinical anatomy and etiology of, 131–133, 132*f*
  decompression in situ for, 135, 138
  diagnostic studies in, 134
  differential diagnosis of, 133
  with elbow dislocation, 254
  full exposure and release of ulnar nerve in, 135–136, 136*f*
  magnetic resonance imaging of, 134
  medial epicondylectomy for, 137, 137*f*
  neurolysis for, 137
  nonoperative treatment of, 134
  operative treatment of, 131, 134–137
    complications in, 138

Cubital tunnel syndrome *(continued)*
    indications and contraindications in, 134–135
    results of, 137–138
    techniques for, 135–137, 136*f*–137*f*
  physical examination in, 133–134
  postoperative management of, 135–137
  postoperative recurrence of, 138
  provocative test for, 50, 50*f*, 134
  radiographic findings in, 134
  sensory examination in, 133–134
  transposition for, 135–137
    intramuscular, 136
    subcutaneous, 136, 136*f*
    submuscular, 136–137
Cubitus valgus, 42
  with lateral condylar fractures, 42, 247, 249–251, 249*f*–251*f*
  with valgus extension overload syndrome, 123
Cubitus varus, 42
  osteotomy for, 239, 241*f*
  with supracondylar fractures, 42, 224*f*, 226, 234, 236, 238–240, 239*f*–241*f*
Curveball pitch, biomechanics of, 33–34, 34*t*, 70
Cutaneous nerves, 1–2, 3*f*
  distribution of, 3*f*
  injury to, with medial and lateral skin incisions, 12
Cybex testing, 110

Deceleration, of arm
  in baseball pitching, 31*f*–33*f*, 35
    muscle activity in, 32*t*
  in football passing, 36
Decompression in situ, for ulnar nerve compression, 135, 138
Deep bursae, 303
Deep fascia of upper limb, 1–2, 4*f*
  in border of cubital fossa, 7, 7*f*
  thickening of, 2, 4*f*
Deep flexor pronator aponeurosis, 133
Dermatofibrosarcoma protuberans, 299
Dermis, as interposition material, 291
Diagnosis, of elbow injury, 41
Diagnostic arthroscopy, 163–169
  complications of, 167–168
  contraindications to, 163
  indications for, 163
  neurologic complications of, 168
  nonneurologic complications of, 168
  results of, 167
  techniques for, 163–167, 165*f*–167*f*
    authors' preferred, 164–167, 165*f*–167*f*
  value of, 163
Diagnostic imaging, 55. *See also specific imaging modalities*
Dialysis elbow, 304
Dicloxacillin, for olecranon bursitis, 305
Direct lateral portal, for arthroscopy, 161*f*, 161–162, 166–167
  in capsular release, for ankylosis, 180
  in radial head excision, 191, 191*f*
Direct posterior portal, for arthroscopy, 162, 166–167
Direct radiographic views, 53
Dislocation, 253–258
  acute, 257
  anterior, 253
    mechanism of injury, 253
  classification of, 253
  closed reduction of, 253, 255*f*–256*f*, 256–257

Dislocation *(continued)*
    complications of, 257
  contractures with, 285
  coronoid process fractures with, 265
  divergent, 253
    mechanism of injury, 254
  lateral, 253
    mechanism of injury, 253–254
    treatment of, 256–257
  with lateral condylar fractures, 246
  magnetic resonance imaging of, 61
  mechanism of injury, 253–254
  medial, 253
    mechanism of injury, 253–254
    treatment of, 256–257
  with medial collateral ligament rupture, 57, 254
  neurovascular injury with, 254
  open reduction of, 257
  physical examination of, 254
  posterior, 253
    closed reduction of, 256f, 256–257
    magnetic resonance imaging of, 60, 60f
    mechanism of injury, 253
    with radial head fractures, 207, 213–214
    radial head fractures with, 255f
    treatment of, 256–257
    true, 253
    varieties of, 253–254
  posterolateral, 253
  posteromedial, 253
  radial head fractures with, 255, 255f
  radiographic findings in, 253, 256
  of radioulnar joint, with radial head fractures, 214–215
  treatment of, 256–257
    authors' preferred method of, 256–257
  ulnar
    with lateral condylar fractures, 246
    proximal, with fracture, 266–269
Displacement, angular, in throwing, 29
Distal humerus
  anatomy of, 195, 196f
  arthroscopy of, 161
  intraosseous blood supply to, 11
  radiography of, 51
  supracondylar region of, clinical anatomy of, 223, 224f
  triangular construct of, 195, 196f
Distal humerus fractures
  bone cement for, 204, 204f, 280–281
  bone graft for, 200–201, 202f, 204
  classification of, 195–197, 196f
  comminution of, 195–196, 196f, 198, 200
    treatment of, 200–201, 201f–202f, 204
  in elderly, 196, 203–204, 204f
  fixation of, 18–19, 195–206
  infected or contaminated, treatment of, 281–282
  low, 196–197
    treatment of, 201–203, 203f
  mobilization in, 200
  nonunion of, 273–276
    complications of, 282
    inadequate fixation and, 273, 274f–275f
    open reduction and internal fixation of, 278–281, 279f–280f
    operative treatment of, 276, 278–283
    severity of initial injury and, 273, 275f
    total elbow arthroplasty for, 276
  order of fracture assembly in, 199
  in osteoporotic bone, 278
    treatment of, 203–206, 204f
  patient positioning in

Distal humerus fractures *(continued)*
    for exposure/treatment, 197–198, 198f, 205
    for radiography, 197, 197f
  physeal, 245. *See also* Lateral condylar fractures
  plates for, selection and positioning of, 199, 200f, 202–203, 206
  postoperative considerations in, 205
  preoperative planning for, 197, 198f, 205
  problem fractures, 195–206
    general principles of treatment in, 195–200
    specific, guidelines for treatment of, 200–205
  radiographic findings in, 51, 196f, 197, 197f–198f, 204–205
  shearing, 196–197, 197f, 203, 203f
  soft tissue management in, 205–206
  surgical approaches to, 198–199
    Bryan and Morrey's, 16, 198, 205
    chevron olecranon osteotomy, 18–19, 19f, 198–199, 199f, 205, 278, 281–282
    Kocher's lateral, 19
    Wadsworth's posterolateral, 14
  symptomatic hardware in, 282
Distention, of elbow, for arthroscopy, 159, 164, 178–179
Distraction interposition arthroplasty, for contractures, 291–292
Distraction, joint, in throwing mechanism, 30–31, 70
Divergent dislocation, 253
  mechanism of injury, 254
Double-hand technique, in tennis, 37
Dynamic elbow suspension splint, 13
Dynamic joint distractor, for complex fracture-dislocation of proximal ulna, 267–269, 268f
  technique for applying, 267–269, 268f
Dynamic splinting, for contractures, 287

Ecchymosis
  with biceps tendon rupture, 109–110, 110f
  with triceps tendon rupture, 109, 119
Edema. *See* Swelling
Eiphysis fractures, magnetic resonance imaging of, 55
Elderly, distal humerus fractures in, 196, 203–204, 204f
Electrodiagnostic studies
  in contractures, 286
  in elbow dislocation, 254
  in median nerve compression (pronator syndrome), 143–144, 146
  in radial nerve compression, 151
  in ulnar nerve compression (cubital tunnel syndrome), 134
Electrolyte levels, in olecranon bursitis, 304
Electromyography, 29
  during baseball pitching, 34, 35f, 90
  in contractures, 286
  in lateral epicondylitis, 318–319
  magnetic resonance imaging with, in entrapment neuropathies, 65
  in median nerve compression (pronator syndrome), 143–144
  in supracondylar fractures, 237–238
  during tennis playing, 37
  in ulnar collateral ligament injuries, 90, 94
  in ulnar nerve compression, 134
  of ulnar neuritis
    with Little League elbow, 73
    with medial epicondylitis, 85

Enchondroma, 299
Endoscopy. *See* Arthroscopy
Endpoint of motion, quality of, 46
Entrapment neuropathies, 131. *See also specific nerves*
  magnetic resonance imaging of, 55, 64–65, 66f
  sensory examination in, 47, 133–134
Eosinophilic granuloma, 296, 299–300, 300f
Epicondylar groove, 132
Epicondyle(s). *See also* Lateral epicondyle; Medial epicondyle
  as arthroscopic landmark, 159, 164
  avulsion fracture of, fluoroscopy of, 53
  in border of cubital fossa, 6–7, 7f
  ossification of, 245
  palpation of, 42–44, 43f, 45f
  radiography of, 51
Epicondylectomy, medial, 10
  for ulnar nerve compression, 137, 137f
Epicondylic release, skin incision for, 13
Epicondylitis, 79–88. *See also* Lateral epicondylitis; Medial epicondylitis
  clinical presentations of, 80
  counterforce bracing in, 81, 81f, 86, 317–318
  extensor carpi radialis brevis as origin of, 48–49, 49f, 58, 80, 82–83, 83f, 85
  magnetic resonance imaging of, 57–60, 58f–60f
  nonoperative treatment of, 59, 80–81, 81f
  operative treatment of, 81–85
    contraindications to, 81
    indications for, 81, 87
    procedures for, 81–85
  palpation of, 43–44, 45f
  pathology of, 79–80
  postoperative management of, 86
  provocative tests for, 48–50, 49f–50f, 80
  radiographic findings in, 82, 82f
  rehabilitation of, 86, 315–318, 318t
  surgical failure in, 87, 87f
  surgical results in, 86–87
Epiphyseal injury, in Little League elbow, 69
Epithelial sarcoma, 299–300
Equipment, for arthroscopy, 157–158, 164–165, 165f
Erythema, inspection for, 42
Erythrocyte sedimentation rate
  in olecranon bursitis, 304
  with tumors of elbow, 295
Essex-Lopresti injuries, 214–215, 219, 267
Ewing's sarcoma, 299
Exercise-tubing drills, 311, 319
Extension, 29
  assessment of, 45, 45f
  in baseball pitching
    during arm acceleration, 34–35
    during arm cocking, 33–34, 35f
    during arm deceleration, 35
  in football passing, 36
  force in, 31
  in javelin throw, 37
  loss of
    with dislocation injury, 256
    injuries causing, 45
  mean torque in, 31
  muscles involved in, 4, 30
    strength testing of, 46
  normal arc of, 29, 45
  palpation during, 42–43, 43f
  passive, of wrist and fingers, in medial epicondylitis, 50
  post-surgery, 13
  in tennis, 36

Extension (continued)
  weakness of, with triceps tendon rupture, 109
Extension injuries, posterior, in young athletes (Little League elbow), 75–76
Extension-type supracondylar fractures, 223–241
  classification of, 226–230, 231f
  clinical presentation of, 223–224
  preferred treatment of, 233–235
Extensor carpi radialis brevis muscle, 8
  action of, 5t, 30
  in baseball pitching, 32t
  fibrous edge of, radial nerve compression by, 150, 150f, 152, 154
  insertion of, 5t
  in joint stabilization, 102, 103f
  nerve supply to, 5t
  origin of, 5t
  palpation of, 43
  strength testing of, 47
Extensor carpi radialis brevis tendon, in epicondylitis, 48–49, 49f, 58, 80, 82–83, 83f, 85
Extensor carpi radialis longus muscle, 8
  action of, 5t, 30
  in baseball pitching, 32t
  insertion of, 5t
  in joint stabilization, 102, 103f
  nerve supply to, 5t, 149
  origin of, 5t
  palpation of, 43
  in provocative test for lateral epicondylitis, 48–49, 49f
  in radial nerve surgery, 155
  strength testing of, 47
Extensor carpi ulnaris muscle
  action of, 5t, 30
  insertion of, 5t
  in joint stabilization, 102, 103f
  in lateral collateral ligament reconstruction, 105
  nerve supply to, 5t
  origin of, 5t
  posterior interosseous nerve compression syndrome and, 150
  strength testing of, 47
Extensor digiti quinti muscle, in joint stabilization, 102, 103f
Extensor digitorum communis muscle
  action of, 5t
  in baseball pitching, 32t
  insertion of, 5t
  in joint stabilization, 102, 103f
  nerve supply to, 5t
  origin of, 5t
  posterior interosseous nerve compression syndrome and, 150
Extensor mechanism overload, 123
Extensor muscle(s)
  in joint stabilization, 101–102, 103f
  major, across elbow, 30
Extensor muscle mass, 259
Extracompartmental tumors, 296, 297t

Fascia lata, as interposition material, 291
Fasciotomy
  Henry's anterior approach in, 24
  in vascular injury, with supracondylar fracture, 238
Fast spin-echo magnetic resonance imaging, 55–56
Fastball pitch, biomechanics of, 33–35, 34t, 70
Fat pad(s), 9, 9f
  radiography of, 9, 52

Fat pad(s) (continued)
  in lateral condylar fractures, 246
  in supracondylar fractures, 225–226, 227f
Fat suppression, in magnetic resonance imaging, 56, 60
Fenestration, of olecranon, 192f–193f
  with arthroscopic radial head excision, 192–193, 192f–193f
  with capsular release, for ankylosis, 180–181
Fibrin adhesive glue, for radial head fracture fixation, 212
Fibrohistiocytic tumors, malignant, 299
Fibromatosis, 299–300
Fibrosarcoma, 299
Fibrous band of tissue, anterior to radiocapitellar joint, radial nerve compression by, 149–150, 150f, 152
Fibrous histiocytoma, malignant, 301f, 302
Figure-of-eight tension-band wiring, 261–262, 262f
Flexibility exercises
  for flexor-pronator tendinitis, 315
  for lateral epicondylitis, 318
  for ulnar neuritis, 313
  for valgus extension overload syndrome, 319
Flexion, 29–30
  assessment of, 45, 45f
  axis of rotation for, 29–30
  in baseball pitching
    during arm cocking, 33–34, 35f
    during stride, 31
    during windup, 31
  and carrying angle, 30
  force in, 31
  in javelin throw, 37
  loss of, injuries causing, 45
  muscles involved in, 30
    strength testing of, 46
  normal arc of, 29, 45
  palpation during, 42f, 42–43
  for radiographic evaluation of distal humerus fractures, 197, 197f
  resisted, testing with
    for medial epicondylitis, 50
    for medial nerve entrapment, 50
  in tennis, 36–37
  in throwing, 29
  in underhand throw (softball pitching), 37
Flexion arc, of forearm, elbow injuries or arthritis and, 1
Flexion contractures
  arthroscopic treatment of, 177–184
    contraindications to, 178
    indications for, 178
    versus open surgical release, 183
    patient positioning for, 178, 179f
    precautions in, 182–183
    results of, 183
    technique for, 178–181, 179f–182f
  with collateral ligament injury, 178
  nonoperative treatment of, 178
  open capsular release for, 287–291
  with osteochondritis of capitellum, 74
  postoperative management of, 182
  posttraumatic, pathogenesis of, 177–178
  soft endpoints with, 46
  with valgus extension overload syndrome, 123–124
Flexion test, for ulnar nerve compression, 50, 50f, 134
Flexion-extension axis, 90, 90f
Flexion-type supracondylar fractures, 223, 239–240, 241f
Flexor(s), across elbow, 30

Flexor carpi radialis muscle
  action of, 5t
  in baseball pitching, 32t
  innervation of, 142
  insertion of, 5t
  nerve supply to, 5t
  origin of, 5t
Flexor carpi ulnaris muscle, 8f
  action of, 5t
  in baseball pitching, 32t
  insertion of, 5t
  nerve supply to, 5t
  origin of, 5t
  ulnar nerve compression at, 132f, 133, 135–136
Flexor digitorum profundus muscle
  action of, 5t
  innervation of, 142
  insertion of, 5t
  nerve supply to, 5t
  origin of, 5t
  strength testing of, 47
Flexor digitorum superficialis muscle
  action of, 5t
  arch, median nerve compression at, 142f, 142–143, 144f, 145–146, 146f
  in baseball pitching, 32t
  insertion of, 5t
  nerve supply to, 5t, 142
  origin of, 5t
Flexor pollicis longus muscle
  innervation of, 142
  strength testing of, 47
Flexor-pronator muscle mass, 259
  palpation of, 43
  splitting of, in ulnar collateral ligament surgery, 95f–96f, 95–98
  in ulnar collateral ligament injuries, 94
  ulnar nerve transposition to, 136f, 136–138
Flexor-pronator strain, with medial tension overload, 57
Flexor-pronator tendinitis, rehabilitation of, 315–316
Flexor-pronator tendonapathy, 42
Fluoroscopy, 51, 53
  in capsular release, for contractures, 289
  of complex fracture-dislocation of proximal ulna, 268
  of lateral condylar fractures, 247, 250
  of supracondylar fractures, 233, 235–236, 235f–236f
Follow-through, in baseball pitching, 31f–33f, 35–36
  muscle activity in, 32t
Football passing
  biomechanics of elbow during, 36, 36f
  injuries with, 69, 123–124
Force(s), 29–31
  in baseball pitching, 32f–33f, 70, 72f
    during arm acceleration, 32f–33f, 34–35
    during arm cocking, 32f–33f, 32–34
    during arm deceleration, 32f–33f, 35
    during follow-through, 32f–33f, 35–36
  in football passing, 36
  in tennis playing, 37
  three-dimensional model for quantifying, 31
  in underhand throw (softball pitching), 37
Forearm pronation
  for protection of posterior interosseous nerve, in surgery, 6, 19–20, 21f, 23–24
  resisted, in medial epicondylitis, 50, 50f
Forearm, proximal, radiography of, 51
Forearm rotation, elbow injuries or arthritis and, 1

Forearm throw, 34
Form molding, for distal humerus fractures, 200
Fractures. *See also specific fractures*
 radiographically occult or equivocal, magnetic resonance imaging of, 55, 60–61, 63*f*
Friction massage, 315–316
Full-thickness skin flaps
 in olecranon fracture surgery, 260
 for protection of cutaneous nerves, 1–2, 12
 in radial nerve surgery, 153
 in ulnar nerve release, 135–136
Fungal infection, olecranon bursitis with, 304
Fusobacterium infection, olecranon bursitis with, 303

Gadolinium enhancement, of magnetic resonance imaging, 56
 in biceps tendon injury, 63
 in osteochondritis dissecans, 61, 62*f*
Ganglion cyst, 299
Gartland classification system, of supracondylar fractures, 226, 239
Giant cell tumor of bone, 295, 299–300, 301*f*
Ginglymus (hinge) joint, 1, 89
Girth measurements, 42
Gliding joints, 1
Global surgical approach, 21, 23–24, 24*f*–25*f*
 indications for, 15*t*
Golfer's elbow, 43, 57, 79. *See also* Medial epicondylitis
Goniometer, 286
Gordon's surgical approach, 18
 indications for, 15*t*
Gradient-echo sequences, in magnetic resonance imaging, avoidance of, after elbow surgery, 56
Grafts
 bone
  for distal humerus fractures, 200–201, 202*f*, 204
  for lateral condylar fractures, 250–251
  for nonunions of elbow, 276–277
  for olecranon fractures, 260
  in tumor treatment, 299–300
 in lateral collateral ligament reconstruction, 105–107, 106*f*–107*f*
 in ulnar collateral ligament reconstruction
  fixation and tensioning of, 96–98, 97*f*–98*f*
  magnetic resonance imaging of, 57, 57*f*, 92, 94*f*
Grasping forceps, for loose body removal, 173, 173*f*
Gravity irrigation, for arthroscopy, 157
Grip strength, measurement of, 46–47
Ground strokes, in tennis, biomechanics of, 36–37
Growth cartilage injury, in Little League elbow, 69
Growth plate(s)
 fractures, magnetic resonance imaging of, 55
 medial epicondylar, delayed closure of, 73
Guyon's canal, ulnar nerve compression at, 133
Gymnast(s), injuries in, 69

Hamstring tendon, strips of, for ulnar collateral ligament reconstruction, 95
Hand disorders, and lymphatics, 2
Hand ischemia, with supracondylar fracture, 238, 238*f*
Hand strength
 assessment of, 46–47
 ulnar nerve compression and, 133–134

Hardware, symptomatic, 269, 282
Haversian fat pads, 9, 9*f*
Healing tissue, overstressing of, avoidance of, in rehabilitation, 309
Hemangioma, 299
Hemarthrosis
 arthrofibrosis with, 177–178
 with radial head fractures, 208–209, 211
Hematoma(s)
 with distal humerus fracture fixation, 205
 with olecranon fractures, 260
 with radial head fractures, 211, 216
 with supracondylar fractures, 225, 233
Henry's anterior surgical approach, 24–26, 25*f*
 complications of, 26
 indications for, 15*t*, 24
 in open capsular release, 287–288
Herbert miniscrews, for radial head fracture fixation, 216
Herbert screws, for distal humerus fractures, 278
Heterotopic ossification, 286–287, 291, 293
High-field magnetic resonance imaging systems, 55
High-speed videography, of throwing, 29
High-voltage galvanic stimulation, 312–313, 315, 317, 319
Hilton's law, 2
Hinge joint, 1, 89
Hinged external fixators, for complex fracture-dislocation of proximal ulna, 267–269, 268*f*
History, 41–42
Hohmann retractors, in radial head fracture surgery, 216
Holmberg classification system, of supracondylar fractures, 226
Hotchkiss' surgical approach, 22–23, 278, 288, 289*f*
 indications for, 15*t*
Humeral metaphysis, 11
Humeroradial joint
 articulation of, and joint stabilization, 30
 flexion and extension at, 29
 force in, 31
Humeroulnar joint
 articulation of, and joint stabilization, 30
 flexion and extension at, 29
 force in, 31
Humerus
 distal
  anatomy of, 195, 196*f*
  arthroscopy of, 161
  intraosseous blood supply to, 11
  radiography of, 51
  supracondylar region of, clinical anatomy of, 223, 224*f*
  triangular construct of, 195, 196*f*
 force transfer to, 31
 radiography of, 52
Humerus fractures
 distal
  bone cement for, 204, 204*f*, 280–281
  bone graft for, 200–201, 202*f*, 204
  classification of, 195–197, 196*f*
  comminution of, 195–196, 196*f*, 198, 200–201, 201*f*–202*f*, 204
  in elderly, 196, 203–204, 204*f*
  fixation of, 18–19, 195–206
  infected or contaminated, treatment of, 281–282
  low, 196–197, 201–203, 203*f*
  mobilization in, 200
  nonunion of, 273–276, 274*f*–275*f*, 278–283, 279*f*–280*f*

Humerus fractures *(continued)*
  order of fracture assembly in, 199
  in osteoporotic bone, 203–206, 204*f*, 278
  patient positioning in, 197, 197*f*, 197–198, 198*f*, 205
  physeal, 245. *See also* Lateral condylar fractures
  plates for, selection and positioning of, 199, 200*f*, 202–203, 206
  postoperative considerations in, 205
  preoperative planning for, 197, 198*f*, 205
  problem fractures, 195–206
  radiographic findings in, 51, 196*f*, 197, 197*f*–198*f*, 204–205
  shearing, 196–197, 197*f*, 203, 203*f*
  soft tissue management in, 205–206
  surgical approaches to, 14, 16, 18–19, 19*f*, 198–199, 199*f*, 205
  symptomatic hardware in, 282
 extra-articular, surgical approaches in, 15
 metaphyseal, surgical approaches in, 15*t*
 supracondylar
  in children, 15, 223–243
  clinical presentation of, 223–224
  closed reduction and external immobilization of, 230–231
  closed reduction and percutaneous pinning of, 233–237, 235*f*–237*f*
  complications of, 237–239
  cubitus varus with, 42, 224*f*, 226, 234, 236, 238–240, 239*f*–241*f*
  extension-type, 223–230, 231*f*, 233–235, 240–241
  flexion-type, 223, 239–240, 241*f*
  lateral condylar fractures with, 239, 240*f*
  magnetic resonance imaging for exclusion of, 61
  nerve injury with, 225–226, 233, 237–238, 240
  nonoperative treatment of, 230–233
  open reduction and internal fixation of, 237
  open reduction of, 233
  operative treatment of, 233, 235–237
  pinning configurations for, 234, 234*f*
  radiographic evaluation of, 224–225, 224*f*–225*f*, 224–226, 225*f*, 227*f*–232*f*, 233–236, 240*f*
  rotational deformity with, 223, 224*f*
  surgical approaches in, 15, 15*t*, 18–19
  traction for, 231–233
  treatment options in, 230–233
  type I (flexion), 239
  type IA, 226, 226*t*, 227*f*, 233
  type IB, 226, 226*t*, 228*f*, 233–234
  type II (flexion), 239
  type IIA, 226*t*, 226–230, 229*f*, 233–234
  type IIB, 226*t*, 230, 230*f*, 233–234
  type III (extension), 226*f*, 226*t*, 230, 231*f*–232*f*, 233–236, 238
  type III (flexion), 239–240, 241*f*
  type IIIA, 226*t*, 230, 231*f*, 233–235
  type IIIB, 226*t*, 226*f*, 230, 232*f*, 233–235
  ulnar nerve injury with, 132
  vascular injury with, 225–226, 226*f*, 238, 238*f*
Hyaline articular cartilage, magnetic resonance imaging of, 56
Hyperextension
 and coronoid process fractures, 265
 and dislocation, 253–254, 256
 and olecranon bursitis, 303
Hypertrophy, of muscles, as diagnostic sign, 42

Iliac crest, bone graft from
　for distal humerus fractures, 200
　preparation for, 276
Ilizarov construct, for stabilization of infected or contaminated distal humerus fractures, 281–282
Immobilization
　after major elbow surgery, 13
　of dislocation injury, 256–257
　inadequate, and nonunion, 271
　of lateral condylar fractures, 246
　in median nerve compression (pronator syndrome), 146
　minimizing effects of, in rehabilitation, 309
　for nonunions, 276
　of olecranon fractures, 259–260
　for osteochondritis dissecans, 316
　in radial nerve compression, 155
　of supracondylar fractures, 230–231
　of ulnar collateral ligament injury, 310–311
Immunoelectrophoresis, for tumors of elbow, 295
Incisions, 12–13
Indomethacin, for olecranon bursitis, 305
Infection, near elbow joint, effect on flexion and extension, 1
Inferior ulnar collateral artery, 8f
　relationship to medial and lateral intermuscular septa, 4f
Injury(ies). *See also specific elbow injuries*
　acute, 41
　chronic, 41
　diagnosis of, history and physical examination for, 41–54
　inspection of, 42, 42f
　loss of extension with, 45
　loss of flexion with, 45
Inspection, 42, 42f
Instability
　arthroscopy of, 163, 167, 167f
　assessment of, 47–48, 47f–49f, 92
　in epicondylitis surgery, 87
　posterior, magnetic resonance imaging of, 60, 60f
　posterolateral rotatory
　　arthroscopy of, 167, 167f
　　assessment of, 48, 48f–49f
　　Boyd's surgical approach and, 17–18
　　clinical presentation of, 102
　　deficiency of lateral ulnar collateral ligament in, 10
　　diagnosis of, 102–104
　　in epicondylitis surgery, 87
　　functional anatomy in, 101–102, 102f–103f
　　history in, 101–102
　　Kocher's lateral approach and, 20
　　lateral collateral ligament reconstruction for, 101–108
　　lateral ulnar collateral ligament injury with, 60
　　magnetic resonance imaging of, 104, 105f
　　palpation in, 103
　　physical findings in, 101
　　provocative test for, 104, 104f
　　radiocapitellar joint degeneration with, 186
　　radiographic findings in, 103–104, 103f–104f
　　surgical repair of, 104–107, 106f–107f
　　radial head fractures and, 214–215, 219
　valgus
　　with radiocapitellar joint degeneration, 187, 189, 190f

Instability *(continued)*
　　with ulnar collateral ligament injuries, 89–92, 99
Internal fixation
　of coronoid process fractures, 260, 265–266, 266f
　of distal humerus fractures, 18–19, 195–206, 278–281, 279f–280f
　of olecranon fractures, 260–264, 277
　of proximal ulnar fractures, 266, 277
　of radial head fractures, 13, 211–213, 215–217, 217f, 255, 255f
　of supracondylar humerus fractures, 237
Interosseous artery, 4f
Interosseous ligament injury, with dislocation, 254
Interosseous membrane, 208
　radial head fractures and, 214–215
Interosseous nerve. *See also* Anterior interosseous nerve; Posterior interosseous nerve
　isolation and protection of, in surgery
　　in Boyd's approach, 17–18
　　in global approach, 23–24
　　in Henry's anterior approach, 26
　　in Kaplan's direct lateral approach, 20, 21f
　　in Kocher's lateral approach, 20
　　in lateral approaches, 6, 19
　　pronation of forearm for, 6, 19–20, 21f, 23–24
Interphalangeal joints, assessment of, in radial nerve compression, 151
Interposition arthroplasty, for contractures, 291–292
Interval throwing program, in rehabilitation, 312, 314t–315t
Intra-articular abnormalities, diagnostic arthroscopy for, 163–169
Intra-articular fracture, radiography of, 52
Intra-articular injury, with ulnar collateral ligament injuries, 95–96
Intra-articular problems, with radiocapitellar joint degeneration, 193
Intracompartmental tumors, 296, 297t
Intralesional surgical margin, 297
Intramedullary compression screws, with tension-band wiring, for olecranon fractures, 262–263, 264f
Intramuscular transposition, of ulnar nerve, 136
Intraosseous blood supply, to distal humerus, 11
Inverse dynamic equations, 29
Iontophoresis, 315, 317
Irrigation systems, for arthroscopy, 157–158, 167
Ischemia
　in compressive neuropathies, 131
　hand, with supracondylar fracture, 238, 238f
　Volkmann's, 231, 238, 269
Isokinetic assessment, in rehabilitation, 309, 310f, 315
Isometric exercises
　for flexor-pronator tendinitis, 315
　for lateral epicondylitis, 318
　for medial epicondylitis, 315
　for osteochondritis dissecans, 317
　for ulnar collateral ligament injury, 311
　for ulnar neuritis, 313
　for valgus extension overload syndrome, 319
Isotonic exercises
　for biceps tendon, 117
　for flexor-pronator tendinitis, 316
　for lateral epicondylitis, 318
　for medial epicondylitis, 316

Isotonic exercises *(continued)*
　for osteochondritis dissecans, 317
　Thrower's Ten program for, 311–312, 312t, 314
　for ulnar collateral ligament injury, 311
　for ulnar neuritis, 313–314
　for valgus extension overload syndrome, 319

Javelin throw
　biomechanics of, 37
　injuries with, 69, 79, 89, 123–124, 309
Jobe's medial utility approach, 23, 23f
Joint contractures. *See* Contracture(s)
Joint distraction, in throwing mechanism, 30–31, 70
Joint effusion, inspection of, 42, 42f
Joint instability. *See* Instability
Joint replacement. *See* Arthroplasty
Joint stability, testing of, 47–48, 47f–49f
Joint stabilization, 30–31, 208, 259
　anconeus muscle in, 4, 30, 34
　in baseball pitching, 34
　functional anatomy in, 101–102, 102f–103f
Joint surface injury, in Little League elbow, 69

Kaplan's direct lateral surgical approach, 20, 21f
Kaposi's sarcoma, 299
Keith needles, in biceps tendon repair, 113, 113f–114f, 115–116, 116f
Key and Conwell's surgical approach, 13t, 21
Kinematics, of throwing, 29, 36, 89
Kinetics, of throwing, 29, 36
Kirschner wires (K-wires)
　for fixation
　　of acute lateral condylar fracture, 247–248, 248t
　　of biceps tendon, 114–116, 115f–116f, 206
　　of distal humerus fracture, 198–199, 201–203, 278, 281
　　in nonunion of proximal ulna, 277
　　of olecranon fractures, 260–262, 260f–263f, 277, 282
　　of radioulnar joint, with radial head fracture surgery, 219
　　of supracondylar fractures, 231–232, 236, 236f
　for osteotomy in cubitus varus, 239
Kissing lesions, 127, 128f, 166, 171
Knee immobilizer, pediatric, 13
Kocher clamp, in biceps tendon repair, 112–113, 113f
Kocher, Theodor, 11
Kocher's lateral surgical approach, 13t, 19–21, 20f, 104
　for dislocation injury, 257
　indications for, 15t, 19
　modifications in, 20–21
　for radial head fractures, 15t, 19–20, 188, 216, 278
Krakauer sutures, in triceps tendon repair, 120

Lacertus fibrosus (bicipital aponeurosis), 2, 4f, 7, 7f, 110
　biceps tendon secured to, in nonanatomic repair of rupture, 111
　magnetic resonance imaging of, 63, 65f
　median nerve compression by, 142f, 142–143, 145–146
　palpation of, 43
Lactic dehydrogenase, serum levels of, with tumors of elbow, 295
Lag-screw fixation
　in coronoid process fractures, 260
　in distal humerus fractures, 200–201, 201f

Langerhan's cell histiocytosis, 300, 300f
Lateral antebrachial cutaneous nerve, isolation and protection of, in surgery, 153
Lateral collateral ligament (radial collateral ligament), 9f–10f, 10, 10f, 101, 186f, 186–187
   arthroscopy of, 165
   functional anatomy of, 101–102, 102f–103f
   injury, with lateral epicondylitis, 59f, 59–60
   in radial head excision, 188, 278
   reconstruction of, 101–108
     Kocher's lateral approach in, 19, 104
     results of, 107
     technique for, 104–107, 106f–107f
   in stability testing, 48
   strength of, 30–31
   in trochlear shear fracture surgery, 203, 203f
Lateral column, of distal humerus, 195, 196f
   reconstruction of, 199
Lateral compartment compression, with valgus extension overload syndrome, 123
Lateral compression injuries
   baseball pitching and, 33, 73–75
   in young athletes (Little League elbow), 73–75
Lateral condylar epiphysis, 11
Lateral condylar fractures
   acute, treatment of, 247f, 247–248, 248f
   atypical patterns of, 246
   bone graft for, 250–251
   chronic, treatment of, 249–250, 249f–251f
   classification of, 245–246
     Milch system of, 245, 246f
     Salter-Harris system of, 245–246
   clinical anatomy in, 245–246
   complications of, 250–251
   cubitus valgus with, 42, 247, 249–251, 249f–251f
   delayed union of, 250–251
   displacement of, 246–248, 247f–248f, 248–249
   magnetic resonance imaging of, 61, 61f, 64
   mechanism of injury in, 245
   Milch type I, 245, 246f
   Milch type II, 245, 246f
   nonoperative treatment of, 246
   nonunion of, 247f, 249–250, 249f–251f
   open reduction and fixation of, 247f–248f, 247–251
   operative treatment of, 247–250
   pediatric, 245–252
   physical examination of, 246
   radiographic findings in, 245–247, 247f–251f
   Salter-Harris type II, 61, 64, 245, 246f
   Salter-Harris type IV, 61, 61f, 245–246, 246f, 247
   semi-acute, treatment of, 248–249
   stage I, 246
   stage II, 246
   stage III, 246
   with supracondylar fractures, 239, 240f
   supracondylar varus osteotomy for, 249–250, 249f–250f
   surgical approaches in
     alternative, 15t
     recommended, 15t
   treatment of, 246–250
   ulnar dislocation with, 246
   ulnar nerve injury with, 132, 249–250
Lateral condylar physis
   clinical anatomy of, 245–246
   versus lateral epicondyle, 245
Lateral condylar physis fracture. See Lateral condylar fractures

Lateral condyle, 11
Lateral cutaneous nerve of forearm, 1, 3f
   protection of, in surgery, in Henry's anterior approach, 25
Lateral decubitus position
   for arthroscopy, 158, 158f, 164, 164f, 190
   in olecranon fractures, 260, 261f
Lateral dislocation, 253
   mechanism of injury, 253–254
   treatment of, 256–257
Lateral elbow instability. See also Posterolateral rotatory instability
   lateral collateral ligament reconstruction for, 101–108
Lateral epicondylar osteotomy, 21
Lateral epicondyle, 11
   as arthroscopic landmark, 159, 164
   in border of cubital fossa, 6–7, 7f
   fracture
     avulsion, with posterolateral rotatory instability, 103, 103f
     radiographic findings in, 245
   lateral condylar physis versus, 245
   ossification of, 245
   palpation of, 42–43, 43f, 44, 45f
   radiography of, 51
Lateral epicondylitis, 37, 186–187
   age and, 79
   chair test for, 49, 49f
   clinical presentation of, 80
   differential diagnosis of, 80
   incidence of, 79
   magnetic resonance imaging of, 58–60, 59f–60f
   nonoperative treatment of, 59, 80–81, 81f
   operative treatment of, 81–85
     arthroscopic technique, 83–85, 84f
     contraindications to, 81
     indications for, 81, 87
     procedures for, 81–85
     technique for, 82–83, 82f–84f
   palpation of, 44, 45f
   pathology of, 79–80
   physical findings in, 80
   postoperative management of, 86
   provocative tests for, 48–49, 49f, 80
   radiographic findings in, 82, 82f
   rehabilitation of, 316–318, 318t
   surgical failure in, 87, 87f
   surgical results in, 86–87
Lateral intermuscular septum, relationship of nerves and arteries to, 2, 4f
Lateral J approach, 11
Lateral ligament complex, 10, 10f
   in Boyd's surgical approach, 17–18
Lateral pivot-shift test, 48, 48f
Lateral portal, for arthroscopy, 160–161, 161f, 165–167
   in capsular release, for ankylosis, 180
   for loose body removal, 173–174, 174f
   in radial head excision, 190–192, 191f
Lateral provocative tests, 48–50
Lateral radiographic views, 51–52, 52f
Lateral soft spot
   inspection of, 42, 42f
   palpation of, 45
Lateral surgical approaches, 11–12, 13t, 19–21
   protection of posterior interosseous nerve in, 6, 19
Lateral symptoms, 41
Leash of Henry, radial nerve compression by, 149–150, 150f, 152–154, 153f
Lesser toe extensor tendons, for ulnar collateral ligament reconstruction, 95

Ligament complexes, 9–10, 10f. See also specific ligaments
   biomechanics of, 30–31
   magnetic resonance imaging of, 55
   in stability testing, 47–48
   strength of, 30–31
Ligament of Struthers
   median nerve compression by, 142f, 142–143
   palpation of, 43
Ligamentous instability, iatrogenic, in epicondylitis surgery, 87
Limitation of motion, assessment of, 46
Limited-contact dynamic compression plates, 277
Lipofibromatous hamartoma of nerve, 299
Lipoma, 299–300
Liposarcoma, 299, 302
Little League elbow, 35, 69–77
   disorders termed, 69
   lateral compression, 73–75
   loose bodies with, 171
   magnetic resonance imaging of, 58
   pain with, 42
   palpation in, 45
   pathogenesis of, 69–70, 70f
   physical examination and treatment of, 69–76
   posterior extension, 75–76
   prevention of, sports guidelines for, 76
   true (medial tension injuries), 71–73
   ulnar neuritis with, 73
Locking and catching, 41, 73, 171–172
Longitudinal instability, radial head fractures and, 214–216, 219
Long-toss program, in rehabilitation, 312, 314t
Loose bodies
   arthrography of, 53
   arthroscopy of, 160, 163, 166–167
   computed tomography of, 172
   with dislocation injury, 256
   firm endpoints with, 46
   fluoroscopy of, 53
   history in, 171
   loss of pronation or supination with, 46
   magnetic resonance imaging of, 56–57, 61–62, 63f, 172, 172f
   nonoperative treatment of, 172
   in olecranon fossa, flexion contracture with, 178
   operative treatment of, 172–175
     complications in, 175
     contraindications to, 172
     indications for, 172
     postoperative management of, 175
     results of, 175
     techniques for, 173–175, 173f–175f
   pain with, 41
   palpation of, 44–45
   physical examination in, 172
   with radiocapitellar joint degeneration, 186–188, 191, 193–194
   radiography of, 171–172
   removal of
     arthroscopic, 171–176, 173f–175f, 191, 193–194
     Kocher's lateral approach in, 19
     Molesworth's medial approach in, 22
   throwing/pitching and, 34–35, 171
   with ulnar collateral ligament injuries, 91–92, 93f, 95
   with valgus extension overload syndrome, 123–125, 124f, 171–172
   in young athletes (Little League elbow), 73, 171

Loupe magnification, in radial nerve
    decompression, 152
Lymphatics, superficial, 1–2
Lymphoma, 299

MacAusland's surgical approach, 19
Magnetic resonance imaging (MRI), 53, 55–68
  advantages of, 55
  of biceps tendon injury, 56, 62–63, 64f–65f
  of biceps tendon rupture, 56, 111
  confounding of, steroid injections and,
      57–59, 58f–59f
  of contractures, 286
  of elbow pathology, 56–66
  of entrapment neuropathies, 64–65, 66f
  of fractures, 55, 60–61, 63f
  improvements in, 55
  of lateral epicondylitis, 58–60, 59f–60f
  of Little League elbow, 58
  of loose bodies, 56–57, 61–62, 63f, 172,
      172f
  of medial (ulnar) collateral ligament, 89
  of medial (ulnar) collateral ligament injuries,
      56–57, 57f, 59f, 59–60, 92, 93f–94f
  of medial epicondylar avulsion, 72
  of medial epicondylar osteochondrosis, 72
  of medial epicondylitis, 57–58, 58f
  of olecranon apophysitis, 75
  of osteochondritis dissecans of capitellum,
      57, 61, 73–74, 74f
  of posterior dislocation injury and instability,
      60, 60f
  of posterolateral rotatory instability, 104,
      105f
  of radial head fractures, 61, 209
  of radial nerve compression, 152
  technique, 55–56
  of triceps tendon injury, 63–64
  of tumors, 296, 297f, 300
  of ulnar nerve compression, 64–65, 66f, 134
Malignant tumors, 299, 301–302
Manual resistance drills, 311, 312f
Marginal surgical margin, 297
Mason classification system, of radial head
    fractures, 209–211
Mason type I fracture, 207, 209, 209f
  treatment of, 211, 216
Mason type II fracture, 208–210, 210f
  treatment of, 211–213, 216–218, 217f
Mason type III fracture, 209–210, 210f
  treatment of, 212–213, 216–218, 217f
Massage, transverse or friction, 315–316
Mayo distraction device, for contractures
  in distraction interposition arthroplasty, 291
  in open capsular release, 289, 290f–291f
MCL. See Medial collateral ligament
Medial antebrachial cutaneous nerve
  protection of, in arthroscopic surgery,
      159–160
  trauma
    with biceps tendon repair, 118
    with ulnar collateral ligament
        reconstruction, 99
    in ulnar nerve decompression, 138
Medial collateral ligament (ulnar collateral
    ligament), 9–10, 10f, 186f, 186–187,
    208
  chronic degeneration of, magnetic resonance
      imaging of, 56–57
  clinical anatomy of, 89–91, 90f–91f
  composition of, 89
  functional anatomy of, 89–91
  injury, with coronoid process fractures,
      265–266

Medial collateral ligament (continued)
  instability, Molesworth's medial approach
      and, 22
  laxity, radiography of, 53
  magnetic resonance imaging of, 89
  olecranon fractures and, 264, 265f
  origin of, 90, 90f
  palpation of, 43, 43f, 91–92
  reconstruction of, 23, 23f, 94–98, 95f–98f
    arthroscopy with, 95–98, 95f–98f
    complications of, 99
    graft assessment in, magnetic resonance
        imaging of, 57, 57f, 92, 94f
    graft fixation and tensioning in, 96–98,
        97f–98f
    magnetic resonance imaging of, 92, 94f
    palmaris longus tendon graft for, 30, 94f,
        95, 97
    rehabilitation after, 98–99
    results of, 99
    with valgus extension overload syndrome,
        126–129
  repair of, 94–95
    with radial head fracture, 219, 255
  rupture/tear of
    acute, 56
    dislocation with, 57, 254
    magnetic resonance imaging of, 56–57
    midsubstance, 56
    rehabilitation in, 310–312
    treatment of, 94
  sprain, 57
    rehabilitation in, 10–312, 310t, 310–312
  in stability testing, 47–48
  strain, treatment of, 92–93
  strength of, 30–31
    ultimate tensile, 30
  and ulnar nerve compression, 132f, 132–133
      132f, 138
  in valgus extension overload syndrome,
      124–125
Medial collateral ligament injuries, 57, 89–100
  acute, 56
  with coronoid process fractures, 265–266
  dislocation with, 57, 254
  with epicondylitis, 59f, 59–60, 80, 85
  history in, 91
  magnetic resonance imaging of, 56–57, 57f,
      59f, 59–60, 92, 93f–94f
  with medial epicondylitis, 57
  nonoperative treatment of, 92–94, 310
  operative treatment of, 94–98
    authors' preferred method of, 95–98,
        95f–98f
    complications of, 99
    contraindications to, 94
    indications for, 94
    results of, 99
    technique for, 94–95
  physical examination in, 91–92
  postoperative management of, 98–99
  radiographic findings in, 92, 93f
  range of motion brace for, 311, 311f
  rehabilitation of, 98–99, 310t, 310–312,
      311f–312f, 312t
    interval throwing program in, 312,
        314t–315t
    long-toss program in, 312, 314t
    off-the-mound throwing program in, 312,
        315t
    plyometric exercise drills in, 311–312,
        312f–314f
    Thrower's Ten program for, 311–312,
        312t

Medial collateral ligament injuries (continued)
  throwing/pitching and, 32–33, 42, 56–57,
      57f, 73, 90–91, 186–187
    return to activity after reconstruction,
        98–100
  in young athletes (Little League elbow), 73
Medial column, of distal humerus, 195, 196f
  reconstruction of, 199
Medial compartment distraction, with valgus
    extension overload syndrome, 123
Medial condylar fracture, Molesworth's medial
    approach in, 22
Medial cutaneous nerve of forearm, 1–2, 3f
Medial dislocation, 253
  mechanism of injury, 253–254
  treatment of, 256–257
Medial epicondylar avulsion, 72–73
  physical findings in, 72
  radiographic findings in, 72, 73f
  surgical repair of, 72–73, 73f
  treatment of, 72–73
Medial epicondylar bursitis, 303
Medial epicondylar growth plate, delayed
    closure of, 73
Medial epicondylar osteochondrosis, 72
  physical findings in, 72
  radiographic findings in, 72
  treatment of, 72
Medial epicondyle
  as arthroscopic landmark, 159, 164
  in border of cubital fossa, 6–7, 7f
  fracture of
    avulsion, fluoroscopy of, 53
    Molesworth's medial approach in, 22
  ossification of, 245
  palpation of, 42–43, 43f
  plate wrapping of, in distal humerus fracture
      fixation, 202
  radiography of, 51
Medial epicondylectomy, 10
  for ulnar nerve compression, 137, 137f
Medial epicondylitis
  baseball pitching and, 32, 57–58, 80
  clinical presentation of, 80
  magnetic resonance imaging of, 57–58, 58f
  nonoperative treatment of, 80–81, 81f
  operative treatment of, 81–82, 85
    contraindications to, 81
    indications for, 81, 87
    planning for, magnetic resonance imaging
        in, 58
    procedures for, 81–82, 85
    technique for, 85, 86f
  palpation of, 43
  pathology of, 79–80
  postoperative management of, 86
  provocative tests for, 50, 50f
  rehabilitation of, 86, 315–316
  surgical failure in, 87
  surgical results in, 86–87
  ulnar nerve injury with, 58, 80, 82, 86–87,
      315
  in young athletes (Little League elbow), 58
Medial force, in baseball pitching, 33, 33f
Medial instability, in epicondylitis surgery,
    87
Medial intermuscular septum, 8f
  relationship of nerves and arteries to, 2, 4f
  ulnar nerve compression at, 132f
  in ulnar nerve exposure and release,
      135–136, 136f
Medial laxity, radiography of, 53
Medial portal, for arthroscopy, 159–160,
    159f–160f, 164–165

Medial portal, for arthroscopy (continued)
    for capsular release, in ankylosis, 179–180, 179f–180f
    in radial head excision, 190–192, 191f
Medial prominence overgrowth, 73
Medial provocative tests, 50, 50f
Medial stability, assessment of, 47f, 47–48
Medial surgical approaches, 11–12, 13t, 22–23
Medial symptoms, 41
Medial tension injuries
    classic history triad of, 71–72
    complications of, 73
    in young athletes (true Little League elbow), 71–73
Medial tension overload, 57, 123
Median nerve, 3f, 7, 7f
    branching pattern of, variable patterns of, 141–142
    clinical anatomy of, 141–142, 142f
    injury
        with elbow dislocation, 254, 256–257
        with supracondylar fractures, 226, 226f, 237
    palsy, with biceps tendon repair, 118
    protection of, in surgery, 22
        arthroscopic, 159–160
Median nerve compression/entrapment, 6, 141–147
    with complex fracture-dislocation of proximal ulna, 269
    diagnostic criteria for, 143
    diagnostic studies in, 143–144
    with elbow dislocation, 254, 256–257
    at flexor digitorum superficialis, 142f, 142–143, 144f
    history in, 141
    at lacertus fibrosus, 142f, 142–143, 145–146
    at ligament of Struthers, 142f, 142–143
    magnetic resonance imaging of, 65
    with medial epicondylitis, 85
    nonoperative treatment of, 144–145
    operative treatment of, 145–146
        complications in, 146
        Henry's anterior approach in, 24
        indications for, 145
        results of, 146
    palpation of, 43, 143
    physical examination in, 143, 144f
    postoperative treatment of, 146
    at pronator teres muscle, 142f, 142–143, 144f, 145–146
    provocative tests for, 50, 143, 144f
    sensory examination in, 47, 143
    sites of, 142, 142f
Mesenchymal syndrome, 79
Metacarpophalangeal joints, assessment of, in radial nerve compression, 151
Metallic radial head prostheses, 214, 219
Metaphyseal humeral fracture, surgical approaches in
    alternative, 15t
    recommended, 15t
Metastatic tumor, 296–299
Methylprednisolone acetate, for olecranon bursitis, 305
Middle finger resistance test, for radial tunnel syndrome, 151
Midfield magnetic resonance imaging systems, 55
Midlateral portal, for arthroscopy, 161f, 161–162
Milch fractures, of lateral condylar, 245
    type I, 245, 246f
    type II, 245, 246f

Milking maneuver, in assessment of ulnar collateral ligament, 91–92
Molesworth's medial surgical approach, 13t, 22–23
    complications of, 22
    indications for, 22
    modifications in, 22–23
Monteggia fracture, surgical approaches in
    Boyd's, 16
    Gordon's, 15t, 18
    recommended, 15t
Monteggia's classification of fracture-dislocations, 266
Motion
    endpoint of, quality of, 46
    limitation of, assessment of, 46
Motion, range of, 29–30
    assessment of, 45–46, 45f–46f
    functional, 29
    intraoperative assessment of, in distal humerus fractures, 205
    normal
        for extension, 29, 45
        for flexion, 29, 45
        for pronation, 29
        for supination, 29
    ulnar nerve compression and, 134
Motor nerve, compression/entrapment of, loss of pronation or supination with, 46
MRI. See Magnetic resonance imaging
Muscle(s). See also specific muscles
    of elbow, 1–6, 5t
        function of, 30
    hypertrophy of, as diagnostic sign, 42
    magnetic resonance imaging of, 55
Muscle activity
    during baseball pitching, 32t
    electromyography of, 29
    during tennis playing, 37
Muscle strength testing, 46–47, 46f–47f
Mycobacterium infection, olecranon bursitis with, 303
Myeloma, 295–296, 299
Myxoid liposarcoma, 302

Needle biopsy/aspiration, 298
Needle electromyography, in median nerve compression (pronator syndrome), 144
Nerve conduction studies
    in contractures, 286
    magnetic resonance imaging with, in entrapment neuropathies, 65
    in median nerve compression (pronator syndrome), 143–144
    in ulnar nerve compression, 134
Nerves, cutaneous, 1–2, 3f
    distribution of, 3f
    injury to, with medial and lateral skin incisions, 12
Neural tunnels, around elbow, 7–9, 8f
Neurilemmoma, 299–300
Neuroblastoma, metastatic, 296
Neurofibroma, 299–300
Neurologic complications, of diagnostic arthroscopy, 168
Neurolysis, of ulnar nerve
    in compression/entrapmenet of nerve, 137
    with surgery for nonunions of distal humerus, 278, 281–283
Neuropathies. See also specific nerves
    compressive/entrapment, 131
        magnetic resonance imaging of, 55, 64–65, 66f
        sensory examination in, 47, 133–134

Nonsteroidal antiinflammatory drugs
    following contracture surgery, 292–293
    for ulnar collateral ligament injuries, 93
    for valgus extension overload syndrome, 125
Nonunions of elbow, 271–284
    arthroplasty for, 276
    complications of, 282–283
    in distal humerus fractures, open reduction and internal fixation of, 278–281, 279f–280f
    history of, 271–276
    in lateral condylar fractures, 247f, 249–250, 250f–251f
    nonoperative treatment of, 276
    in olecranon fractures, 272
    operative treatment of, 276–282
        contraindications to, 276
        general principles in, 271
        indications for, 276
        patient positioning for, 276, 277f
        results of, 281–282
        techniques for, 276–281, 277f
    physical examination in, 276
    in proximal radial fractures, 272–273, 274f
        operative treatment of, 277–278, 281
    in proximal ulnar fractures, 272, 272f–273f
        open reduction and internal fixation of, 277
    radiographic findings in, 247f, 249f–251f, 272f–275f, 279f–280f
    stiffness with, 282
    symptomatic hardware in, 282
    time for determination of, 276
    ulnar nerve injury with, 271, 275f, 278, 281–283

Oblique ligament, 10
Off-speed pitches, biomechanics of, 33, 34t
Off-the-mound throwing program, in rehabilitation, 312, 315t
Olecranon
    as arthroscopic landmark, 159, 164
    arthroscopy of, 162, 166
    baseball pitching and, 34–35, 75–76
    fenestration of, 192f–193f
        with arthroscopic radial head excision, 192–193, 192f–193f
        with capsular release for ankylosis, 180–181
    ossification of, 245
    osteophytes in
        with ankylosis, arthroscopic removal of, 180–182, 181f–182f
        arthroscopic inspection for, 166
        with bursitis, 305f–306f, 305–307
        with radiocapitellar joint degeneration, 193
    posteromedial, impingement in, with valgus extension overload syndrome, 123
    radiography of, 51–52
    spurring of, with ulnar collateral ligament injury, 92, 93f
    trauma, and dislocation, 253
Olecranon apophysitis
    physical findings in, 75
    radiographic findings in, 75
    treatment of, 75–76
    in young athletes (Little League elbow), 75–76
Olecranon bursa, 2, 6f
    clinical anatomy of, 6f, 303
    collar shaped, 305
    palpation of, 44, 44f
Olecranon bursitis, 303–307
    concomitant conditions with, 304

Olecranon bursitis *(continued)*
   versus distal biceps tendinitis, 303
   etiology of, 303–304
      infectious, 303–304
      inflammatory, 304
      traumatic, 303
   history and physical examination in, 304–305, 304*f*–305*f*
   laboratory findings in, 304
   nonoperative treatment of, 305
      complications in, 305
   operative treatment of, 305–307
      arthroscopic/endoscopic, 306*f*, 306–307
      authors' preferred technique for, 306–307
      complications in, 307
      open technique for, 306
   osteophytes with, 305*f*–306*f*, 305–307
   palpation of, 44
   septic, 304–307
   swelling with, 42, 304, 304*f*
   throwing/pitching and, 303
   triceps tendon rupture with, 118, 305
Olecranon coronoid ligament (transverse ligament of Cooper), 10, 10*f*
Olecranon excision, for chronic bursitis, 306
Olecranon fossa, 9*f*, 223
   arthroscopy of, 162
   debridement of, with capsular release for ankylosis, 180
   fat pad within, 9*f*
   loose bodies in, flexion contracture with, 178
   maintaining free from obstruction, in distal humerus fracture fixation, 200, 205
   in mechanical strength of distal humerus, 195, 196*f*
Olecranon fractures, 259–264
   avulsion, 264–265*f*
   bicortical screw fixation of, 263–264, 264*f*
   bone graft for, 260
   classification of, 259
   comminution of, 259–260
   contoured plating technique for, 264, 265*f*
   with coronoid process fractures, 259
   displaced, problems with, 259
   and medial collateral ligament, 264, 265*f*
   nondisplaced, 259
   nonunion of, 272, 272*f*
      open reduction and internal fixation of, 277
      operative treatment of, 276
      total elbow arthroplasty for, 276
   oblique
      complications of, 76
      physical findings in, 76
      in young athletes (Little League elbow), 76
   olecranon excision and triceps tendon repair in, 264, 264*f*–265*f*
   open reduction and internal fixation of, 260–264
   operative treatment of, 259–264
      patient positioning for, 260, 261*f*
      techniques in, 260–264
   patterns of, 259
   with proximal ulnar fracture-dislocation, 259, 264, 265*f*, 266–267
   radiographic findings in, 76, 261
   stress, pain with, 41
   tension-band wiring for, 259–263, 260*f*
      with intramedullary compression screws, 262–263, 264*f*
      with parallel K-wires, 260–262, 261*f*–263*f*
      problems with, 282
   triceps tendon/injury repair with, 259–260, 260*f*, 262, 262*f*

Olecranon osteotomy approach, 18–19, 19*f*
   complications of, 19
   for distal humerus fractures, 18–19, 19*f*, 198–199, 199*f*, 205, 278, 281–282
   indications for, 15*t*, 18
   modifications in, 19
Olecranon osteotomy nonunion, 19
Olecranon screw, for traction, in supracondylar fracture, 232
Olive wires, for stabilization of infected or contaminated distal humerus fractures, 281
One-hand baseball throw plyometric exercise drill, 311–312, 313*f*
Open biopsy, 298–299, 298*f*–299*f*
Open reduction
   of complex fracture-dislocation of proximal ulna, 267
   of coronoid process fractures, 260, 265–266, 266*f*
   of dislocation, 257
   of distal humerus fractures, nonunited, 278–281, 279*f*–280*f*
   of lateral condylar fractures, 247*f*–248*f*, 247–251
   of nonunions in proximal ulnar fractures, 277
   of olecranon fractures, 260–264
      nonunited, 277
   of proximal ulnar fracture, 260
   of radial head fractures, 211–213, 215–217, 217*f*, 255, 255*f*
   of supracondylar fractures, 233, 237
Operating room setup
   for arthroscopy, 157–158, 158*f*, 173, 173*f*
   for closed reduction and percutaneous pinning of supracondylar fracture, 235, 235*f*
Os supra trochleare dorsale, 11
Osborne's ligament, and ulnar nerve compression, 132, 132*f*
Ossification centers, 10–11, 11*f*, 69, 70*f*, 223, 245
Ossification, heterotopic, 286–287, 291, 293
Osteoarthritis
   arthroscopic radial head excision for, 189
   olecranon osteotomy and, 19
   radiocapitellar joint degeneration with, 185, 187, 189
Osteoarthrosis, loose bodies with, 171
Osteoblastoma, 299
Osteochondral chip fractures, of radiocapitellar joint, baseball pitching and, 33
Osteochondral fracture, magnetic resonance imaging of, 56
Osteochondritis dissecans
   baseball pitching and, 33, 42, 73–74, 74*f*
   of capitellum
      arthroscopic radial head excision for, 188
      arthroscopy of, 74, 171, 172*f*, 174
      complications of, 74
      loose bodies with, 171, 172*f*
      magnetic resonance imaging of, 57, 61, 73–74, 74*f*
      pain with, 41
      versus Panner's disease, 61
      physical findings of, 73
      radiographic findings of, 73, 74*f*
      rehabilitation of, 316–317, 317*t*
      staging of, 74
      treatment of, 74
      with ulnar collateral ligament injuries, 93*f*, 95
      in young athletes (Little League elbow), 42, 45, 73–74, 74*f*

Osteochondritis dissecans *(continued)*
   magnetic resonance imaging of, 61, 62*f*
   palpation in, 45
   of radial head, magnetic resonance imaging of, 57
Osteochondroma, 299
Osteochondrosis
   of capitellum (Panner's disease)
      loose bodies with, 171–172
      versus osteochondritis dissecans, 61
      palpation in, 45
      radiographic findings in, 75, 75*f*
      in young athletes (Little League elbow), 74–75, 75*f*
   medial epicondylar, 72
   radial head, in young athletes (Little League elbow), 75
Osteogenesis imperfecta, triceps tendon rupture with, 118
Osteoid osteoma, 299
Osteology, 10–11, 11*f*
Osteomyelitis, magnetic resonance imaging of, 55
Osteophyte(s)
   in coronoid process
      arthroscopic inspection for, 166, 166*f*
      with radiocapitellar joint degeneration, 193
   firm endpoints with, 46
   in olecranon
      with ankylosis, arthroscopic removal of, 180–182, 181*f*–182*f*
      arthroscopy of, 166
      with bursitis, 305*f*–306*f*, 305–307
      with radiocapitellar joint degeneration, 193
   palpation of, 44
   with radiocapitellar joint degeneration, 186–187
      arthroscopic removal of, 192–194
   with ulnar collateral ligament injury, 92, 93*f*
   with valgus extension overload syndrome, 123–130, 124*f*
      arthroscopic removal of, 126–128, 127*f*–128*f*, 175, 175*f*
      radiography of, 124–125, 125*f*
      recurrence of, after surgery, 129
Osteoporotic bone, distal humerus fractures in, treatment of, 203–206, 204*f*
Osteosarcoma, 299
Osteotomy
   chevron olecranon, 18–19, 19*f*
      complications of, 19
   for distal humerus fractures, 18–19, 19*f*, 198–199, 199*f*, 205, 278, 281–282
      indications for, 15*t*, 18
      modifications in, 19
   for cubitus varus, 239, 241*f*
   lateral epicondylar, 21
   for nonunion of radial head/neck fractures, 278
   proximal olecranon, repair of, 262–263
   supracondylar varus, for chronic (nonunited) lateral condylar fractures, 249–250, 249*f*–250*f*
Outerbridge-Kashiwagi procedure, 180–181, 189, 192
Overhead throwing. *See also* Baseball pitching
   injuries from, rehabilitation of, 309–320
Overload training, 36
Overuse injury, 31, 70, 76

Pain
   characterization of, for diagnosis, 41–42
   diagnostic approach in, imaging in, 55

Pain *(continued)*
  localization of, for diagnosis, 41
  patient's reaction to, arthrofibrosis with, 177–178
  referred, reflex assessment in, 47
Palmar flexion, resisted, in medial epicondylitis, 50
Palmaris longus muscle
  action of, 5t
  innervation of, 142
  insertion of, 5t
  nerve supply to, 5t
  origin of, 5t
Palmaris longus tendon
  harvesting of, 97
  for lateral collateral ligament reconstruction, 107
  strength of, 30
  for ulnar collateral ligament reconstruction, 30, 94f, 95, 97
Palpation, 42–45, 43f
  of biceps tendon rupture, 43, 110–111
  during extension, 42–43, 43f
  during flexion, 42–43, 43f
  of median nerve compression (pronator syndrome), 43, 143
  order for, 43
  of posterolateral rotatory instability, 103
  of radial head fractures, 45, 208–209
  in radial nerve compression, 44–45, 151
  of radiocapitellar joint degeneration, 187
  of triceps tendon rupture, 109
  of ulnar collateral ligament, 43, 43f, 91–92
  of valgus extension overload syndrome, 44, 124
Pankovich's surgical approach, 21, 22f
Panner's disease, 74–75
  loose bodies with, 171–172
  versus osteochondritis dissecans, 61
  palpation in, 45
Paralytic contractures, 285
Paresthesia, with compressive neuropathies, 131
Patella cubiti, 11
Patient positioning
  for arthroscopy, 158, 158f, 164, 164f, 173, 173f, 178, 179f, 190, 306
  for closed reduction and percutaneous pinning of supracondylar fracture, 235, 235f
  for dislocation treatment, 256–257
  in distal humerus fractures
    for exposure/treatment, 197–198, 198f, 205
    for radiography, 197, 197f
  in olecranon fractures, 260, 261f
  for surgery, 12
  for triceps tendon repair, 119f, 119–120
Patterson's surgical approach, 21
Pediatric knee immobilizer, 13
Percutaneous extensor tenotomy, for epicondylitis, 82
Percutaneous pinning
  of lateral condylar fractures, 248
  of supracondylar fracture, technique for, 235–237, 235f–237f
  of supracondylar fractures, 233–234
    configurations of, 234, 234f
Pericervical anastomotic ring, 208
Peripheral nerves, compression/entrapment of, 131
Phalen test, for median nerve compression (pronator syndrome), 143
Phonophoresis, 315, 317, 319

Physeal injury
  fractures
    classification of, 245–246
    lateral condylar, 245–252
  growth, injury to, 69–70
  magnetic resonance imaging of, 61
Physical examination, 41–54
Physical therapy, for epicondylitis, 81
Pinning
  of olecranon fractures, 261–262, 261f–263f
  percutaneous
    of lateral condylar fractures, 248
    of supracondylar fracture, 233–237, 234f–237f
Pitcher's elbow, 57. *See also* Medial epicondylitis
Pitching. *See* Baseball pitching; Softball pitching
Pivot-shift test, 48, 48f
Plantaris tendon, for ulnar collateral ligament reconstruction, 95
Plate(s)
  contoured technique with, 264, 265f, 277, 279–280, 280f
  for distal humerus fractures
    nonunited, 279–280, 280f
    selection and positioning of, 199, 200f, 202–203, 206
  for lateral condylar fractures, 249–250, 249f–250f
  for nonunion of proximal ulna, 277
  for olecranon fractures, 264, 265f
  for proximal ulnar fractures, 260, 266
  symptomatic, removal of, 282
Plate wrapping
  for distal humerus fractures, 202, 206
  for segmental fractures of proximal ulna, 264
Pleomorphic liposarcoma, 302
Plica
  prominent posterolateral, debridement of, with capsular release for ankylosis, 180, 181f
  thickened and symptomatic, with radiocapitellar joint degeneration, 186–187, 193
Plyometrics, 311–312, 312f–314f
  for osteochondritis dissecans, 317
  for ulnar collateral ligament injuries, 311–314f
  for ulnar neuritis, 314
  for valgus extension overload syndrome, 319
Polyglycolide pins
  for lateral condylar fractures, 248
  for radial head fractures, 212
Polymethyl methacrylate bone cement, for distal humerus fractures, 204, 204f, 280–281
Popeye arm, 110, 110f
Portals, for arthroscopy, 158–162, 164
  for capsular release, in ankylosis, 179–181, 179f–182f
  lateral, 160–161, 161f, 165–167
  for loose body removal, 173–175, 173f–175f
  medial, 159–160, 159f–160f, 164–165
  midlateral or direct lateral, 161f, 161–162
  in olecranon bursectomy, 306–307
  posterior, 161f, 162, 166–167, 166f–167f
  in radial head excision, 190–192, 191f
  soft spot, 166–167, 167f
    in capsular release, for ankylosis, 180
    in radial head excision, 191, 191f
Positioning, of patient
  for arthroscopy, 158, 158f, 164, 164f, 173, 173f, 178, 179f, 190, 306

Positioning, of patient *(continued)*
  for closed reduction and percutaneous pinning of supracondylar fracture, 235, 235f
  in dislocation injury, 256–257
  in distal humerus fractures
    for exposure/treatment, 197–198, 198f, 205
    for radiography, 197, 197f
  in olecranon fractures, 260, 261f
  for surgery, 12
  for triceps tendon repair, 119f, 119–120
Posterior bundle, of ulnar collateral ligament, 9–10, 10f, 89
  clinical anatomy of, 89–90, 90f
  strength of, 30
Posterior compartment impingement, with valgus extension overload syndrome, 123–130
Posterior cutaneous nerve of forearm, 3f
Posterior dislocation, 253
  closed reduction of, 256f, 256–257
  magnetic resonance imaging of, 60, 60f
  mechanism of injury, 253
  with radial head fractures, 207, 213–214
  radial head fractures with, 255f
  treatment of, 256–257
  varieties of, 253–254
Posterior extension injuries, in young athletes (Little League elbow), 75–76
Posterior instability, magnetic resonance imaging of, 60, 60f
Posterior interosseous artery, relationship to medial and lateral intermuscular septa, 4f
Posterior interosseous nerve, 7f, 7–8
  iatrogenic injury to, 6
  in radial head fracture surgery, 215–216
  innervation of supinator muscle by, 4, 6
  isolation and protection of, in surgery
    arthroscopic, 160–161
    in Boyd's approach, 17–18
    in global approach, 23–24
    in Henry's anterior approach, 26
    in Kaplan's direct lateral approach, 20, 21f
    in Kocher's lateral approach, 20
    in lateral approaches, 6, 19
    pronation of forearm for, 6, 19–20, 21f, 23–24
  palsy, weakness with, 47
Posterior interosseous nerve compression syndrome, 8, 47, 149–156
  clinical anatomy in, 149–150, 150f
  clinical presentation of, 150
  incomplete, 151
  motor deficits with, 150
  nonoperative treatment of, 152
  operative treatment of, 152–155
    anterior approach in, 152–153, 152f–154f
    brachioradialis splitting approach in, 154
    brachioradialis-extensor carpi radialis longus interval approach in, 155
    complications in, 156
    posterior approach in, 154, 154f–155f
    results of, 156
  palpation in, 45, 151
  physical examination in, 151f, 151–152
  postoperative management of, 155–156
  sites involved in, 149–150, 150f
Posterior midline skin incisions, 12–13
Posterior portal, for arthroscopy, 161f, 162, 166–167, 166f–167f
  for loose body removal, 174–175, 174f–175f
Posterior provocative tests, 51

Posterior surgical approaches, 11–19, 13t, 15f
   to distal humerus fracture, 198–199, 199f
   to posterior interosseous nerve, 154, 154f–155f
Posterocentral portal, for arthroscopy, for capsular release, in ankylosis, 180
Posterolateral dislocation, 253
Posterolateral gutter, 186
Posterolateral portal, for arthroscopy, 161f, 162, 166, 166f
   for capsular release, in ankylosis, 180–181, 181f–182f
   for loose body removal, 174–175, 174f–175f
Posterolateral rotatory instability
   arthroscopy of, 167, 167f
   assessment of, 48, 48f–49f
   Boyd's surgical approach and, 17–18
   clinical presentation of, 102
   deficiency of lateral ulnar collateral ligament in, 10
   diagnosis of, 102–104
   in epicondylitis surgery, 87
   functional anatomy in, 101–102, 102f–103f
   history in, 101–102
   Kocher's lateral approach and, 20
   lateral collateral ligament reconstruction for, 101–108
   lateral ulnar collateral ligament injury with, 60
   magnetic resonance imaging of, 104, 105f
   palpation in, 103
   physical findings in, 101
   provocative test for, 104, 104f
   radiocapitellar joint degeneration with, 186
   radiographic findings in, 103–104, 103f–104f
   surgical repair of, 104–107, 106f–107f
Posterolateral rotatory instability test, 104, 104f
Posteromedial dislocation, 253
Probenecid, for olecranon bursitis, 305
Profunda brachii artery, relationship to medial and lateral intermuscular septa, 2, 4f
Pronation
   acceptable norms for, 45
   assessment of, 45–46, 46f
   functional arc of, 45–46
   loss of, 46
      causes of, 46
      with radiocapitellar joint degeneration, 185–186
   mean torque in, 31
   muscles involved in, 30
      strength testing of, 46–47
   for protection of posterior interosseous nerve, in surgery, 6, 19–20, 21f, 23–24
   range of motion for, 29
      normal, 29
   resisted
      in medial epicondylitis, 50, 50f
      in medial nerve entrapment, 50
   in tennis, 36
   ulnar abduction in, anconeus muscle in, 4
Pronation-supination sign, in radial tunnel syndrome, 49–50
Pronator quadratus muscle
   action of, 30
   innervation of, 142
Pronator syndrome, 141–147. *See also* Median nerve compression/entrapment
   clinical anatomy in, 141–142, 142f
   diagnostic criteria for, 143
   diagnostic studies in, 143–144
   history in, 141
   nonoperative treatment of, 144–145
   operative treatment of, 145–146

Pronator syndrome *(continued)*
   complications in, 146
      Henry's anterior approach in, 24
      indications for, 145
      results of, 146
   palpation in, 43, 143
   physical examination in, 143, 144f
   postoperative treatment of, 146
   provocative tests for, 143, 144f
   sensory examination in, 47, 143
Pronator teres muscle, 6
   action of, 5t, 30
   in baseball pitching, 32t
   in border of cubital fossa, 7, 7f
   insertion of, 5t
   median nerve compression by, 142f, 142–143, 144f, 145–146
   nerve supply to, 5t, 142
   origin of, 5t
   palpation of, 43
   in tennis playing, 37
Prone position
   for arthroscopy, 158, 164, 178, 179f, 190, 306
   for dislocation treatment, 257
Proprioception, enhancement of, in ulnar collateral ligament injury, 311–312
Proton-density magnetic resonance imaging, 55, 60
Provocative tests, 48–51
   for epicondylitis, 48–50, 49f–50f, 80
   for median nerve compression (pronator syndrome), 50, 143, 144f
   for posterolateral rotatory instability, 104, 104f
   for radial nerve compression, 49–50, 151
   for ulnar nerve compression, 50, 50f, 134
   for valgus extension overload syndrome, 51, 124, 125f
Proximal medial portal, for arthroscopy, 159f, 159–160, 164–165
Proximal radial fractures
   nonunion of, 272–273, 274f
   nonunions of elbow, 272–273, 274f
      operative treatment of, 277–278, 281
Proximal radioulnar joint, 1, 2f
   degeneration of
      arthroscopic radial head excision for, 185–194
      history in, 185–186
      nonoperative treatment of, 188
      operative treatment of, 188–194
   fractures of, 259
   pronation and supination at, 29
Proximal ulnar complex fracture-dislocation, 266–269
   classification of, 266–267
   compass elbow hinge for, technique for applying, 268f, 269
   complications of, 269
   dynamic joint distractor for, 267–269, 268f
      technique for applying, 267–269, 268f
   hinged external fixators for, 267–269, 268f
Proximal ulnar fractures, 259
   coronoid process fractures with, 264, 265f, 266–267
   nonunion of, 272, 272f–273f
      open reduction and internal fixation of, 277
   olecranon fractures with, 259, 264, 265f, 266–267
   segmental
      contoured plating technique for, 264, 265f
      open reduction and fixation of, 260

Proximal ulnar tumors, 296
Pulling, force in, 31
Pulse, absent or dimmed, with supracondylar fractures, 238, 238f
Pulsed irrigation system, for arthroscopy, 157–158

Quadrate ligament, 10

Radial artery
   recurrent branch of, 4f, 8, 149–150, 208
      in Henry's anterior approach, 26
      relationship to medial and lateral intermuscular septa, 4f
Radial bicipital bursa, 303
   enlargement of, magnetic resonance imaging of, 63, 64f–65f
   and radial nerve entrapment, 65
Radial collateral artery, 149
Radial collateral ligament (lateral collateral ligament), 9f–10f, 10, 10f, 101, 186f, 186–187
   arthroscopy of, 165
   functional anatomy of, 101–102, 102f–103f
   injury, with lateral epicondylitis, 59f, 59–60
   in radial head excision, 188, 278
   reconstruction of, 101–108
      Kocher's lateral approach in, 19, 104
      results of, 107
      technique for, 104–107, 106f–107f
   in stability testing, 48
   strength of, 30–31
   in trochlear shear fracture surgery, 203, 203f
Radial fossa, 9f, 165
Radial fracture, with triceps tendon rupture, 118
Radial head
   as arthroscopic landmark, 159, 164–165, 165f
   arthroscopy of, 160–162, 165, 167
   clinical anatomy of, 186–187, 207–208
   functions of, 207
   ossification of, 245
   osteochondritis dissecans of, magnetic resonance imaging of, 57
   osteochondrosis or deformation of, in young athletes (Little League elbow), 75
   palpation of, 45
   radiography of, 51–52, 52f
   subluxation of, loss of pronation or supination with, 46
   vascular supply to, 208
Radial head arthroplasty, Kocher's lateral approach in, 19
Radial head dislocation, palpation of, 45
Radial head excision
   arthroscopic, 181, 185–194
      complications in, 193–194
      contraindications to, 190
      inadequately performed, 194
      indications for, 188–189
      versus open excision, 188
      for radial head fractures, 189, 215
      results of, 193
      technique for, 190–193, 191f–193f
   chronic proximal migration of radius with, 215
   and longitudinal instability, 214–215
   prostheses use after, 207, 211, 214–216, 218f, 219, 255
   for radial head fractures, 189, 207, 211–214, 217–219
      with coronoid process fractures, 265–266
      delayed, 213

Radial head excision *(continued)*
    with elbow dislocation, 255
    nonunited, 276–278, 281
    partial, 212
Radial head fractures, 207–222, 259
    age and, 207
    arthrosopy of, 160
    borderline cases in, 210
    chronic proximal migration of radius with, 215
    classification of, 209–211
    clinical findings in, 208–209
    comminution of, 209–210, 210*f*, 212, 216, 217*f*, 267, 273
    in complex fracture-dislocation of proximal ulna, 266–267
    with complex injuries, treatment of, 213–214, 218*f*, 218–219
    with coronoid process fractures, 218*f*, 219, 265–266
    with elbow dislocation, 255, 255*f*
    flexion contracture with, 178
    incidence of, 207
    and longitudinal instability, 214–216, 219
    magnetic resonance imaging of, 61, 209
    malunited
        arthroscopic radial head excision for, 189
        radial nerve injury with, 193–194
        radiocapitellar joint degeneration with, 185–186, 189
    mechanism of injury in, 208
    nonunion of, 272–273, 274*f*
        operative treatment of, 276–278, 281
    open reduction and internal fixation for, 13, 211–213, 215–217, 217*f*, 255, 255*f*
    pain with, 41
    palpation of, 45, 208–209
    radial head excision for, 189, 207, 211–214, 217–219, 277–278
        arthroscopic, 189, 215
        delayed, 213
        with elbow dislocation, 255
        partial, 212
        prostheses use after, 207, 211, 214–216, 218*f*, 219, 255
    radiocapitellar joint degeneration with, 185–186
        arthroscopic radial head excision for, 188–194
        nonoperative treatment of, 188
    radiographic findings in, 209, 209*f*–210*f*, 217*f*–218*f*, 255*f*
    surgical approaches in
        alternative, 15*t*
        Boyd's, 16
        global, 15*t*, 23
        Kocher's lateral, 15*t*, 19–20, 188, 216, 278
        recommended, 15*t*
    treatment of
        arthroscopic, 189, 215, 219
        authors' preferred technique of, 216–219
        complications in, 215–216
        nonoperative, 211–212, 215–216
        results of, 212
        review of, 211–215
    with triceps tendon rupture, 118
    type I, 207–209, 209*f*
        treatment of, 211, 216
    type II, 208–210, 210*f*
        treatment of, 211–213, 216–218, 217*f*
    type III, 209–210, 210*f*
        treatment of, 212–213, 216–218, 217*f*
    type IV, 210, 213–214

Radial head prostheses, 207, 211, 214–215, 218*f*, 219, 255
    complications with, 216
Radial neck fractures
    with elbow dislocation, 255, 255*f*
    incidence of, 207
    nonunion of, 272–273, 274*f*
        operative treatment of, 277–278, 281
    with triceps tendon rupture, 118
Radial nerve, 7, 7*f*, 8, 118. *See also* Posterior interosseous nerve
    clinical anatomy of, 149–150, 150*f*
    injury, with supracondylar fractures, 226, 237
    protection of, in surgery, 26, 153, 193–194
        arthroscopic, 160–161, 165–166
    relationship to medial and lateral intermuscular septa, 2, 4*f*
    superficial branch of, 3*f*, 8, 26, 149, 153
Radial nerve compression/entrapment, 8, 149–156. *See also* Posterior interosseous nerve compression syndrome; Radial tunnel syndrome
    by arcade of Frohse, 65, 150, 150*f*, 152, 154
    clinical presentation of, 150–151
    with complex fracture-dislocation of proximal ulna, 269
    diagnostic studies in, 151–152
    by distal edge of supinator muscle, 150, 150*f*, 152, 154, 154*f*
    by fibrous band of tissue anterior to radiocapitellar joint, 149–150, 150*f*, 152
    by fibrous edge of extensor carpi radialis brevis muscle, 150, 150*f*, 152, 154
    with lateral epicondylitis, 80
    by leash of Henry, 149–150, 150*f*, 152–154, 153*f*
    magnetic resonance imaging of, 65
    mimicking or accompanying lateral epicondylitis, 60
    nonoperative treatment of, 152
    operative treatment of, 152–155
        anterior approach in, 24, 152–153, 152*f*–154*f*
        brachioradialis splitting approach in, 154
        complications in, 156
        Henry's anterior approach in, 24
        posterior approach in, 154, 154*f*–155*f*
        results of, 156
    operative treatment of, brachioradialis-extensor carpi radialis longus interval approach in, 155
    palpation in, 44–45, 151
    physical examination in, 151*f*, 151–152
    postoperative management of, 155–156
    provocative tests for, 49–50, 151
    sites of, 149–150, 150*f*
Radial tuberosity, 186, 303
    reattachment of ruptured biceps tendon to, 112*f*–117*f*, 112–118
Radial tunnel, 8
Radial tunnel syndrome, 47, 149–156
    clinical anatomy in, 149–150, 150*f*
    clinical presentation of, 150–151
    nonoperative treatment of, 152
    operative treatment of, 152–155
        complications in, 156
        results of, 156
    palpation in, 44, 151
    physical examination in, 151–152
    postoperative management of, 155–156
    provocative test for, 49–50, 151
    sites involved in, 149–150, 150*f*
Radical surgical margin, 297

Radiocapitellar compression test, 50
Radiocapitellar joint, 1, 2*f*
    arthroscopy of, 165, 165*f*, 173–174
    chondromalacia of, with valgus extension overload syndrome surgery, 126
    degenerative changes in, with ulnar collateral ligament injuries, 92
    and distal humerus stability, 195
    fibrous band of tissue anterior to, radial nerve compression by, 149–150, 150*f*, 152
    force transfer through, 31
    injuries, in young athletes (Little League elbow), 42
    inspection of, in epicondylitis surgery, 83
    in lateral epicondylitis, 80
    osteochondral chip fractures of, baseball pitching and, 33
    palpation of, 45
    provocative tests of, 50
    radiography of, 51
Radiocapitellar joint degeneration
    arthroscopic radial head excision for, 185–194
    history in, 185–186
    nonoperative treatment of, 188
    operative treatment of, 188–194
        complications in, 193–194
        contraindications to, 190
        indications for, 188–189
        results of, 193
        technique for, 190–193, 191*f*–193*f*
    palpation of, 187
    physical examination in, 187–188
    radiographic findings in, 187*f*, 187–188
Radiocapitellar osteochondritis, loss of pronation or supination with, 46
Radiographic evaluation, 51–53
    anteroposterior, 51, 51*f*
    axial, 52–53, 53*f*
    of biceps tendon rupture, 109, 111
    of contractures, 286
    direct, 53
    of dislocation, 253, 256
    of distal humerus fractures, 51, 196*f*, 197, 197*f*, 204–205
        patient positioning for, 197, 197*f*
        traction views in, 197, 198*f*
    of epicondylitis, 82, 82*f*
    lateral, 51–52, 52*f*
    of lateral condylar fractures, 245–247, 247*f*–251*f*
    of lateral epicondyle fractures, 245
    of loose bodies, 171–172
    of medial epicondylar avulsion, 72, 73*f*
    of medial epicondylar osteochondrosis, 72
    of nonunions, 247*f*, 249*f*–251*f*, 272*f*–275*f*, 279*f*–280*f*
        in lateral condylar fractures, 247*f*, 250*f*–251*f*
    of olecranon apophysitis, 75
    of olecranon fractures, 76, 261
    of osteochondritis dissecans of capitellum, 73, 74*f*
    of osteochondrosis of capitellum (Panner's disease), 75, 75*f*
    of posterolateral rotatory instability, 103–104, 103*f*–104*f*
    radial head, 51–52, 52*f*
    of radial head fractures, 209, 209*f*–210*f*, 217*f*–218*f*, 255*f*
    of radial nerve compression, 151
    of radiocapitellar joint degeneration, 187*f*, 187–188

Radiographic evaluation *(continued)*
 routine views in, 51–53
 of supracondylar fractures, 224–226, 225f, 227f–232f, 233–236, 240f
  angles and lines for, 224–225, 224f–225f
 of triceps tendon rupture, 109, 119
 of tumors, 295–296, 296f–298f, 300f–301f, 300–302
 of ulnar collateral ligament injuries, 92, 93f
 of ulnar nerve compression, 134
 of valgus extension overload syndrome, 52–53, 123–125, 125f
 intraoperative, 127, 128f
Radiographically occult fractures, magnetic resonance imaging of, 55, 60–61
Radioulnar joint
 arthroscopy of, 165f, 167, 167f
 distal, dislocation of, with radial head fractures, 214–215, 219
 proximal, 1, 2f
  degeneration of, 185–194
  fractures of, 259
  pronation and supination at, 29
Radioulnar synostosis
 Boyd's surgical approach and, 17–18
 proximal
  anconeus muscle in, 4
  with biceps tendon repair, 118
  surgical approaches in, 15t, 17
Radius, chronic proximal migration of, with radial head fractures, 215
Range of motion, 29–30
 assessment of, 45–46, 45f–46f
 functional, 29
 intraoperative assessment of, in distal humerus fractures, 205
 normal
  for extension, 29, 45
  for flexion, 29
  for pronation, 29
  for supination, 29
 ulnar nerve compression and, 134
Range of motion brace, for ulnar collateral ligament injury, 311, 311f
Recurrent branch of radial artery, 4f, 8, 149–150, 208
 in Henry's anterior approach, 26
Recurrent posterior interosseous artery, relationship to medial and lateral intermuscular septa, 4f
Referred pain, reflex assessment in, 47
Reflection
 lateral, of triceps mechanism, 13, 15f, 16
 medial, of triceps mechanism, 13, 15f, 19–21
Reflexes, assessment of, 47
Rehabilitation
 after arthroscopy, 127–128, 128t
 basic principles of, 309
 in biceps tendon repair, 116–117, 117t
 in epicondylitis
  lateral, 316–318, 318t
  medial, 86, 315–316
 interval throwing program in, 312, 314t–315t
 isokinetic assessment in, 309, 310f, 315
 in lateral pathology, 316–319
 long-toss program in, 312, 314t
 in loose body removal, 175
 in medial pathology, 310–316
 in median nerve compression (pronator syndrome), 146
 off-the-mound throwing program in, 312, 315t
 in osteochondritis dissecans, 316–317, 317t
 of overhead-throwing injuries, 309–320

Rehabilitation *(continued)*
 overview of, 309
 plyometrics in, 311–312, 312f–314f, 314, 317, 319
 in posterior pathology, 319
 in radial nerve compression, 155–156
 sport-specific, determining readiness for, 309
 team approach in, 309
 Thrower's Ten program for, 311–312, 312t, 314
 in triceps tendon repair, 121
 in ulnar collateral ligament injury, 98–99, 310t, 310–312, 311f–314f, 312t, 315t–316t
 in ulnar nerve compression, 135–137
 in ulnar neuritis, 312–315, 316t
 in valgus extension overload syndrome, 127–128, 128t, 319
Repetitive trauma injury, 31
Replacement, of joint. *See* Arthroplasty
Resisted flexion, 50
Resisted palmar flexion, 50
Resisted pronation, 50, 50f
Retraction, of triceps mechanism, 13, 15f, 23–24
Rhabdomyosarcoma, 299
Rheumatoid arthritis
 arthroscopic radial head excision for, 188–189
 classification of, 188–189
 as contraindication to operative treatment of nonunions, 276
 olecranon bursitis with, 304, 306
 radiocapitellar joint degeneration with, 185, 188–189
Rheumatoid factor, in olecranon bursitis, 304
Rhythmic stabilization drills, 311, 311f, 319
Rotation
 center of, 90, 90f
 three-dimensional center, variance in, 29
Rotation, of forearm, elbow injuries or arthritis and, 1
Rotational deformity, with supracondylar fractures, 223, 224f
Round cell liposarcoma, 302

Sagittal plane, magnetic resonance imaging in, 56
Salter-Harris fractures, of lateral condylar fracture, type IV, 247
Salter-Harris fractures, of lateral condyle, 245–246
 type II, 245, 246f
  magnetic resonance imaging of, 61, 64
 type IV, 245–246, 246f
  magnetic resonance imaging of, 61, 61f
Sarcoma, 299, 301–302
Schanz screws, for stabilization of infected or contaminated distal humerus fractures, 281
Schwannoma, malignant, 299
Screw fixation
 of coronoid process fractures, 265–266, 266f
 of distal humerus fractures, 199–201, 200f–201f, 278
  augmentation of, with bone cement, 204, 204f, 280–281
  infected or contaminated, 281
  nonunited, 279–280
 of lateral condylar fractures, 250
 in nonunion of proximal ulna, 277
 of olecranon fractures, 260, 260f, 262–263, 264f
  bicortical, 263–264, 264f

Screw fixation *(continued)*
 of proximal ulnar fractures, 260
 of radial head fractures, 216–217, 217f
Self-reinforced polyglycolic acid pins, for lateral condylar fractures, 248
Self-retaining tenaculum, in coronoid process reduction and fixation, 266
Semiconstrained implant arthroplasty, for distal humerus fractures, 204, 204f
Sensory examination, 47
 in median nerve compression (pronator syndrome), 47, 143
 in ulnar nerve compression (cubital tunnel syndrome), 47, 133–134
Septic arthritis, olecranon bursitis with, 304
Septic olecranon bursitis, 304–307
Serum values, with tumors of elbow, 295
Serve, in tennis, biomechanics of, 37
Shear fractures, of trochlear, 196–197, 197f
 treatment of, 203, 203f
Short TI inversion recovery sequences (STIR), in magnetic resonance imaging, 55–57, 60
Side throw plyometric exercise drill, 311–312, 314f
Side-to-side throw, two-hand, in plyometric exercise drill, 311–312, 313f
Silastic radial head prostheses, 214–216
Silicone radial head implants, 214
Skin incisions, 12–13
Slider pitch, biomechanics of, 33–35, 34t
Sliding extensor mechanism, 16
Small round cell tumors, 299
Snapping triceps tendon, 2
Soccer throw, two-hand overhead, in plyometric exercise drill, 311–312, 312f
Soft spot(s)
 distention of elbow through, for arthroscopy, 159, 164
 inspection of, 42, 42f
 palpation of, 45
Soft spot portal, for arthroscopy, 166–167, 167f
 in capsular release, for ankylosis, 180
 in radial head excision, 191, 191f
Soft tissue contractures, 285–286
 soft endpoints with, 46
Soft tissue management
 with contractures, 286
 in fractures, 259
  of distal humerus, 205–206
  of radial head, 208, 214
 in nonunions of elbow, 276
Soft tissue masses, magnetic resonance imaging of, 55
Soft tissue release
 for ankylosis of elbow, 178
 surgical approaches in
  alternative, 15t
  Bryan and Morrey's extensive posterior, 15t
  combined medial and lateral, 15t
  global, 15t, 23
  Kocher's lateral, 15t, 19
  recommended, 15t
Soft tissue trauma, arthrofibrosis with, 177–178
Soft tissue tumors, 295–302
Softball pitching
 biomechanics of, 37
 injuries with, 37
Spin-echo magnetic resonance imaging, 55–56
Spiral groove, 118
Spiral tomography, of contractures, 286
Splinting
 after major elbow surgery, 13

Splinting *(continued)*
  of biceps tendon, 116
  of complex fracture-dislocation of proximal ulna, 269
  for contractures, 286f, 286–287, 293
  of dislocation injury, 256–257
  of epicondylitis, 317
  of lateral condylar fractures, 246
  in median nerve compression (pronator syndrome), 146
  for nonunions, 276
  of olecranon fractures, 260
  of supracondylar fractures, 232–234, 240
Splitting
  of brachialis muscle, in coronoid process reduction and fixation, 266
  of brachioradialis muscle, in radial nerve surgery, 154
  of flexor-pronator mass, in ulnar collateral ligament surgery, 95f–96f, 95–98
  of triceps mechanism, 13–14, 15f
  for osteotomy in cubitus varus, 239
Sporothrix infection, olecranon bursitis with, 304
Spur formation
  with medial tension overload, 57
  with ulnar collateral ligament injuries, 92, 93f, 95
  with valgus extension overload syndrome, 123
Stability testing, 47–48, 47f–49f
Stabilization, joint, 30–31, 208, 259
  anconeus muscle in, 4, 30, 34
  in baseball pitching, 34
  functional anatomy in, 101–102, 102f–103f
Staging, of tumors, 296–297, 297t, 298f
Staphylococcus aureus infection, olecranon bursitis with, 303–304
Staphylococcus epidermidis infection, olecranon bursitis with, 303–304
Static-progressive splinting, for contractures, 286f, 286–287
Steinmann pins, for olecranon fractures, 261–262, 261f–263f
Step-cut (Z) incision, of annular ligament, in modification of Kocher's lateral approach, 21
Steroid injections
  confounding of magnetic resonance imaging by, 57–59, 58f–59f
  for epicondylitis, 59, 81
  hypopigmentation with, 81, 81f
  for olecranon bursitis, 305
Stiffness. *See* Ankylosis, of elbow; Contracture(s)
Strength, based on in vitro studies, 30–31
Strength testing, 46–47, 46f–47f
Strengthening exercises, in rehabilitation
  Thrower's Ten program for, 311–312, 312t, 314
  in ulnar collateral ligament injury, 311–312
  for ulnar neuritis, 313
  in valgus extension overload syndrome, 319
Streptococcal infection, olecranon bursitis with, 303–304
Stress injury, in Little League elbow, 72
Stride, in baseball pitching, 31, 31f–33f
  muscle activity in, 32t
Subcutaneous plane, 1–2, 3f
Subcutaneous transposition, of ulnar nerve, 136, 136f
Subcutaneous veins, 1, 3f
Submuscular transposition, of ulnar nerve, 136–137

Superficial branch of radial nerve, 3f, 8, 149
  protection of, in surgery, 26, 153
Superficial bursae, 303–304
Superficial lymphatics, 1–2
Superior ulnar collateral artery, 8f
  relationship to medial and lateral intermuscular septa, 4f
Supination
  acceptable norms for, 45
  assessment of, 45–46, 46f
  functional arc of, 45–46
  loss of, 46
    causes of, 46
    with radiocapitellar joint degeneration, 185–186
  muscles involved in, 30
    strength testing of, 46–47
  range of motion for, 29
    normal, 29
  weakness of, with biceps tendon rupture, 109–110
Supinator muscle, 4–6
  action of, 5t, 6, 30
  in baseball pitching, 32t
  distal edge of, radial nerve compression by, 150, 150f, 152, 154, 154f
  insertion of, 5t
  nerve supply to, 4, 5t, 6
  origin of, 5t
Supine position
  for arthroscopy, 158, 164, 173, 306
  for closed reduction and percutaneous pinning of supracondylar fracture, 235, 235f
  for dislocation treatment, 256
  in olecranon fractures, 260, 261f
Supracondylar fractures
  in children, 15, 223–243
  clinical presentation of, 223–224
  closed reduction and external immobilization of, 230–231
  closed reduction and percutaneous pinning of, 233–234
    technique for, 235–237, 235f–237f
  complications of, 237–239
  cubitus varus with, 42, 224f, 226, 234, 236, 238–240, 239f–241f
  extension-type, 223–241
    classification of, 226–230, 231f
    preferred treatment of, 233–235
  flexion-type, 223, 239–240, 241f
  lateral condylar fractures with, 239, 240f
  magnetic resonance imaging for exclusion of, 61
  nerve injury with, 225–226, 233, 237–238, 240
  nonoperative treatment of, 230–233
  open reduction and internal fixation of, 237
  open reduction of, 233
  operative treatment of, 233
    techniques for, 235–237
  pinning configurations for, 234, 234f
  radiographic evaluation of, 224–226, 225f, 227f–232f, 233–236, 240f
    angles and lines for, 224–225, 224f–225f
  rotational deformity with, 223, 224f
  surgical approaches in
    alternative, 15t
    chevron olecranon osteotomy, 15t, 18–19
    recommended, 15t
    Van Gorder's, 15
  traction for, 231–233
  treatment options in, 230–233
  type I (flexion), 239

Supracondylar fractures *(continued)*
  type IA, 226, 226t, 227f
    treatment of, 227f, 233
  type IB, 226, 226t, 228f
    treatment of, 228f, 233–234
  type II (flexion), 239
  type IIA, 226t, 226–230, 229f
    treatment of, 229f, 233–234
  type IIB, 226t, 230, 230f
    treatment of, 230f, 233–234
  type III (extension), 226f, 226t, 230, 231f–232f, 233–236, 238
  type III (flexion), 239–240, 241f
  type IIIA, 226t, 230, 231f
    treatment of, 231f, 233–235
  type IIIB, 226t, 226f, 230, 232f
    treatment of, 232f, 233–235
  ulnar nerve injury with, 132
  vascular injury with, 225–226, 226f, 238, 238f
Supracondylar process, 11, 12f
Supracondylar region, of distal humerus, clinical anatomy of, 223, 224f
Supracondylar ridge, palpation of, 43
Supracondylar varus osteotomy, for chronic (nonunited) lateral condylar fractures, 249–250, 249f–250f
Supracondyloid process, in median nerve compression (pronator syndrome), 142f, 143, 145
Surface coil, in magnetic resonance imaging, 55–56
Surgery
  art of, 1
  skin incisions for, 12–13
Surgical approaches, 1, 11–21
  anterior, 11–12, 13t, 15t, 24–26
    in open capsular release, 287–288
    to radial nerve, 152–154, 152f–154f
  Boyd-Anderson, in biceps tendon repair, 112
  Boyd's, 13t, 15t, 16–18, 18f
    modifications in, 18
  Bryan and Morrey's extensive posterior, 13t, 15t, 16, 17f, 198
    modifications in, 16
  Cadenat's, 20–21
  Campbell's posterolateral, 13t, 13–14, 15t, 16f
  classification of, 11–12
  combined medial and lateral, 11–12, 13t, 23–24
  global, 15t, 21, 23–24, 24f–25f
  Gordon's, 18
  Henry's anterior, 15t, 24–26, 25f
    in open capsular release, 287–288
  Hotchkiss,' 15t, 22–23, 278, 288, 289f
  Jobe's medial utility, 23, 23f
  Kaplan's direct lateral, 20, 21f
  Key and Conwell's, 13t, 21
  Kocher's lateral, 13t, 15t, 19–21, 20f, 104
    for dislocation injury, 257
    modifications in, 20–21
    for radial head fractures, 15t, 19–20, 188, 216, 278
  lateral, 11–12, 13t, 19–21
    protection of posterior interosseous nerve in, 6
  lateral J, 11
  MacAusland's, 19
  medial, 11–12, 13t, 22–23
  Molesworth's medial, 22–23
    modifications in, 22–23
  olecranon osteotomy, 15t, 18–19, 19f, 198–199, 199f
    modifications in, 19

Surgical approaches *(continued)*
    Pankovich's, 21, 22f
    Patterson's, 21
    posterior, 11–19, 13t, 15f
        to posterior interosseous nerve, 154, 154f–155f
    preferred, 15t
    transepicondylar, 21
    understanding, cross section through elbow for, 14f
    Van Gorder's, 13t, 15, 15t, 16f
    Wadsworth's posterolateral, 13t, 14–15, 15t, 16f
        modifications in, 15, 16f
Surgical failure
    algorithm for evaluation of, 87, 87f
    in epicondylitis, 87, 87f
    type I, 87
    type II, 87
Surgical margins, of metastatic tumors, 297–298
Swelling
    assessment of, 41–42
    in compressive neuropathies, 131
    with olecranon bursitis, 42, 304, 304f
    with radial head fractures, 208
    with triceps tendon rupture, 109
Swenson's technique, of closed reduction and pinning, of supracondylar fractures, 233
Switching sticks, for arthroscopy, 157, 174, 179
Synovectomy, in rheumatoid arthritis, 189
Synovial bursae, 303
Synovial fistula, in epicondylitis surgery, 87
Synovial membrane, 9f, 9–10
    arthroscopy of, 163, 165
    inflamed/thickened
        loose body formation with, 171
        mimicking loose bodies, in magnetic resonance imaging, 61–62, 63f
        with radiocapitellar joint degeneration, 187, 194
        with rheumatoid arthritis, 189
Synovial proliferation, inspection of, 42, 42f
Synovial sarcoma, 299, 301

Tardy ulnar palsy, 132
Team approach, in rehabilitation, 309
Technetium bone scan, for tumors of elbow, 295–296
Telangiectatic osteosarcoma, 295, 300
Tendons. *See also specific tendons*
    magnetic resonance imaging of, 55
Tendo-osseous junction, triceps tendon rupture at, 118
Tennis
    biomechanics of elbow in, 36–37
    injuries with, 37, 69, 79, 89, 124, 309
        rehabilitation of, 318–319
    Little League elbow with, 69
Tennis elbow, 37, 79. *See also* Lateral epicondylitis
    medial, 57. *See also* Medial epicondylitis
Tension-band wiring
    for distal humerus fractures, 198–199, 199f, 202–203, 206
    figure-of-eight, 261–262, 262f
    for olecranon fractures, 259–263, 260f
        with intramedullary compression screws, 262–263, 264f
        with parallel K-wires, 260–262, 261f–263f
        problems with, 282
Textbook of Operative Surgery (Kocher), 11
Thomas splints, 13, 232

Thompson test, for triceps tendon rupture, 119, 119f
Thomsen maneuver, 80
Three-joint concept, clinical significance of, 1
Thrower's Ten program, 311–312, 312t, 314
Throwing
    physical adaptations with, 42
    in plyometric exercise drills, 311–312, 312f–314f
    poor technique of, and injury, 69
Throwing injuries, 37, 51, 80
    lateral compression, 33, 73–75
    magnetic resonance imaging of, 56–58, 57f–58f
    medial tension, 71–73
    olecranon bursitis, 303
    pain with, 42
        localization and characterization of, for diagnosis, 42
    palpation in, 45
    posterior extension, 75–76
    radiography of, 52–53
    rehabilitation of, 309–329
        basic principles of, 309
        interval throwing program in, 312, 314t–315t
        isokinetic assessment in, 309, 310f, 315
        in lateral pathology, 316–319
        long-toss program in, 312, 314t
        in medial pathology, 310–316
        off-the-mound throwing program in, 312, 315t
        overview of, 309
        plyometrics in, 311–312, 312f–314f, 314, 317, 319
        in posterior pathology, 319
        sport-specific, determining readiness for, 309
        team approach in, 309
        Thrower's Ten program for, 311–312, 312t, 314
    of ulnar collateral ligament, 32–33, 42, 56–57, 57f, 73, 89–100, 186–187. *See also* Ulnar collateral ligament injuries
    ulnar nerve injury with, 132–133
    valgus extension overload, 123–130. *See also* Valgus extension overload syndrome
    in young athletes (Little League elbow), 69–77. *See also* Little League elbow
Throwing mechanism
    in baseball pitching, 31–36
    biomechanics of elbow and, 29–39
    in football passing, 36
    in javelin throw, 37
    kinematics in, 29
    kinetics in, 29
    in tennis playing, 36–37
    underhand (softball pitching), 37
Time of repetition sequence, in magnetic resonance imaging, 56
Tinel sign, in median nerve compression (pronator syndrome), 143
Tinel's test, 43–44, 50, 92, 124
Titanium radial head prostheses, 219
Tomography, 53. *See also* Computed tomography
    of lateral condylar fractures, 246–247
    of medial epicondylar avulsion, 72
    of olecranon oblique fracture, 76
    of osteochondritis dissecans of capitellum, 73
    of radial head fractures, 209
Tongue approach, for triceps mechanism, 13–15, 15f–16f

Too much, too soon training phenomenon, 69
Topographical anatomy, marking of, for arthroscopy, 159, 164
Torque(s), 29–31
    in baseball pitching, 32f–33f, 90, 310
        during arm acceleration, 32f–33f, 34–35
        during arm cocking, 32f–33f, 32–34, 35f
        during arm deceleration, 32f–33f, 35
        during follow-through, 32f–33f, 35–36
    in football passing, 36
    mean extension, 31
    mean pronation, 31
    in tennis playing, 37
    in underhand throw (softball pitching), 37
Total elbow arthroplasty
    for nonunions
        of distal humerus, 276
        of olecranon, 276
    surgical approaches in, 15t
        Bryan and Morrey's extensive posterior, 15t, 16
        Campbell's posterolateral, 13, 15t
        Kocher's lateral, 15t, 19
        Wadsworth's posterolateral, 14, 15t
Traction
    for dislocation injury, 256–257
    for supracondylar fractures, 231–233
Traction radiographic views
    of distal humerus fractures, 197, 198f
    of supracondylar fractures, 224
Transepicondylar approach, 21
Transposition, of ulnar nerve, 135–137
    in distal humerus fracture fixation, 200, 202
    intramuscular, 136
    with lateral condylar fracture surgery, 249–250
    subcutaneous, 136, 136f
    submuscular, 136–137
Transverse bundle, of ulnar collateral ligament, 89
Transverse ligament of Cooper, 10, 10f
Transverse massage, 315–316
Triceps avulsion injury, palpation of, 44, 44f
Triceps brachii muscle, 2, 6f, 8f
    action of, 5t, 30
    in baseball pitching, 32t, 33–34
    insertion of, 2, 5t, 6f
    medial head, ulnar nerve compression at, 132–133
    nerve supply to, 5t, 149
    origin of, 2, 5t, 6f
    strain, in young athletes (Little League elbow), 75–76
    strength testing of, 46, 47f
    in tennis playing, 37
    work capacity of, 30
Triceps mechanism
    rupture of, 16
    surgical options for, 13, 15f
        in lateral collateral ligament reconstruction, 104–107, 106f–107f
        in osteotomy for cubitus varus, 239
        reflect laterally, 13, 15f, 16
        reflect medially, 13, 15f, 19–21
        retraction, 13, 15f, 23–24
        in shear fractures of trochlea, 203, 203f
        split, 13–14, 15f, 239
        tongue, 13–15, 15f–16f
Triceps reflex, assessment of, 47
Triceps tendinitis
    pain with, 41
    palpation of, 44, 44f
Triceps tendon, 259
    clinical anatomy of, 118

Triceps tendon (continued)
  injury
    magnetic resonance imaging of, 63–64
    with olecranon fracture, 259–260, 260f, 262, 262f, 264, 264f
  palpation of, 44, 44f
  repair of, 119–121, 120f–121f
    anatomic, 109
    complications in, 121
    with olecranon excision, 264, 264f
    patient positioning for, 119f, 119–120
    postoperative management of, 121
    results of, 121
Triceps tendon rupture, 109, 118–121
  disorders associated with, 118
  mechanism of injury, 118
  nonoperative treatment of, 119
  with olecranon bursitis, 118, 305
  operative treatment of, 119–121
    author's preferred technique for, 119–121, 120f–121f
    complications in, 121
    indications for, 119
    patient positioning for, 119f, 119–120
    results of, 121
    techniques for, 119
  palpation of, 109
  physical examination in, 118–119, 119f
  postoperative management of, 121
  radiographic findings in, 109, 119
  at tendo-osseous junction, 118
Trispiral tomography, of distal humerus fractures, 197
Trocars, blunt-tipped, for arthroscopy, 157, 164
Trochlea, 9f, 11, 12f
  arthroscopy of, 160–161, 166, 166f, 173
  in axis of rotation, 90, 90f
  chondromalacia of, with valgus extension overload syndrome, 127, 128f
  comminution of, treatment of, 201, 202f
  in mechanical strength of distal humerus, 195, 196f
  medial aspect of, impingement in, with valgus extension overload syndrome, 123
  ossification of, 245
Trochlear fractures, 259
  intra-articular shear, 196–197, 197f
  treatment of, 203, 203f
Trochlear physis, 11
Tuberculosis, olecranon bursitis with, 304
Tubing exercises, 311, 319
Tumor extension, magnetic resonance imaging of, 55
Tumors of elbow, 295–302
  benign, 299–300
    staging of, 296–297, 298f
  biopsy of
    complications related to, 297–298
    needle, 298
    open, 298–299, 298f–299f
    principles of, 297–299, 302
  differential diagnosis of, 295
  evaluation of, 295–296
  laboratory findings in, 295
  magnetic resonance imaging of, 296, 297f, 300
  malignant, 299, 301–302
    staging of, 296, 297t
  operative treatment of, 299
  radiographic findings of, 295–296, 296f–298f, 300f–301f, 300–302
  staging of, 296–297, 297t, 298f
  surgical margins of, 297
Turnbuckle splint, for contractures, 287, 287f, 293

T1-weighted magnetic resonance imaging, 55, 60
T2*-weighted gradient-echo sequences, in magnetic resonance imaging, 56, 60
T2-weighted magnetic resonance imaging, 55, 57, 60
Two-hand chest pass plyometric exercise drill, 311–312, 313f
Two-hand overhead soccer throw plyometric exercise drill, 311–312, 312f
Two-hand side-to-side throw plyometric exercise drill, 311–312, 313f
Type I surgical failure, 87
Type II surgical failure, 87

UCL. See Ulnar collateral ligament
Ulnar abduction, in pronation, anconeus muscle in, 4
Ulnar artery, relationship to medial and lateral intermuscular septa, 4f
Ulnar collateral artery
  relationship to medial and lateral intermuscular septa, 2, 4f
  in vascular supply to radial head, 208
Ulnar collateral ligament (medial collateral ligament), 9–10, 10f, 186f, 186–187, 208
  chronic degeneration of, magnetic resonance imaging of, 56–57
  clinical anatomy of, 89–91, 90f–91f
  composition of, 89
  functional anatomy of, 89–91
  injury, with coronoid process fractures, 265–266
  instability, Molesworth's medial approach and, 22
  laxity, radiography of, 53
  magnetic resonance imaging of, 89
  olecranon fractures and, 264, 265f
  origin of, 90, 90f
  palpation of, 43, 43f, 91–92
  reconstruction of, 23, 23f, 94–98, 95f–98f
    arthroscopy with, 95–98, 95f–98f
    complications of, 99
    graft assessment in, magnetic resonance imaging of, 57, 57f, 92, 94f
    graft fixation and tensioning in, 96–98, 97f–98f
    magnetic resonance imaging of, 92, 94f
    palmaris longus tendon graft for, 30, 94f, 95, 97
    rehabilitation after, 98–99
    results of, 99
    with valgus extension overload syndrome, 126–129
  repair of, 94–95
    with radial head fracture, 219, 255
  rupture/tear of
    acute, 56
    dislocation with, 57, 254
    magnetic resonance imaging of, 56–57
    midsubstance, 56
    rehabilitation in, 310–312
    treatment of, 94
  sprain, 57
    rehabilitation in, 310t, 310–312
  in stability testing, 47–48
  strain, treatment of, 92–93
  strength of, 30–31
    ultimate tensile, 30
  and ulnar nerve compression, 132f, 132–133, 132f, 138
  in valgus extension overload syndrome, 124–125
Ulnar collateral ligament injuries, 57, 89–100
  acute, 56

Ulnar collateral ligament injuries (continued)
  with coronoid process fractures, 265–266
  dislocation with, 57, 254
  with epicondylitis, 59f, 59–60, 80, 85
  history in, 91
  magnetic resonance imaging of, 56–57, 57f, 59f, 59–60, 92, 93f
  with medial epicondylitis, 57
  nonoperative treatment of, 92–94, 310
  operative treatment of, 94–98
    authors' preferred method of, 95–98, 95f–98f
    complications of, 99
    contraindications to, 94
    indications for, 94
    results of, 99
    technique for, 94–95
  physical examination in, 91–92
  postoperative management of, 98–99
  radiographic findings in, 92, 93f
  range of motion brace for, 311, 311f
  rehabilitation of, 98–99, 310t, 310–312, 311f–312f, 312t
    interval throwing program in, 312, 314t–315t
    long-toss program in, 312, 314t
    off-the-mound throwing program in, 312, 315t
    plyometric exercise drills in, 311–312, 312f–314f
    Thrower's Ten program for, 311–312, 312t
  throwing/pitching and, 32–33, 42, 56–57, 57f, 73, 90–91, 186–187
  return to activity after reconstruction, 98–100
  in young athletes (Little League elbow), 73
Ulnar dislocation, with lateral condylar fractures, 246
Ulnar fracture-dislocation
  complex proximal, 266–269
  proximal complex, 266–269
    classification of, 266–267
    compass elbow hinge for, 268f, 269
    complications of, 269
    dynamic joint distractor for, 267–269, 268f
    hinged external fixators for, 267–269, 268f
Ulnar fractures, proximal, 259
  coronoid process fractures with, 264, 265f, 266–267
  nonunion of, 272, 272f–273f, 277
  olecranon fractures with, 259, 264, 265f, 266–267
  segmental, 260, 264
    contoured plating technique for, 264, 265f
  open reduction and fixation of, 260
Ulnar nerve, 3f, 7–8, 8f
  as arthroscopic landmark, 164
  in distal humerus fracture fixation, handling of, 198, 200, 202
  hypermobility of, 44, 44f, 132
  injury
    with elbow dislocation, 254
    iatrogenic, 20, 99, 233
    with lateral condylar fractures, 132, 249–250
    with nonunion of fractures, 271, 275f, 278, 281–283
    with supracondylar fractures, 226, 233, 237, 240
  isolation and protection of, in surgery, 13, 22, 95, 99, 126, 138
    arthroscopic, 160, 162, 182

Ulnar nerve *(continued)*
    in capsular release, for contractures, 289
    in fixation of distal humerus fractures, 198
        for olecranon fractures, 261
        for supracondylar fractures, 237
    palpation of, 44, 44f
    palsy, with cubitus valgus, 42
    relationship to medial and lateral intermuscular septa, 2, 4f
    subluxation of, 8, 41, 44, 44f, 132, 134, 138
        medial epicondylar bursitis with, 303
Ulnar nerve compression/entrapment, 8, 131–139
    classic presentation of, 133
    clinical anatomy and etiology of, 131–133, 132f
    common sites of, 131–133, 132f
    with complex fracture-dislocation of proximal ulna, 269
    decompression in situ for, 135, 138
    diagnostic studies in, 134
    differential diagnosis of, 133
    with elbow dislocation, 254
    full exposure and release for, 135–136, 136f
    magnetic resonance imaging of, 64–65, 66f, 134
    mass lesions and, 132
    medial epicondylectomy for, 137, 137f
    with medial epicondylitis, 80, 82, 85–87, 315
    with medial tension overload, 57
    neurolysis for, 137
    nonoperative treatment of, 134
    operative treatment of, 134–137
        complications in, 138
        indications and contraindications in, 134–135
        results of, 137–138
        techniques for, 135–137, 136f–137f
    physical examination in, 133–134
    pitching/throwing and, 132–133
    postoperative management of, 135–137
    postoperative recurrence of, 138
    provocative tests for, 50, 50f, 134
    radiographic findings in, 134
    sensory examination in, 47, 133–134
    transposition for, 135–137
        in distal humerus fracture fixation, 200, 202
        intramuscular, 136
        in lateral condylar fracture fixation, 249–250
        subcutaneous, 136, 136f
        submuscular, 136–137
    with ulnar collateral ligament injury, 92, 96, 315
    with valgus extension overload syndrome, 123–124
Ulnar neuritis
    with Little League elbow, 73
    magnetic resonance imaging of, 64–65, 66f
    with medial epicondylitis, 58, 80, 82, 85–87, 315
    palpation of, 44
    physical examination in, 134
    pitching/throwing and, 42
    rehabilitation of, 312–315, 316t
        Thrower's Ten program for, 312t, 314
    treatment of, 73
    triceps tendon rupture with, 118
    with ulnar collateral ligament injury, 92, 96
    with ulnar collateral ligament reconstruction, 99

Ulnar neuritis *(continued)*
    with valgus extension overload syndrome, 123–124
Ulnar recurrent artery, relationship to medial and lateral intermuscular septa, 4f
Ulnar shortening, for chronic proximal migration of radius, 215
Ulnar traction spurring, with medial tension overload, 57
Ulnar tumors, proximal, 296
Ulnar tunnel(s), in lateral collateral ligament reconstruction, 105–107, 106f–107f
Ulnar tunnel syndrome, 133
Ulnohumeral angle, for radiography, of supracondylar fracture, 224–225, 225f
Ulnohumeral arthroplasty, 181, 189, 192
Ulnohumeral joint, 29, 89
    as arthroscopic landmark, 166, 166f
    arthroscopy of, 162, 166, 173, 174f
    degenerative changes in, with ulnar collateral ligament injuries, 92
    radiocapitellar joint degeneration and, 193
Ulnotrochlear joint, 1, 2f
    force transfer through, 31
Underhand throw (softball pitching)
    biomechanics of, 37
    injuries with, 37
Unicameral bone cyst, 299
Unossified cartilage, magnetic resonance imaging of, 55
Uric acid, serum levels of, in olecranon bursitis, 304

Vacuum phenomenon, in magnetic resonance imaging, 61
Valgus angle, 29
Valgus deformity, ulnar nerve compression with, 132
Valgus extension overload syndrome, 92, 123–130
    arthroscopic treatment of, 123, 125–128, 127f–128f, 171–172, 175, 175f
    diagnosis of, 124–125
    history in, 123
    loose bodies with, 123–125, 124f, 171–172
    magnetic resonance imaging of, 57
    nonoperative treatment of, 125
    olecranon bursitis with, 303
    operative treatment of, 123, 125–128
        authors' preferred technique for, 126–128, 127f–128f
        complications of, 129
        contraindications to, 125–126
        indications for, 125–126
        results and expectations of, 128–129
        techniques for, 126, 126f
    osteophytes with, 123–130, 124f
        radiography of, 124–125, 125f
        recurrence of, after surgery, 129
    pain with, 41–42, 124–125
    palpation in, 44, 124
    pathophysiology of, 123–124
    physical examination in, 124–125, 125f
    postoperative management of, 127–128, 128t
    provocative tests for, 51, 124, 125f
    radiographic findings in, 52–53, 123–125, 125f
        intraoperative, 127, 128f
    rehabilitation of, 127–128, 128t, 319
    relevant anatomy in, 123–124
    throwing/pitching and, 35, 123
Valgus extension snap maneuver, 51, 124, 125f

Valgus gravity radiograph, 53
Valgus instability/stability
    assessment of, 47f, 47–48, 92
    in medial epicondylitis, 85
    with radiocapitellar joint degeneration, 187, 189, 190f
    with ulnar collateral ligament injuries, 89–92, 99
Valgus stress
    and dislocation, 253–254
    resistance to, 30–31, 89
        anterior bundle in, 90, 90f
        in baseball pitching, 34–35, 90
        radial head in, 207–208
Valgus stress test, 124
Valgus torque
    in overhead throwing, 32–33, 310
    in underhand throw (softball pitching), 37
Van Gorder's surgical approach, 13t, 15, 15t, 16f
Varus instability, assessment of, 48
Varus stress
    in lateral condylar fractures, 245
    resistance of, 30–31
Varus stress test, 48
Varus torque
    in baseball pitching, 32–33, 32f–33f, 90
    in football passing, 36
    in underhand throw (softball pitching), 37
Vascular insufficiency, with supracondylar fracture, 238, 238f
Veins, subcutaneous, 1, 3f
Velocity, angular
    in baseball pitching, 34
    in javelin throw, 37
    in tennis, 36
Velocity, in throwing, 29
Verbrugge clamp, in coronoid process reduction and fixation, 266, 266f
Volkmann's ischemia, 231, 238, 269
Vulpius Achilles tendon lengthening technique, 121

Wadsworth's posterolateral surgical approach, 13t, 14–15
    indications for, 14, 15t
    modifications in, 15, 16f
Wall dribble plyometric exercise drill, 311–312, 314f
Whirlpool, 312–313, 315
Wide surgical margin, 297–298
Windup, in baseball pitching, 31, 31f–33f
    muscle activity in, 32t
Wissinger rods, for arthroscopy, 157, 160, 161f, 174f, 179
Wolfe and Ranawat's surgical approach, 16
Worker's compensation cases
    of epicondylitis, 81, 87
    of radial nerve compression, 156
Wound management, in distal humerus fractures, 205–206
Wrist extension plyometric exercise drill, 311–312, 313f

X-rays. *See* Radiographic evaluation

Y-type plate, for distal humerus fixation, 199

Z incision, of annular ligament, in modification of Kocher's lateral approach, 21
Zone of hypertrophy, 69

ISBN 0-387-98905-6

9 780387 989051